医道寓园

Medical Philosophy from Campus

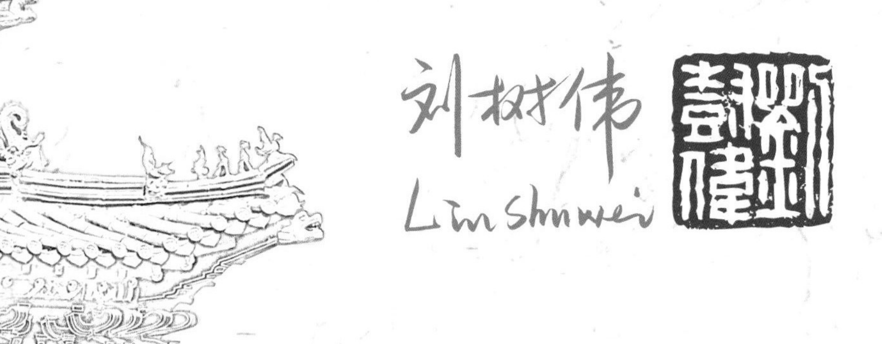

山东大学出版社
SHANDONG UNIVERSITY PRESS

图书在版目（CIP）数据

医道寓园 / 刘树伟著. — 济南 : 山东大学出版社,
2024.1
ISBN 978-7-5607-7299-8

Ⅰ. ①医… Ⅱ. ①刘… Ⅲ. ①山东大学齐鲁医学院－
校史 Ⅳ. ①R-40

中国版本图书馆 CIP 数据核字（2021）第 268636 号

责任编辑：徐　翔
英文翻译：刘　静
摄　　影：刘树伟
封面设计：张　荔

医道寓园	印　刷：山东蓝海文化科技有限公司
出版发行：山东大学出版社	版　次：2024 年 1 月第 1 版
社　址：山东省济南市历下区山大南路 20 号	印　次：2024 年 1 月第 1 次印刷
邮　编：250100	规　格：787mm×1092mm　1/8
发行热线：（0531）88363008	42 印张　200 千字
经　销：新华书店	定　价：498.00 元

序

自我 1962 年来到这个校园攻读六年制医学本科，已经有 60 个年头了。60 年沧桑岁月时光荏苒，我从一个意气风发的小伙子变成了一位白发苍苍的老者，唯一不变的是我对山东大学齐鲁医学院的感情。这是我学习、工作和生活的地方，我成长于斯，奋斗于斯，将来终老于斯，她就是我永远的家。

目前，尽管我已赋闲在家，但这个校园的一草一木、一人一事，都时刻牵动着我的心。最近，基础医学院解剖学与神经生物学系刘树伟教授将他的新作《医道寓园》初稿送我，并邀我作序。我仔细看了全稿，感到十分高兴。这是一本以“博施济众，广智求真”为灵魂，以历史为主线，以建筑为依托，以花草树木为背景，展示山东大学齐鲁医学院悠久历史、重大事件、代表人物和关键成果的画册。该书第一次以中英文注释的画册形式系统地介绍了山东大学齐鲁医学院的悠久历史和百年校园，因此具有显著的资料价值和历史意义。该书语言优美，采用了原创的散文和诗词形式，图片精良且均系作者原创（历史性照片除外），因此在艺术上具有一定的创新性。我相信它的出版发行不仅对于保存、研究和传播山东大学齐鲁医学院的悠久历史具有重要意义，而且一定能达到睹物励志、启迪心灵的效果，对充分发挥校园隐性课程的教育作用，培养优秀的医学人才和创建“双一流”大学也具有重要的现实意义。因此，我欣然为之作序，并热情地向广大读者推荐。

难能可贵的是这本优秀的专著竟然出自一位解剖学教授之手。刘树伟教授是 1989 年华西医科大学毕业来我校工作的，曾在美国肯塔基大学医学院解剖学与神经生物学系做过访问学者。他主要从事人体解剖学教学和断层影像解剖学研究，由于成绩突出，破格晋升为教授。他先后担任过山东医科大学基础医学院副院长、山东大学医学院副院长和山东大学研究生院常务副院长，对学校的情况十分熟悉。因此，由他完成这样的著作可谓适得其人。

最后，我衷心祝贺这本书的出版，也希望大家能保护好和利用好这个校园，将“敢为人先，心系天下，仁心仁术，文理兼修”的齐鲁医学精神传承下去，并不断发扬光大。

原山东医科大学校长

2021 年 11 月 8 日 王琪璧

Foreword

It has been 60 years since I came to this campus in 1962 to study for a six-year undergraduate medical course. Over the past 60 years, I have changed from a young man with high spirits to an old man with white hair. The only thing that remains unchanged is my feelings for Cheeloo College of Medicine of Shandong University. This is where I study, work and live. I grew up here, worked here, and will spend my remaining years here. She is my eternal home.

Although I have retired now, everything on campus always affects my feeling. Recently, Professor Liu Shuwei of the Department of Anatomy and Neurobiology of the School of Basic Medical Sciences sent me the first draft of his new book *Medical Philosophy from Campus*, and invited me to make a foreword. I read the whole draft carefully and felt very happy. With the soul of "relieving the public by providing extensive medical assistance and seeking truth via continuing study", this picture book shows the long history, major events, representative figures and key achievements of Cheeloo College of Medicine through taking history as the main line, buildings as the support, and flowers and trees as the background. This is the first book that systematically introduces the long history and century-old campus of Cheeloo College of Medicine of Shandong University in the form of a picture book with Chinese and English introductions, so it has remarkable data value and historical significance. With beautiful language, original prose and poetry, excellent pictures originally taken by the author (except historical photos), this book has a certain degree of artistic innovation. I believe that its publication is not only of great significance to preserve, study and disseminate the long history of Cheeloo College of Medicine of Shandong University, but also inspiring and enlightening. It is also of great practical significance to give full play to the educational role of the campus, to cultivate excellent medical talents and to establish a first-class university and a first-class discipline. Therefore, I am pleased to make a foreword to it and warmly recommend it to the vast number of readers.

What is commendable is that this excellent monograph is written by an anatomy professor. Professor Liu Shuwei came to work in Shandong Medical University after graduating from West China Medical University in 1989 and he once served as a visiting scholar in the Department of Anatomy and Neurobiology, Medical College, University of Kentucky, USA. He is mainly engaged in the teaching of human anatomy and the research on sectional image anatomy. Due to his outstanding achievements, he was promoted to professor as an exception. He once served as vice dean of the School of Basic Medical Sciences of Shandong Medical University, vice dean of the Medical School of Shandong University and executive vice dean of the Graduate School of Shandong University successively. Therefore, he is very familiar with the university and it is appropriate for him to complete such a work.

Finally, I want to express my heartfelt congratulations on the publication of this book, and I also hope that everyone can protect and make good use of this campus, and carry forward the spirit of "dare to be the first, keep the world in heart, have benevolent mind and heart, and practise both liberal arts and sciences".

Wang Yanbi

President of former Shandong Medical University

8 November 2021

前 言

当我完成本书的最后一页时，东方已露出了晨曦。我迎着朝霞，掩卷而思，心中感到欣慰、解脱和遗憾。欣慰的是作为教师和校文化委员会委员，终于为校园文化建设做了一点实实在在的工作。解脱的是我从齐鲁医学文化的汪洋大海中暂时上岸了，在几个月的苦苦挣扎之后可以平静呼吸了！遗憾的是本人才疏学浅，若一小小蜻蜓，在浩渺无垠的齐鲁医学天空中，只能窥其一鳞半爪，本书定有挂一漏万和流于肤浅之弊。

本书不是全面系统地介绍山东大学齐鲁医学院历史的专著，也不是简简单单的校园风光画册，而是以历史文化为主线、楼宇建筑为依托、花草树木为背景，试图将我校医科知名人物、重大事件和重要成果融入校园风光的作品。它有十章六十节，每节由 1 ~ 8 个单元组成，每个单元包括中英文对照的一段介绍性文字和 3 ~ 6 幅照片。我希望它能成为一个向导，在欣赏百年齐鲁遗存的过程中，轻松愉快地感知她的风采、风格和风度，不知不觉中领悟她的精神、道理和教诲，春雨润物般提升我们的品质、情怀和志趣。本书是第一本以中英文注释的画册形式简要地介绍山东大学齐鲁医学院悠久历史和百年校园的画册，我不知道这 20 万文字和 655 幅图片，是否诠释了百年学院“博施济众，广智求真”的灵魂？只能留待广大读者予以评判了。

齐鲁医学院校园，林木茂密，花草繁盛，建筑瑰丽，中西合璧，被老舍赞为“非正式的公园”。她是花的海洋，沐浴其中，每个基因都表达着馥郁的气息。她是绿的世界，苍翠扑面，定使人脑清目明，精神倍增。她是铁的熔炉，置身其里，能使你百炼成钢，终成擎天立柱。我本无意撰写此书，但她的优雅神韵，驱使我不由得留墨纸上；她的美丽身姿，逼迫我自主地举起了相机。我赞叹前人的创造力，感谢他们为今天留下的一座座丰碑。我祈盼来者的超越力，希望他们开辟更加美好的未来。我也感慨今天对文物保护的欠缺，如果老的经典在不断消失，那么我们创造今天的奇迹又有何意义呢？我盼望这本书在历史的霞光中能发出几声呐喊，要让这些已经列入国家重点保护文物的楼舍能真正焕发青春，永远不要让这些前人创造的伟大建筑艺术在新的瓦砾中哭泣！

在本书即将付梓之即，我要衷心感谢山东大学宣传部、齐鲁医学院、基础医学院和齐鲁医院的领导，他们的鼓励和支持是我力量的无穷源泉；我要衷心感谢原山东医科大学校长王琰璧教授，他为本书撰写了序言并给予了许多指导；我要衷心感谢山东大学校友、毕业于外国语学院的山东财经大学外国语学院刘静博士，她出色地完成了本书的英文翻译工作；我要衷心感谢山东大学趵突泉校区管理办公室和各学院所给予的配合和支持；我要衷心感谢齐鲁医院田道正教授、基础医学院王怀经教授和体育学院谢飞教授等所给予的帮助和支持；我要衷心感谢潍坊医学院蒋吉英教授和于丽教授、潍坊护理职业学院崔书田书记和李茂松教授，在他们的帮助下我顺利获得了齐鲁大学的早期历史资料；我还要衷心感谢山东大学出版社陈斌社长和医学分社徐翔社长，他们的耐心、帮助和支持是本书得以顺利完成不可或缺的保障。本书历史性图片主要来自 Charles Hodge Corbett 所著 *Shantung Christian University (Cheeloo)*，在编写过程中，除参考了书末参考文献中列出的公开出版发行的著作外，还参阅了大量内部资料和网络资料，在此也向上述资料的原作者表示衷心感谢！

精雕细琢方为器，千锤百炼始成钢。恳望读者及时告知本书的不足乃至错误，以便再版时参考。

2021 年，是中国共产党建党 100 周年、山东大学建校 120 周年和原齐鲁大学医科于济南建校 110 周年。谨将本书献给伟大的中国共产党和慈爱的母校！

刘树伟

2021 年 11 月 10 日

Preface

By the time I have finished the last page of the manuscript, the first rays of the morning sun have begun to shine in the east. Facing the morning glow, I cover the manuscript and feel gratified, relieved and regretful. It is gratifying that as a teacher and member of the Cultural Committee of the university, I have finally done some real work for the construction of the campus culture. The relief is that I have temporarily landed from the ocean of Qilu medical culture, and can breathe calmly after several months of struggle. It's a pity that with limited knowledge I can only have a limited view in the vast sky of Qilu medicine.

This book is not a comprehensive and systematic introduction to the history of Cheeloo College of Medicine of Shandong University, nor is it a simple picture album of the campus scenery, but a work that tries to integrate well-known medical figures, major events and important achievements of the university into the campus scenery through taking history and culture as the main line, buildings as the support, and flowers and trees as the background. It consists of 10 chapters subdivided into 60 sections, each section consists of 1-8 units, and each unit includes an introductory text in Chinese and English and 3-6 pictures. I hope it can become a guide so that we can easily and happily perceive her elegant demeanour, style and manner, and unconsciously understand her spirit, truth and teaching in the process of appreciating the remains of the century-old Cheeloo University, which can enhance our quality, feelings and interests like spring rain. This book is the first picture album with Chinese and English annotations to briefly introduce the long history and century-old campus of Cheeloo College of Medicine of Shandong University. It is up to the readers to decide whether these 200,000 or so words and 655 pictures interpret the spirit of the century-old university, that is, "We practice medicine for the welfare of all the people; we do research to pursue truth and enlightenment."

On campus of Cheeloo College of Medicine, there are dense trees, luxuriant flowers and plants, and magnificent buildings, with a combination of Chinese and Western styles. The campus was praised by Lao She as "an informal park". She is a sea of flowers; bathed in it, you can find each gene exudes a strong fragrance. She is a green world; the verdant view will make quick at thinking and seeing, vigorous and energetic. She is the melting furnace of iron, in which you can be refined into steel and eventually become a tower of strength. At first I had no intention of writing this book, but the elegant charm of the campus drove me to leave it on paper and her beautiful posture compelled me to raise the camera voluntarily. I admire the creativity of my predecessors and thank them for the monumental works they have left behind today. I look forward to the transcendence of those incoming people and hope that they will open up a better future. I also have a pity for the deficiency in cultural relics protection. If the classics continue to disappear, then what is the point of the miracle we have created today? I hope this book can help these buildings which have been listed as key cultural relics under national protection truly glow with youth. Never let these great architectural arts created by predecessors cry in the new rubble.

As this book is about to be published, grateful thanks are due to the following people: the leaders of the Publicity Department of Shandong University, Cheeloo College of Medicine, School of Basic Medical Sciences and Qilu Hospital for their encouragement and support which are the endless source of my strength; Professor Wang Yanbi, former president of Shandong Medical University, for writing the foreword and giving many instructions to this book; Dr. Liu Jing, a graduate of School of Foreign Languages and Literature of Shandong University, for her English translation of this book; the Management Office and schools of Baotuquan Campus of Shandong University for their cooperation and support; Professor Tian Daozheng of Qilu Hospital, Professor Wang Huaijing of School of Basic Medical Sciences, Professor Xie Fei of School of Physical Education and others for their help and support; Professor Jiang Jiying and Professor Yu Li of Weifang Medical University, and Secretary Cui Shutian and Professor Li Maosong of Weifang Nursing Vocational College, for their helping me to have successfully obtained the early historical materials of Cheeloo University; Chen Bin, director of Shandong University Press, and Xu Xiang, head of the Medical Branch, for their patience, help and support which are indispensable for the completion of this book. The historical pictures in this book are mainly from *Shantung Christian University (Cheeloo)* written by Charles Hodge Corbett. In addition to the public publications listed in the references at the end of this book, I have also referred to a large number of internal and online materials in the process of writing this book. I would like to express my heartfelt thanks to the original authors of these materials.

The instrument needs to be carefully carved and refined; the steel needs to be severely trained and hammered. We sincerely hope that readers will inform us of the deficiencies and even errors of this book in time for reference in reprint.

2021 marks the 100th anniversary of the founding of the Communist Party of China, the 120th anniversary of the founding of Shandong University and the 110th anniversary of the founding of the former Medical School of Cheeloo University in Jinan. I would like to dedicate this book to the great Communist Party of China and my loving alma mater.

Liu Shuwei

10 November 2021

医道寓园

刘树伟

2017 年 10 月 18 日

在今年暑期的一个中午，我在趵突泉校区中心花园见到了齐鲁医院普外科 82 岁高龄的王占民教授。相互问候之后，他不无自豪地微笑着说："树伟啊，我经常来这里坐坐。你看，古色古香的教学楼，满目苍翠的花木，这炙热的阳光和凉爽的夏风，到哪里去找？我坐在这里有种神仙般的感觉。"的确，这样优美的校园在国内实为翘楚，她是原齐鲁大学的校园。校园设计精巧，办公楼（原名麦考密可楼）坐北朝南，居中轴线北端，与南端的教学八楼（原为康穆堂）遥相呼应。花园中心为喷泉绕山，四块长方形草坪终年常绿。花园两侧由北向南依次有柏根楼与考文楼相望，葛罗神学院楼与教学七楼（原为奥古斯丁图书馆）对视。校园风光应四季而变。春风来袭，二月兰氤氲梦幻，丁香花如云似烟；夏日烈炎，绿色连天，静坐听蝉；秋枝萧瑟，青檐与红藤共舞，黄叶与白云齐飞；冬雪飘洒，银装素裹，笑语声声，宛入童话。

二十八年前，我第一次来到这个校园，首先映入眼帘的是悬挂着"山东医科大学"校名的大门。这个建于 1924 年的飞檐式牌楼，远看颇像繁体的"齐"字，是原齐鲁大学的标志性建筑。后来才知道，它是众多校友捐资所建，其南面的"校友门"题字古朴厚重，为清末状元王寿彭先生的手笔。多少年来，我一直埋头于学习与工作，没有去深究每一座建筑的来龙去脉，实在愧对齐鲁医学的百年历史。后来有一次机会，改变了我的认识。那是 1995 年秋天，我迎来了我的恩师、著名解剖学家、华西医科大学王永贵教授。原来，王老师 1940 年就毕业于齐鲁大学医学院，当时被齐鲁大学和多伦多大学分别授予医学学士与医学博士学位。老人家回到阔别经年的母校自然是感慨万千，首先来到齐鲁医院新兴楼与共合楼，在楼周围，他绕了几圈，举起相机拍了又拍。然后对我说："新兴楼是齐鲁大学最早的大楼，建于 1911 年，我的解剖课就是在这里完成的。"我又陪着他参观了广智院、求真楼和景蓝斋等，还在四百号院他当年住过的宿舍前留了影。但给我印象最为深刻的是，他老人家仰望校友门，久久凝视，两行热泪滚滚而下。我此时默默地躲到他的身后，不知道眼前这位年逾八旬依然风度翩翩的齐鲁学子，面对母校的大门，在想些什么？从此以后，我便开始关注和收集齐鲁大学的历史，越来越感到她博大精渊，深不可测。

我想两位王先生深爱母校校园，并不仅仅是睹物思人，定是被某种精神所吸引，所激励。那一定是"博施济众，广智求真"的齐鲁医学精神，这才是齐鲁大学最大的遗产。

前几天，我又见到了坐在中心花园里的王占民先生。他举目环顾，一片黄叶落到了头上而浑然不知。也许他在想，这金秋之后，又要踏雪寻梅了。是的，葛罗神学院楼前的蜡梅又快开放了。拂去历史的尘埃和冰雪，齐鲁大学就像那梅花一样，依然散发出阵阵幽香，永远给人以无穷的魅力和前进的勇气。有词为证：

《临江仙·咏梅》

朵朵寒梅花放蕊，嫣然欢送严冬。面朝大地悄无声。飞雪遮不住，暗香透长空。

万丈梅香枝叶炼，凝集雨绿阳红。根深何惧彤云冷？冰雪融化日，依旧笑春风。

Medical Philosophy from Campus

Liu Shuwei

18 October 2017

One day this summer, I met Professor Wang Zhanmin at noon in the Central Garden on Baotuquan Campus. He is 82 years old and once worked in the General Surgery Department of Qilu Hospital. After greeting each other, he smiled proudly and said: "Shuwei, I often come here to have a sit. The ancient teaching buildings, the luxuriant flowers and trees, the hot sun and cool summer wind are rare. Sitting here, I feel like an immortal." Indeed, such a beautiful campus is really an outstanding one in China. She is the campus of former Cheeloo University. The design of the campus is exquisite; the Office Building (former McCormick Hall) faces south and is located at the north end of the central axis, echoing the Eighth Teaching Building (former Kumler Chapel) at the south end. There is a fountain surrounded by the rockwork in the center of the garden, and four rectangular lawns are evergreen all the year round. On both sides of the garden from north to south, there are Bergen Hall and Calvin Mateer Hall facing each other, and the Building of Gotch-Robinson Theological College and the Seventh Teaching Building (former Augustine Library) facing each other. The scenery on campus changes during the four seasons. When the spring breeze blows, there are dense flowers of Orychophragmus violaceus and lilac flowers like clouds. On hot summer days, you can sit and listen to cicadas chirping around the green scenery. In autumn, besides bleak branches, there are also blue eaves and red vines, yellow leaves and white clouds. When the winter snow falls, the snow-covered surroundings and laughter make you feel like you are in a fairy tale world.

When I first came to this campus twenty-eight years ago, the first thing that came into view was the gate with the name of "Shandong Medical University". Built in 1924, the archway with overhanging eaves looks like the traditional Chinese character "Qi" from a distance and it is the landmark building of the former Cheeloo University. Later, I learned that it was built with donations from many alumni. The simple and decorous inscription of "Xiao You Men" on the south side was written by Mr. Wang Shoupeng, the Number One Scholar in the late Qing Dynasty. For many years, I have been immersed in study and work, and then I feel guilty about not going deep into the ins and outs of each building which is part of the century-old history of Qilu Medicine. Later, there was a chance that changed my mind. In the autumn of 1995, I met my mentor Professor Wang Yonggui, a famous anatomist of West China Medical University. Professor Wang graduated from the Medical School of Cheeloo University in 1940, and he was awarded a Bachelor of Medicine and a Doctor of Medicine by Cheeloo University and the University of Toronto respectively. When he returned to his alma mater after many years, all sorts of feelings well up in his mind. First, he came to the Xinxing Building and Gonghe Building of Qilu Hospital, and walked around them to take pictures. Then he said to me, "Xinxing Building is the earliest building of Cheeloo University. It was built in 1911, and this is the place where I attended my anatomy classes." Then I accompanied him to visit Tsinanfu Institute, Qiuzhen Building and Jinglan Building, and also took a photo in front of the dormitory where he lived in the Courtyard. But what impressed me most was that he looked up at the Alumni Gate and stared for a long time, then two lines of tears rolled down his face. At this time, I silently hid behind him. I don't know what he was thinking in the face of the gate of his alma mater as a graduate of Cheeloo University who is still elegant in his 80s. Since then, I have begun to notice and collect materials about the history of Cheeloo University, and more and more feel that she is broad and profound.

I think Mr. Wang Zhanmin and Mr. Wang Yonggui deeply love the campus of their alma mater not only because seeing the things on campus makes them think of the people. They must be attracted and inspired by some kind of spirit. That must be the spirit of Qilu medicine, that is, "We practice medicine for the welfare of all the people; we do research to pursue truth and enlightenment." It is the greatest legacy of Cheeloo University.

A few days ago, I met Mr. Wang Zhanmin sitting in the Central Garden. He looked around and didn't notice a yellow leaf falling on his head. Perhaps he was thinking that it would be the time to look for plum flowers while treading on snow after this golden autumn. The wintersweet in front of the Building of Gotch-Robinson Theological College is about to open again. Cheeloo University, like the plum blossom, still emits bursts of fragrance, always giving people infinite charm and courage to move forward. Here is a *ci* to prove it.

Lin Jiang Xian: Ode to the Plum Blossom

The plum blossoms bloom in the cold, sweetly sending off the severe winter. They bloom silently on the earth. The flying snow can not cover the delicate fragrance through the sky.

The fragrance comes from the refinement of branches and leaves which absorb the rain and sunshine. The plum blossoms with deep roots do not fear the cold clouds. When the ice and snow melt, they still smile to welcome the spring breeze.

目 录

第一章 Chapter One

1917 年之前的齐鲁大学老建筑

Old Buildings of Cheeloo University Before 1917

01 登州文会馆

Tengchow College

登州文会馆由美北长老会传教士狄考文于 1864 年创办，始于蒙养学堂。1882 年纽约长老会总部批准以 Tengchow College 为学校英文名称，这标志着中国第一所教会大学的诞生。它为齐鲁大学的创始阶段，也是中国最早的现代大学。1904 年，登州文会馆迁至潍县，与英国浸礼会在青州创办的广德书院合并，更名为广文学堂。1947 年，登州文会馆被当地国民党政府拆除。至 1904 年，登州文会馆共有正式毕业生 208 人，其中从事教育工作的多达 60%，为中国早期高等学堂输送了大批师资力量。他们分布于全国 16 个省份，先后任教于 200 多所学校，如上海圣约翰大学、山西大学堂、京师大学堂（今北京大学）、山东大学堂、上海南洋公学（今上海交通大学）、金陵大学、浙江高等学堂（今浙江大学）等。

Tengchow College was founded by Calvin Wilson Mateer, a missionary of the American Presbyterian Missions, North in 1864, the predecessor of which is Tengchow Boy's Boarding School. In 1882, the headquarters of the Presbyterian Church in New York approved Tengchow College as the English name of this college, which marked the birth of the first missionary university in China. It is the founding stage of Cheeloo University and the earliest modern university in China. In 1904, Tengchow College moved to Weixian and merged with Tsingchow Kwang Teh Shu Yun founded by the English Baptist Missionary Society to change its name to Wei Hsien Arts and Science College. In 1947, Tengchow College was demolished by the local Kuomintang government. By 1904, Tengchow College had a total of 208 formal graduates, of whom as many as 60% were engaged in education, sending a large number of teachers to early colleges and universities in China. They were distributed in 16 provinces and had taught in more than 200 schools, such as St. John's University in Shanghai, Shanxi University, Imperial University of Peking (now Peking University), Shandong University, Shanghai Nanyang Public College (now Shanghai Jiao Tong University), University of Nanking, Zhejiang Academy of Higher Education (now Zhejiang University) and so on.

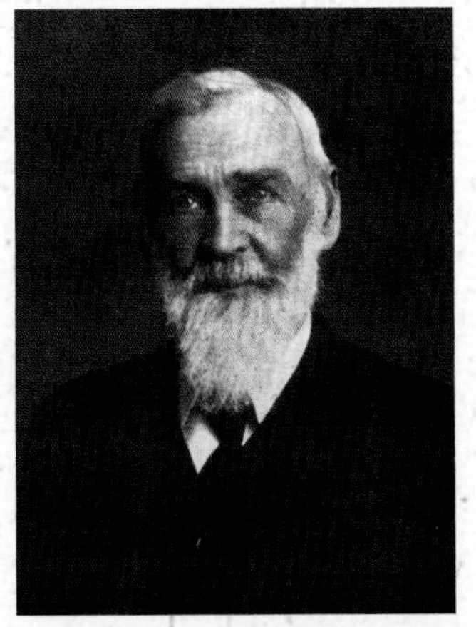

图 1 狄考文（Calvin Wilson Mateer,1836~1908），美国宾夕法尼亚人，神学和法学博士，基督教美北长老会传教士，著名教育家，近代中西文化交流的先驱。1908 年病逝于青岛，葬于烟台毓璜顶美国长老会墓地。

Fig. 1 Calvin Wilson Mateer (1836-1908), born in Pennsylvania in the United States, Doctor of Divinity and Laws, was a missionary of the American Presbyterian Missions, North. He was also a famous educator and pioneer of modern cultural exchange between China and Western countries. He died of illness in Qingdao in 1908 and was buried in the cemetery of the Presbyterian Church, USA in Yuhuangding, Yantai.

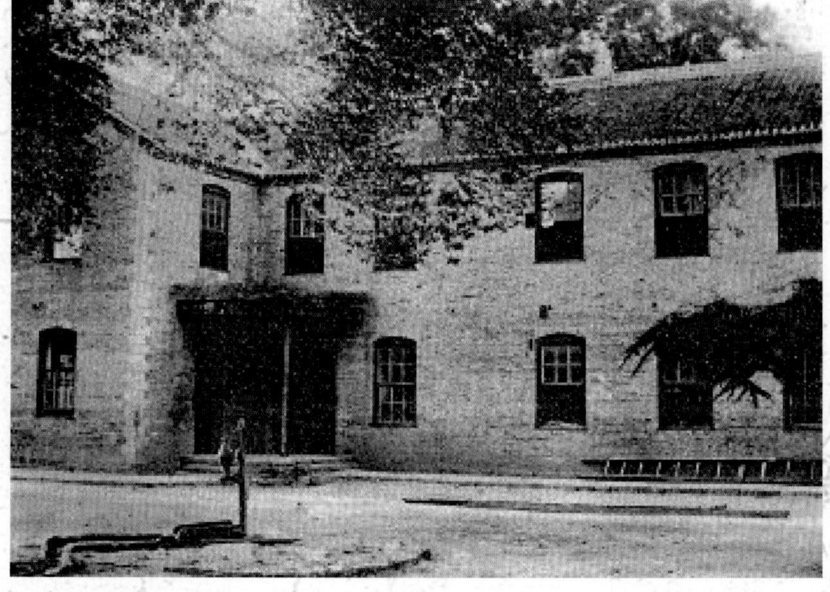

图 2 登州文会馆讲堂

Fig. 2 The Lecture Hall of Tengchow College

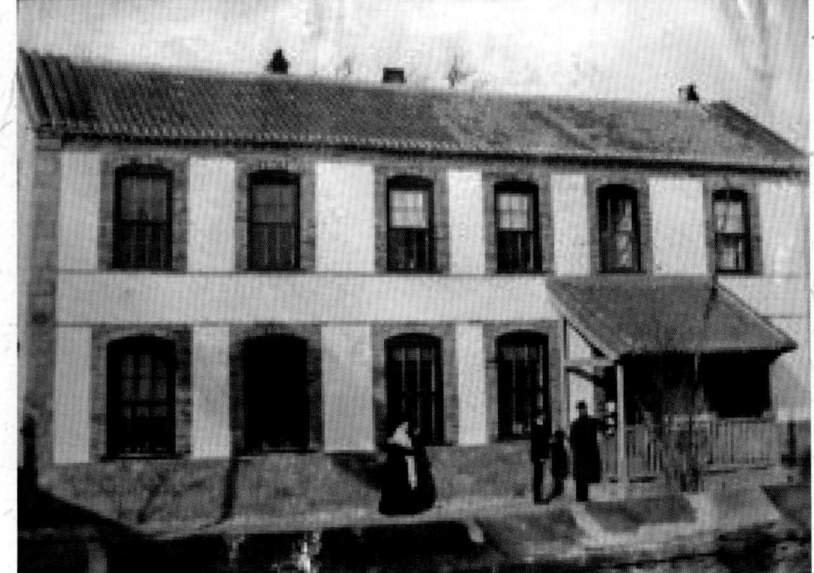

图 3 登州文会馆外国教习宿舍

Fig. 3 Dormitory of foreign teachers in Tengchow College

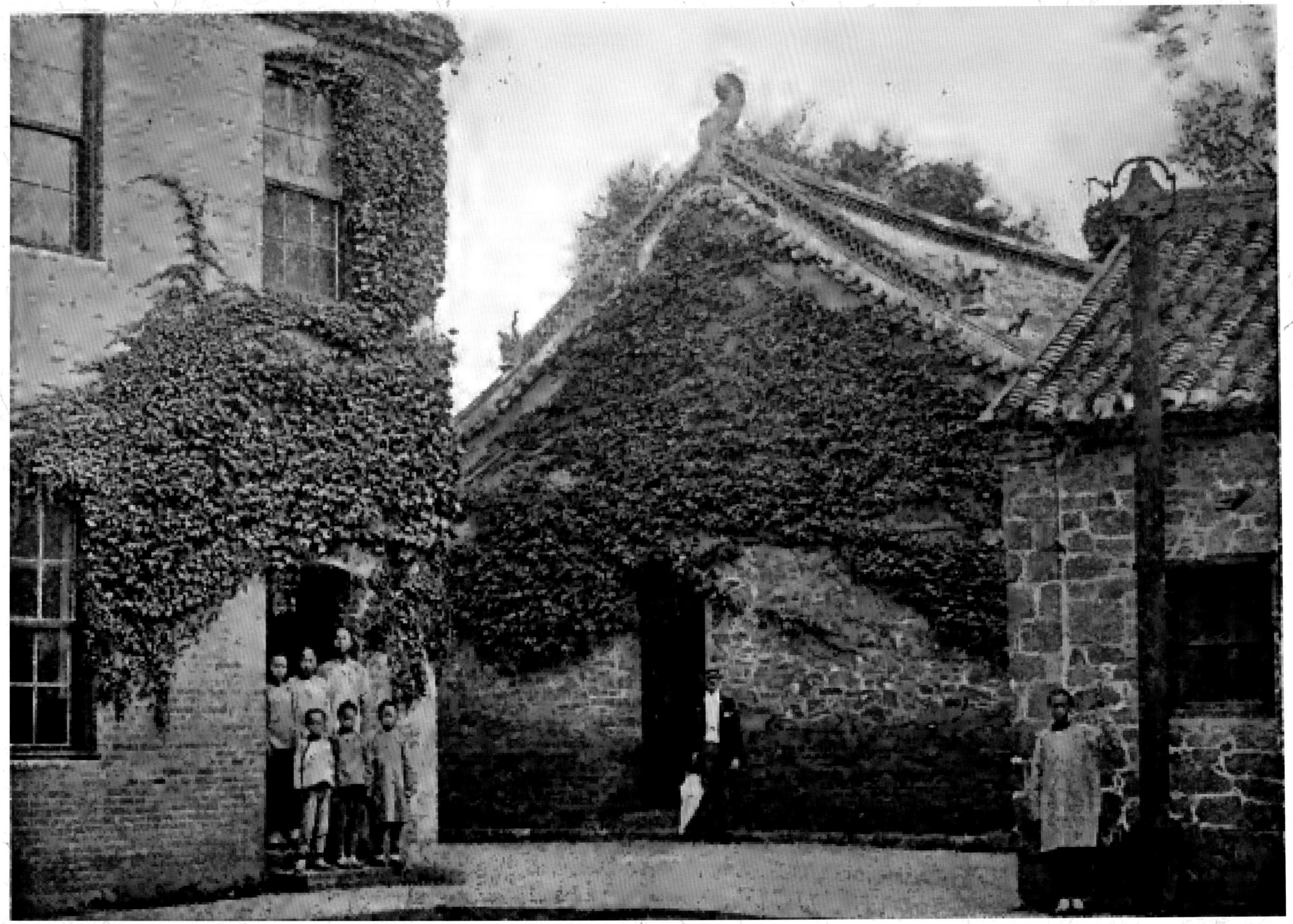

图4 登州文会馆教学楼（左）、小教室（中）、校铃和备斋小教室

Fig. 4 Teaching building (left), small classroom (middle), bell and small classroom for preparing food of Tengchow College

02 华美医院和医校

Sino-American Hospital and Medical School

1890 年，美国北长老会传教医师聂会东夫妇奉命从登州来到济南，协助开展教会医务工作。他们在狭小的原有教会诊所——文璧诊所基础上扩建成华美医院，这就是齐鲁医院的前身。华美医院院址位于济南市青龙桥北，兴华街（原华美街）中段，现济南五中对面。1891 年，医院添建病房，并创建了华美医院医校，开办西医教育。该医校于 1903 年与英国浸礼会在青州及邹平所办的医学堂、美北长老会在沂州创办的医学堂合并，建成山东共合医道学堂，此学堂后来成为著名的齐鲁大学医学院，聂会东为首任院长。1937 年，日本侵略军占领济南，早已成为齐鲁医院分部的华美医院遂告停办。1948 年，华美医院毁于战火。

In 1890, James Boyd Neal, a missionary doctor of the American Presbyterian Missions, North, was ordered to come to Jinan from Dengzhou with his wife to assist in the medical work of the church. They expanded the small original church clinic to Sino-American Hospital, the predecessor of Qilu Hospital. Sino-American Hospital was located in the middle of Xinghua Street (former Huamei Street), North of Qinglongqiao, Jinan City and opposite Jinan No.5 Middle School. In 1891, the hospital built additional wards and established the Medical School of Sino-American Hospital to provide Western medicine education. In 1903, the medical school merged with the hospitals run by the English Baptist Missionary Society in Qingzhou and Zouping to form Shandong Union Medical College, which later became the famous Medical School of Cheeloo University, with James Boyd Neal as the first dean. In 1937, the Japanese invaders occupied Jinan, and Sino-American Hospital, which had long become a branch of Qilu Hospital, was suspended. In 1948, Sino-America Hospital was destroyed in war.

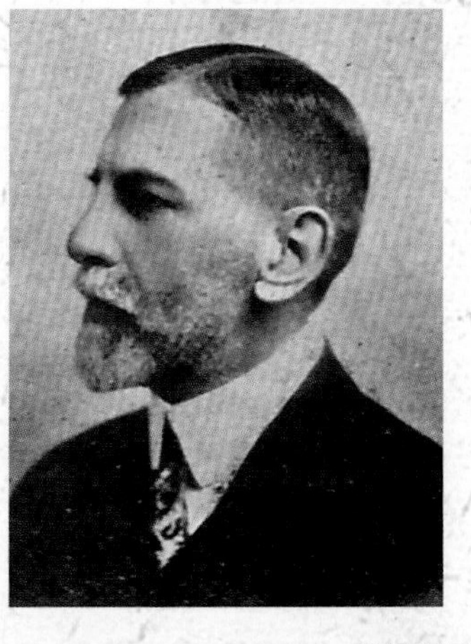

图 5 聂会东（James Boyd Neal,1855~1925），美国基督教北长老会传教医师。山东大学齐鲁医院主要创建者，齐鲁大学医学院首任院长，1919 年任齐鲁大学第二任校长。1922 年因病返美，1925 年病逝。

Pic 5. James Boyd Neal (1855-1925), a missionary doctor of the American Presbyterian Missions, North, was the main founder of Qilu Hospital of Shandong University. He was the first dean of the Medical School of Cheeloo University. In 1919, he became the second president of Cheeloo University. He returned to the United States in 1922 due to illness and died in 1925.

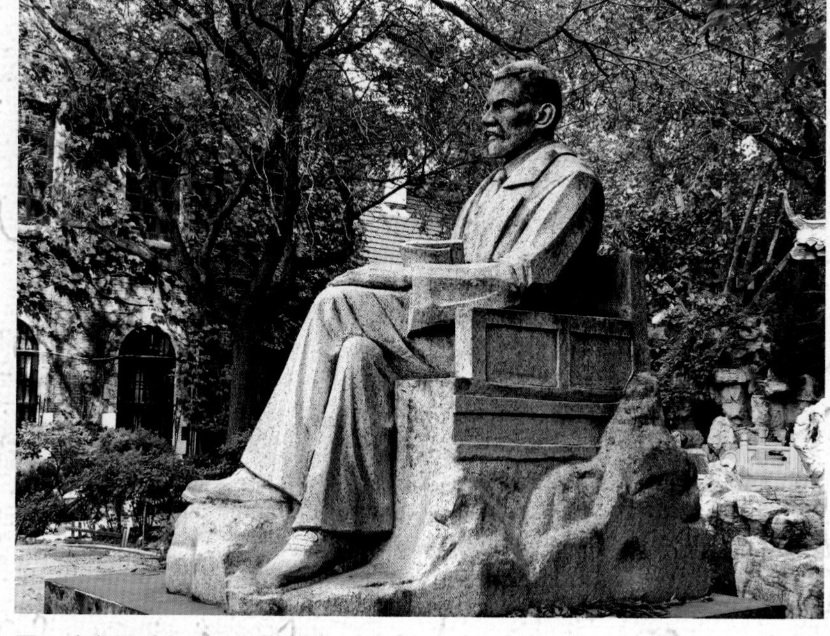

图 6 齐鲁医院内的聂会东塑像

Fig. 6 Statue of James Boyd Neal in Qilu Hospital

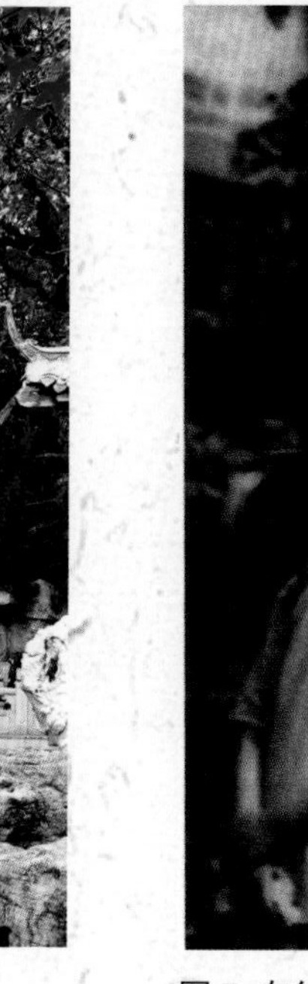

图 7 在华美医院工作的女职工

Fig. 7 Female employees working in Sino-American Hospital

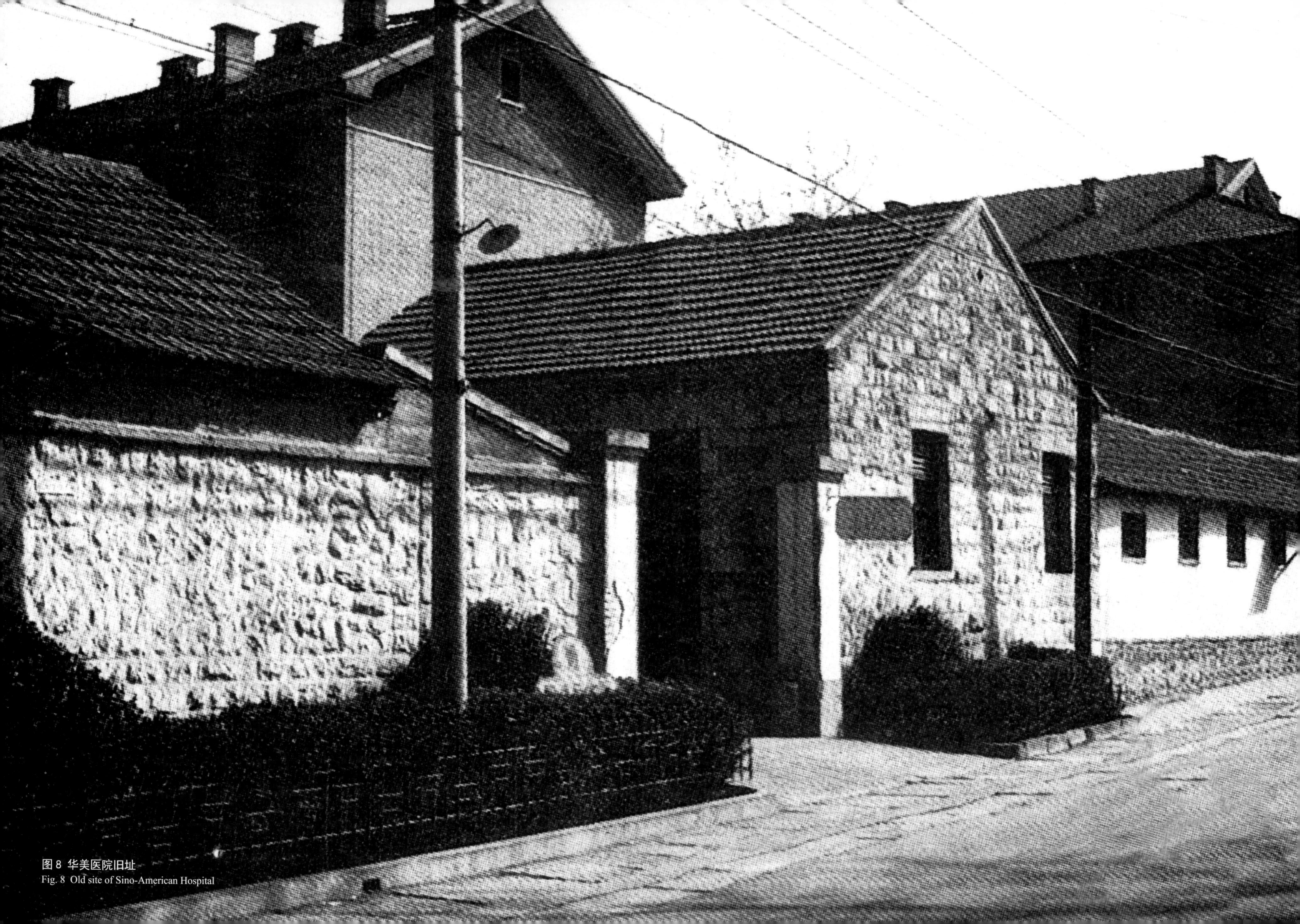

图 8 华美医院旧址
Fig. 8 Old site of Sino-American Hospital

03 青州广德医院和医学堂

Tsingchow Kwang Teh Hospital and the Medical School

1875年，英国基督教浸礼会传教士李提摩太，由登州至青州传教布道。1877年，青州连逢干旱，李提摩太遂设立粥场，开办施医所，免费施粥施药，以扩大传教范围。1885年，英国基督教浸礼会医学传教士武成献夫妇奉命来到青州，开始扩建施医所。1892年，历尽周折医院终于建成，拥有一座616平方米的办公楼，门诊、药房、病房、教室等平房共105间。医院定名为青州广德医院，同时成立青州医学堂，当时是山东最大的医院和医学堂。1911年，医学堂迁至济南，与华美医院医校等合并为山东共合医道学堂，原校更名为青州广德医院护士学校，几经变迁，今为潍坊护理职业学院，广德医院现为益都中心医院。

In 1875, Timothy Richard, a missionary of the English Baptist Missionary Society, came from Dengzhou to Qingzhou to preach. In 1877, Qingzhou suffered from drought; Timothy Richard set up a porridge farm and opened a clinic to give porridge and medicine free of charge in order to expand the scope of his missionary work. In 1885, James Russell Watson, a medical missionary of the English Baptist Missionary Society, was ordered to come to Qingzhou with his wife and began to expand the clinic. In 1892, the hospital was finally completed after all the twists and turns, with a 616-square-meter office building and 105 bungalows of outpatient services, pharmacies, wards, classrooms and so on. The hospital was named Tsingchow Kwang Teh Hospital and the Medical School was established at the same time. They were the largest hospital and medical school in Shandong Province at that time. In 1911, the Medical School moved to Jinan and merged with the Medical School of Sino-American Hospital to become Shandong Union Medical College. The original school was renamed Nursing School of Tsingchow Kwang Teh Hospital. After several changes, it has become now Weifang Nursing Vocational College. Kwang Teh Hospital is now Yidu Central Hospital.

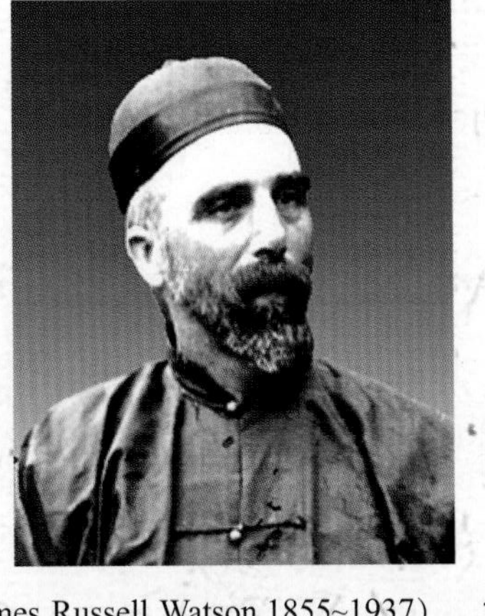

图9 武成献（James Russell Watson,1855~1937），1855年出生于苏格兰阿伯丁，医学学士、理学硕士、哲学博士，基督教英国浸礼会传教士，齐鲁大学医学院的创始人之一。1937年3月15日在济南辞世，安葬在齐鲁大学校园内。

Fig. 9 James Russell Watson (1855-1937) was born in Aberdeen, Scotland in 1855. He was a Bachelor of Medicine, a Master of Science and a Doctor of Philosophy. He was a missionary of the English Baptist Missionary Society and one of the founders of the Medical School of Cheeloo University. He died in Jinan on 15 March 1937 and was buried on campus of Cheeloo University.

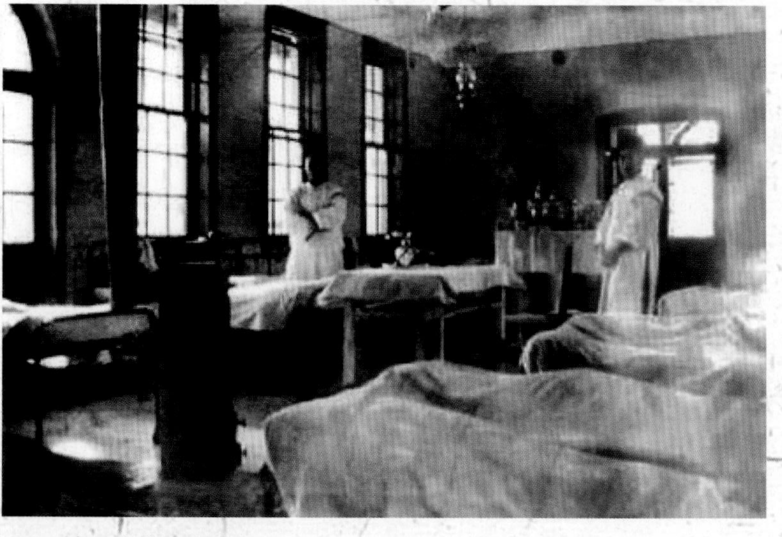

图10 青州广德医院病房

Fig. 10 Ward of Tsingchow Kwang Teh Hospital

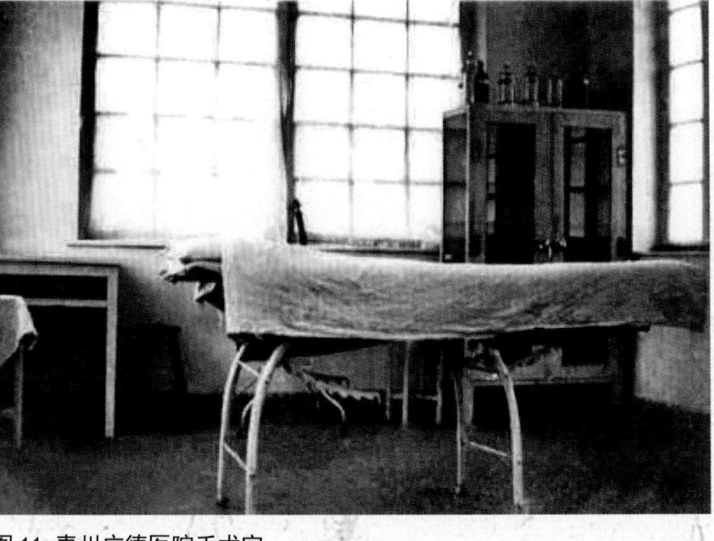

图11 青州广德医院手术室

Fig. 11 Operating room of Tsingchow Kwang Teh Hospital

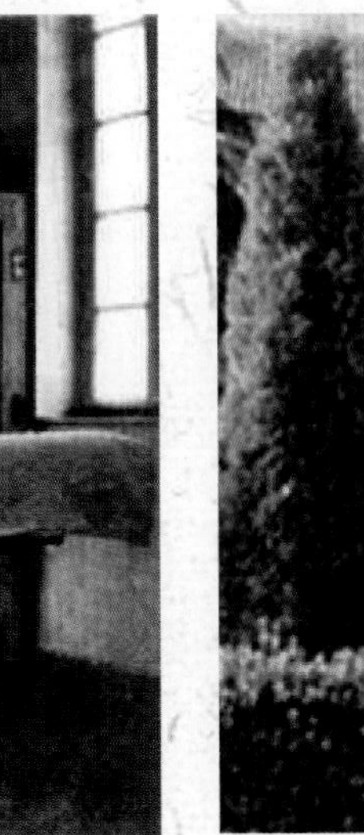

图12 青州广德医院和医学堂旧址

Fig. 12 Old site of Tsingchow Kwang Teh Hospital and the Medical School

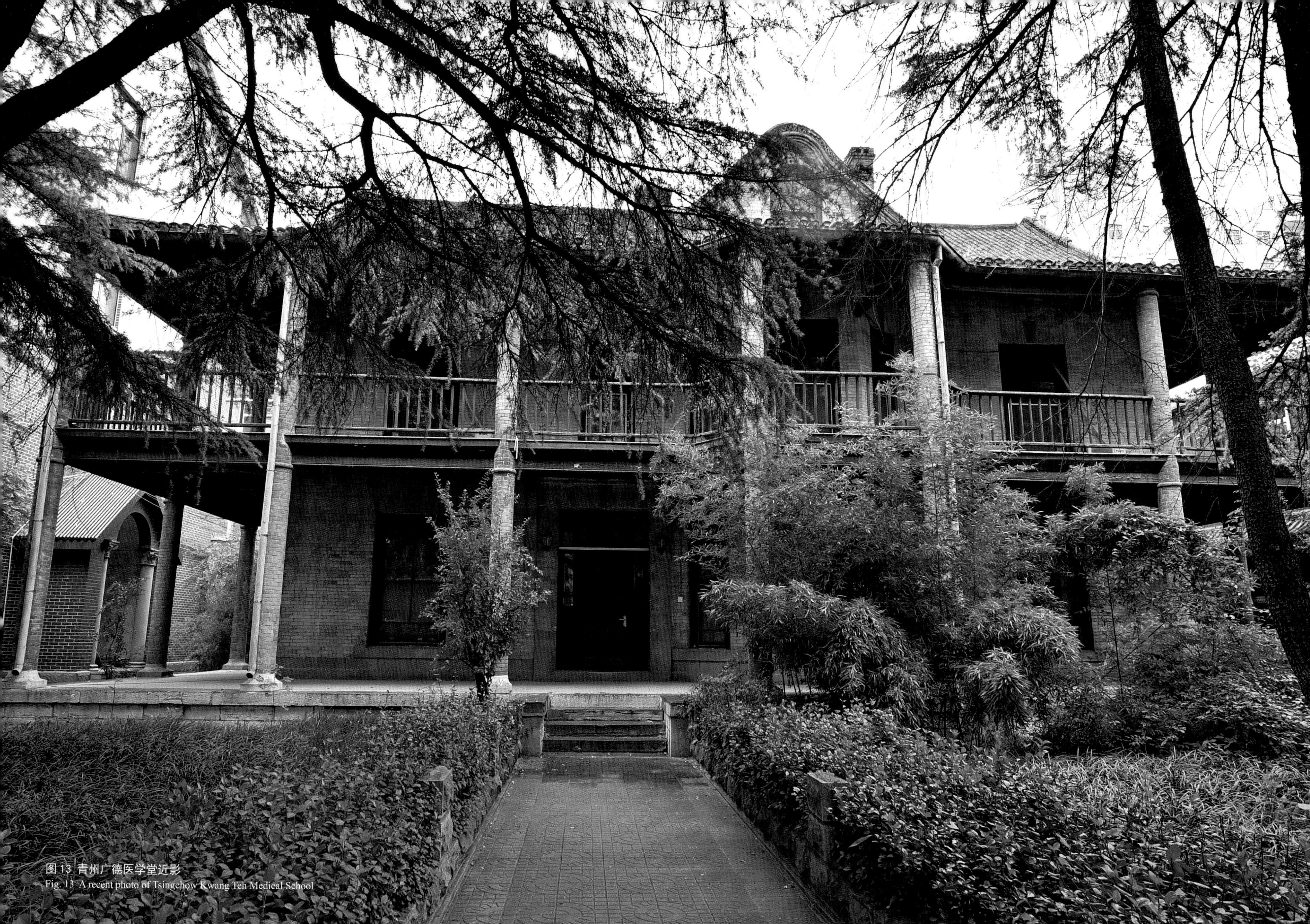
图 13 青州广德医学堂近影
Fig. 13 A recent photo of Tsingchow Kwang Teh Medical School

04 潍县广文学堂

Wei Hsien Arts and Science College

1904 年，青州广德书院大学部和登州文会馆大学部的文理科合并，分别由青州和登州迁往潍县乐道院，作为山东新教大学的文理学院，取名“广文学堂”，又称“广文大学”（Wei Hsien Arts and Science College）。合并后的学生中 84 人来自登州，30 人来自青州，教员中有 10 名中国人，4 名西方人，柏尔根被选为校长。1917 年，广文学堂迁往济南，乐道院仍是长老会的中心。珍珠港事变爆发后，日本侵略军使它成为臭名昭著的潍县集中营，专门关押盟国侨民。广文学堂曾被美国人称为“中国哈佛”和“现代教育的温床”，现为潍坊市人民医院和广文中学驻地。

In 1904, the Department of Arts and Science of Tsingchow Kwang Teh Shu Yun and that of Tengchow College merged, and they moved from Qingzhou and Dengzhou to the Courtyard of the Happy Way in Weixian respectively. As the School of Arts and Science of Shantung Protestant University, it was named “Wei Hsien Arts and Science College”. Of the merged students, eighty-four were from Dengzhou and thirty were from Qingzhou. Among the faculty were ten Chinese and four Westerners. Bergen was elected president. In 1917, Wei Hsien Arts and Science College moved to Jinan, and the Courtyard of the Happy Way was still the center of the Presbyterian Church. After the Pearl Harbor Incident, the Japanese invaders made the Courtyard of the Happy Way a notorious concentration camp which held allied nationals. Wei Hsien Arts and Science College was once called “Harvard in China” and “hotbed of modern education” by Americans. It is now the residence of Weifang People’s Hospital and Guangwen Middle School.

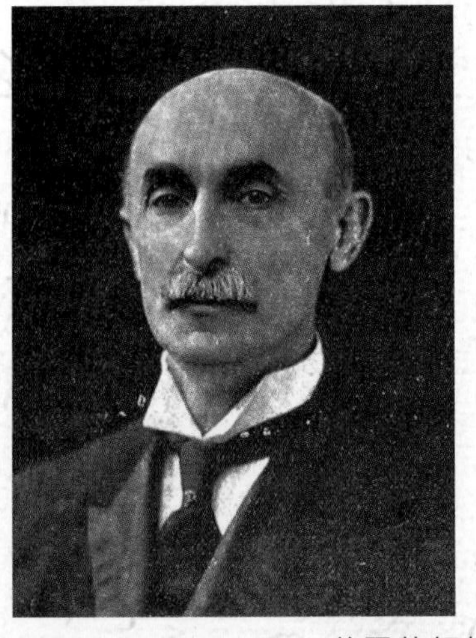

图 14 柏尔根（Paul D. Bergen,1860~1915），美国基督教北长老会传教士，1893 年到登州文会馆任教，1901 年接替赫士出任监督（校长），1904 年随文会馆一起迁往潍县，1915 年病逝于潍县。

Fig. 14 Paul D. Bergen (1860-1915), a missionary of the American Presbyterian Missions, North, taught in Tengchow College in 1893 and succeeded Watson Mcmillen Hayes as supervisor (president) in 1901. He moved to Weixian with Tengchow College in 1904 and died of illness there in 1915.

图 15 潍县广文学堂为狄考文庆祝 70 寿辰

Fig. 15 Wei Hsien Arts and Science College celebrating Calvin Wilson Mateer’s 70th birthday

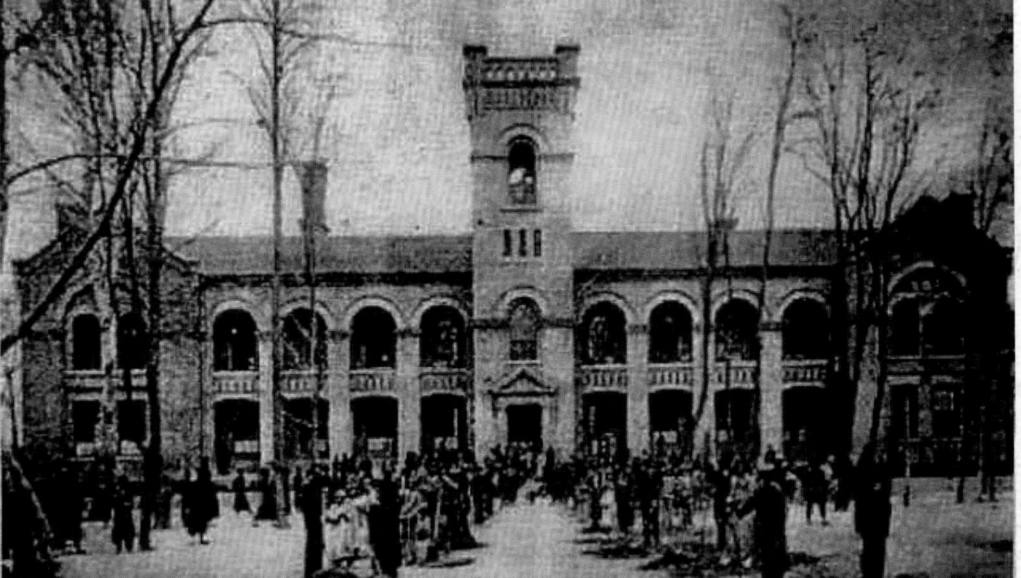

图 16 潍县广文学堂旧址

Fig. 16 Old site of Wei Hsien Arts and Science College

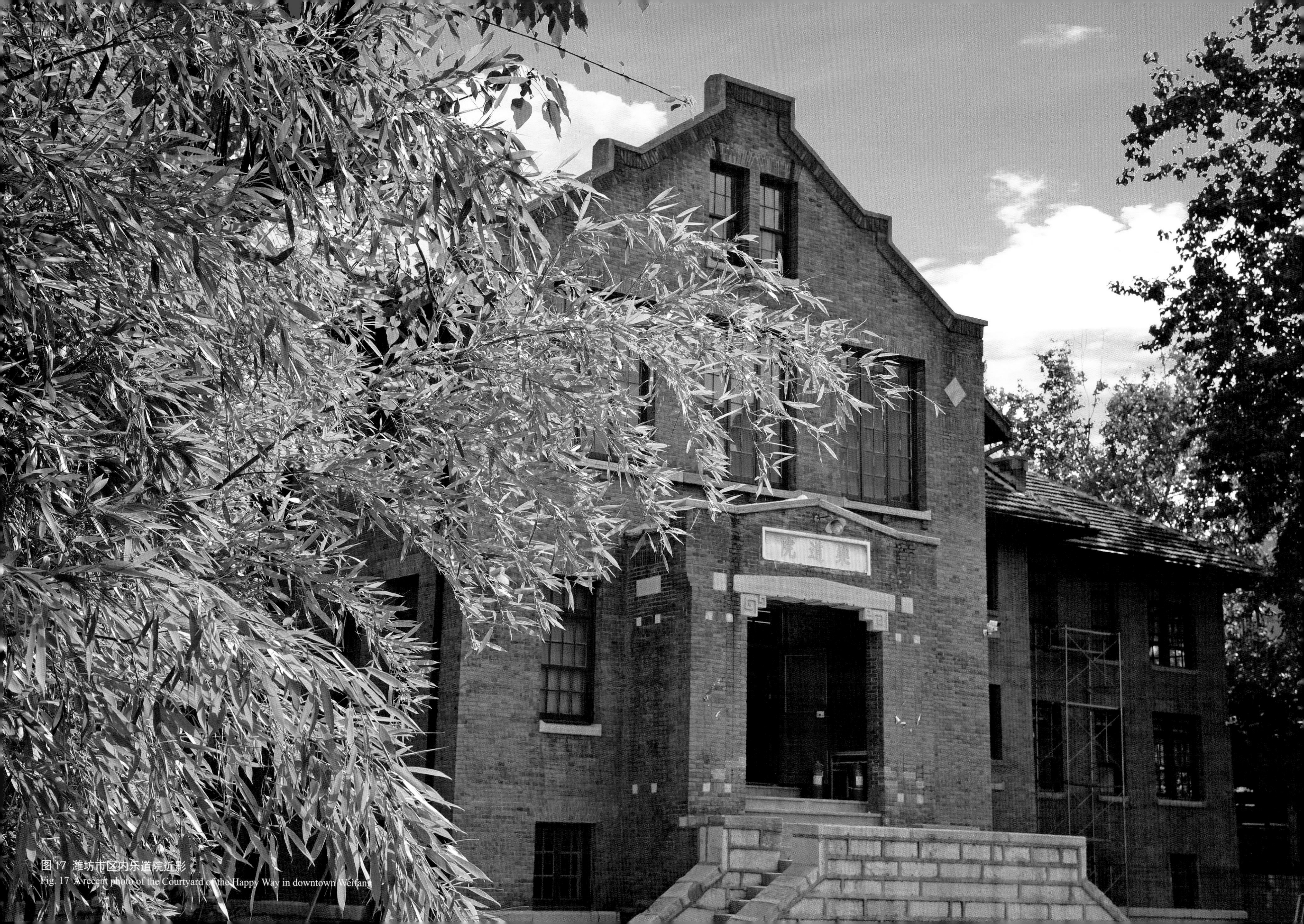

图 17 潍坊市区内乐道院近影
Fig. 17 A recent photo of the Courtyard of the Happy Way in downtown Weifang

05 济南广智院（1）

Tsinanfu Institute (1)

济南广智院是山东省首座博物馆，也是中国最早的博物馆之一，其前身为青州博物堂，由英国基督教浸礼会传教士怀恩光(John Sutherland Whitewright，1858 ~ 1926)创办。1879年神学院毕业后，怀恩光被派到山东青州传教。1887年，他在青州创建了一座称为“博物堂”的展览馆，参观者每年达7万人之多。1904年，胶济铁路通车后，济南的重要性大增，怀恩光便将博物堂迁到济南，并扩大至2万余平方米，定名为“广智院”，取“广其智识”之意。广智院由怀恩光之子设计，既有中国传统庙宇特色又有西方建筑风格。1905年11月6日，广智院落成，时任山东巡抚杨士骧率大批文武官员参加了典礼。广智院后来成为齐鲁大学社会教育科，1954年划归山东省博物馆，现为山东大学齐鲁医院的医学博物馆和图书馆。

Tsinanfu Institute is the first museum of Shandong Province and one of the earliest museums in China, the predecessor of which was Tsingchowfu Museum. It was founded by John Sutherland Whitewright (1858-1926), a missionary of the English Baptist Missionary Society. After graduating from a theological college in 1879, John Sutherland Whitewright was sent to Qingzhou, Shandong Province to preach. In 1887, he set up an exhibition hall in Qingzhou called “Tsingchowfu Museum”, attracting as many as 70,000 visitors a year. In 1904, after the Qingdao-Jinan Railway was opened to traffic, Jinan’s importance increased greatly. Then John Sutherland Whitewright moved the museum to Jinan and expanded it to more than 20,000 square meters. It was named “Tsinanfu Institute” with the meaning of “broadening the wisdom and knowledge”. Designed by the son of John Sutherland Whitewright, Tsinanfu Institute had both the characteristics of traditional Chinese temples and Western architectural style. On 6 November 1905, Tsinanfu Institute was completed. Yang Shixiang, then governor of Shandong Province, led a large number of civil and military officials to attend the dedication. Tsinanfu Institute later became the Department of Social Education of Cheeloo University. It was transferred to Shandong Museum in 1954 and is now the medical museum and library of Qilu Hospital of Shandong University.

图18 济南广智院大门

Fig. 18 Gate of Tsinanfu Institute

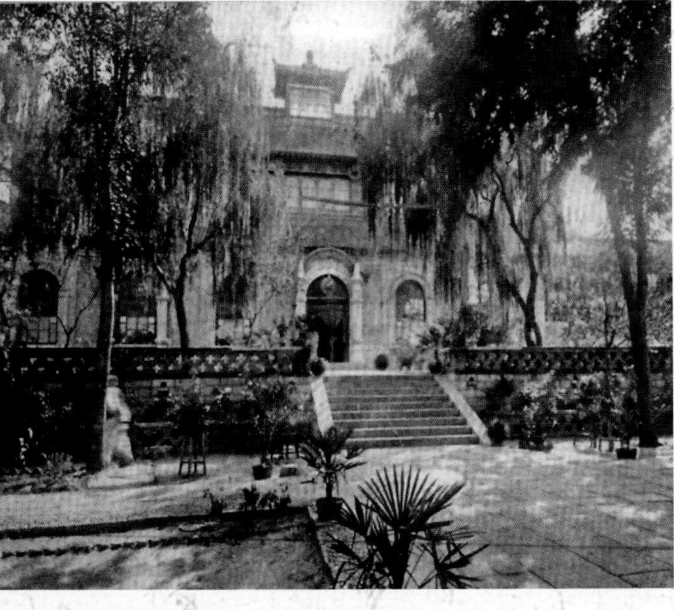

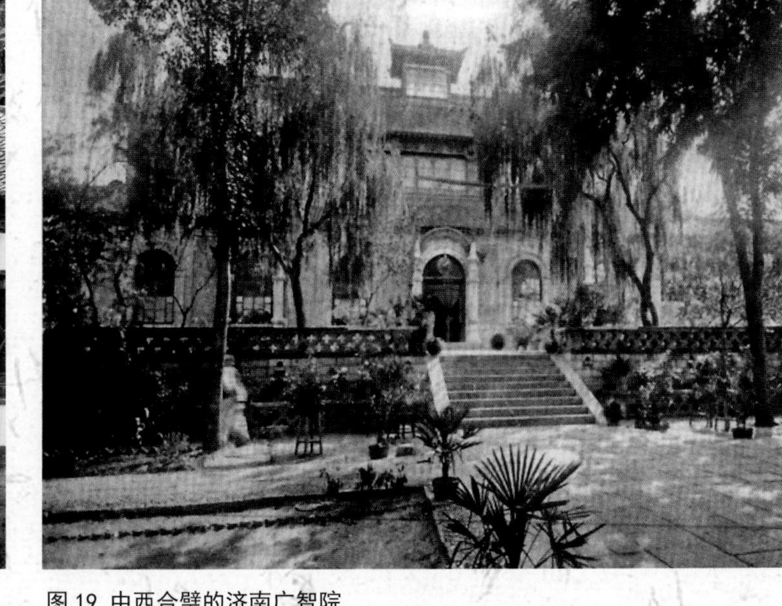

图19 中西合璧的济南广智院

Fig. 19 Tsinanfu Institute with the combination of Chinese and Western styles

图20 济南广智院旧影

Fig. 20 An old photo of Tsinanfu Institute

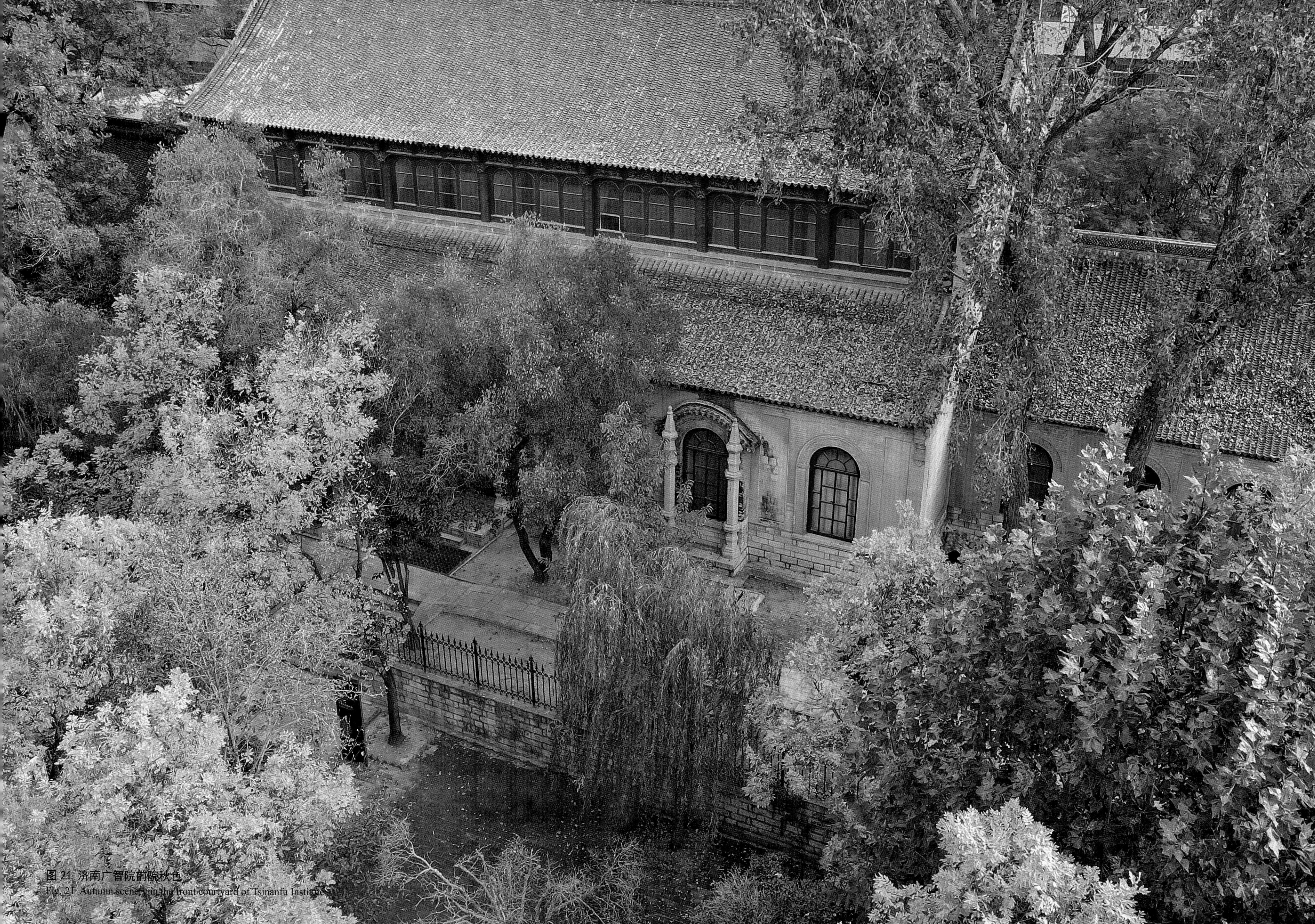

图 21 济南广智院前院秋色

Fig. 21 Autumn scenery in the front courtyard of Tsinanfu Institute

05 济南广智院（2）

Tsinanfu Institute (2)

广智院是一所综合性博物馆，有展品万余件，分为动物、植物、矿物、天文、地理、机工、卫生、生理、农产、文教、艺术、历史、古物等 13 个门类，采用展橱、镜框、挂图等方式，分为 2000 余组，常年开展。展览分为经常展览和特别展览，前者以启发民智为主，后者多侧重社会急需，如农村事业展览会、卫生事业展览会等。广智院还有声有色地举办演讲会，每礼拜日下午举行，内容多以科学、卫生、哲学、宗教、道德等为主题。为广泛开拓观众群，针对不同阶层，设立参观日、学堂和协修会，放映当时令国人最感新鲜的幻灯和电影。由于其教会背景，广智院理所当然地成为了那个时期一个科学与宗教的汇集地，也给百年前封闭的国民打开了一扇通往外部世界的窗口。

Tsinanfu Institute is a comprehensive museum with more than 10,000 exhibits, including 13 categories of animals, plants, minerals, astronomy, geography, mechanics, health, physiology, agriculture, culture and education, art, history and antiquities. These exhibits were divided into more than 2,000 groups by means of display cabinets, picture frames and wall charts. Tsinanfu Institute was open all year round. The exhibitions were divided into regular ones and special ones. The former focused on inspiring people's wisdom, while the latter focused on urgent social needs, such as rural undertakings exhibitions, health undertakings exhibitions and so on. Tsinanfu Institute also held lectures on science, health, philosophy, religion and morality every Sunday afternoon. In order to broaden the audience, visiting days, schools and fellowship meetings were set up for different classes to show the most fresh slides and films of the time. Because of its church background, Tsinanfu Institute naturally became a gathering place for science and religion at that time, and opened a window to the outside world for the people who were closed a hundred years ago.

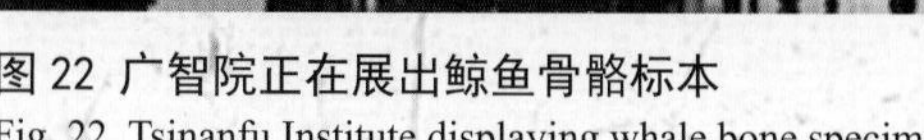

图 22 广智院正在展出鲸鱼骨骼标本
Fig. 22 Tsinanfu Institute displaying whale bone specimens

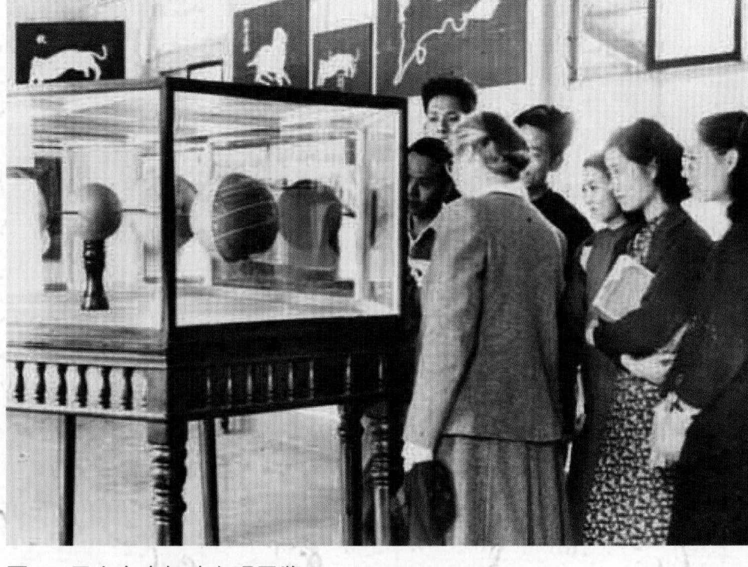

图 23 民众在广智院参观展览
Fig. 23 People visiting the exhibition at Tsinanfu Institute

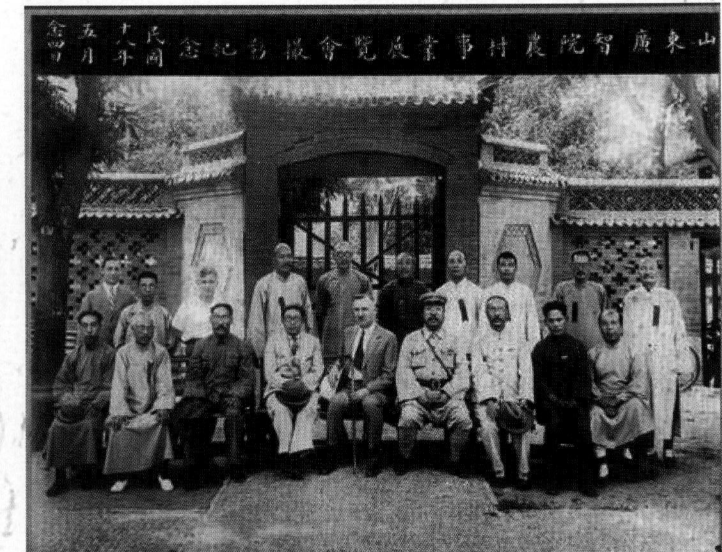

图 24 1929 年当地官员出席农村事业展览会
Fig. 24 Local officials attending the rural undertakings exhibition in 1929

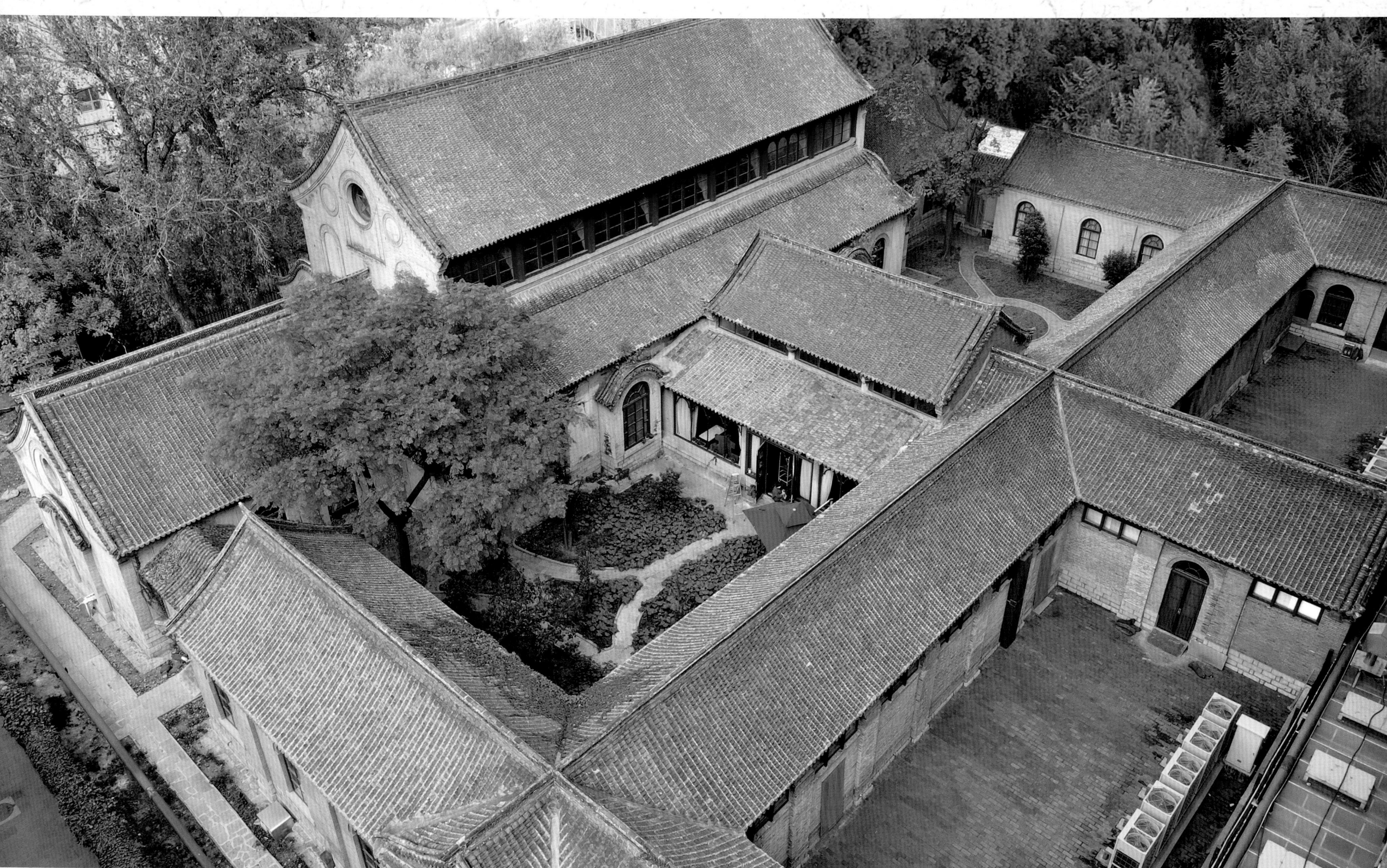

图 25 济南广智院后院近影
Fig. 25 A recent photo of the backyard of Tsinanfu Institute

05 济南广智院（3）

Tsinanfu Institute (3)

广智院当时社会影响很大，参观者来自 30 多个国家。据 1924 年《齐鲁大学社会学系调查》的统计：“参观广智院的人每年 50 多万，济南人常到这里来，也吸引了外地参观者到济南来。在广智院里，人们可以看到涉及一个先进社会所有方面的有教育意义的逼真展览品。”1914 年，黄炎培先生在专访记录中对广智院的盛况赞叹不已。1922 年，胡适先生参观广智院后，其兴奋之心情均记录在当天的日记里。民国作家倪锡瑛曾在其《都市地理小丛书：济南》中写道：“去济南的人，山水的胜景少领略一点倒不要紧，可是广智院是不能不去参观一下的。”曾在齐鲁大学任教的老舍先生专门写了《广智院》一文。广智院对中国的博物馆事业也产生了积极影响，1922 年创立的天津广智馆、1949 年陈嘉庚先生建立的鳌园，均深受广智院的启发。

Tsinanfu Institute had a great social impact at that time and its visitors came from more than 30 countries. According to the *Survey of the Department of Sociology of Cheeloo University* in 1924, “More than 500,000 people visit Tsinanfu Institute every year. People in Jinan often come here and it also attracts visitors from other places to Jinan. In Tsinanfu Institute, one can see the educational and realistic exhibits covering all aspects of an advanced society.” In 1914, Mr. Huang Yanpei praised the grand occasion of Tsinanfu Institute in the interview. In 1922, Mr. Hu Shi visited Tsinanfu Institute and his excitement was recorded in his diary on that day. Ni Xiying, a writer of the Republic of China, wrote in his *Urban Geography Series: Jinan*, “It doesn’t matter if people who go to Jinan have a little less appreciation of the scenery of mountains and rivers, but Tsinanfu Institute is a must to visit.” Mr. Lao She, who once taught at Cheeloo University, wrote a special article entitled “Tsinanfu Institute”. Tsinanfu Institute has also had a positive impact on China’s museum undertakings. Tianjin Guangzhi Museum founded in 1922 and the Kah Kee Park founded by Mr. Chen Jiageng in 1949 were deeply inspired by Tsinanfu Institute.

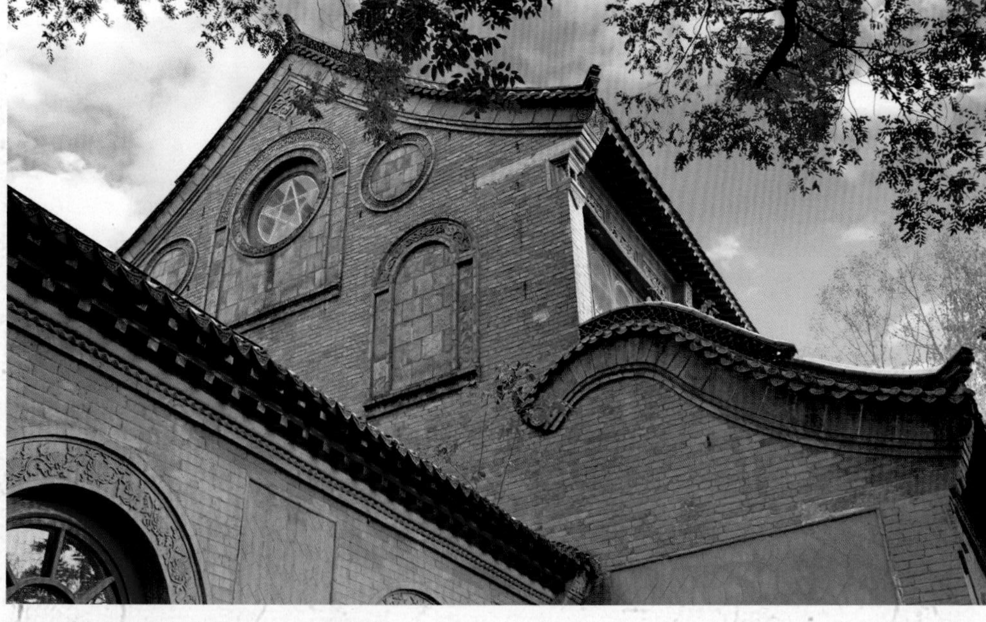

图 26 济南广智院主楼屋山（东面观）

Fig. 26 Gable of the main building of Tsinanfu Institute (the east view)

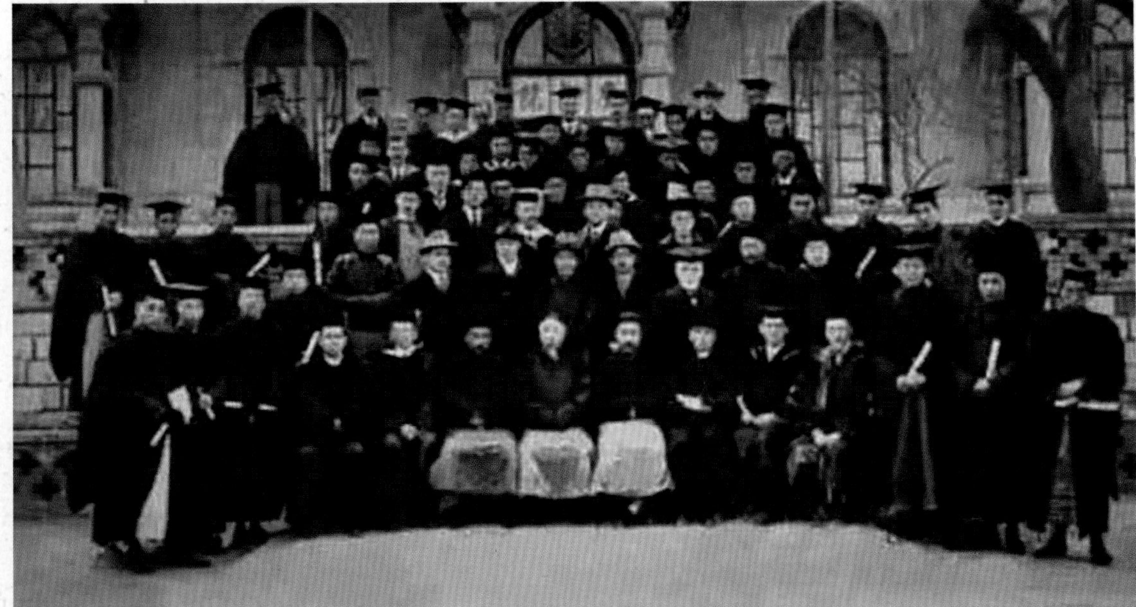

图 27 齐鲁大学毕业生在广智院留影

Fig. 27 Graduates of Cheeloo University taking photos at Tsinanfu Institute

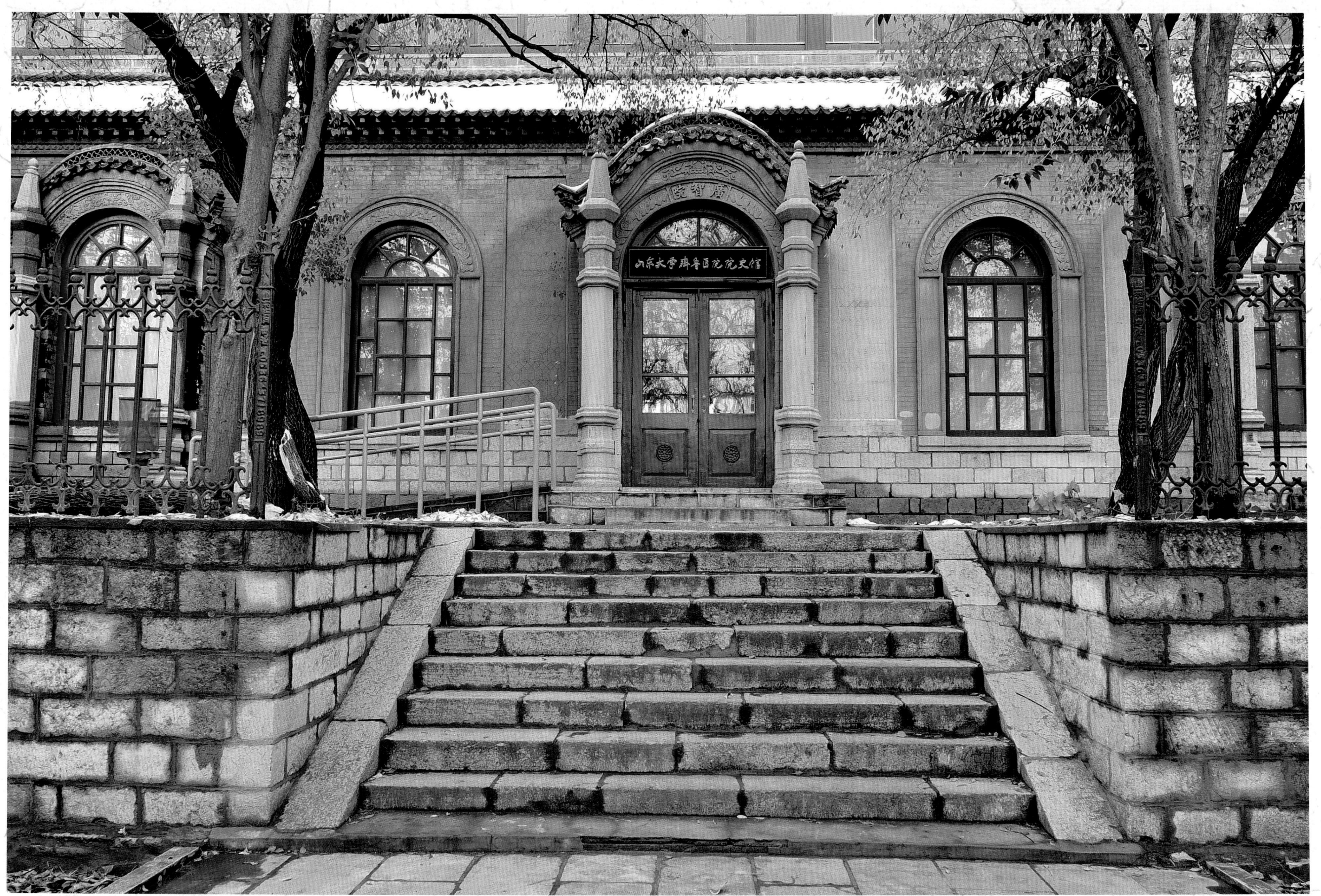

图 28 济南广智院主楼大门

Fig. 28 Gate of the main building of Tsinanfu Institute

06 南关教堂

Nanguan Church

南关教堂始建于 1905 年，是英国浸礼会的礼拜堂，也是齐鲁大学神学院的一部分。教堂东临广智院，坐南朝北，建筑面积 600 多平方米。灰砖墙体，青瓦檐头，双坡顶，哥特式建筑，融会中国传统建筑风格。现教堂已改变用途，成为齐鲁医院的临床技能培训中心。

Nanguan Church, founded in 1905, was the chapel of the English Baptist Missionary Society and part of the School of Theology of Cheeloo University. Facing north, the church was adjacent to Tsinanfu Institute in the east, with a construction area of more than 600 square meters. With grey brick walls, green tile eaves and double-slope top, Nanguan Church was a fusion of Gothic architecture and traditional Chinese architecture. Now the church has changed to become the Training Center for Clinicnl Skills of Qilu Hospital.

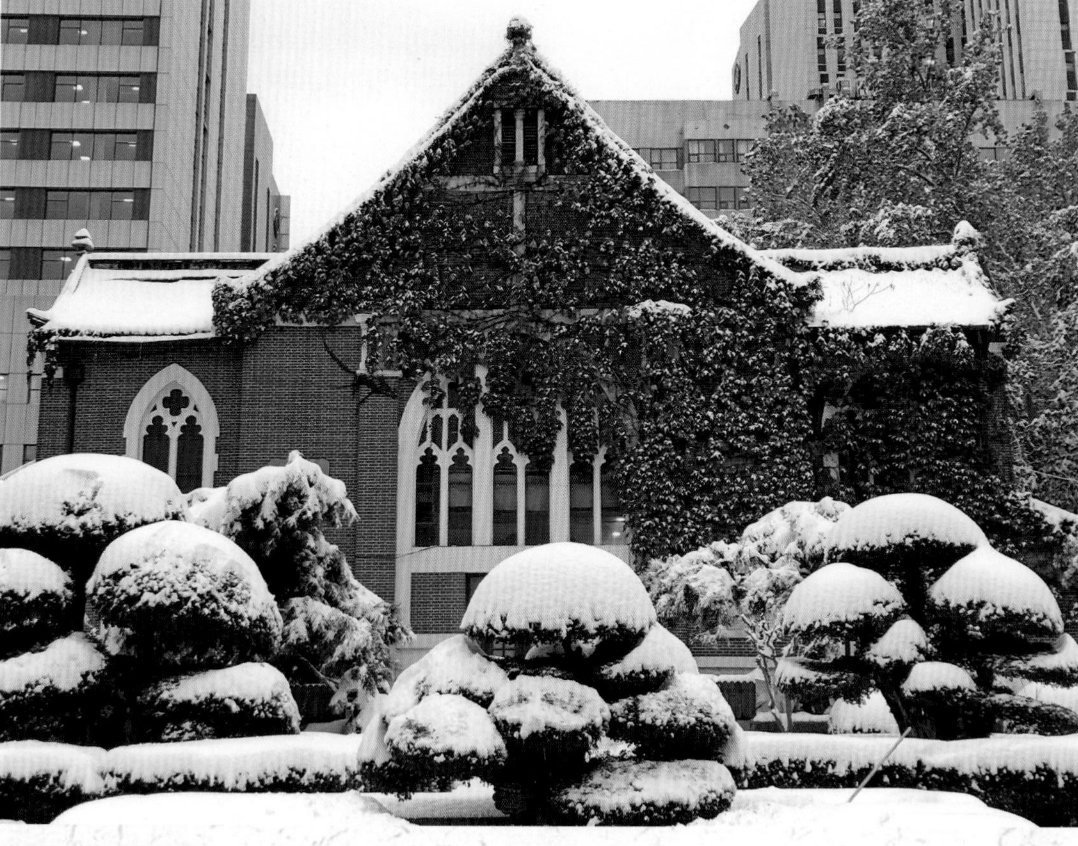

图 29 南关教堂雪景
Fig. 29 Snow view of Nanguan Church

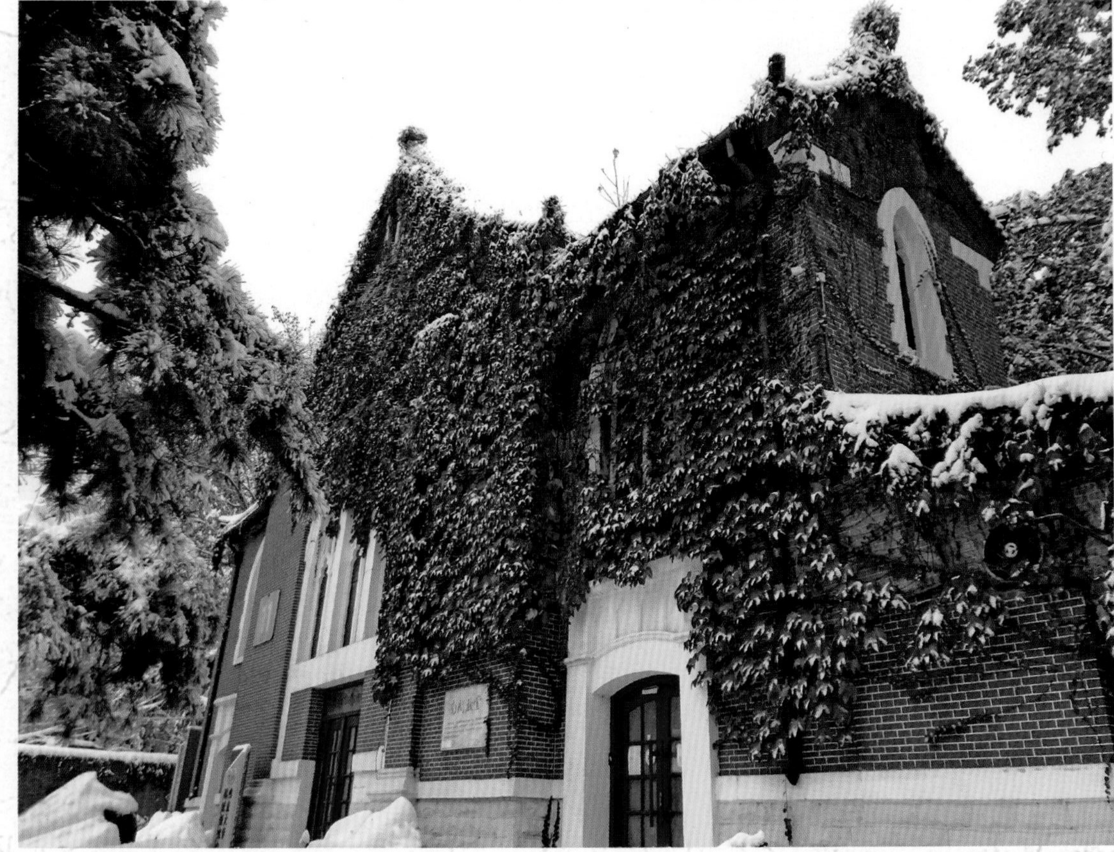

图 30 南关教堂冬景
Fig. 30 Winter view of Nanguan Church

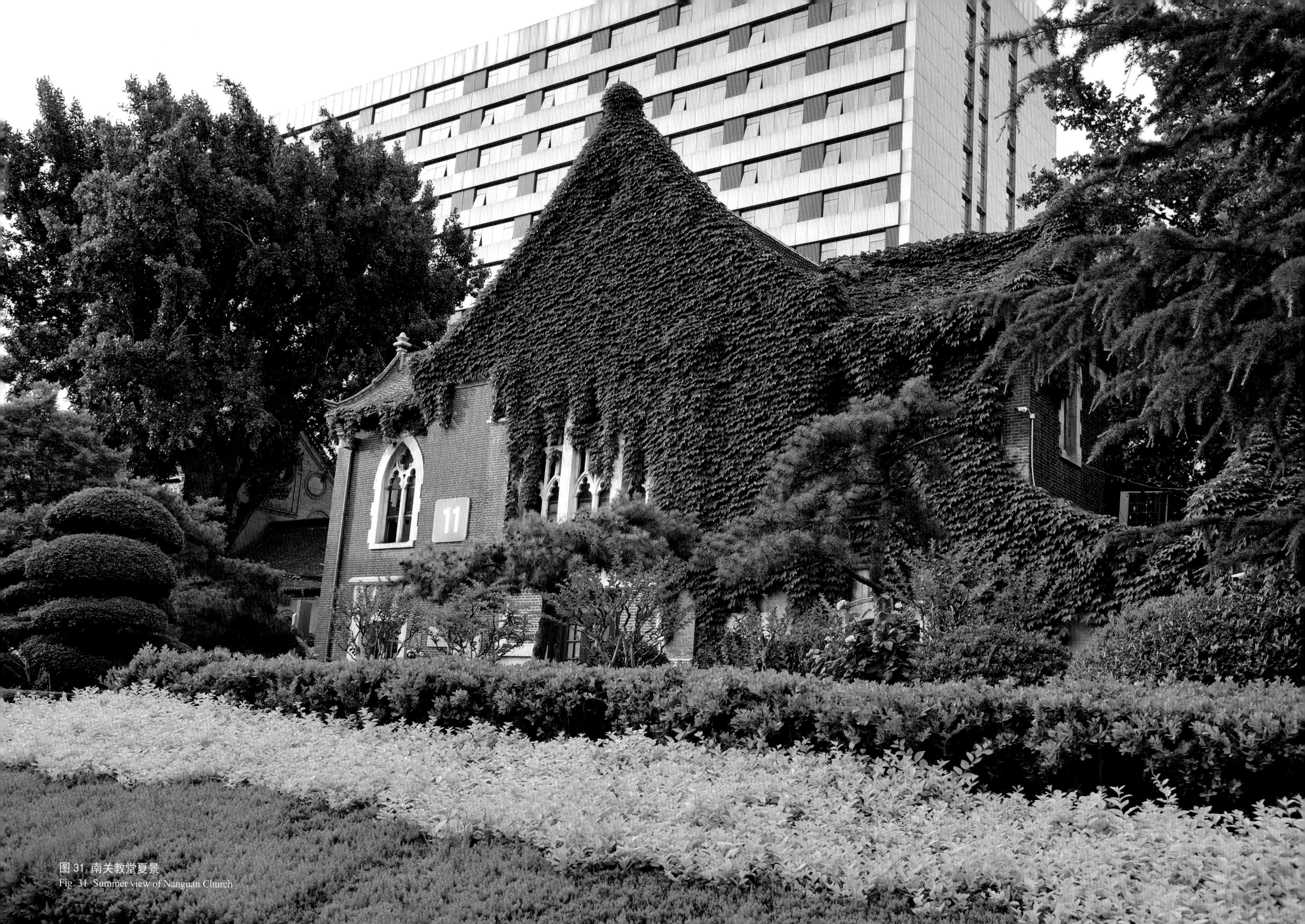

图 31 南关教堂夏景
Fig. 31 Summer view of Nanguan Church

07 新兴楼（医学大讲堂）（1）

Xinxing Building (The Medical Lecture Hall) (1)

1902 年 6 月 13 日，美北长老会和英国浸礼会商定，联合成立“山东基督教共合大学”，并成立董事会，学校分为文理科、神学科和医科，各科在省内不同地区办学。1903 年董事会决定将济南、青州、邹平和沂州的医校合并，成立“山东共合医道学堂”（Shantung Union Medical College），武成献任校长，学制四年，在各教学点进行教学和轮流实习。至此，山东省第一所正规现代西医高等学校诞生。

1907 年，英国浸礼会收到英国阿辛顿基金会的 9000 英镑捐款，美国北长老会也募集到部分资金。1908 年，浸礼会在趵突泉南侧购买了 16 英亩土地并开工建设医学新校区。为配合新校区建设，聂会东同时在现南新街 85 号开设了济南共合医院。在医学大讲堂（新兴楼）和诊病所（求真楼）竣工后，于 1911 年 4 月 17 日举行庆典，宣布山东共合医道学堂更名为“山东基督教共合大学医科”，科长为聂会东，共合医院院长为英国传教医师、外科教授巴慕德（Harold Balme）。这一天被定为齐鲁大学医学院建院日和山东医科大学建校日。时任清政府山东巡抚的孙宝琦出席典礼并捐赠白银千两（相当于 7 万美元）。至此，山东基督教共合大学医科有了固定的办学地点，青州、邹平和沂州的医校也陆续迁来济南。

On 13 June 1902, the American Presbyterian Missions, North and the English Baptist Missionary Society agreed to jointly establish Shantung Christian University and set up a board of directors. The university had Arts and Science, Theology and Medicine in different regions of the province. In 1903, the board of directors decided to merge the medical schools in Jinan, Qingzhou, Zouping and Yizhou to establish Shantung Union Medical College, with James Russell Watson as the president. The university had a four-year schooling system with teaching and rotating internships at various teaching sites. So far the first formal modern university of Western medicine was born.

In 1907, the English Baptist Missionary Society received a £9,000 donation from the Ashington Foundation in Britain, and the American Presbyterian Missions, North also raised some money. In 1908, the English Baptist Missionary Society purchased 16 acres on the south side of Baotu Spring and began the construction of a new medical campus. In order to cooperate with the construction of the new campus, James Boyd Neal opened Jinan Union Medical Hospital at No. 85 Nanxin Street. After the completion of the Medical Lecture Hall (Xinxing Building) and the clinic (Qiuzhen Building), a celebration was held on 17 April 1911, announcing that Shantung Union Medical College was renamed “Medical Department of Shantung Christian University”, with James Boyd Neal as the chief and Harold Balme, an English missionary doctor and professor of surgery, as the president of the hospital. This day was designated as the founding day of the School of Medicine of Cheeloo University and that of Shandong Medical University. Sun Baoqi, then Shandong Governor of the Qing Government, attended the dedication and donated 1,000 taels of silver (equivalent to $70,000). So far, the Medical Department of Shantung Christian University had a fixed location, and the medical schools in Qingzhou, Zouping and Yizhou had also moved to Jinan one after another.

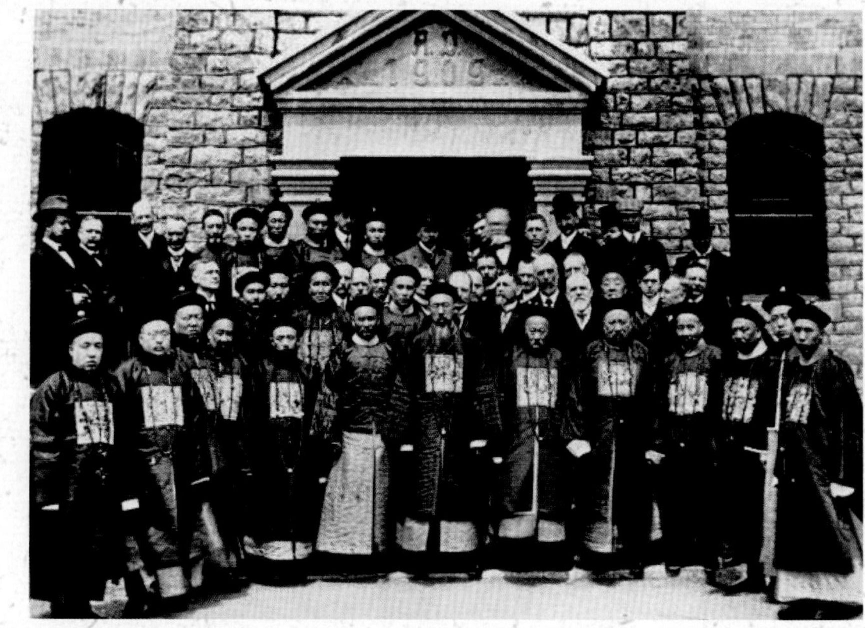

图 32 山东巡抚孙宝琦（前排中）出席医学大讲堂落成典礼
Fig. 32 Shandong Governor Sun Baoqi (middle of the front row) attending the dedication of the Medical Lecture Hall

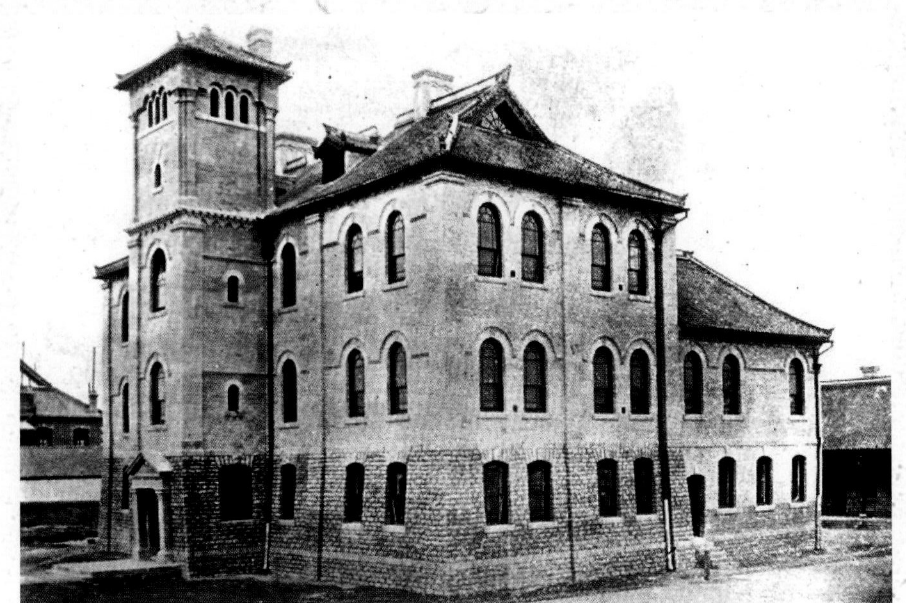

图 33 医学大讲堂旧影
Fig. 33 An old photo of the Medical Lecture Hall

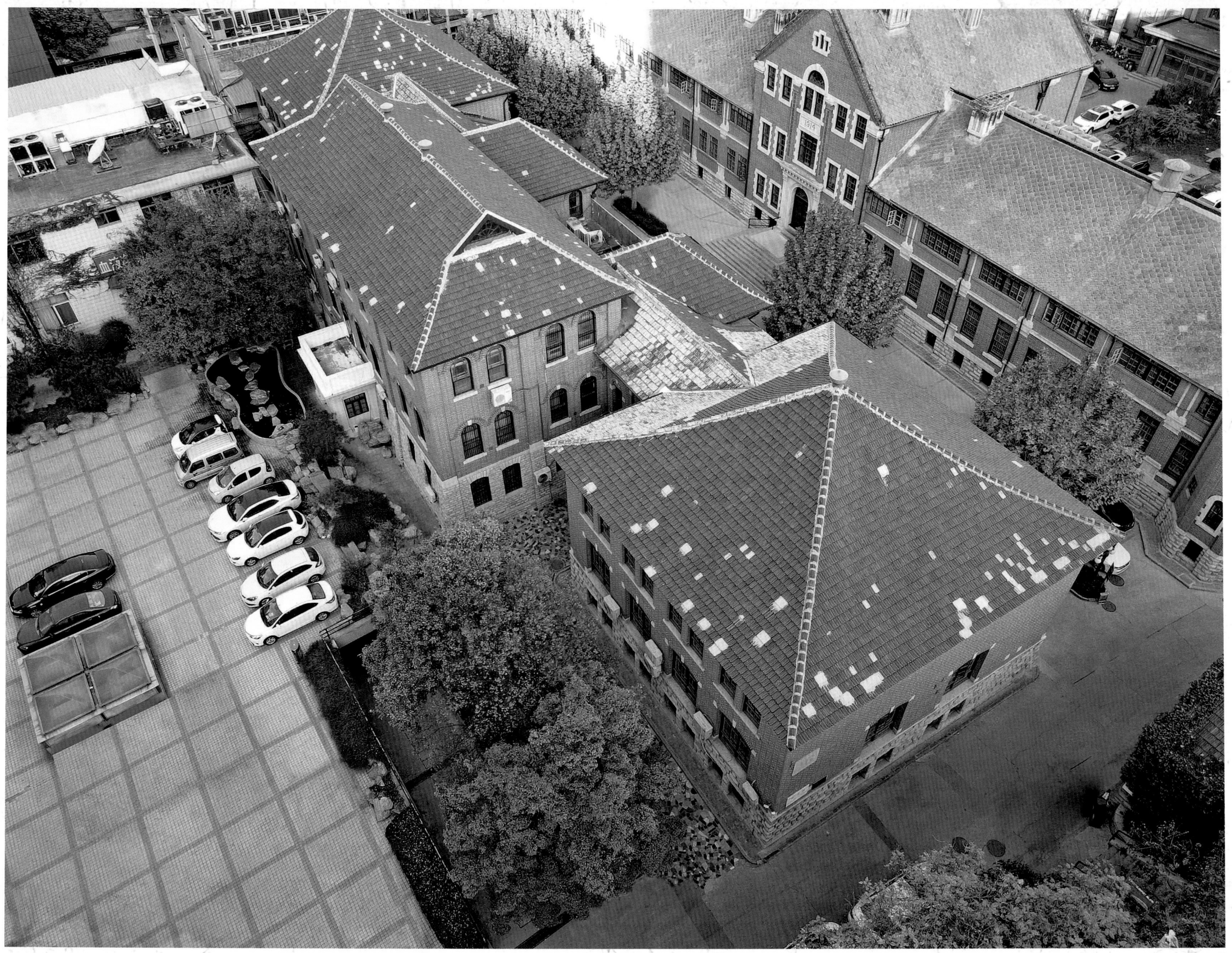

图 34 新兴楼全景
Fig. 34 Panorama of Xinxing Building

07 新兴楼（医学大讲堂）（2）

Xinxing Building (The Medical Lecture Hall) (2)

新兴楼（医学大讲堂）为山东共合医道学堂的主体建筑，当时俗称“大主楼”。新兴楼由东、西翼楼和中楼三部分组成，但并非一次建成。中楼主体三层，设有半地下室，始建于 1909 年，1911 年落成。东、西翼楼为方形二层，带有半石砌地下室，为后来增建。中楼屋顶为仿中式歇山顶，翼楼为四角攒尖顶。整座楼地下室部分皆由蘑菇石砌成，上为清水砖墙。屋顶、墙面、窗户均造型别致，不拘一格。这个体形比较大的三层楼房，曾经建有一座塔楼，在后来改建时被拆除。但即便没了起画龙点睛作用的塔楼，这座造型相对复杂的大楼仍是充满无限魅力、不可多得的建筑佳作。整座建筑富于变化美感，与共合楼、求真楼一起组成环境氛围和谐统一的近代建筑群。

Xinxing Building (The Medical Lecture Hall) was the main architecture of Shantung Union Medical College, which was then commonly known as the Main Building. The Xinxing Building consisted of three parts, that is, the east wing, the west wing and the middle building, which were not a one-time completion. The main body of the middle building had three floors, with a semi-basement. It was built in 1909 and completed in 1911. The east and west wings were square two-storey buildings, with semi-basements of stone which were built later. The roof of the middle building was an imitation of the Chinese gable and hip roof, and that of the wing buildings was pyramidal roof. The basement of the whole building was all made of mushroom stone, with fair-faced brick wall. The roof, wall and windows were unique in shape and not limited to one type. This large three-storey building once had a tower which was demolished during a later renovation. But even without the tower that made the finishing touch, the relatively complex building was still a rare piece of architecture full of infinite charm and changing beauty. This building, together with Gonghe Building and Qiuzhen Building, formed a modern complex with harmonious and unified ambience.

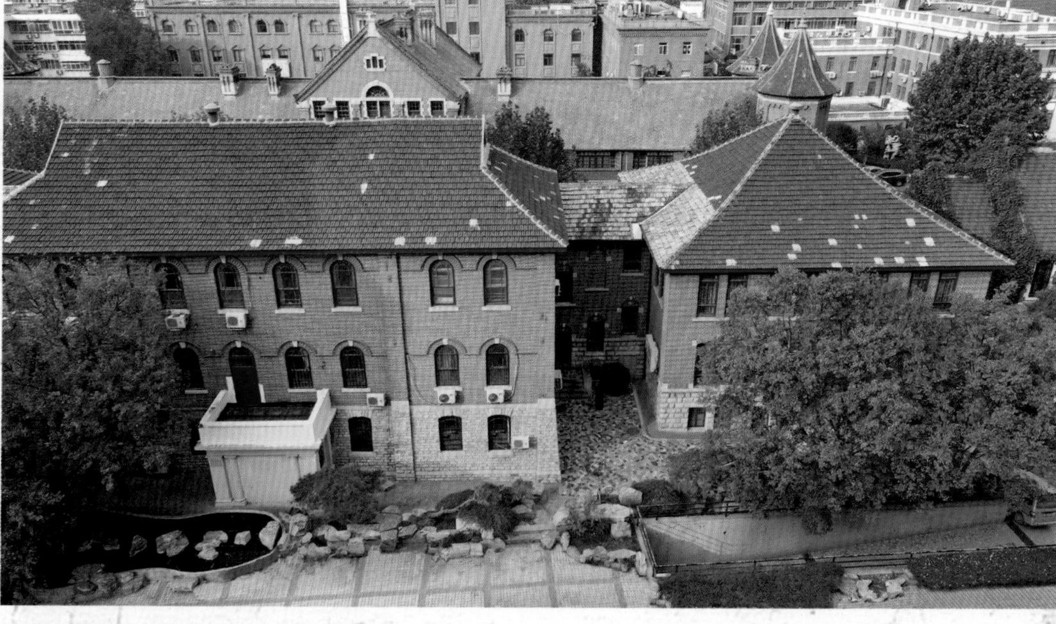

图 35 新兴楼（医学大讲堂）连接部
Fig. 35 Connection of Xinxing Building (The Medical Lecture Hall)

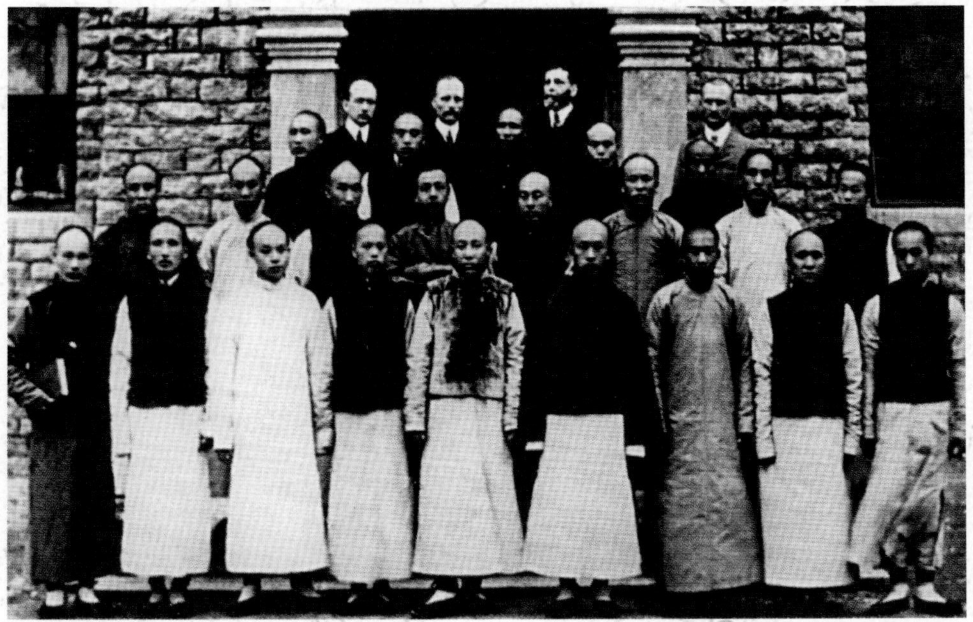

图 36 山东共合医道学堂师生在新兴楼前合影
Fig. 36 Teachers and students of Shantung Union Medical College taking photos in front of Xinxing Building

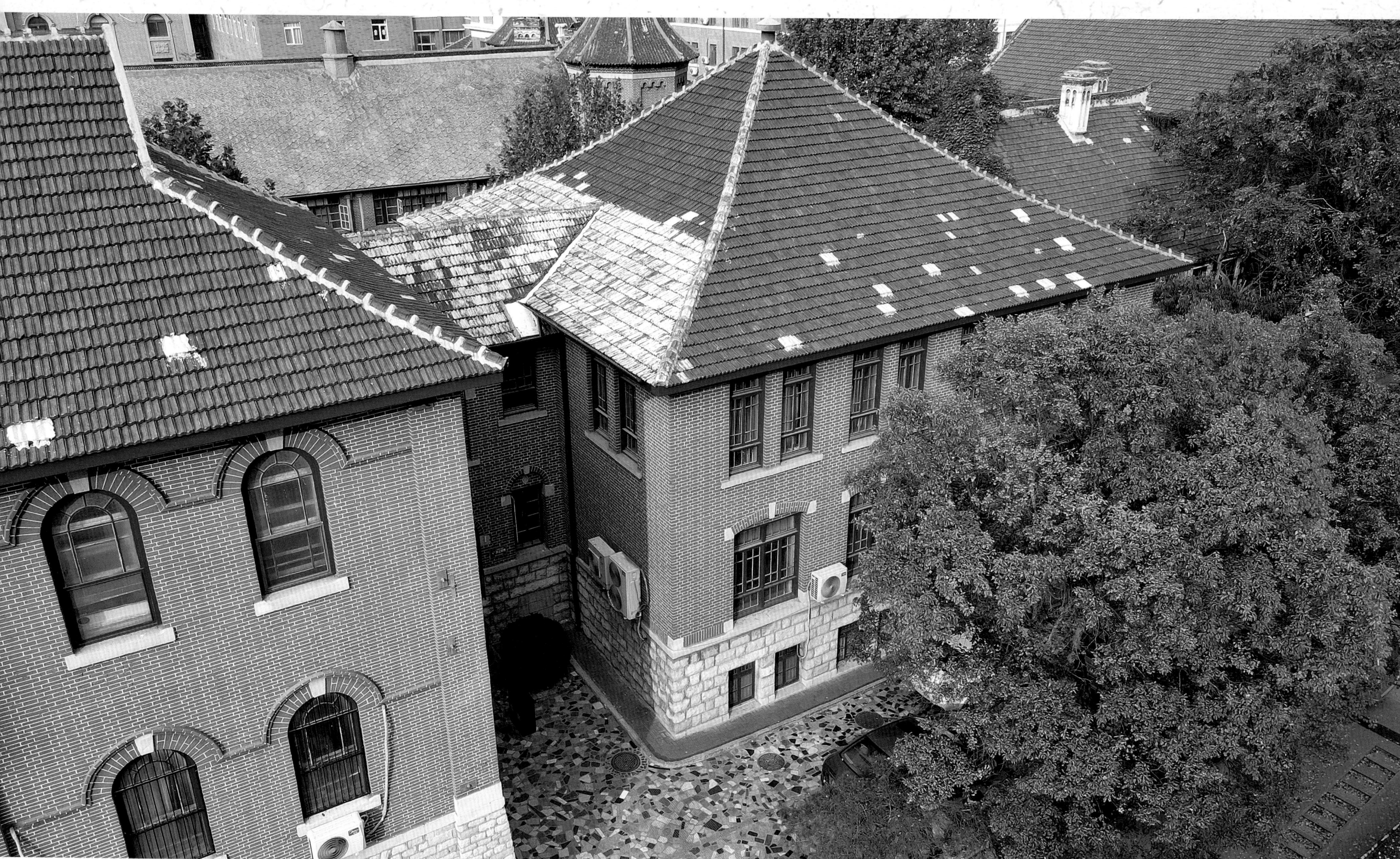

图 37 新兴楼（医学大讲堂）东翼
Fig. 37 The east wing of Xinxing Building (The Medical Lecture Hall)

07 新兴楼（医学大讲堂）（3）

Xinxing Building (The Medical Lecture Hall) (3)

新兴楼建筑面积为 3016 平方米，当时楼内有会计室、教室、可容纳百余名学生的大会堂，有设有阶梯形座位的手术室以及解剖学、组织学、药理学、生理学、病理学和临床等各类实验室。一层还有部分高级病房。当时山东基督教共合大学医科科长聂会东的办公室以及医学编译馆、图书室也在此楼内。新兴楼现在是齐鲁医院办公二楼。

位于新兴楼内的医学编译馆，全称为“中国博医会驻济编译部”。1932 年中华医学会与中国博医会合并，其会刊《中华医学杂志》编辑部也因经费拮据，而由上海迁至济南，与齐鲁大学医学院《齐鲁医刊》合并。编译馆成员由少量专职人员和齐鲁大学教授组成，翻译和编辑了大量医学著作，有力促进了中国医学事业的发展。新中国成立后，编译馆迁至北京参与组建人民卫生出版社，其副主任鲁德馨出任人民卫生出版社副总编辑。

Xinxing Building has a construction area of 3,016 square meters. At that time, the building had the accounting room, the classroom, the great hall capable of accommodating more than 100 students, the operating room with stepped seats, and various laboratories of anatomy, histology, pharmacology, physiology, pathology and clinical practice. There were also some advanced wards on the first floor. At that time, the office of James Boyd Neal, chief of the Medical Department of Shantung Christian University, the Medical Compilation and Translation Hall and the library were also in this building. Xinxing Building is now the Second Office Building of Qilu Hospital.

The full name of the Medical Compilation and Translation Hall located in Xinxing Building is “Compilation and Translation Department of China Medical Missionary Association in Jinan”. In 1932, the Chinese Medical Association merged with China Medical Missionary Association, and the editorial department of its Journal *National Medical Journal of China* moved from Shanghai to Jinan due to financial straits and merged with *The Tsinan Medical Review* of the Medical School of Cheeloo University. The Compilation and Translation Hall, composed of a small number of full-time staff and professors of Cheeloo University, had translated and edited a large number of medical works, effectively promoting the development of the medical cause in China. After the founding of the People’s Republic of China, the Compilation and Translation Hall moved to Beijing to participate in the establishment of the People’s Medical Publishing House, and Lu Dexin, deputy director of the Compilation and Translation Hall, became deputy editor-in-chief of the People’s Medical Publishing House.

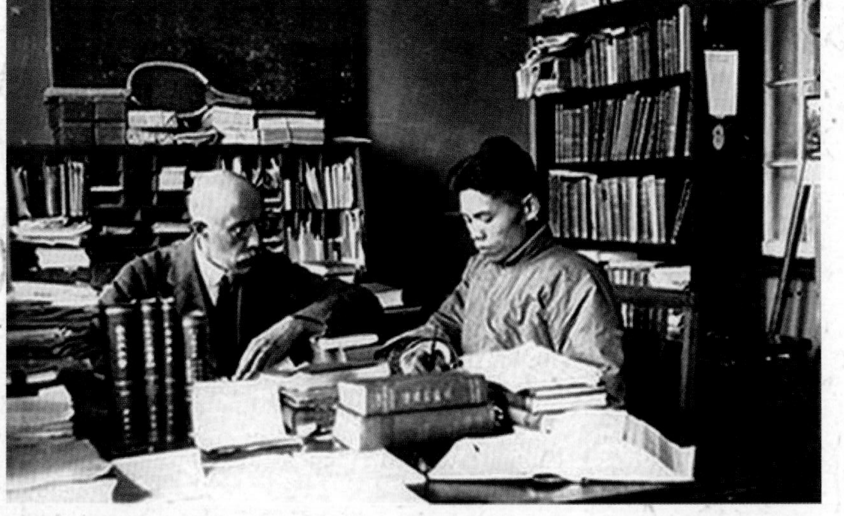

图 38 编译馆主任孟合理（Percy Lonsdale McAll）（左）与副主任鲁德馨（右）在一起工作

Fig. 38 Percy Lonsdale McAll (left), director of the Compilation and Translation Hall, working with Lu Dexin (right), deputy director of the Compilation and Translation Hall

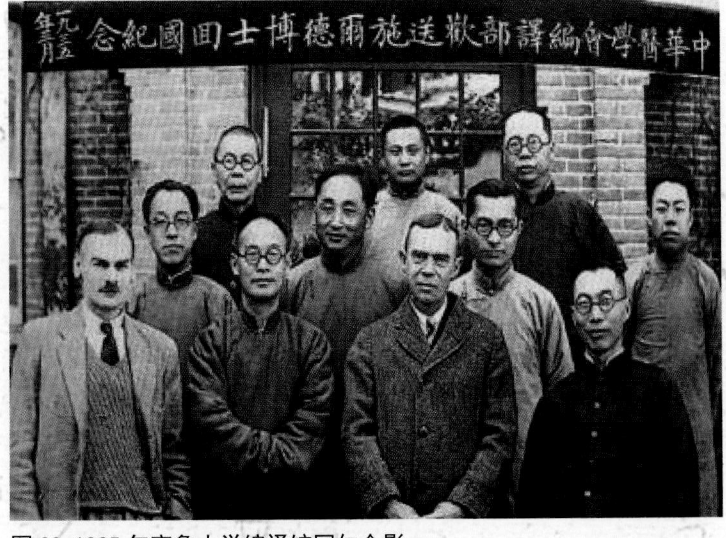

图 39 1935 年齐鲁大学编译馆同仁合影

Fig. 39 Group photo of colleagues in the Compilation and Translation Hall of Cheeloo University in 1935

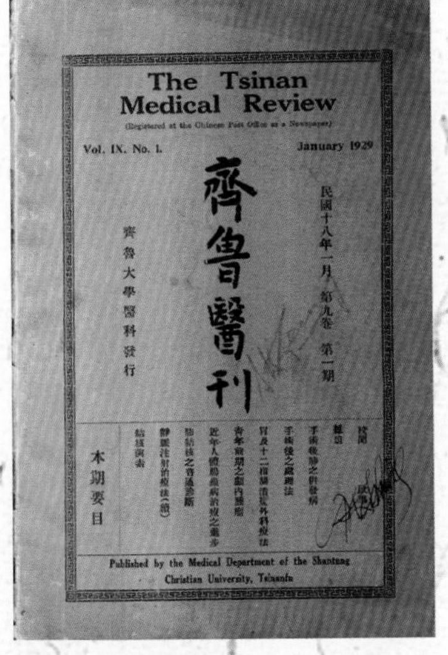

图 40 齐鲁医刊

Fig. 40 *The Tsinan Medical Review*

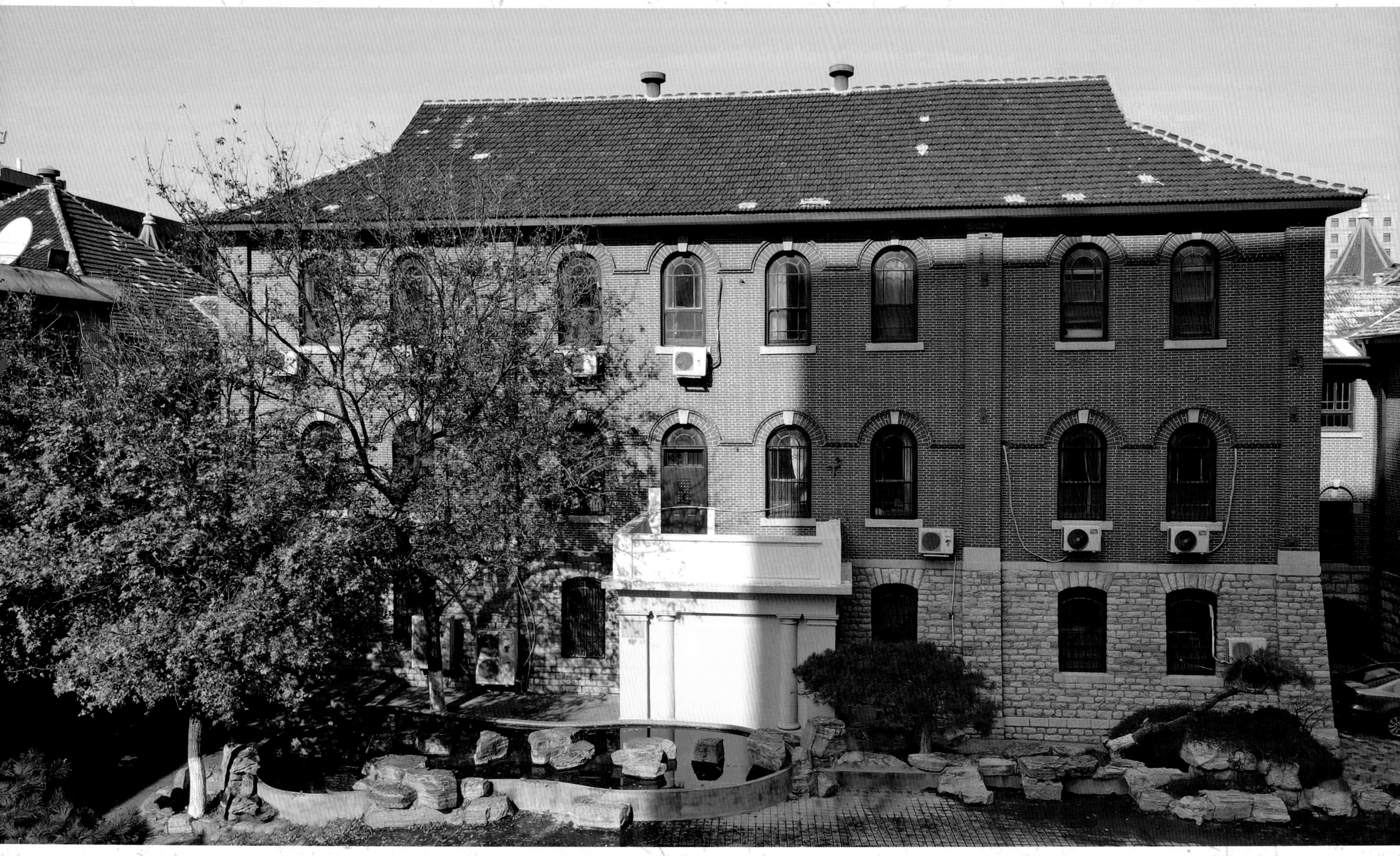

图 41 新兴楼（医学大讲堂）主楼
Fig. 41 Main building of Xinxing Building (The Medical Lecture Hall)

08 求真楼（1）

Qiuzhen Building (1)

求真楼建成于 1911 年，位于新兴楼东面，始建时为诊病所（门诊部）。求真楼是一座坐南朝北的砖石建筑，建筑面积 1034 平方米。平面结构分三部分，中间主体部分前后方向突出，两层，兼有地下室。东西两翼进深缩小，为单层坡面平房。左右对称，略有变化。东侧平房南门建有柱廊，高柱座，圆柱身、柱头都由青砖砌成。建筑的墙体也是青砖砌成，但门窗有石头外套，做隅石状处理。整体看来，屋顶、屋脊、硬山墙为中国风格，门窗、柱廊、墙面细部及烟囱则是欧洲风格。中西合璧，而又和谐统一。

Qiuzhen Building was built in 1911, located in the east of Xinxing Building. It was originally built as a clinic (outpatient department). Qiuzhen Building is a brick-and-stone building, facing north and with a construction area of 1,034 square meters. The plane of the building is divided into three parts, and the main part in the middle protrudes in the front and back directions, with two floors and a basement. The east and west wings are single-storey slope bungalows with reduced length. They are symmetrical, but slightly different. The south gate of the bungalow on the east side has a colonnade with high column base, and the column body and capital are made of black bricks. The walls of the building are also made of black bricks, but the doors and windows have stone coats and are treated in the shape of corner stones. On the whole, the roof, ridge and gable are in Chinese style, while the doors and windows, colonnades, wall details and chimneys are in European style. The combination of Chinese and Western styles is of harmonious unity.

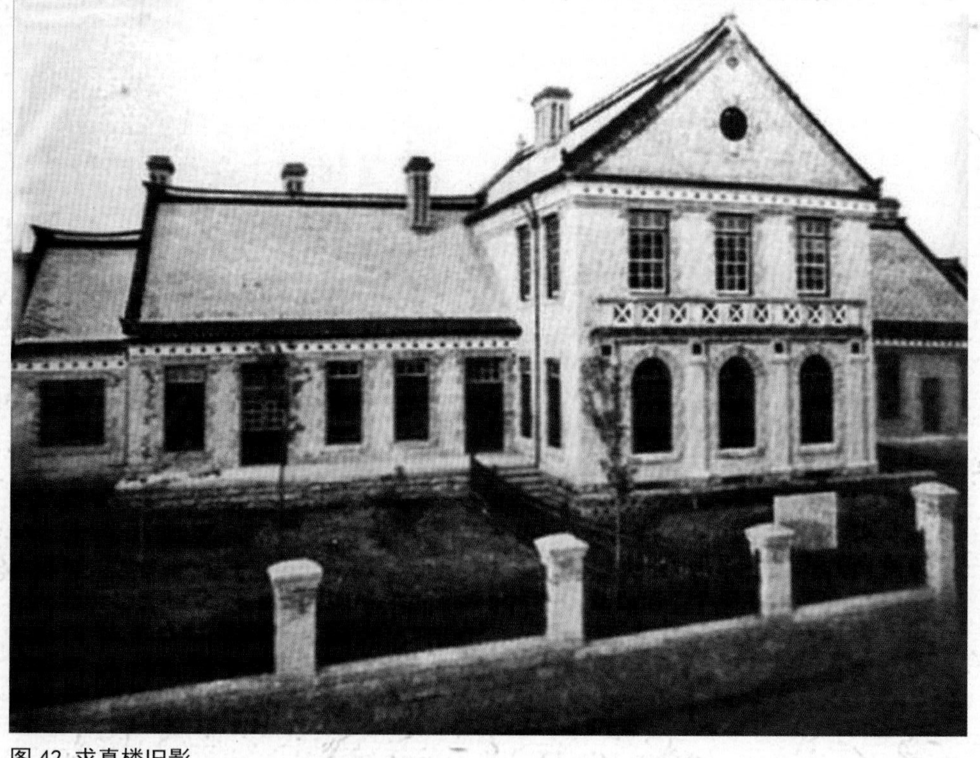

图 42 求真楼旧影

Fig. 42 An old photo of Qiuzhen Building

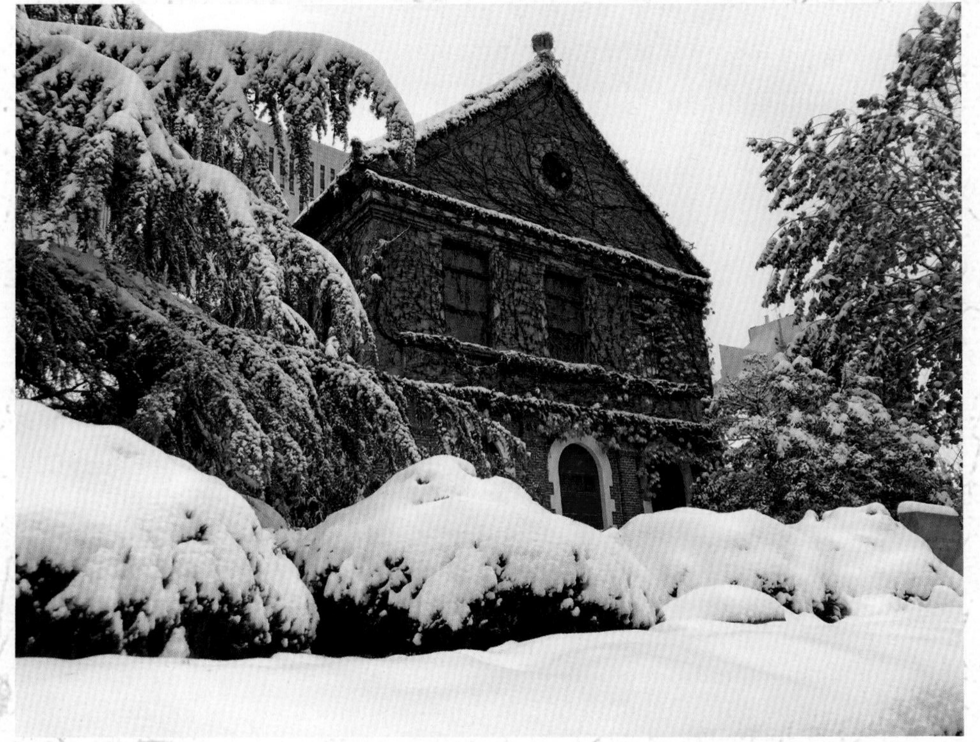

图 43 求真楼雪景

Fig. 43 Snow view of Qiuzhen Building

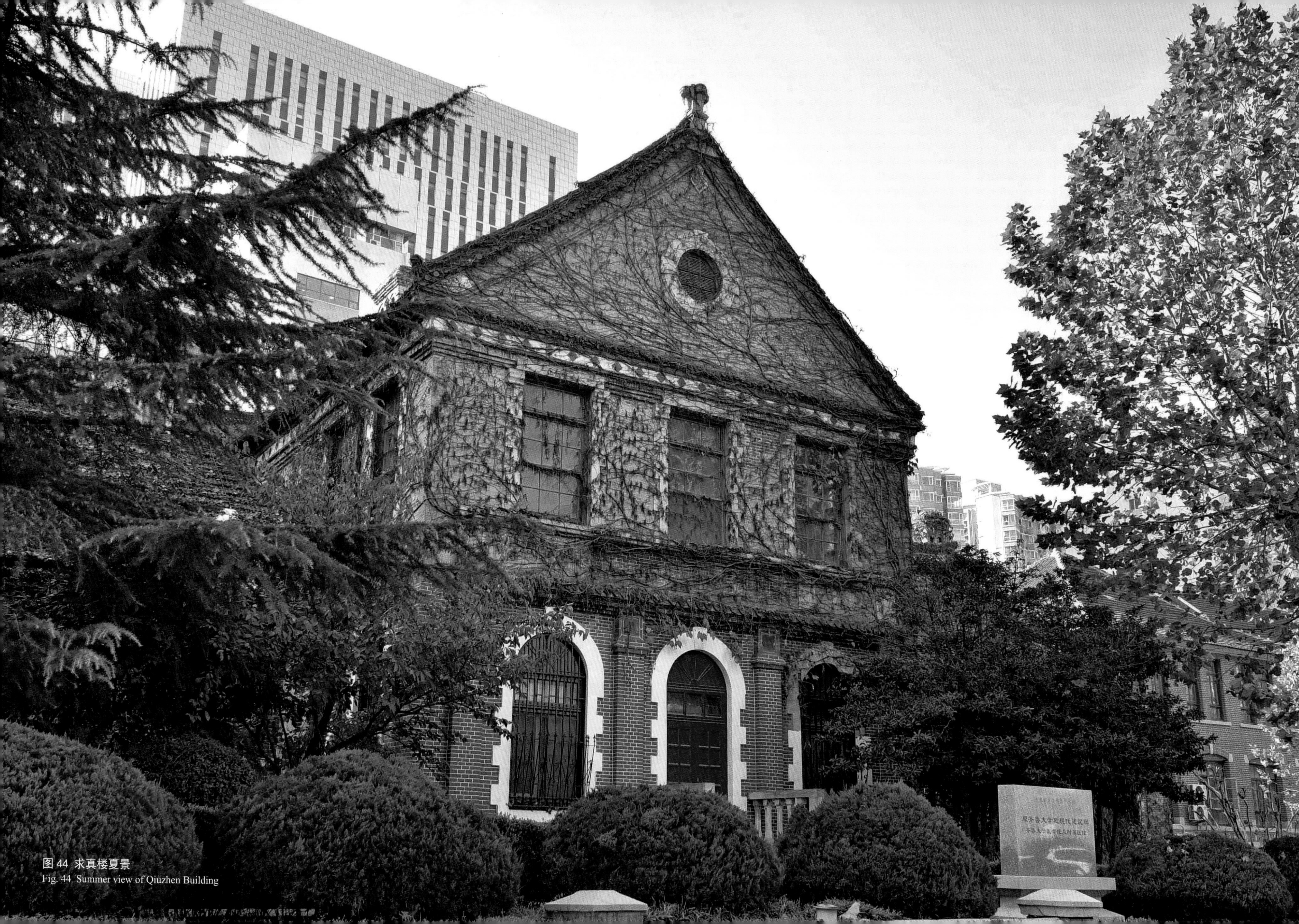

图 44 求真楼夏景
Fig. 44 Summer view of Qiuzhen Building

08 | 求真楼（2）

Qiuzhen Building (2)

求真楼原是医院的诊病所（门诊部）。地下室有挂号室、X 光室和锅炉房等。一层东面是手术室和外科门诊；中间是大候诊室，候诊室内设有讲台，供传教士向病人布道，还设有内科和耳鼻喉科诊室；一层西侧为药房、药品仓库和眼科、皮肤科的诊疗室。二层主要是观察病房和护士用房。求真楼曾作为齐鲁大学附属医院的医生宿舍楼，也做过生化及生理系用房。1950 年后成为山东医学院附属医院和山东医科大学附属医院的办公楼，现为临床技能模拟训练中心。

Qiuzhen Building was originally the clinic (outpatient department) in the hospital. The basement had the registration room, X-ray room, boiler room and so on. On the east side of the first floor were the operating rooms and surgical clinics. In the middle was a large waiting room provided with a podium for missionaries to preach to patients, and there were also clinics of internal medicine and otolaryngology. On the west side of the first floor were pharmacies, drug warehouses and clinics of ophthalmology and dermatology. On the second floor there were mainly the observation wards and the nurses' rooms. Qiuzhen Building was once used as the doctors' dormitory of the hospital affiliated to Cheeloo University and also used as the rooms of the Department of Biochemistry and Physiology. After 1950, it became the office building of the hospitals affiliated to Shandong Medical College and Shandong Medical University respectively, and now is the Simulation Training Center for Clinical Skills.

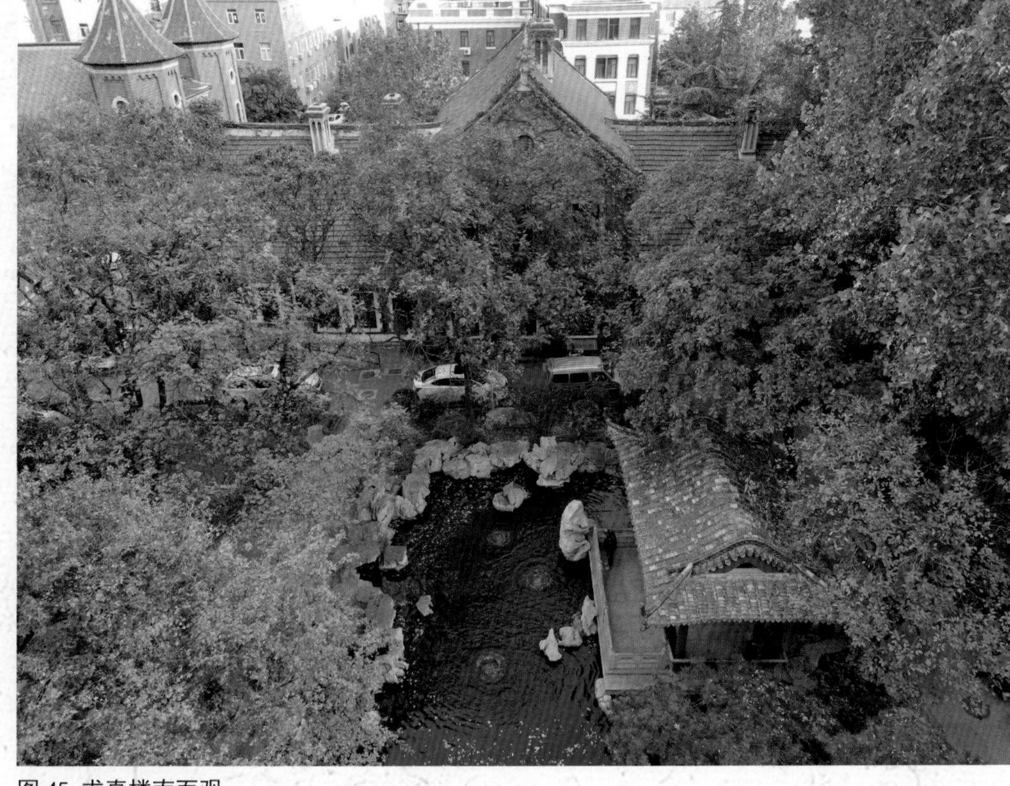

图 45 求真楼南面观
Fig. 45 The south view of Qiuzhen Building

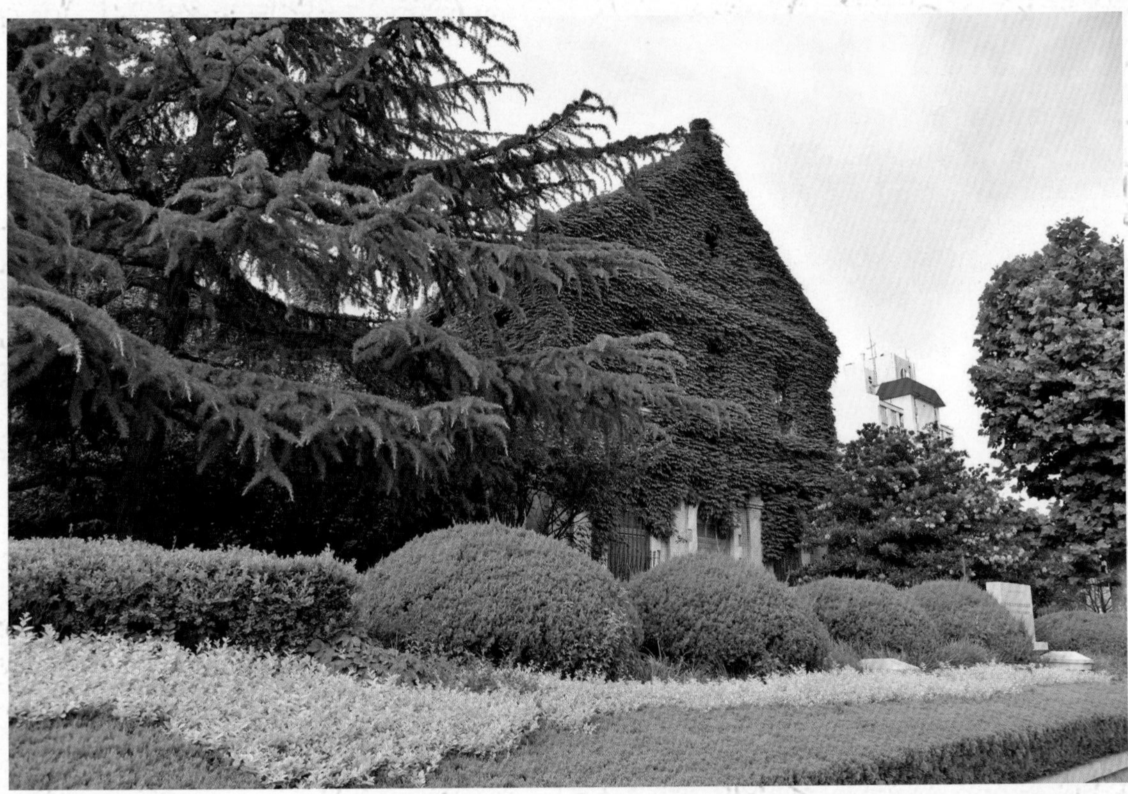

图 46 求真楼夏景
Fig. 46 Summer view of Qiuzhen Building

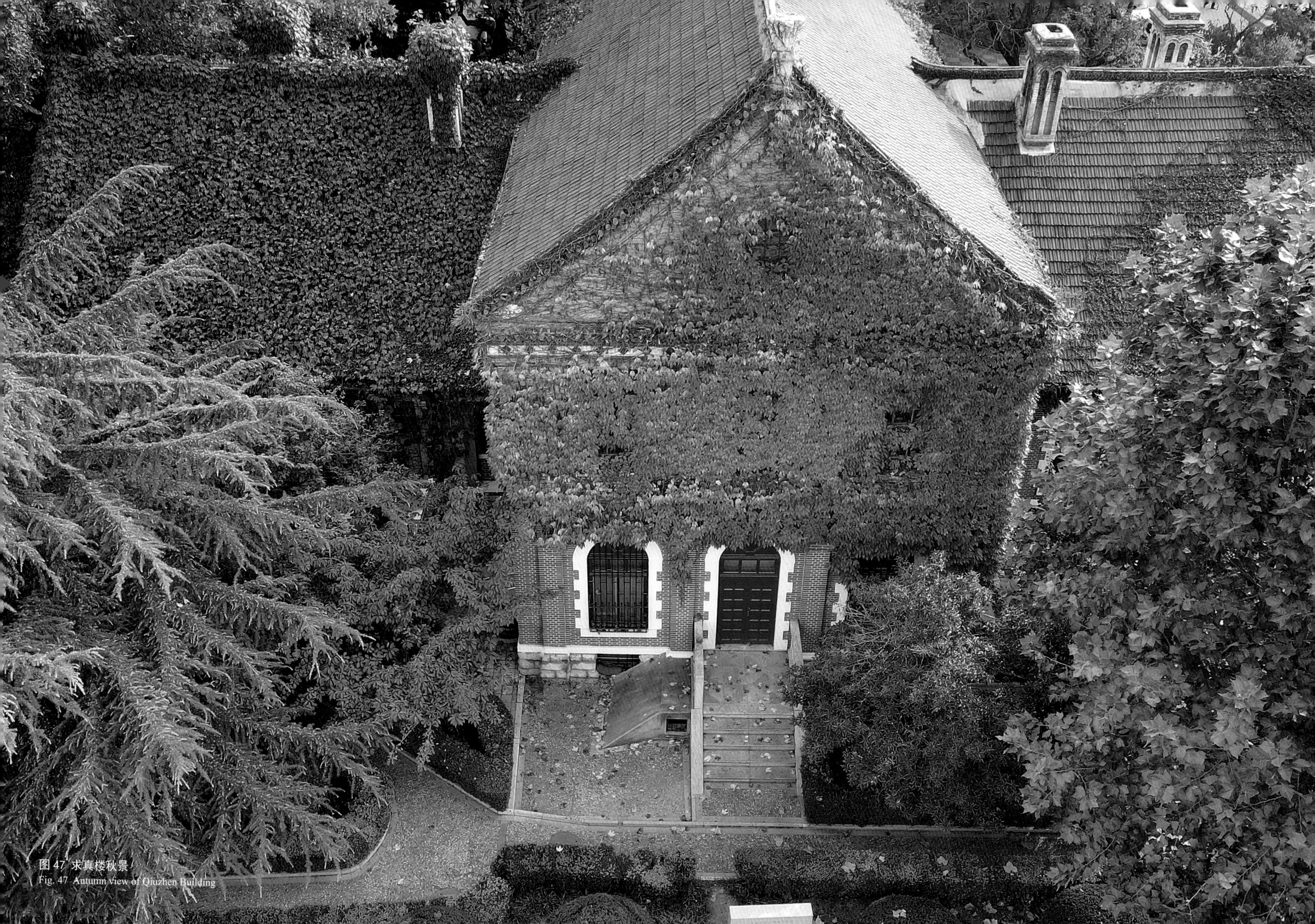

图 47 求真楼秋景
Fig. 47 Autumn view of Qiuzhen Building

09 共合楼（养病所）（1）

Gonghe Building (The Infirmary) (1)

共合楼，原名齐鲁大学养病所，1914 年在英国浸礼会资助下兴建，次年竣工。1915 年 9 月 27 日，共合楼落成典礼，时任北洋政府山东督军的靳云鹏（此后曾任国务总理）亲临祝贺，并亲书“共合医院五月初八日即救主降世一千九百一十四年，山东都督靳云鹏率众行开工礼”奠基碑。此奠基碑今嵌在共合楼一楼门厅的北墙上，碑文用中英两种文字书写。

Gonghe Building, formerly known as the Infirmary of Cheeloo University, was built in 1914 funded by the English Baptist Missionary Society and was completed the following year. On 27 September 1915, at the dedication of Gonghe Building, Jin Yunpeng, then Shandong Military Governor of the Beiyang Government (later served as Prime Minister of the State), gave congratulations in person and wrote the following words on the foundation stone: “On 8 May 1914 in the lunar calendar when the Savior has been born for 1914 years, Jin Yunpeng, Shandong Military Governor, led the people to start the opening ceremony.” This foundation stone is now embedded in the north wall of the entrance hall on the first floor of Gonghe Building. The inscription is written in Chinese and English languages.

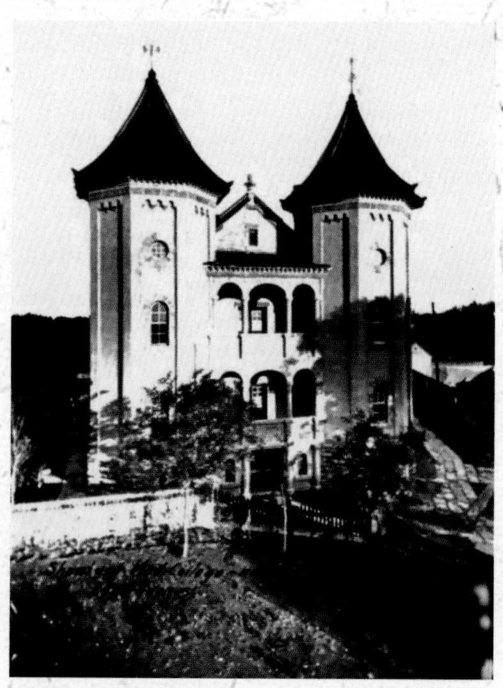

图 48 共合楼塔楼

Fig. 48 Tower of Gonghe Building

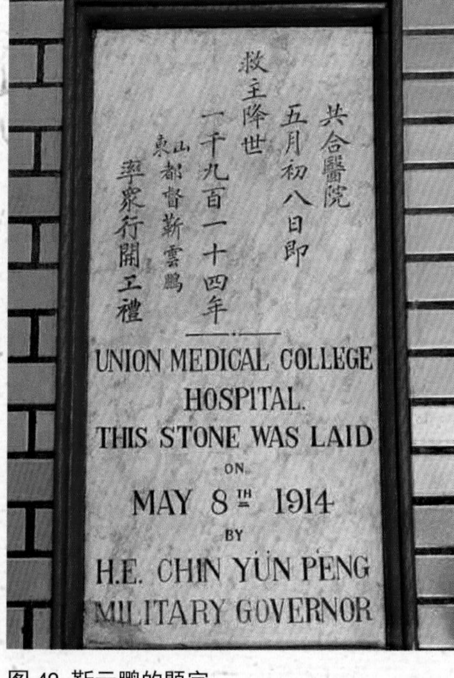

图 49 靳云鹏的题字

Fig. 49 Inscription of Jin Yunpeng

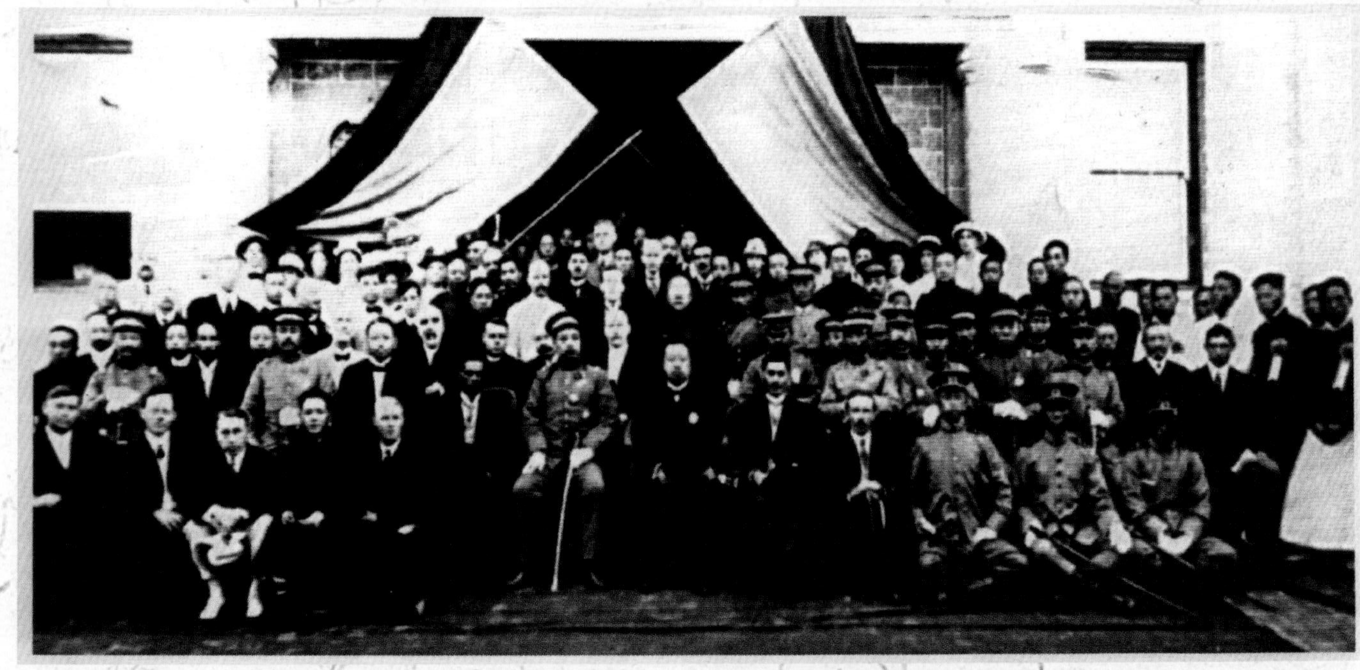

图 50 1915 年 9 月 27 日，时任北洋政府山东督军靳云鹏（前排中间持军刀者）出席共合楼落成典礼

Fig. 50 On 27 September 1915, Jin Yunpeng, then Shandong Military Governor of the Beiyang Government (with a military knife in the middle of the front row), attended the dedication of Gonghe Building

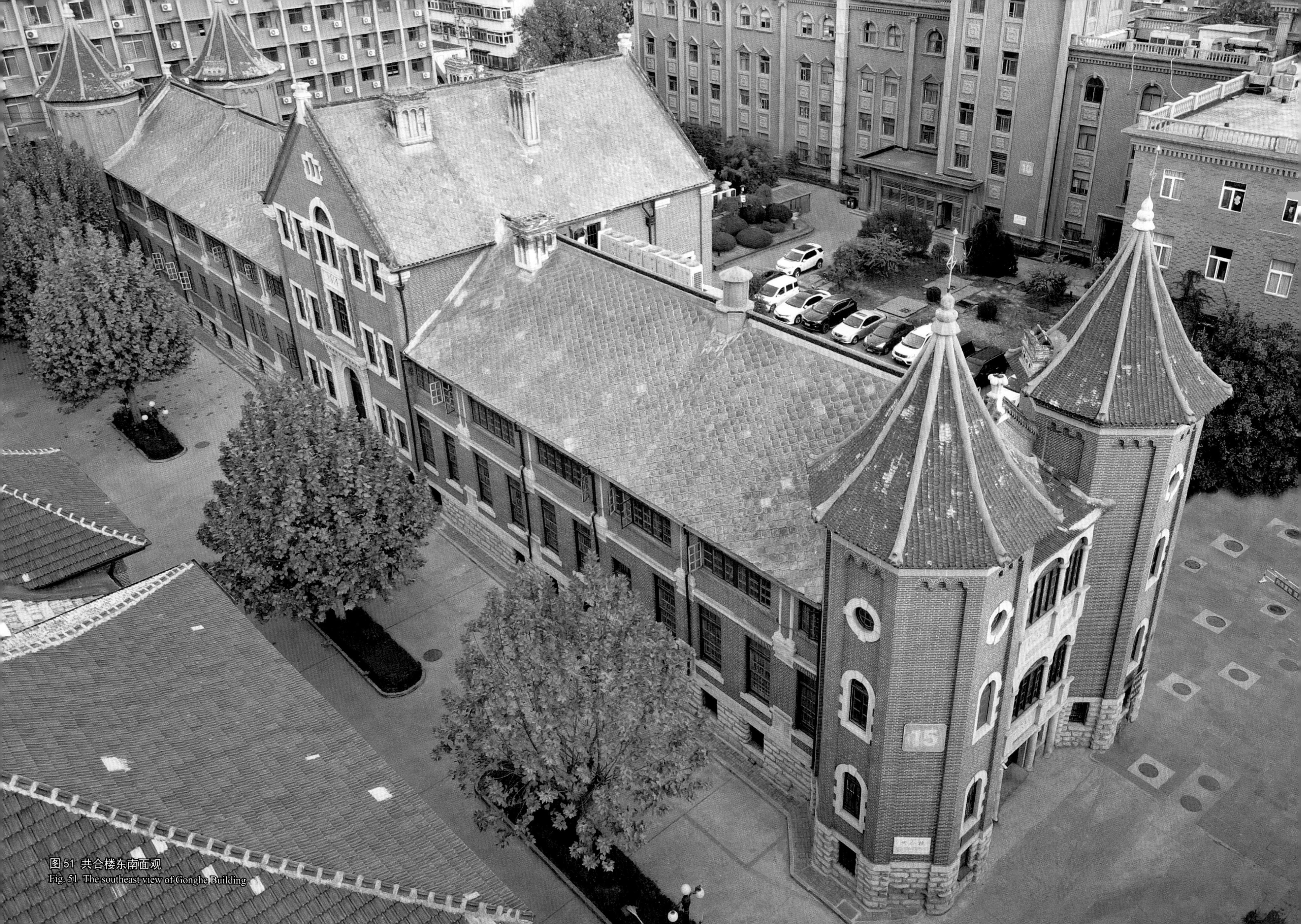

图 51　共合楼东南面观

Fig. 51　The southeast view of Gonghe Building

09 共合楼（养病所）（2）

Gonghe Building (The Infirmary) (2)

共合楼平面布局对称，整个建筑呈哑铃状。中间部分突出，南部是主入口，门前有石砌台阶，大门为欧洲古典券柱式，二层窗户上嵌有一块石匾，上书“1914”；北部墙上两层窗户中间，刻有“齐鲁大学养病所”字样。两翼为两层，东西延伸，尽端南北各有一座塔楼，东西对称，两塔楼间夹三开间次出入口。塔楼为三层，顶为六边形小青瓦覆顶的攒尖顶，建筑使用了叠落的圆石柱、连续的券形门窗等手法。窗下有精美的花卉石雕，所有门窗外套都用石头作原料，做隅石状处理。整个建筑为欧式风格，四个塔楼高高耸立，远远望去，气势非凡。

The plane layout of Gonghe Building is symmetrical, and the whole building is in the shape of a dumb bell. The middle part is prominent and the main entrance is in the south. There are stone steps in front of the gate and the gate is a type of classical European arch. The window on the second floor is embedded with a stone plaque with the words “1914” on it. In the middle of the two windows on the northern wall, the words “The Infirmary of Cheeloo University” are engraved. The two wings have two floors, extending to the east and west, with towers in the south and north at the end respectively that are of east-west symmetry. The two towers are sandwiched with secondary entrances and exits of three rooms. The tower is a three-storey building with a hexagonal small grey tile-covered pyramidal roof. The building uses stacked round stone columns, continuous arch doors and windows and other techniques. There are exquisite stone carvings of flowers under the window, and all the door and window coats are made of stone which are treated as cornerstones. The whole building is in European style with four towers standing high and looking magnificent from afar.

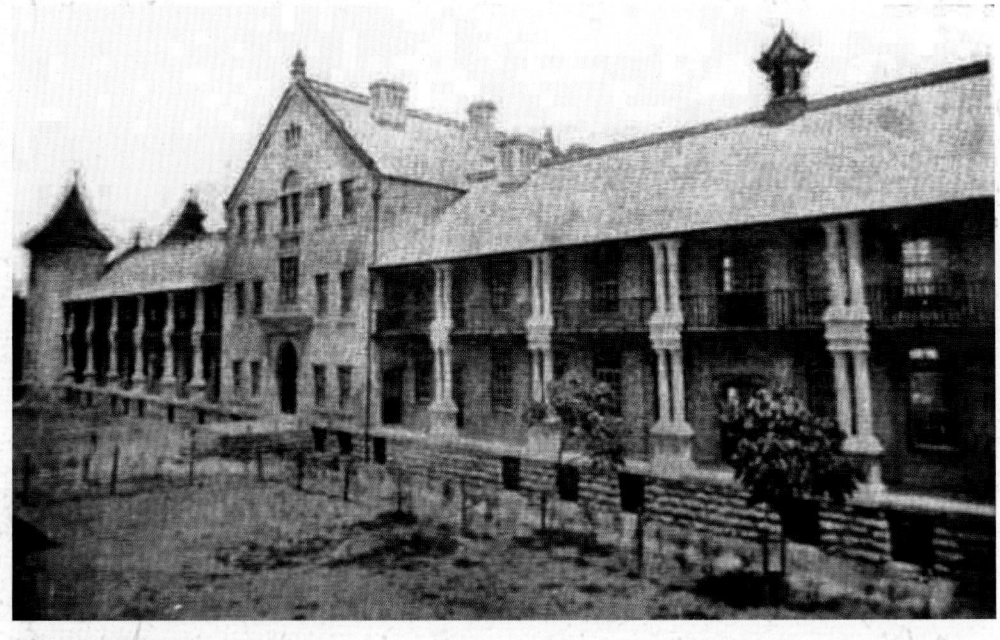

图 52 共合楼旧影
Fig. 52 An old photo of Gonghe Building

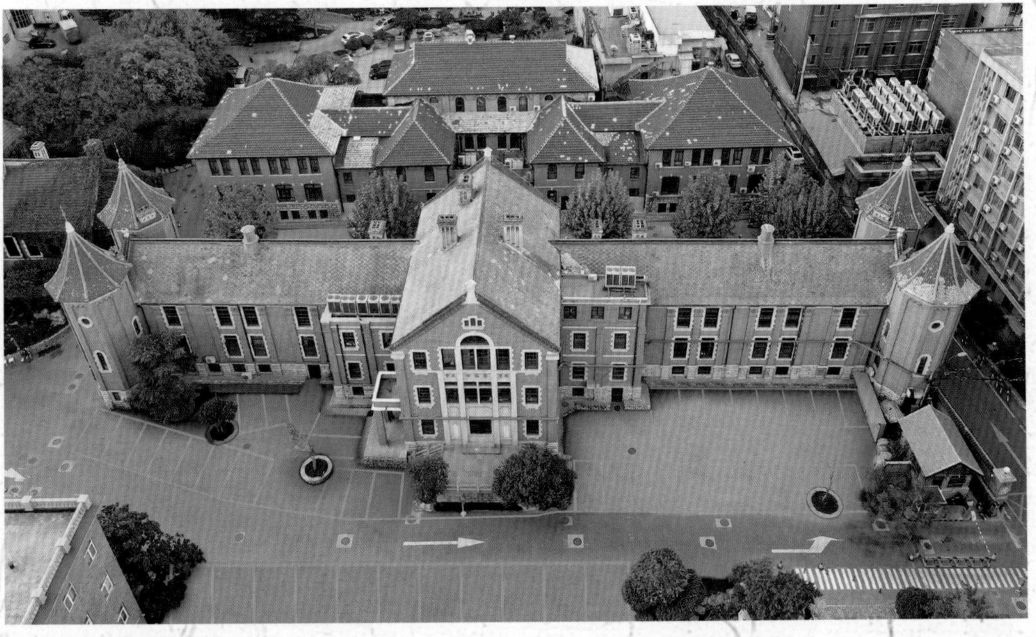

图 53 共合楼北面观
Fig. 53 The north view of Gonghe Building

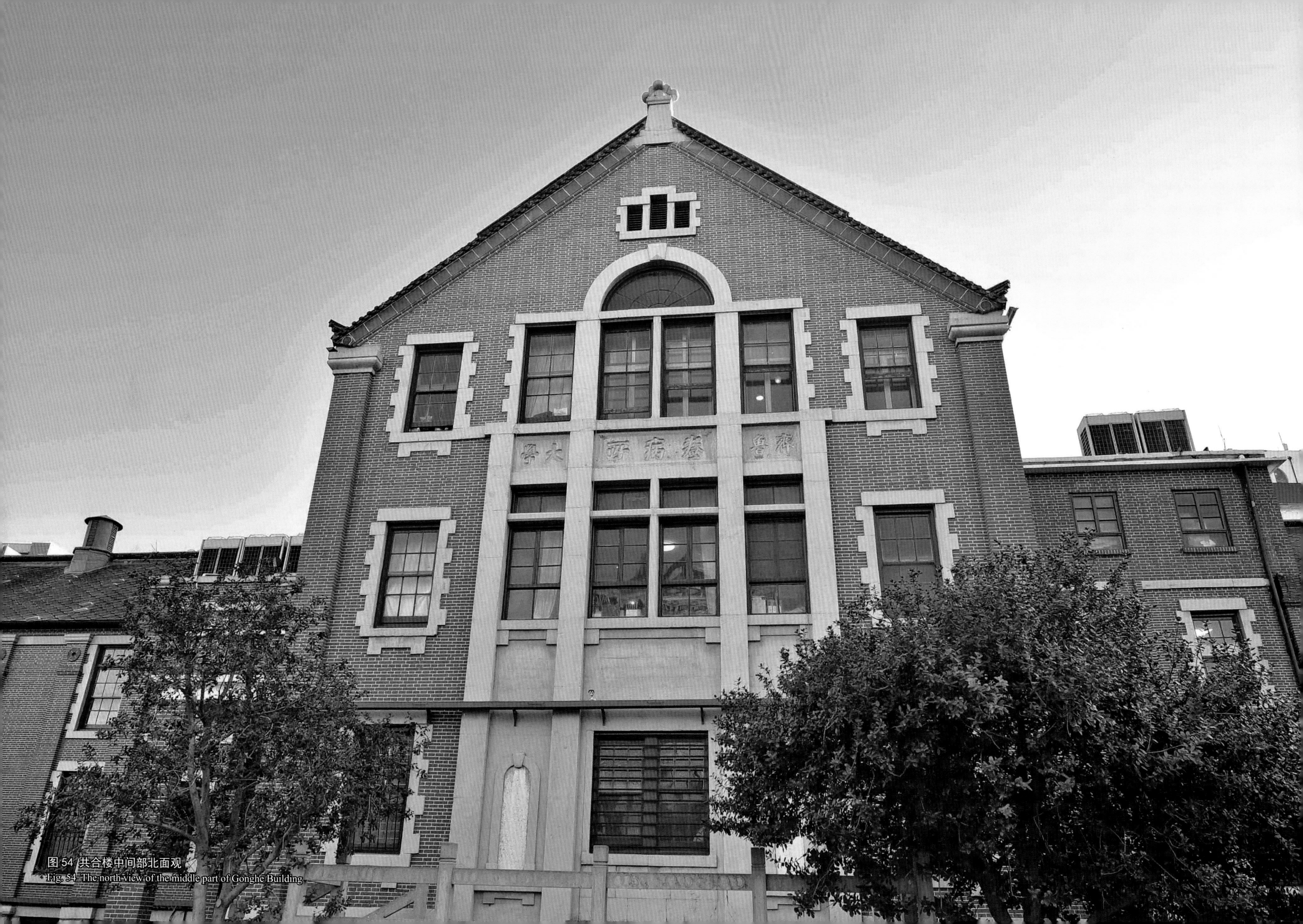

图 54 共合楼中间部北面观

Fig. 54 The north view of the middle part of Gonghe Building

09 共合楼（养病所）（3）

Gonghe Building (The Infirmary) (3)

共合楼是当时医院内单体最大的建筑物，共三层砖混结构，建筑面积 3171 平方米。楼内有院长办公室、护士长办公室等，有普通病房 10 间、隔离及加护病房数间，有病床 115 张，分男女养病室，收治内、外、妇产、小儿、眼、耳鼻喉、皮肤、牙科等患者，此外还有割症房（手术室）、化验室、X 光室、配药室等。1952 年以后，这里曾经作为山东医学院附属医院和山东医科大学附属医院的口腔科和眼科病房，现为山东大学齐鲁医院的办公一楼。

Gonghe Building was the largest single building in the hospital at that time, with a total of three floors of brick-concrete structure and a construction area of 3,171 square meters. The building had the dean's office, the head nurse's office, ten general wards, a few isolation and intensive care wards, and 115 sickbeds divided into male and female ones. It received and cured patients of internal medicine, surgery, gynaecology and obstetrics, paediatrics, ophthalmology, otolaryngology, dermatology, dentistry and so on. In addition, there were the operating room, laboratory, X-ray room, pharmacy room and so on. After 1952, it was used to be wards of stomatology and ophthalmology of the hospitals affiliated to Shandong Medical College and Shandong Medical University respectively, and is now the First Office Building of Qilu Hospital of Shandong University.

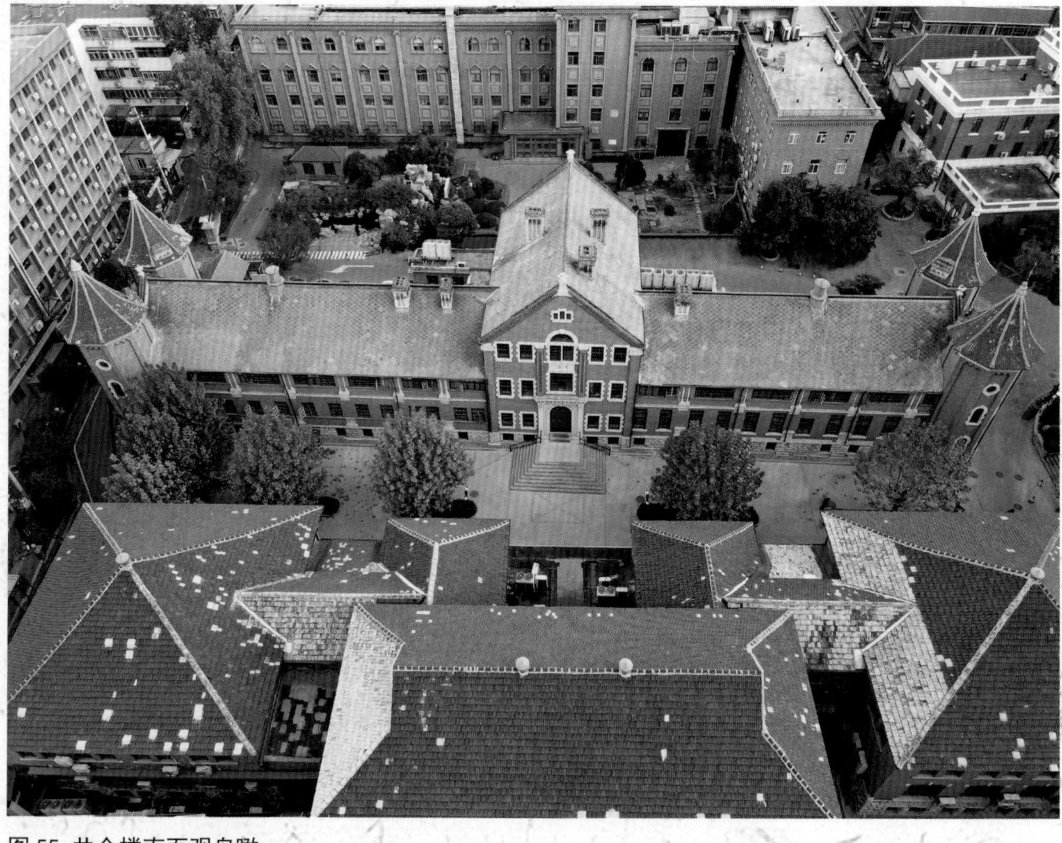

图 55 共合楼南面观鸟瞰
Fig. 55 A bird's-eye view of the south side of Gonghe Building

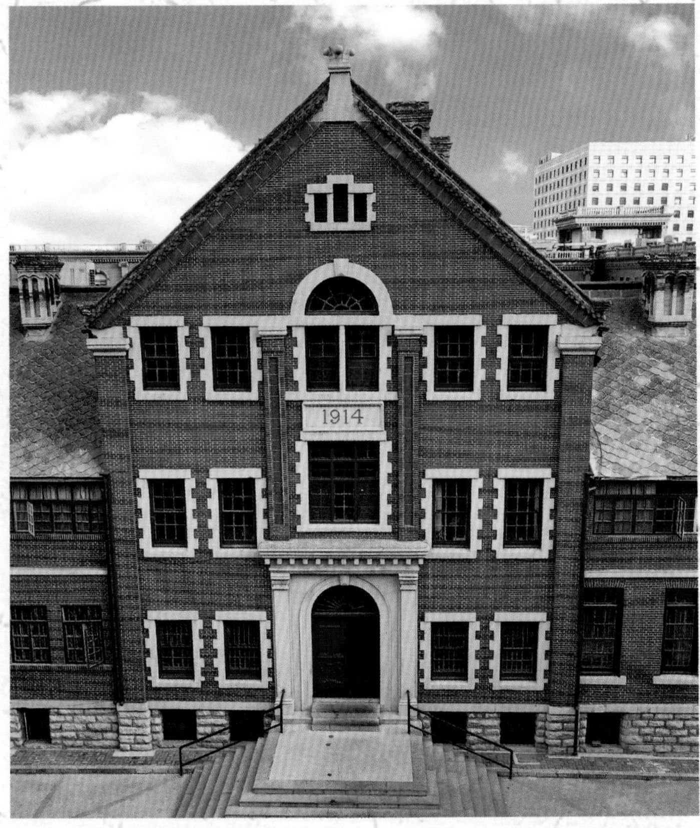

图 56 共合楼中间部南面观
Fig. 56 The south view of the middle part of Gonghe Building

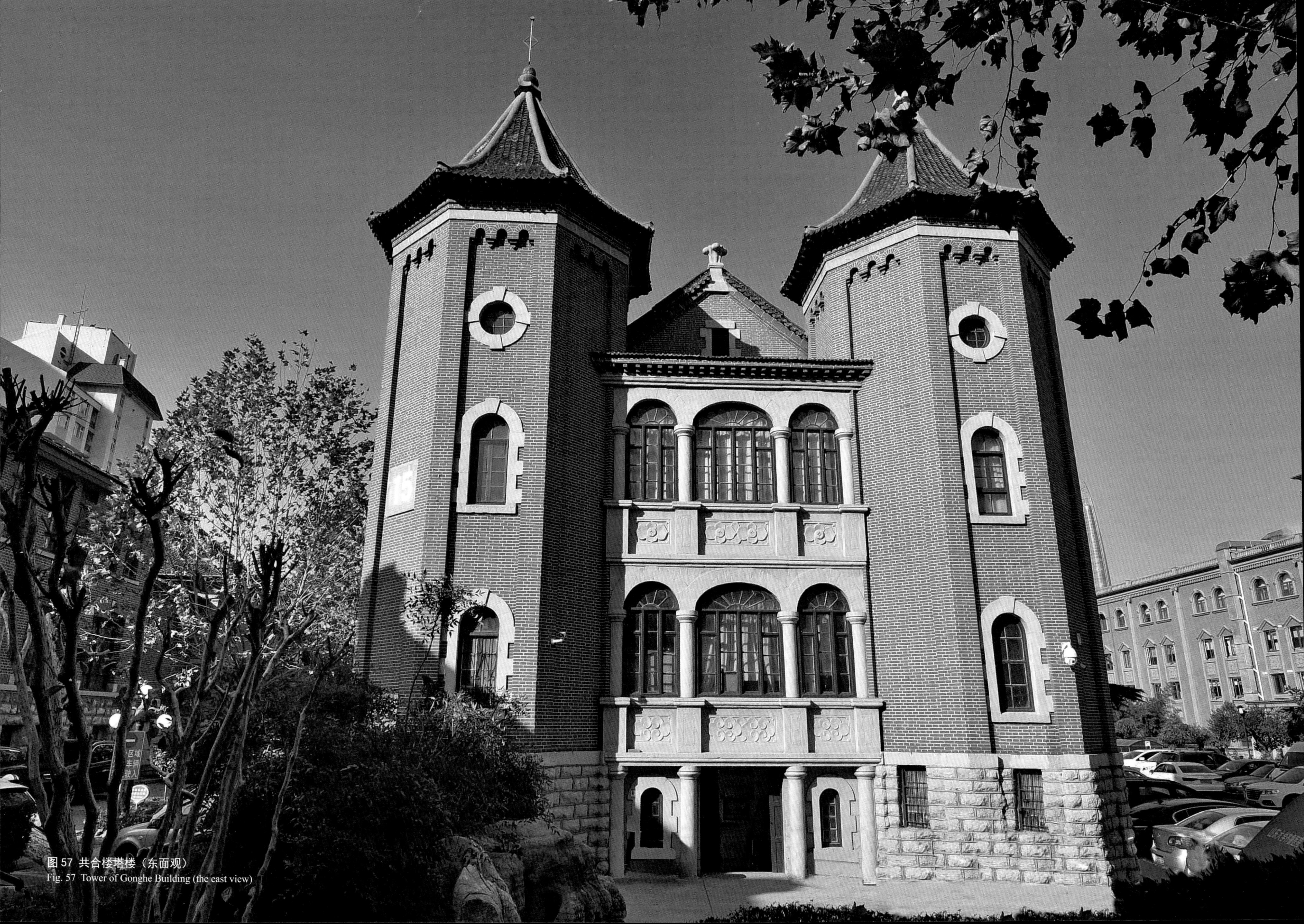

图 57 共合楼塔楼（东面观）
Fig. 57 Tower of Gonghe Building (the east view)

10 和平楼

Heping Building

和平楼建于1915年，原为山东共合医道学堂附设护士养成学校所在地，现供齐鲁医院党委宣传统战部、临床药理基地使用。护士养成学校由英国浸礼会劳根女士于1914年创办（初期为护士班），学制四年，男女生皆收。1917年，该校成为齐鲁大学医科的护理专科。1929年，护理科独立设置，由四年制改为五年制（预科三年、正科两年），入学时应试资格与医科相同。1952年，五年制护理本科班停办。

劳根（Margaret Faiconer Logan），1908年毕业于英国格拉斯哥皇家医院，此后在那里当了一年护士。1909年，她受英国浸礼会派遣来青州工作。次年，青州广德医院护士学校成立。这是山东共合医道学堂护理教育的起点。1913年，劳根来济南工作。劳根是山东护理教育的开拓者，为山东省乃至全国培养了一大批医德修养好、业务水平高的护理骨干人才。

Heping Building was built in 1915 and it was originally the site of the Nurse Cultivation School attached to Shantung Union Medical College. It is now the location of the Publicity and United Front Work Department of the Party Committee of Qilu Hospital and the Clinical Pharmacology Base. The Nurse Cultivation School was founded in 1914 by Ms. Margaret Faiconer Logan of the English Baptist Missionary Society (initially a nursing class). It had a four-year schooling for both male and female students. In 1917, the school became a nursing specialty in the Medical School of Cheeloo University. In 1929, the Nursing Department was set up independently, changing from a four-year system to a five-year system (three years for preparatory courses and two years for formal courses), and the admission qualification was the same as that of the Medical School. In 1952, the five-year nursing undergraduate class was suspended.

Margaret Faiconer Logan graduated from the Royal College of Glasgow, UK in 1908 and worked there for a year. In 1909, she was sent to Qingzhou by the English Baptist Missionary Society to work. The following year, the Nursing School of Tsingchow Kwang Teh Hospital was established, which was the starting point of the nursing education in Shantung Union Medical College. In 1913, Logan came to Jinan to work. Logan was a pioneer of the nursing education in Shandong Province and she had trained a large number of backbone talents of nursing with good medical ethics and high professional level for Shandong Province and even the whole country.

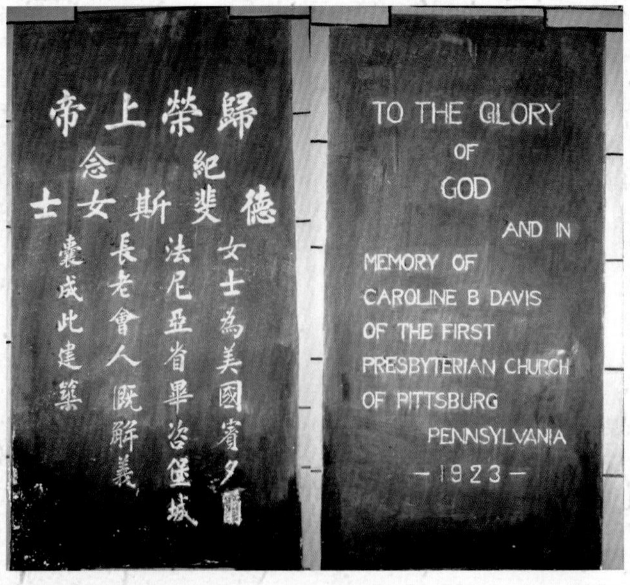

图58 和平楼上的题字
Fig. 58 The inscription on Heping Building

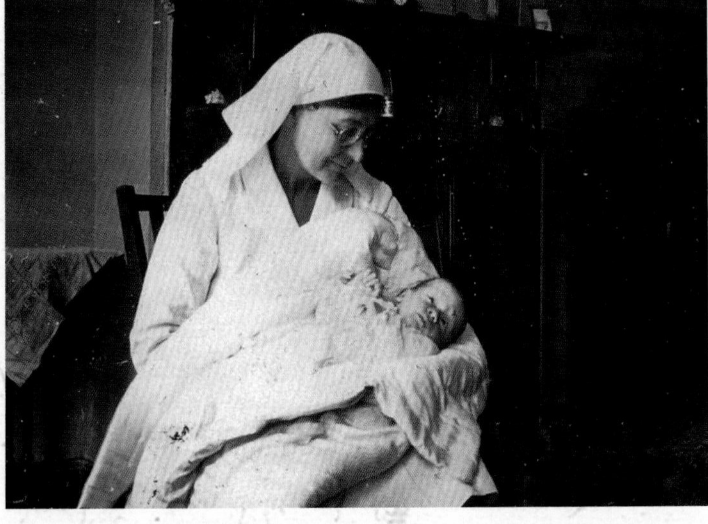

图59 山东护理教育的先驱——劳根女士
Fig. 59 A pioneer of the nursing education in Shandong Province—Ms. Logan

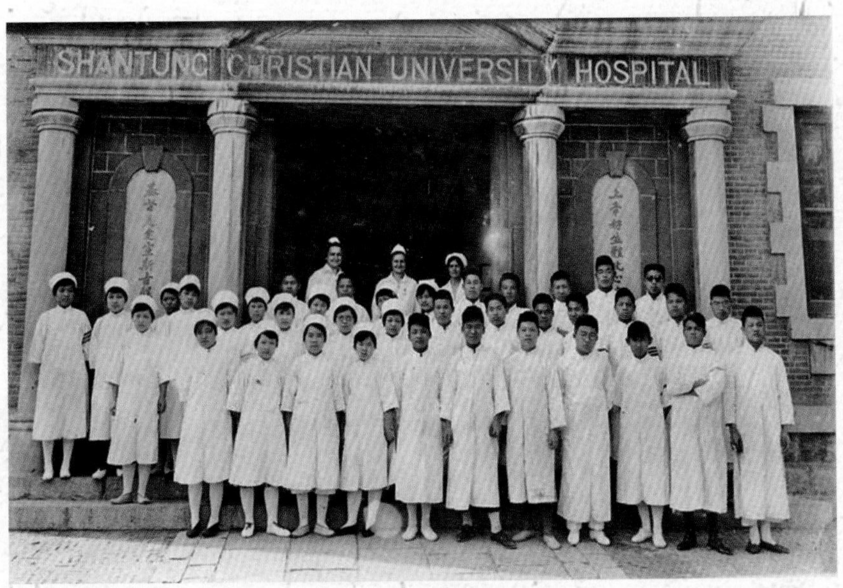

图60 护士养成学校毕业生与教师合影
Fig. 60 Group photo of graduates and teachers of the Nurse Cultivation School

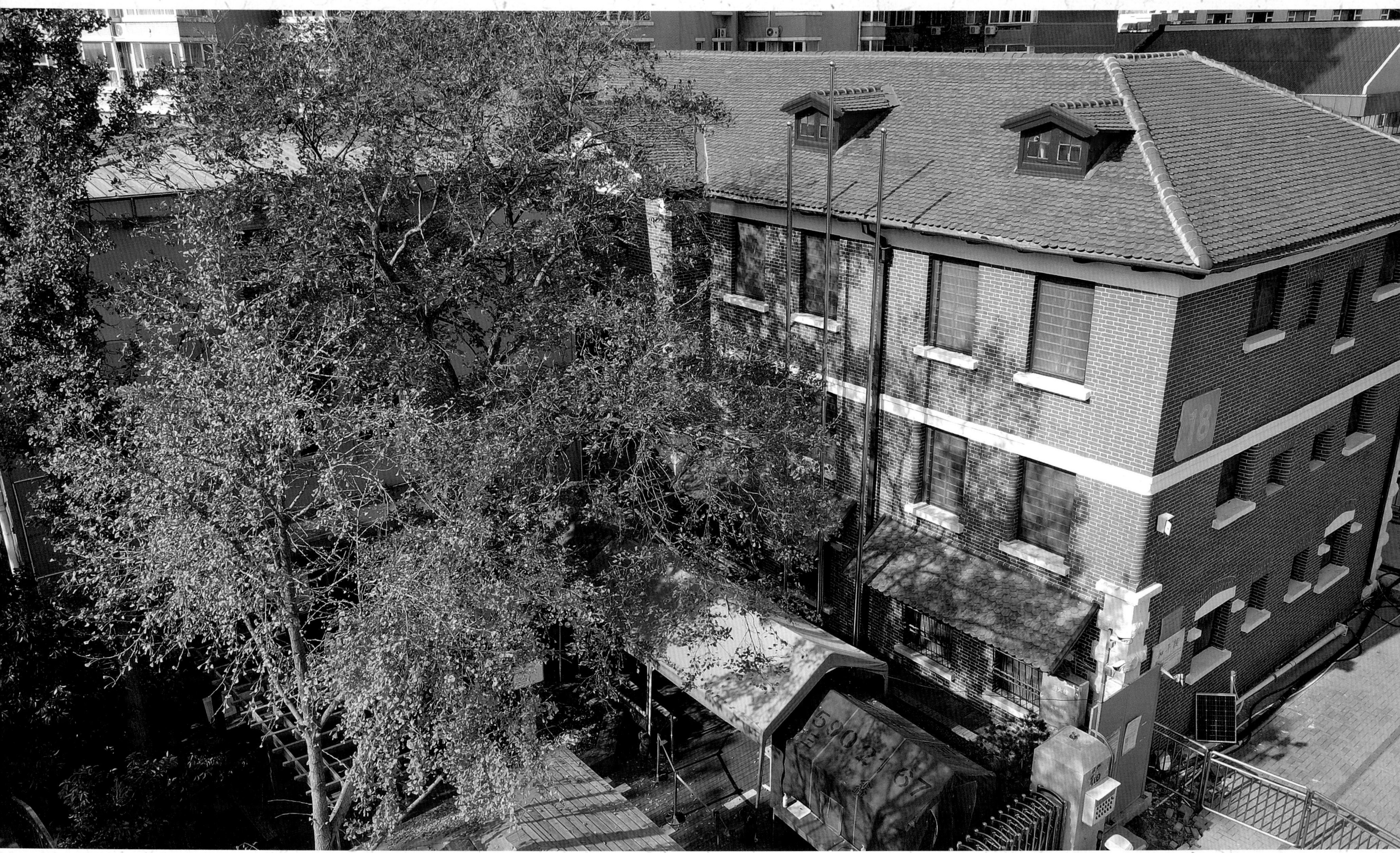

图 61 和平楼近影
Fig. 61 A recent photo of Heping Building

11 校园规划图纸

Planning Drawings of the Campus

建立山东基督教共合大学济南共同校区的建议是由芝加哥大学巴顿（Ernest D. Burton）教授提出的。当时，他担任美国东方教育委员会的主席，于 1909 年访问了中国。1912 年，教会征得中华民国时期第一任山东都督周自齐同意后，在济南南圩子门外名为永租实为强购 600 余亩土地用作建立新校区。这要归因于怀恩光先生的不懈努力。募集建设资金的功劳首推路思义（Henry W. Luce），其长子鲁斯为美国《时代》周刊的创始人。校园整体规划方案的设计由芝加哥珀金斯（Perkins）、法罗斯（Fellows）和汉密尔顿（Hamilton）公司负责，但后来由于资金问题未能实现全部设计目标。1917 年 9 月，潍县的文理学院和青州的神学院、师范学校迁来济南校区，并以“齐鲁大学”为正式校名举行了开学典礼。此时，英国浸礼会牧师卜道成（Joseph Percy Bruce, 1861~1934）为校长，路思义为副校长。

The proposal to establish a common campus of Shantung Christian University in Jinan was put forward by professor Ernest D. Burton of the University of Chicago who was then Chairman of the American Council on Eastern Education and visited China in 1909. In 1912, with the consent of Zhou Ziqi, the first governor of Shandong Province during the Republic of China, the church forcibly purchased more than 600 *mu* of land at the Nanweimenwai Street in Jinan under the name of permanent rent for the construction of a new campus, which was due to Mr. John Sutherland Whitewright's unremitting efforts. Henry W. Luce contributed the most to the raising of construction funds and his eldest son Henry R. Luce was the founder of the American magazine *Time*. The companies from Chicago, Perkins, Fellows and Hamilton, were responsible for the overall plan of the campus, but not all the design objectives had been achieved due to financial problems. In September 1917, Wei Hsien Arts and Science College and the Theological College and Normal College in Qingzhou moved to Jinan, and held the opening ceremony under the official name of "Cheeloo University". Joseph Percy Bruce (1861-1934), pastor of the English Baptist Missionary Society, was the president, and Henry W. Luce was the vice president.

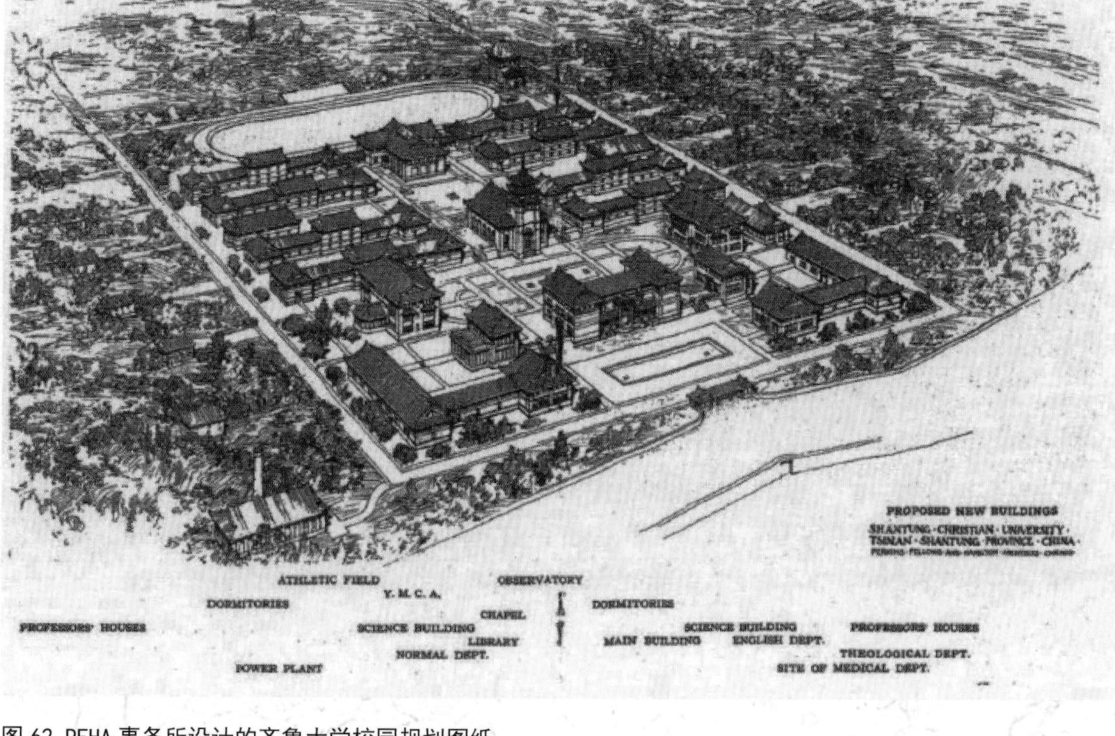

图 62 PFHA 事务所设计的齐鲁大学校园规划图纸
Fig. 62 The planning drawings of the campus of Cheeloo University designed by PFHA

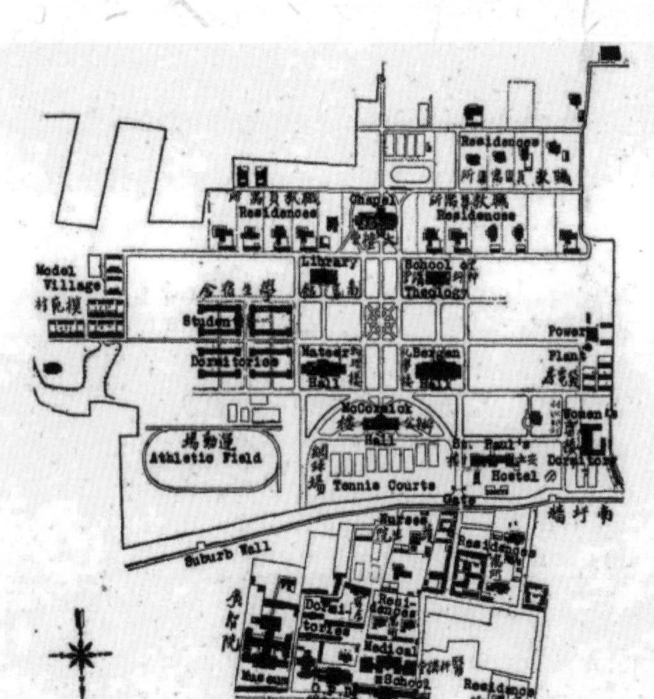

图 63 1924 年后的齐鲁大学校园布局
Fig. 63 Campus layout of Cheeloo University after 1924

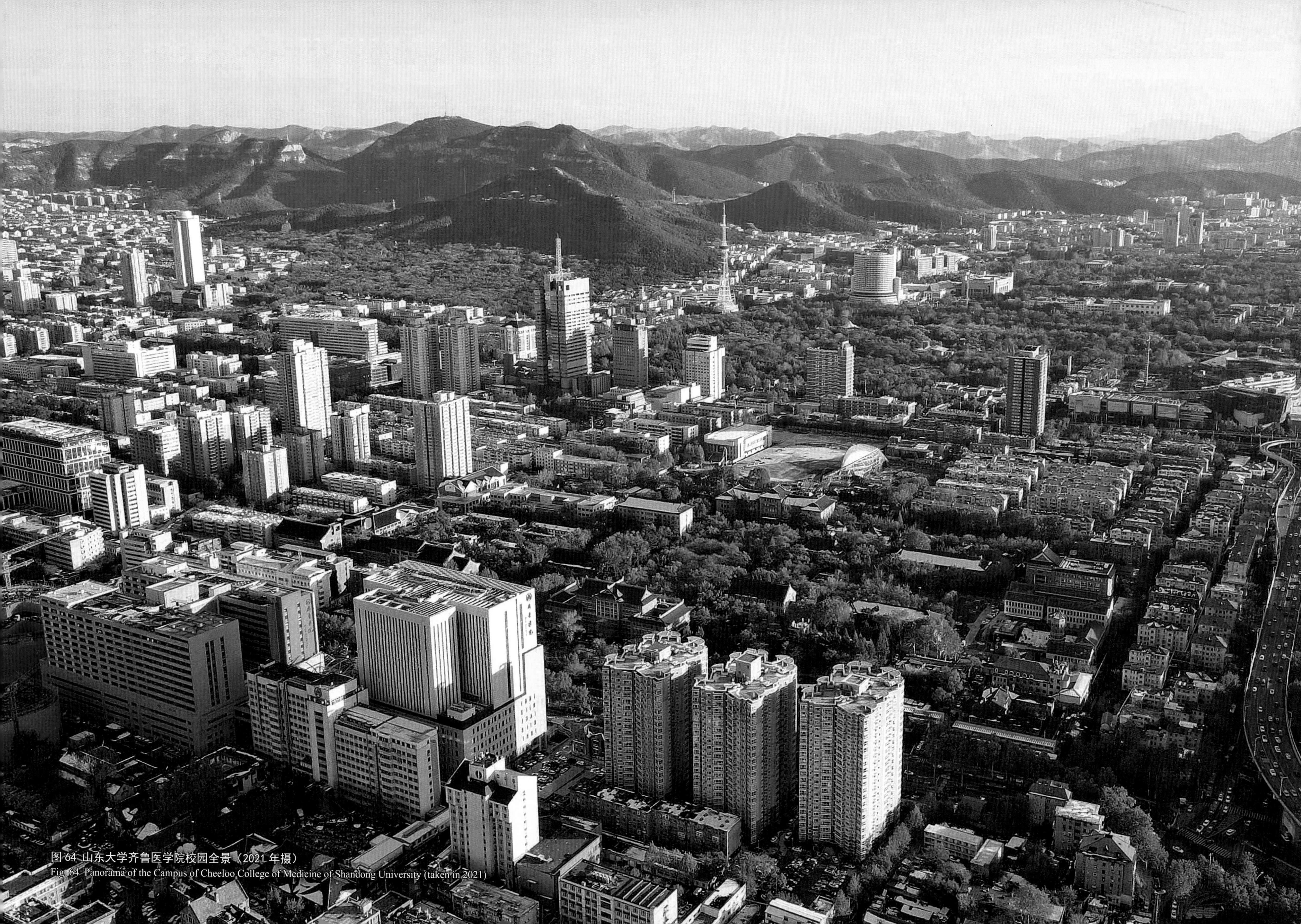

图 64 山东大学齐鲁医学院校园全景（2021 年摄）
Fig. 64 Panorama of the Campus of Cheeloo College of Medicine of Shandong University (taken in 2021)

12 校园全景（1）

Panorama of the Campus (1)

齐鲁医学院建筑中西合璧，校园布局精巧，用齐鲁大学早期学生的一句妙语来说：“四条交叉大道把校园安排得恰到好处。”中轴线上，综合楼（以前为麦考密可楼）和教学八楼（以前为康穆堂）北南呼应，两者中间为中心花园。中轴线两厢，各有三排建筑整齐分列。西厢，教学三楼（柏根楼）与教学四楼（葛罗神学院楼）在近中轴线的第一排上默默相视，第二排有电镜楼、教学一楼（解剖楼）和教学二楼北南排列；最西边的第三排由北向南座列着景蓝斋、桐荫阁与国家卫健委耳鼻咽喉科学重点实验室、美德楼、水塔、实验动物中心和国家糖工程中心。东厢，在近中轴线的内侧排上教学五楼（考文楼）与教学七楼（原为奥古斯丁图书馆）顾盼生情，中间排上由北向南可见教学九楼（公共卫生楼）、教学六楼、号院和图书馆，最东边的外侧排上有令人神往且韵律十足的国家生殖医学中心、口腔楼、护理楼、食堂和梦迪音乐厅。学校大门称“校友门”，并不位于中轴线上，而是耸立于北侧偏东，其西侧为圣保罗楼和小教堂。教学八楼的两侧为别墅群，南侧是体育场，其东南侧原为麻风病院（图 65 中的 27），现为学生宿舍和青年教师公寓。

The architecture of Cheeloo College of Medicine is a combination of Chinese and Western styles, and the layout of the campus is exquisite. Here is to quote a witticism from the early students of Cheeloo University, “The four intersecting avenues have arranged the campus just right.” On the central axis, the Comprehensive Building (former McCormick Hall) and the Eighth Teaching Building (former Kumler Chapel) echo each other in the north and south, with the Central Garden in the middle. The two wings of the central axis have three rows of buildings in order. In the west wing, the Third Teaching Building (Bergen Hall) and the Fourth Teaching Building (Gotch-Robinson Theological Building) silently face each other in the first row near the central axis. The second row has the Building of Electron Microscopy, the First Teaching Building (Anatomy Building) and the Second Teaching Building arranged from north to south. In the westernmost third row, from north to south, there are Jinglan Building, Tongyin Pavilion, Key Laboratory of Otorhinolaryngology of the Ministry of Health, Miner Building, Water Tower, the Laboratory Animal Center and National Glycoengineering Research Center. In the east wing, on the inner side near the central axis, there are the Fifth Teaching Building (Calvin Mateer Hall) and the Seventh Teaching Building (formerly Augustine Library) looking at each other. In the middle row, there are the Ninth Teaching Building (Public Health Building), the Sixth Teaching Building, the Courtyard and the library from north to south. On the outer side of the easternmost row, there are the fascinating and rhythmic National Reproductive Medicine Center, the Building of Stomatology, the Nursing Building, the canteen and the Mengdi Concert Hall. The school gate, also known as the Alumni Gate, is not located on the central axis, but stands east-north, with the Stom atological Building and the Chapel on its west side. On both sides of the Eighth Teaching Building are villa groups, on the south side is the stadium, and on the southeast side is the Leprosy Hospital (27 in Fig. 65), which is now the student dormitory and the young teacher’s apartment.

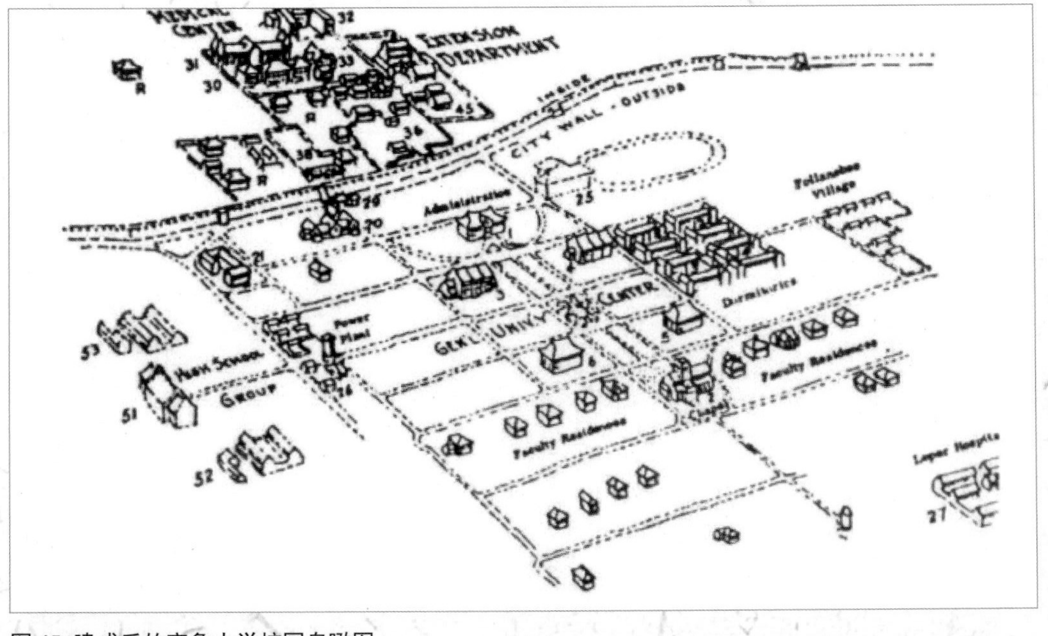

图 65 建成后的齐鲁大学校园鸟瞰图

Fig. 65 A bird’s-eye view of the campus of Cheeloo University after completion

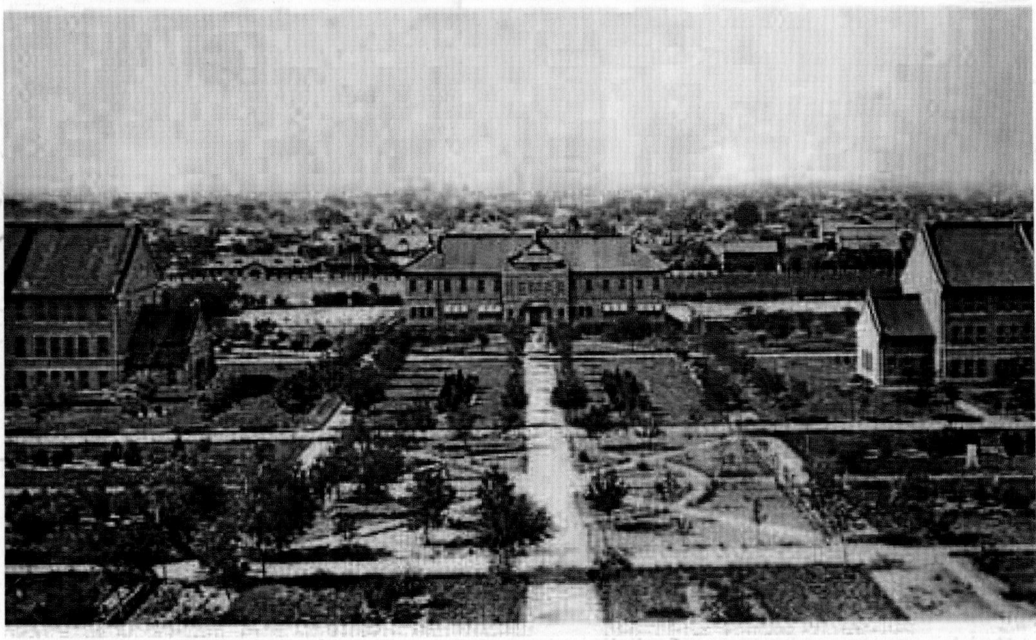

图 66 齐鲁大学校园旧影

Fig. 66 An old photo of the campus of Cheeloo University

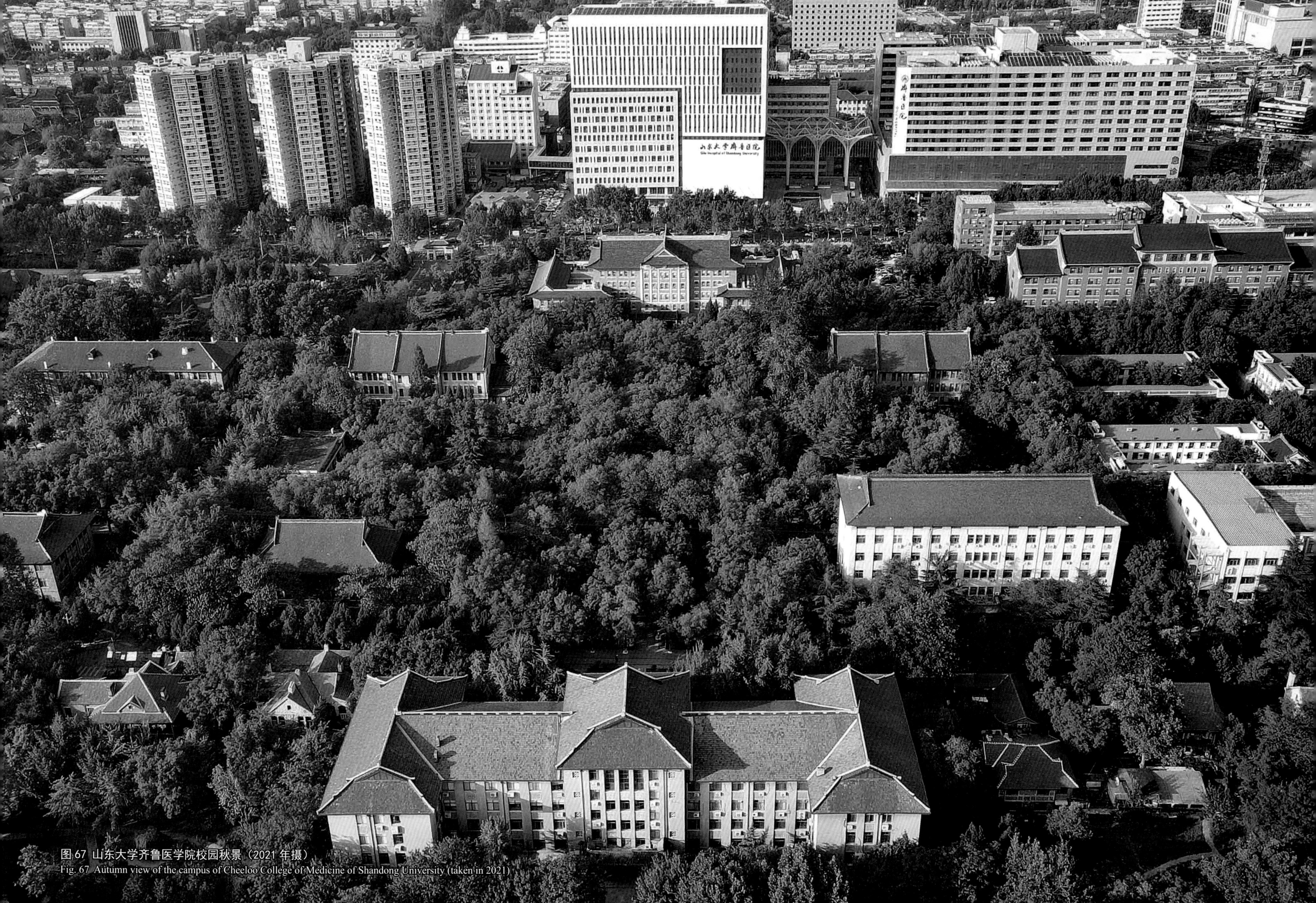

图 67 山东大学齐鲁医院学院校园秋景（2021 年摄）

Fig. 67 Autumn view of the campus of Cheeloo College of Medicine of Shandong University (taken in 2021)

12 校园全景（2）
Panorama of the Campus (2)

我们今天不得不佩服齐鲁大学先辈们选择校址的独特眼光和建设校园的奇妙构思。它北邻日夜喷涌的趵突泉，南靠连绵起伏的千佛山，地理位置十分优越。校园内，建筑飞檐灵动，中西合璧，错落有致；花木绿冠成荫，蜂蝶共舞，鸟虫和鸣。徜徉其中，就像著名外科圣手王占民先生所说的那样："我坐在这里有种神仙般的感觉。"20 世纪 30 年代，曾两度在齐鲁大学文学院任教的老舍先生十分喜爱这个校园，把它称为"非正式的公园"。他在这篇散文中娓娓写道："拐过礼堂，你看见南面的群山，绿的。山前的田，绿的。一个绿海，山是那些高的绿浪。礼堂的左右，东西两条绿径，树阴很密，几乎见不着阳光。顺着这绿径走，不论是往西往东，你看见些小的楼房，每处有个小花园。园墙都是矮松做的。"这就是一代文学大师笔下的齐鲁大学校园，这就是我们学习的圣殿、工作的桃源和生活的乐土。

Today, we have to admire the unique vision of Cheeloo University's ancestors in choosing the campus site and their wonderful idea of the campus construction. It is adjacent to the Baotu Spring gushing day and night in the north and the Qianfo Hill rolling continuously in the south. The geographical location is very superior. On campus, the buildings of Chinese and Western styles are well arranged with flexible cornices. Flowers and trees are shaded by green crowns; bees and butterflies dance; birds and insects sing. Wandering on campus, you will have the feeling of what the skilled surgeon Mr. Wang Zhanmin once said, "I'm sitting here feeling like a fairy." In the 1930s, Mr. Lao She who twice taught at the School of Literature of Cheeloo University liked the campus very much and called it "an informal park". In the essay "The Informal Park", Lao She wrote eloquently: "Turn around the auditorium, you will see the lush mountains in the south and the green fields in front of the mountains. The mountains are those high green waves of a green sea. On the left and right of the auditorium, there are two green paths in the east and west respectively. The dense shade of trees almost blocks the sunlight. Follow the green path, and you will see small buildings whether in the west or in the east, each with a small garden, and the walls of of the gardens are made of dwarf pines." This is the campus of Cheeloo University in the works of a literary master. This is the temple of our study, the paradise of our work and the happy land of our life.

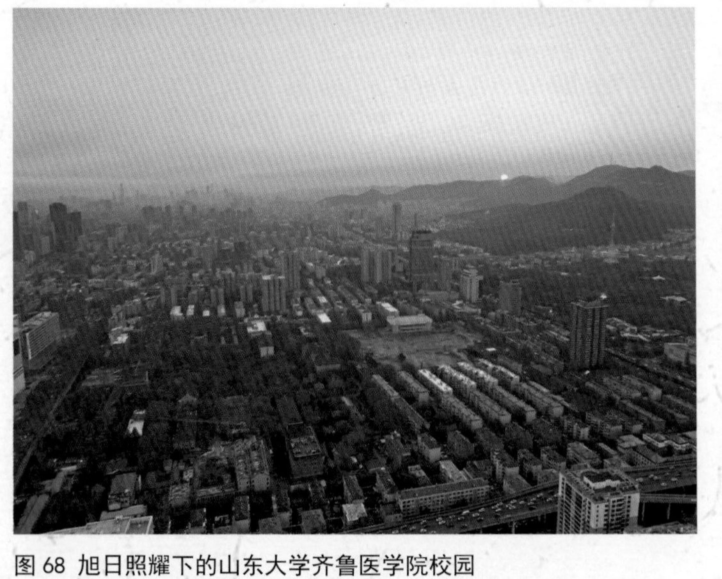

图 68 旭日照耀下的山东大学齐鲁医学院校园
Fig. 68 Campus of Cheeloo College of Medicine of Shandong University under the rising sun

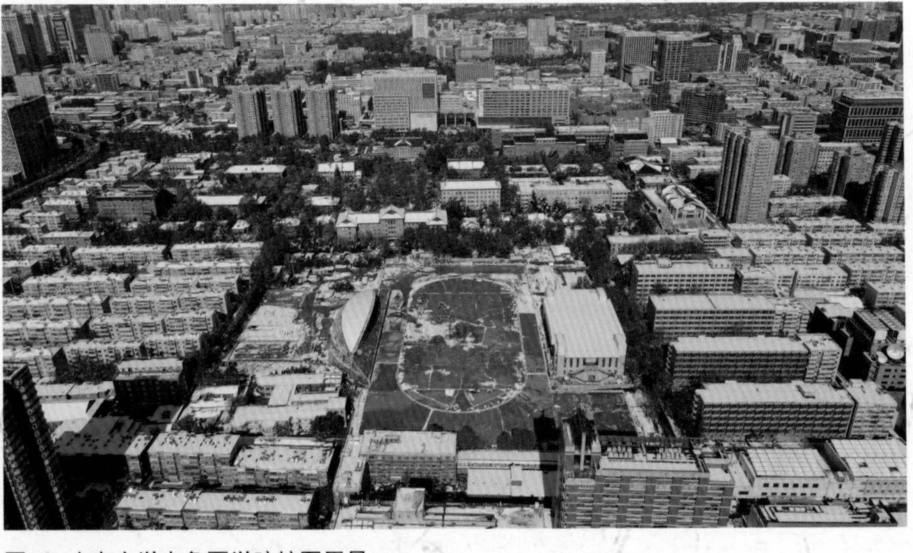

图 69 山东大学齐鲁医学院校园雪景
Fig. 69 Snow view of the campus of Cheeloo College of Medicine of Shandong University

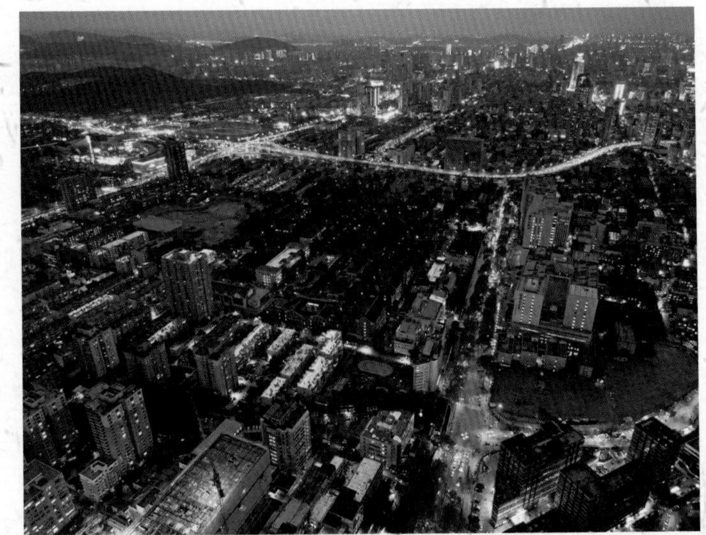

图 70 山东大学齐鲁医学院夜景
Fig. 70 Night view of Cheeloo College of Medicine of Shandong University

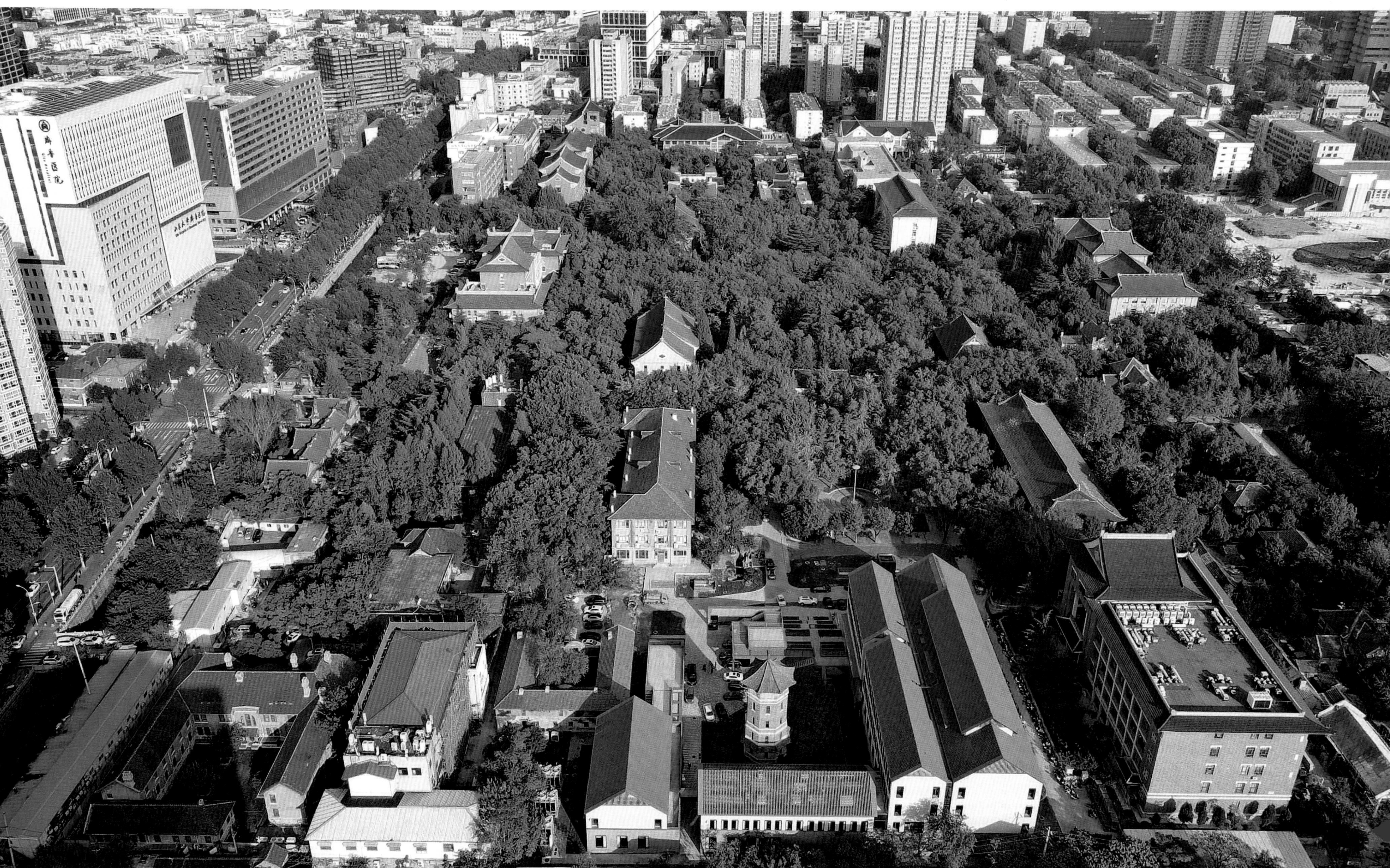

图 71 山东大学齐鲁医学院校园核心区域

Fig. 71 Core area of the campus of Cheeloo College of Medicine of Shandong University

第三章 Chapter Three

校友门 Alumni Gate

13 | 校友门（1）

Alumni Gate (1)

山东大学齐鲁医学院校门亦称校友门，是原齐鲁大学校门，由千名校友集资 2000 银元兴建。1924 年 6 月 17 日，齐鲁大学举行了校友门落成典礼。她既是原齐鲁大学也是现山东大学齐鲁医学院的标志性建筑，见证了学校的合合分分与发展历程。

The gate of Cheeloo College of Medicine of Shandong University, also known as the Alumni Gate, is the former gate of Cheeloo University. It was built by thousands of Cheeloo University graduates raising 2,000 yuan of silver. On 17 June 1924, Cheeloo University held the dedication of the Alumni Gate. She is the landmark building of both the former Cheeloo University and Cheeloo College of Medicine, which has witnessed the university's integration and development.

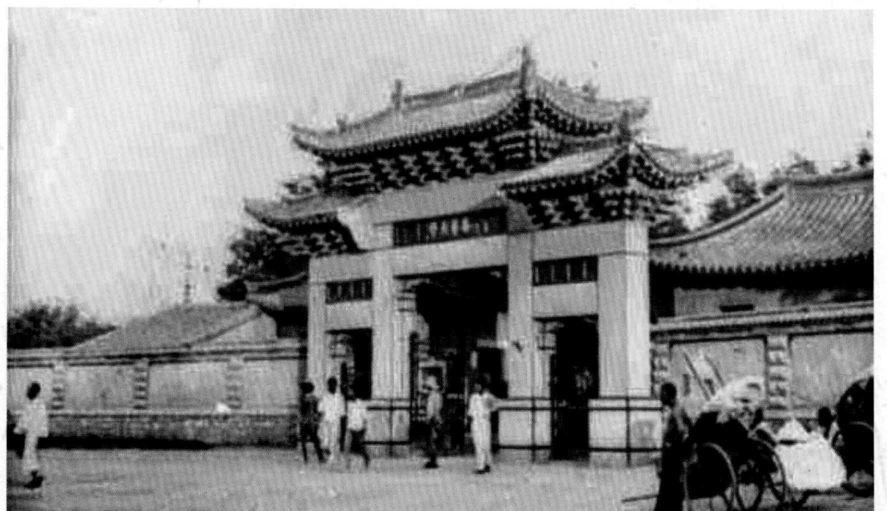

图 72 齐鲁大学时期的校友门
Fig. 72 Alumni Gate of Cheeloo University

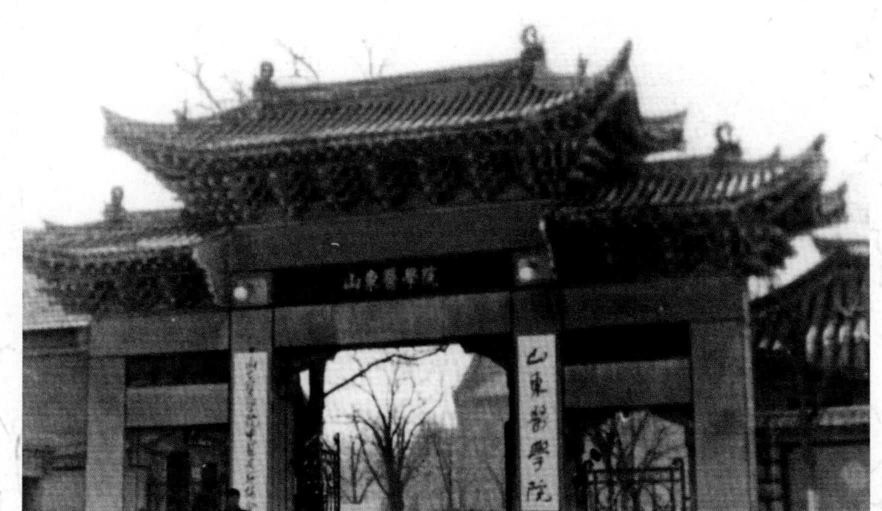

图 73 1952 年院系调整后的山东医学院大门
Fig. 73 Gate of Shandong Medical College after the adjustment of schools and departments in 1952

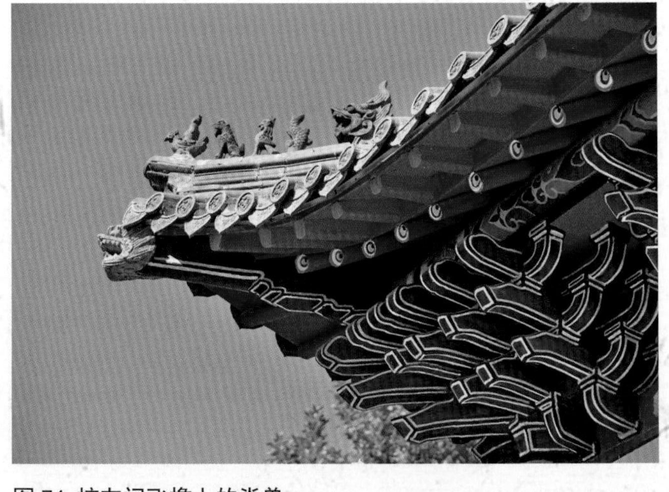

图 74 校友门飞檐上的脊兽
Fig. 74 Beast ornaments on the cornice of the Alumni Gate

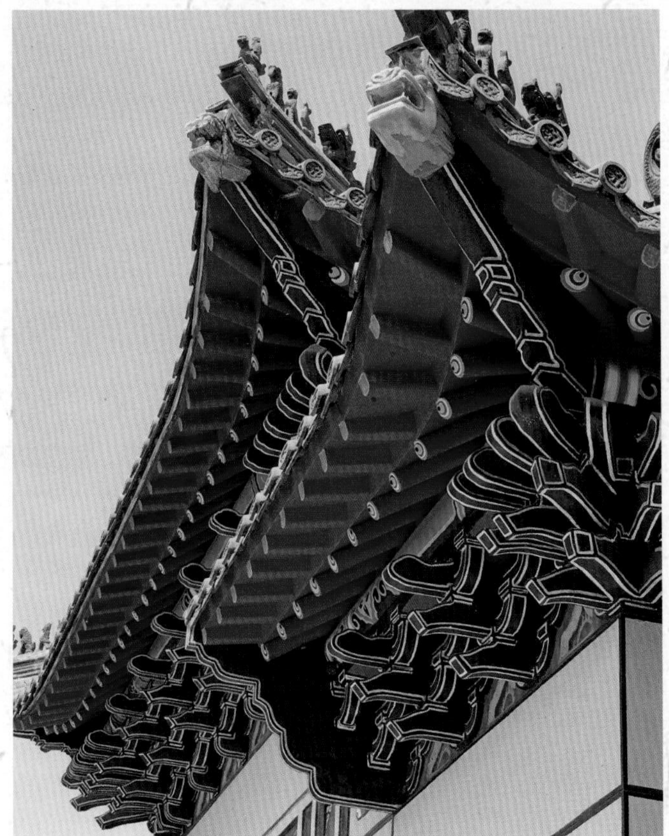

图 75 校友门的飞檐
Fig. 75 Cornice of the Alumni Gate

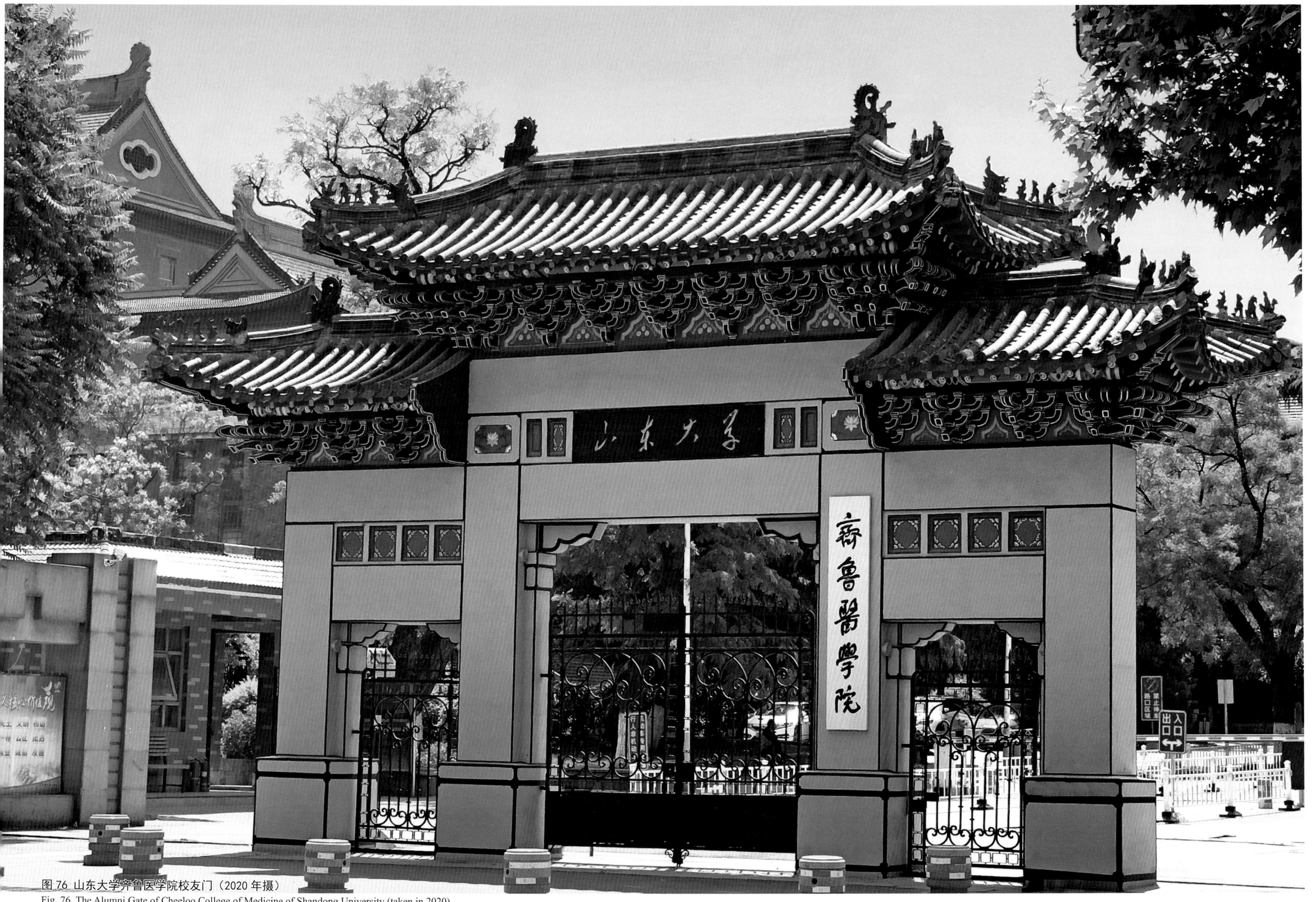

图 76 山东大学齐鲁医学院校友门（2020 年摄）
Fig. 76 The Alumni Gate of Cheeloo College of Medicine of Shandong University (taken in 2020)

13 校友门（2）

Alumni Gate (2)

校友门外面刻有“齐鲁大学”四字，内面刻有“校友门”三字，均为清末状元、教育家、书法家、民国时期曾任山东省教育厅厅长及山东大学校长的王寿彭先生手书。校友门外面“齐鲁大学”四字上面，1952 年覆盖以舒同同志手书“山东医学院”匾，1985 年替换为舒同同志手书“山东医科大学”匾，2000 年后改为毛泽东主席手书“山东大学”匾。王寿彭手书的“校友门”三字一直未变。

舒同（1903 ~ 1998），江西抚州人，1954 年 8 月至 1960 年 10 月，任中共山东省委第一书记兼济南军区第一政委。舒同是当代自成一体的书法大师，创立了著名的“舒体”，是中国书法家协会创始人和第一届主席。毛泽东主席赞扬他是“红军书法家、党内一枝笔”。

The outside of the Alumni Gate is engraved with the four characters “Qi Lu Da Xue” and the inside is engraved with the three characters “Xiao You Men”. These characters were all written by Mr. Wang Shoupeng, the No. 1 scholar of the late Qing Dynasty, educator, calligrapher, and former director of Shandong Provincial Education Department and president of Shandong University during the Republic of China. In 1952, the plaque of “Shan Dong Yi Xue Yuan” written by Comrade Shu Tong covered the four characters “Qi Lu Da Xue” on the outside of the Alumni Gate. In 1985, it was replaced by the plaque of “Shan Dong Yi Ke Da Xue” written by Comrade Shu Tong. After 2000, it was changed to the plaque of “Shan Dong Da Xue” written by Chairman Mao Zedong. The three characters “Xiao You Men” written by Wang Shoupeng have not changed ever since.

Shu Tong (1903-1998), a native of Fuzhou, Jiangxi Province, was the First Secretary of the Shandong Provincial Party Committee and the First Political Commissar of the Jinan Military Region from August 1954 to October 1960. Shu Tong is a contemporary calligrapher of his own style, and he created the famous “Style of Shu”. He is the founder and the first president of the Chinese Calligraphers Association. Chairman Mao Zedong praised him as “a calligrapher of the Red Army and a pen within the party”.

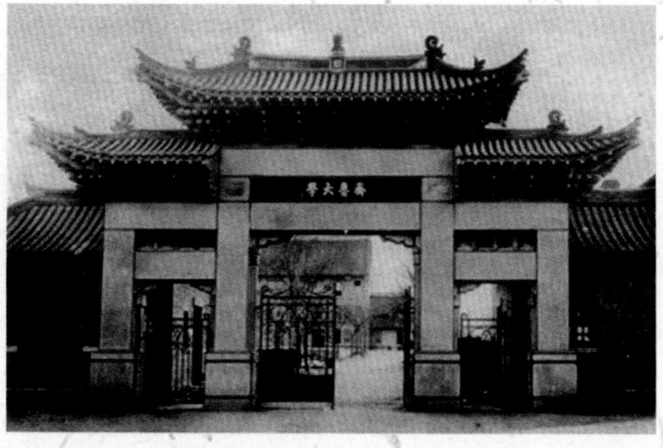

图 77 齐鲁大学时期的校友门
Fig. 77 Alumni Gate of Cheeloo University

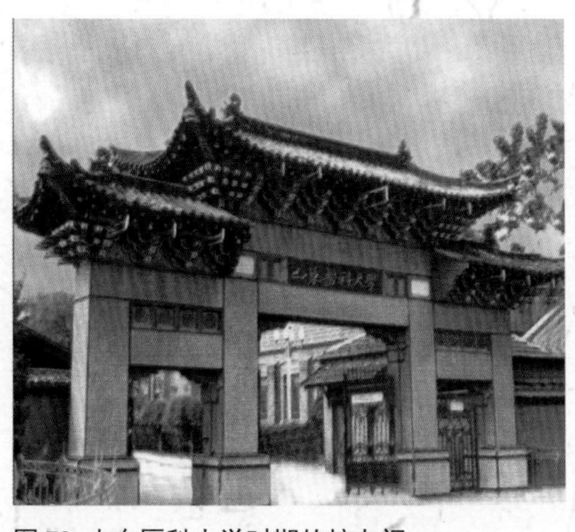

图 78 山东医科大学时期的校友门
Fig. 78 Alumni Gate of Shandong Medical University

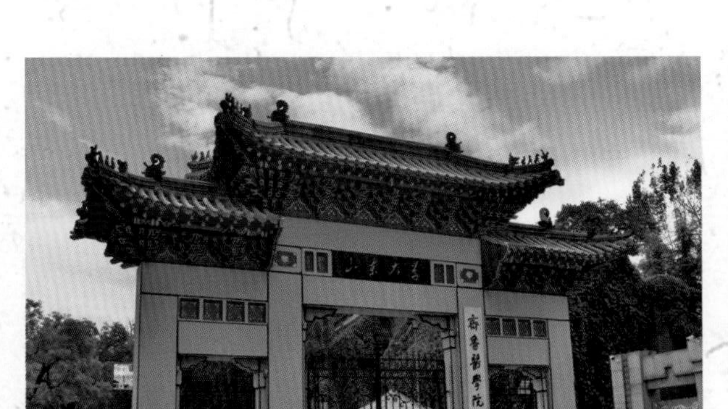

图 79 山东大学时期的校友门
Fig. 79 Alumni Gate of Shandong University

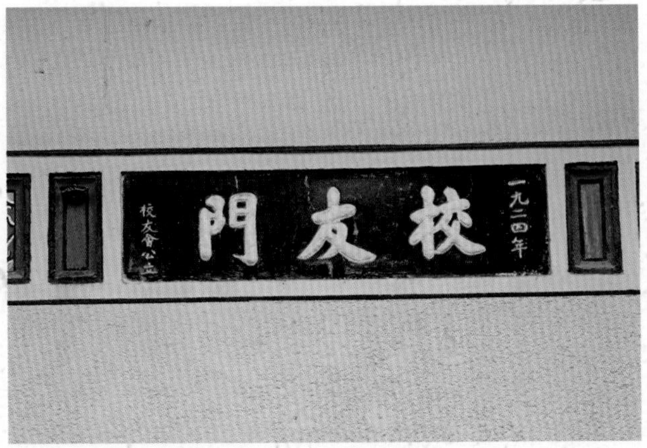

图 80 清末状元王寿彭书写的“校友门”三字
Fig. 80 The three characters of “Xiao You Men” written by Wang Shoupeng, the No. 1 scholar in the late Qing Dynasty

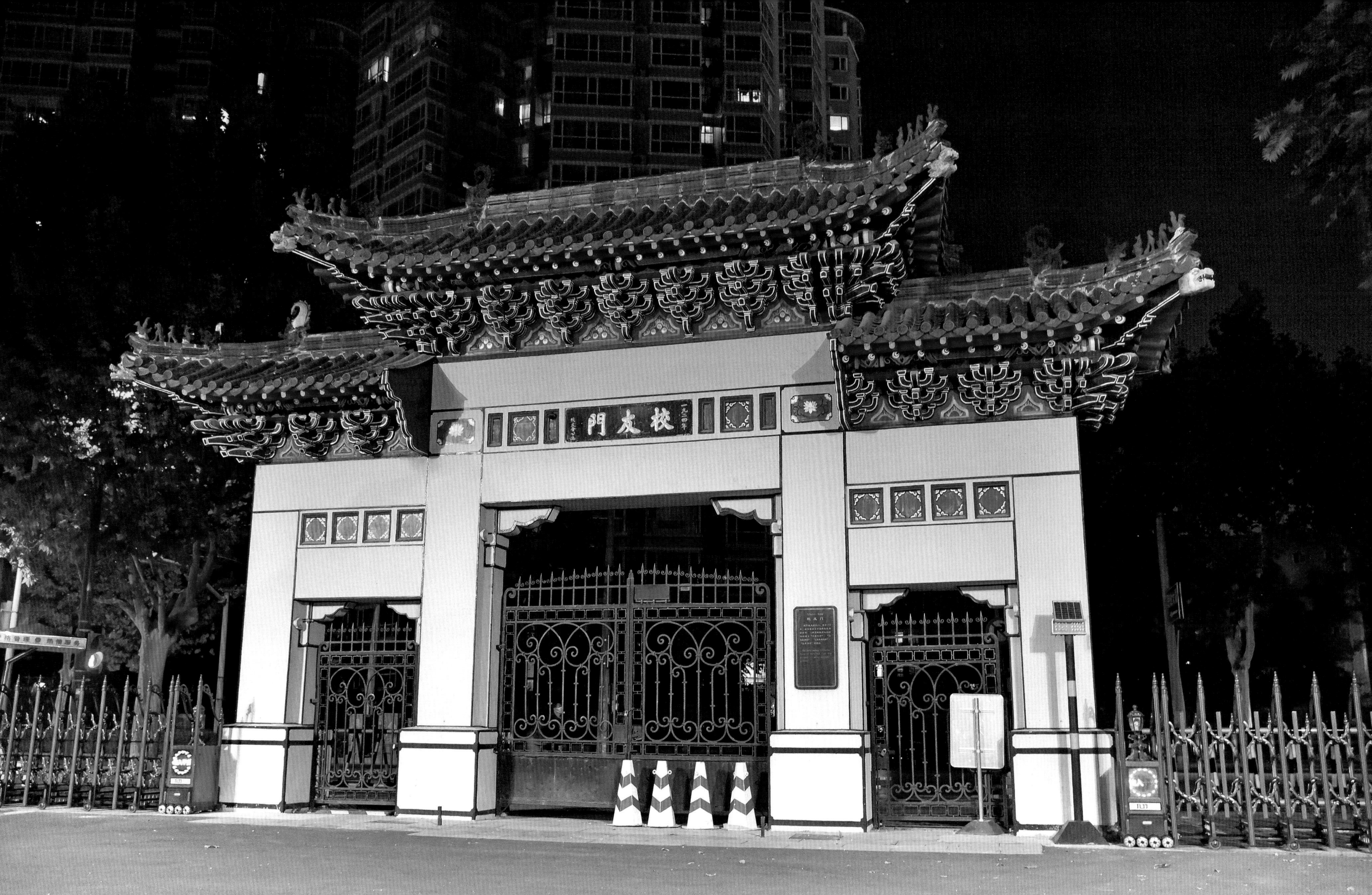

图 81 夜色中的校友门（2020 年摄）
Fig. 81 Alumni Gate in the night (taken in 2020)

13 | 校友门（3）

Alumni Gate (3)

校友门采用中国传统的三间三叠式的牌楼造型。大门牌楼主门顶较高，两侧门顶稍矮，形成一个“山”字形，支撑立柱是典型的现代建筑，中西合璧，浑然一体。整个大门颇像繁体“齐”字，特别是左右侧的两层飞檐，给人一种展翅凌霄之感，寓意深厚。历代师生均选择在校友门前合影留念，以寄托对母校的留恋之情。

The Alumni Gate is of the traditional Chinese style of three-room three-fold archway. The main top of the archway is higher and the tops on both sides are slightly lower, forming the shape of the Chinese character “Shan”. The supporting columns are typical modern architecture of integrated Chinese and Western styles. The whole gate is quite like the traditional Chinese character “Qi”. The two layers of cornices on the left and right sides give people a sense of soaring into the sky, implying profound meanings. Generations of teachers and students have chosen to take photos in front of the Alumni Gate to express their nostalgia for their alma mater.

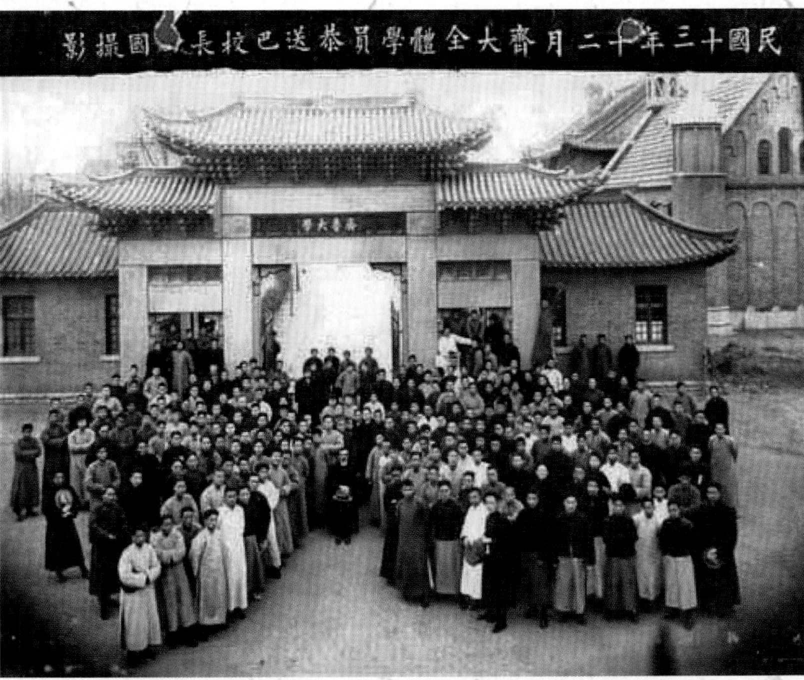

图 82 1924 年齐鲁大学师生在校友门前为巴慕德校长送行

Fig. 82 Teachers and students of Cheeloo University seeing President Harold Balme off in front of the Alumni Gate in 1924

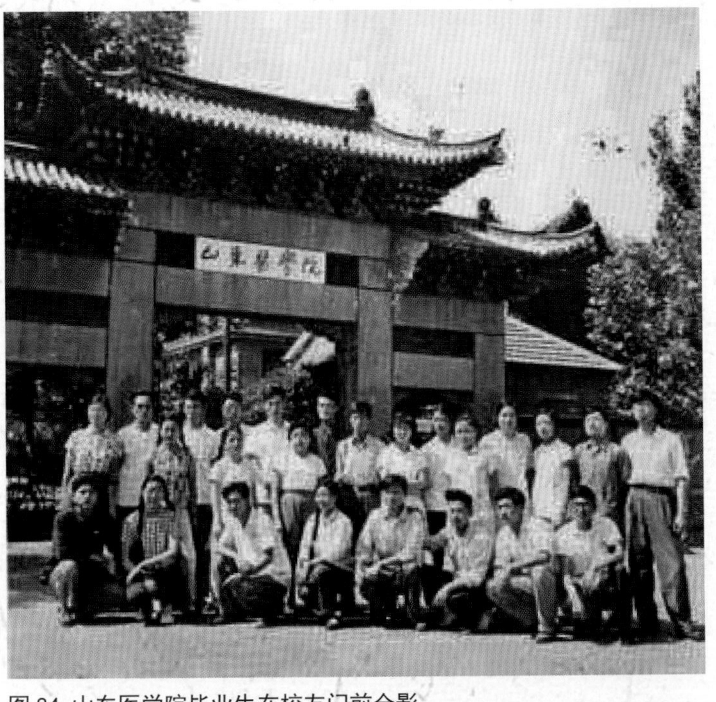

图 84 山东医学院毕业生在校友门前合影

Fig. 84 Graduates of Shandong Medical College taking a photo in front of the Alumni Gate

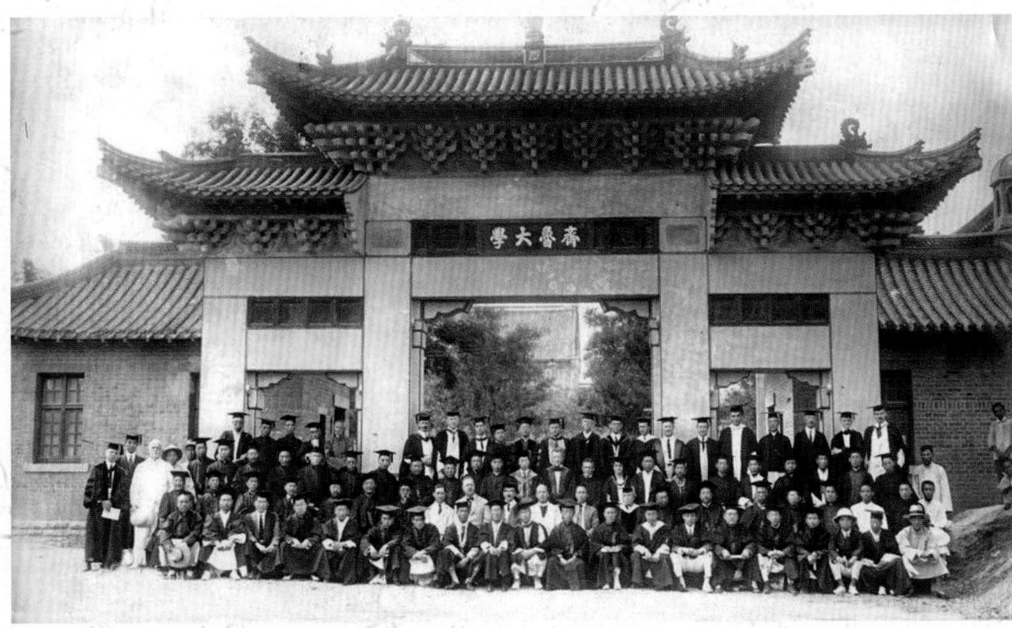

图 83 齐鲁大学毕业生在校友门前合影

Fig. 83 Graduates of Cheeloo University taking a photo in front of the Alumni Gate

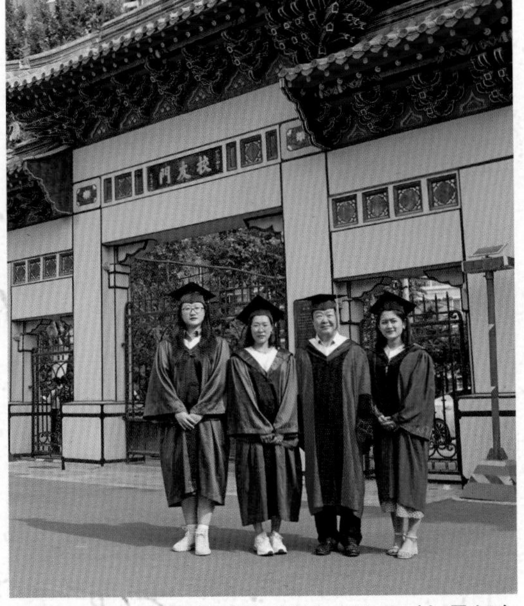

图 85 山东大学齐鲁医学院研究生毕业时与导师在校友门前合影

Fig. 85 Graduate students of Cheeloo College of Medicine of Shandong University taking a photo with their tutor in front of the Alumni Gate

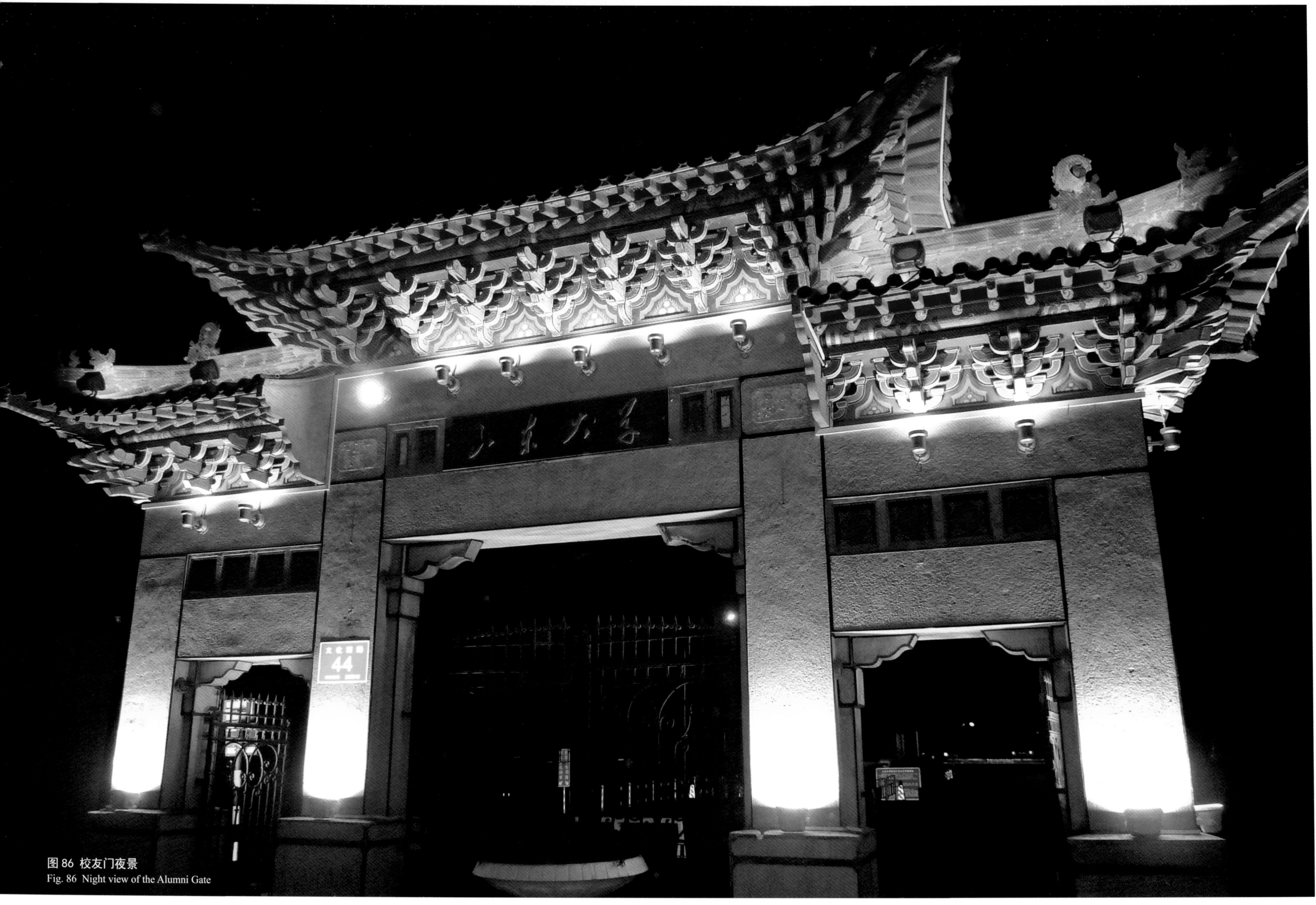

图 86 校友门夜景
Fig. 86 Night view of the Alumni Gate

第四章 Chapter Four

中心花园 The Central Garden

14 中心花园之春（1）

Spring in the Central Garden (1)

春天总是令人惊喜的，中心花园是最早感受到春回信息的地方。不用说葛罗神学院楼和考文楼前飘若绯云的桃花，也不用说花园中心假山上自愿报春的迎春花，就说水池边那只重新返回的鸭子，它扑闪着翅膀、摇着尾巴、不时引颈高歌的情景是最令人感动的。因为水池里的冰消融了，它又可以自由自在地在里面游泳了。春天一来，最忙的是那些花儿，一会儿丁香花洒满了清香，一会儿鸢尾花恍若精灵，那一片油菜花黄灿灿的，这几树樱花粉嘟嘟的……真是令人目不暇给！恰如这首诗描写的那样："好景无边刻刻新，杏花才放碧桃跟。含红嫩叶需春雨，待绿老枝供夏荫。翠柳斜飞风细细，繁樱飘落雪纷纷。迷离三月芳菲梦，谁比蜂蝶醉意深？"

Spring is always a pleasant surprise, and the Central Garden is the first place to feel the spring. Besides the peach flowers floating like clouds in front of the Gotch-Robinson Theological Building and Calvin Mateer Hall and the winter jasmine heralding the spring voluntarily on the rockery in the center of the garden, the returning duck singing from time to time by the pool, with its wings fluttering and tail wagging, is the most moving scene. As the ice in the pool has melted, it is free to swim in it again. Spring comes, and the flowers are the busiest: the lilacs full of fragrance, the elf-like irises, the bright yellow rape flowers, and the pink cherry blossoms. All of these are really dizzying, just as the poem describes: "The good scene is boundless and constantly updated; the apricot and peach blossoms bloom successively. The red tender leaves need spring rain; the old branches waiting to turn green supply the summer shade. The green willows swing in the gentle winds; the cherry blossoms fall in the drifting snow. In the blurred dream of flowers in March, who's more drunk than a bee and a butterfly?"

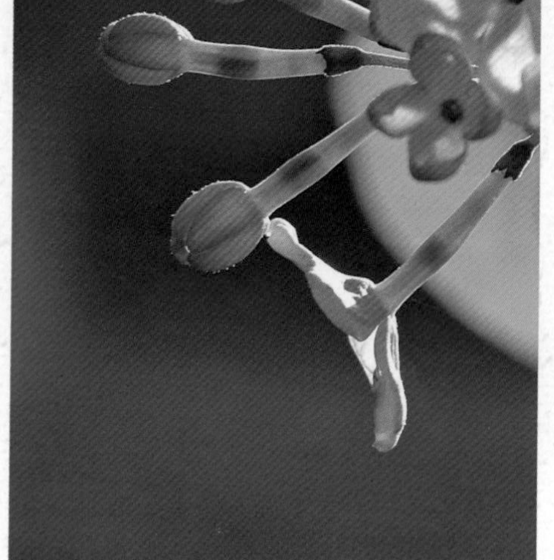

图 87 丁香花
Fig. 87 Lilacs

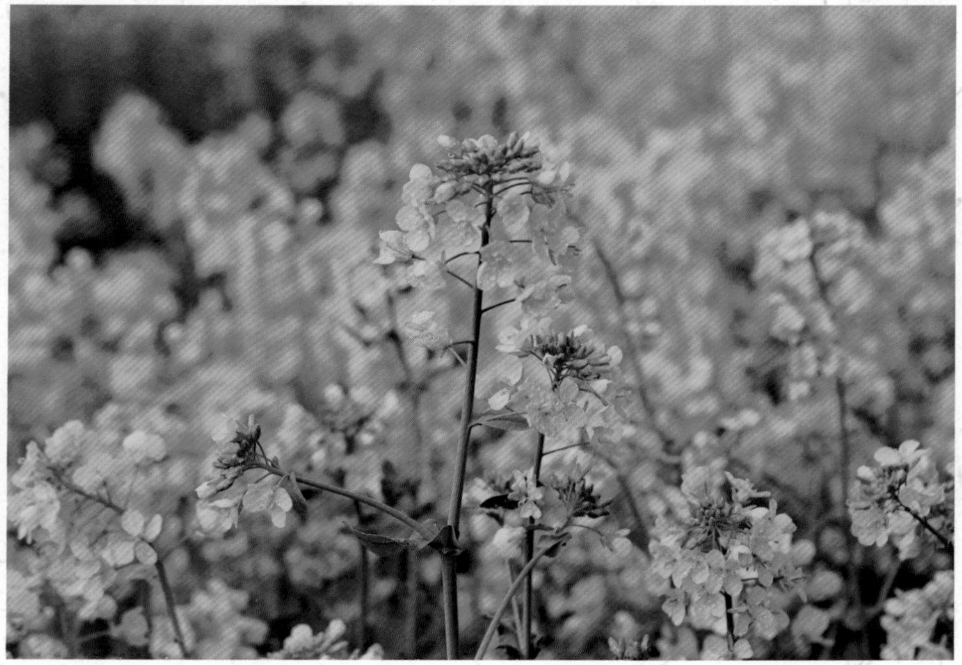

图 88 油菜花
Fig. 88 Rape flowers

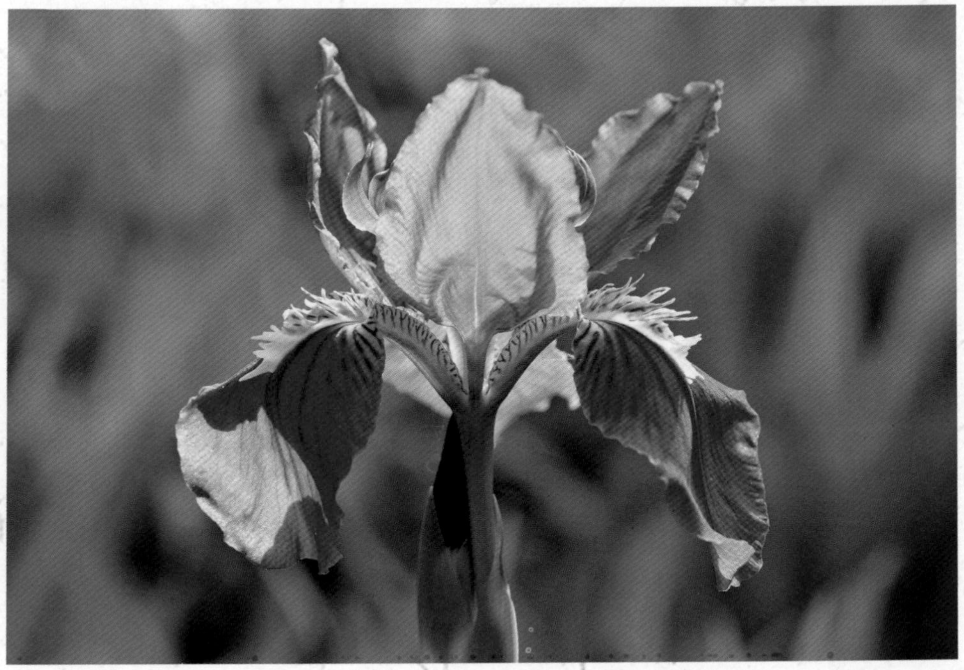

图 89 鸢尾花
Fig. 89 Irises

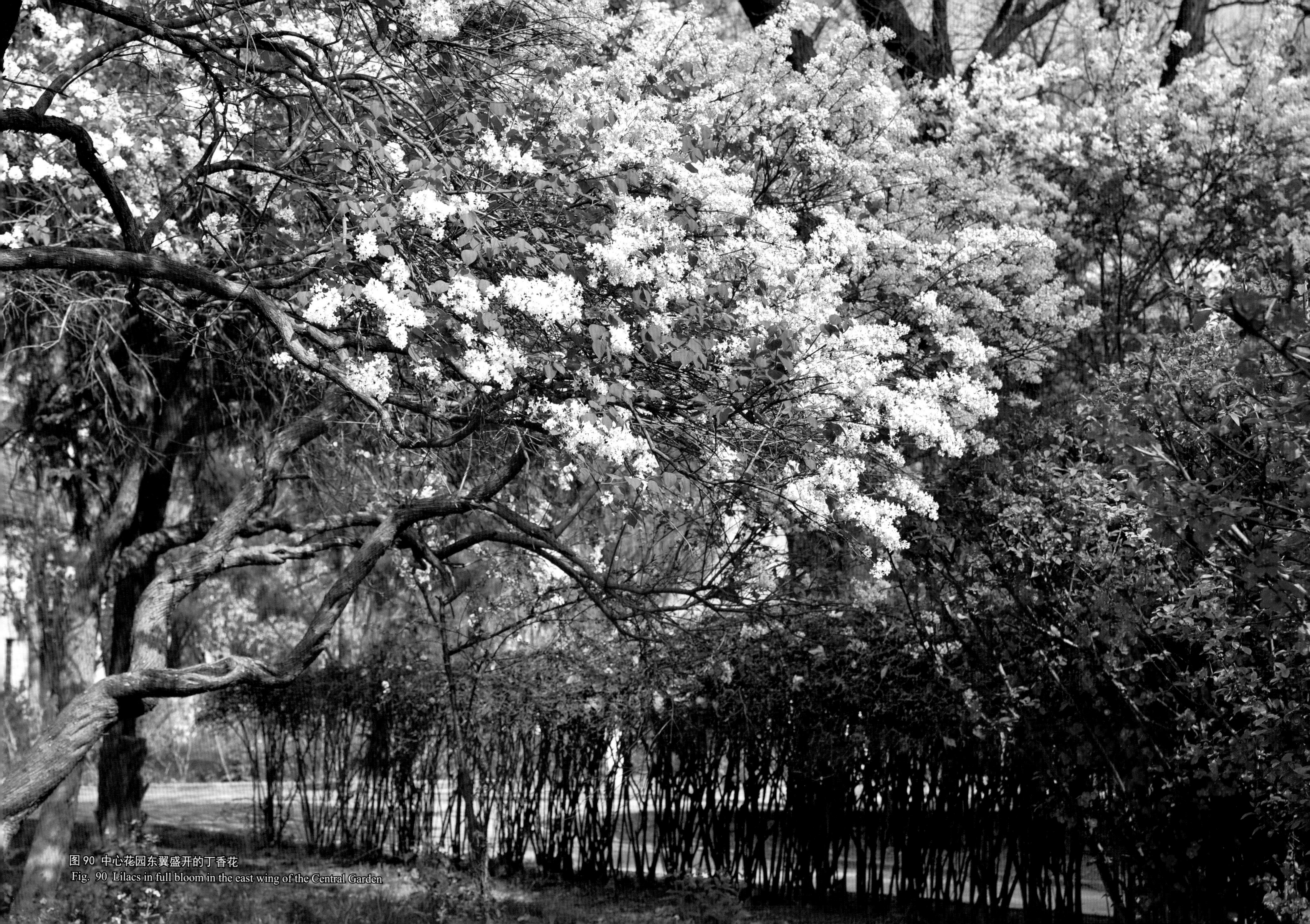

图 90 中心花园东翼盛开的丁香花
Fig. 90 Lilacs in full bloom in the east wing of the Central Garden

14 中心花园之春（2）

Spring in the Central Garden (2)

春天，于中心花园，开得最热烈奔放的要数贴梗海棠。这种花的种植面积大，历史悠久，尽管每年都剪枝削头，但花树还是长到了两米多。春天一来，这些树枝先吐绿芽，接着便冒出无数的花骨朵儿。一夜酣睡醒来，突然发现中心花园变成了红色的海洋。我不得不佩服贴梗海棠的集体主义精神，试想一下，若是一朵一朵抑或一枝一枝地开花，就不会有这样震撼的效果了。贴梗海棠的另一种品质是拼命开放，它倾尽所有来绽放红色，似乎要实现“止于至善”的目标，真是曾子的好学生。

In spring, the quinces bloom in profusion in the Central Garden. With a large planting area and a long history, the trees have grown to more than two meters despite being cut every year. As soon as spring comes, green buds sprout from the branches and then countless flower buds emerge. When you wake up overnight, you will suddenly find that the Central Garden has become a red ocean. I can't help admiring the collectivist spirit of the quinces. There will not be such a shocking effect if the quinces bloom one by one. Another quality of the quinces is their full bloom in profusion. They put forth the red flowers at full split, seeming to achieve the “aim of absolute perfection”, which proves a good student of Zeng Zi.

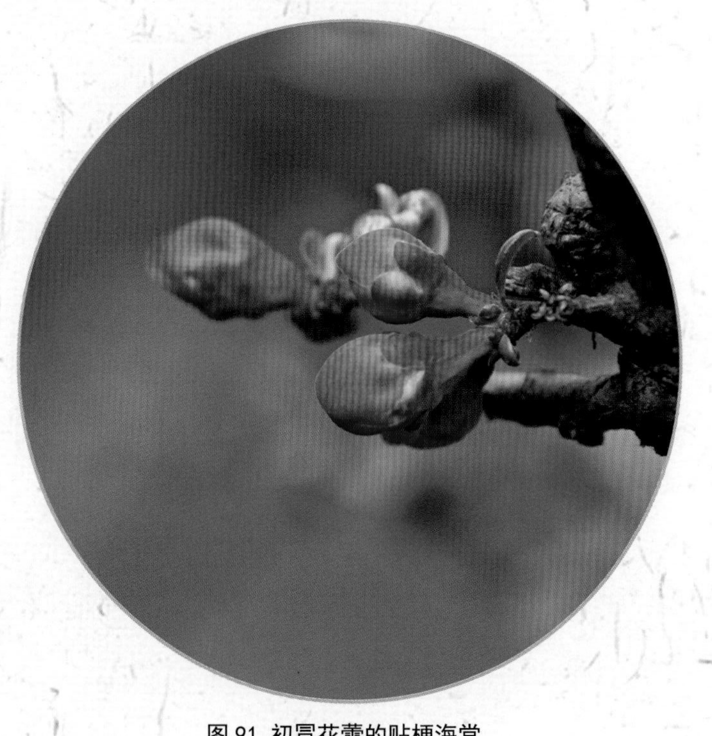

图 91 初冒花蕾的贴梗海棠
Fig. 91 Budding quinces

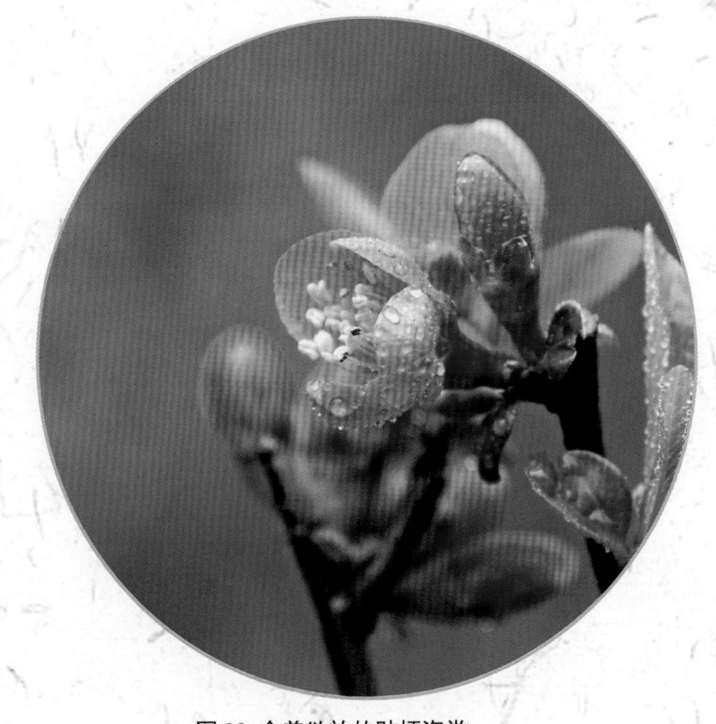

图 92 含羞欲放的贴梗海棠
Fig. 92 Quinces about to bloom

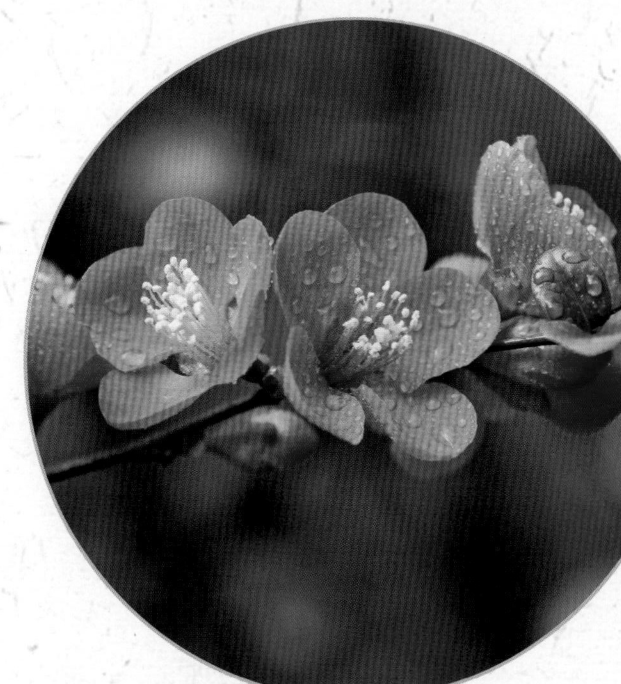

图 93 春风中怒放的贴梗海棠
Fig. 93 Quinces in full bloom in spring breeze

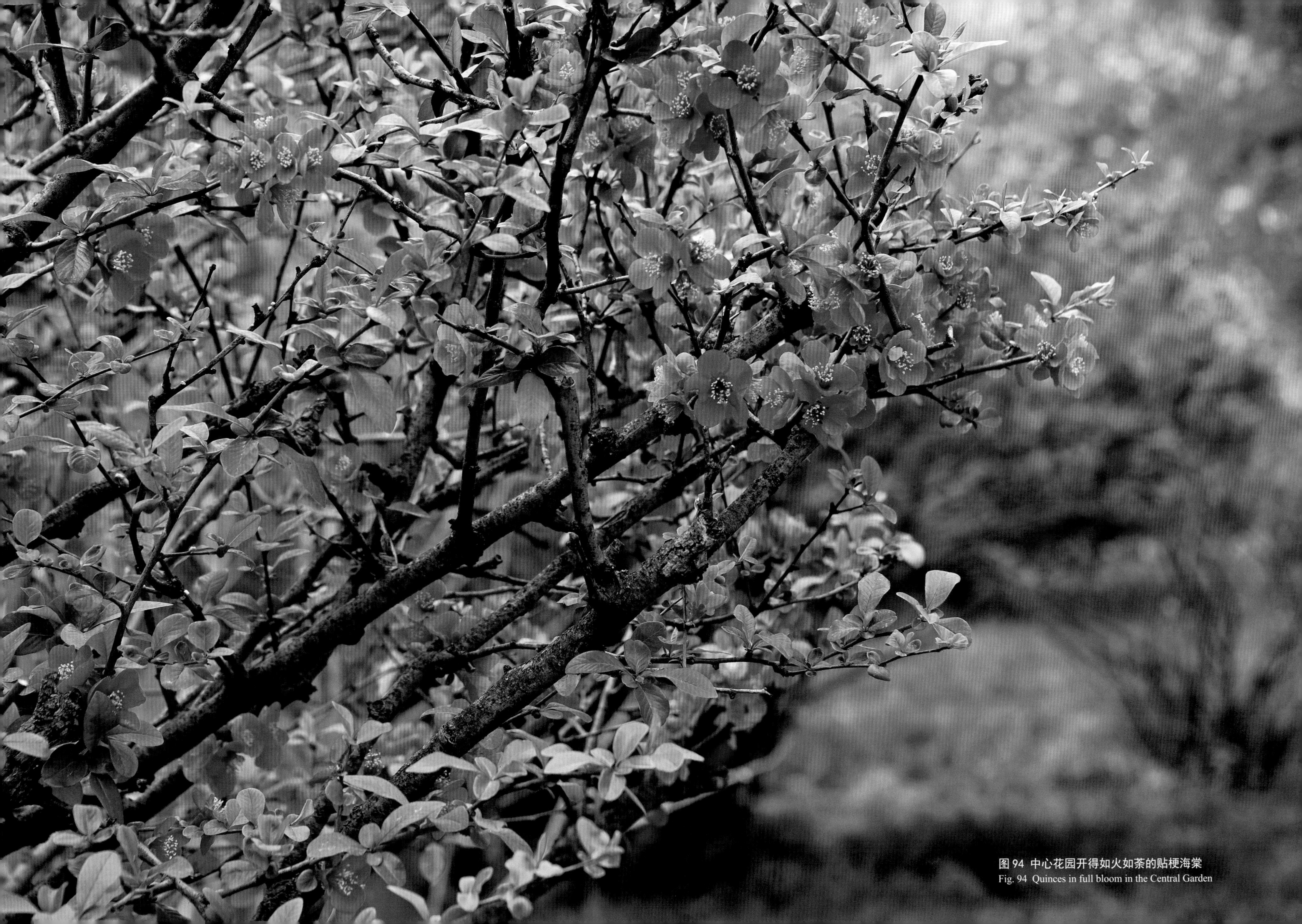

图 94 中心花园开得如火如荼的贴梗海棠
Fig. 94 Quinces in full bloom in the Central Garden

15 中心花园之夏（1）

Summer in the Central Garden (1)

夏天，中心花园的主色调只有一个“绿”字。绒坦的草坪是绿的，茂密的树林是绿的，挂满爬山虎的屋山是绿的，就连那只鸭子的羽毛都泛着绿光。在烈日炎炎的夏日，来中心花园石桌旁一坐是十分惬意的。这里大树遮天蔽日，满目苍翠，温度自然比校外低几度。如果有微风吹拂，送来月季花的香味，那心中的爽快便又增加了许多。坐在这里，举首远望红檐青瓦在树叶中忽隐忽现，低头近观绿草兰花于阳光下熠熠生辉。此起彼伏的蝉鸣从树上传来，有低调的，有高音的，交织成一支支优美的交响曲。正是“百年绿树历峥嵘，青瓦红檐世纪风。林下把书迎月夜，花前阔论震晨空。千声鸟语无人动，一阵蝉鸣万木訇。碧叶莽苍连岱岳，新枝更比老枝浓”。

In summer, the main color of the Central Garden is “green”. The lawn is green, the dense wood is green, the gable walls covered with creepers are green, and even the duck’s feathers show green light. It’s nice to sit at the stone table in the Central Garden on a hot summer day. Here, the trees can shade the sun and you can have an eyeful of verdant view. Thus the temperature here is naturally several degrees lower than that outside the university. Moreover, the breeze floating with the fragrance of rose will make you more refreshed. Sitting here, you can look up at the red eaves and grey tiles flickering among the leaves, and look down at the green grass and orchids shining in the sun. You can hear the chirping of the cicadas coming from the trees, with the low keys and high keys interwoven into a beautiful symphony. All of these can be expressed by a poem: “The century-old green trees have gone through the extraordinary times; the grey tiles and red eaves live out a century. You can read books in the wood to meet the moonlight; you can discuss with people before the flowers in the morning. The birdsong cannot alarm anyone; the chirping of cicadas can alarm the whole forest. The boundless green leaves seem to stretch to Mount Tai; the new branches are greener than the old ones.”

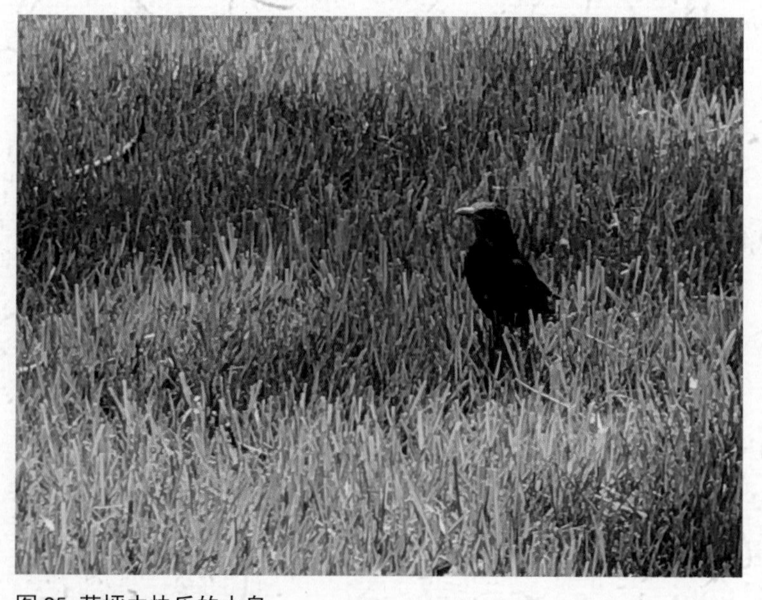

图 95 草坪中快乐的小鸟

Fig. 95 A happy bird in the lawn

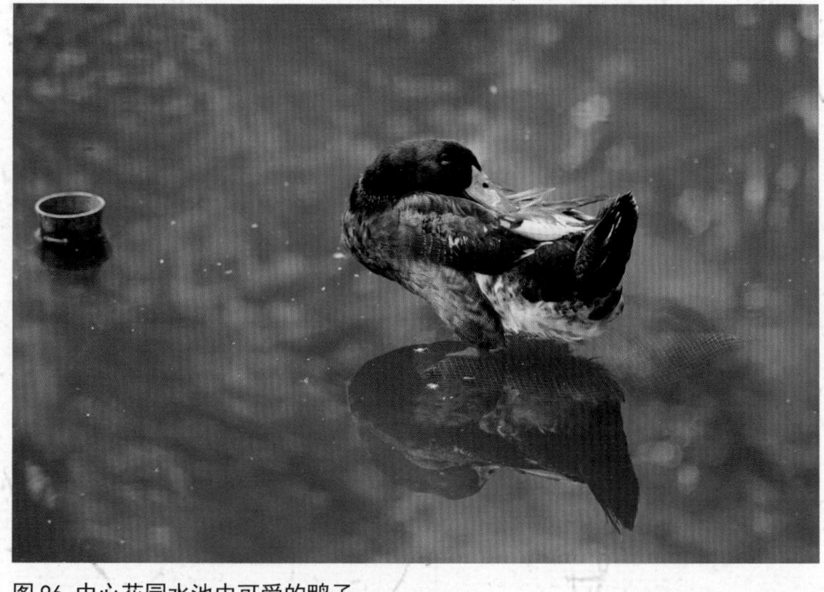

图 96 中心花园水池中可爱的鸭子

Fig. 96 A lovely duck in the pool of the Central Garden

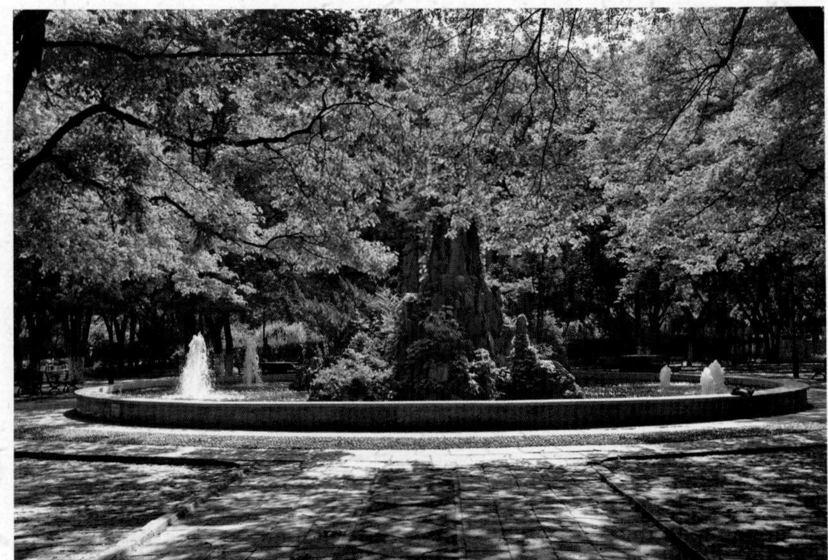

图 97 茂密的枫林环绕中心花园中央的水池与假山

Fig. 97 Dense maple forest surrounding the pool and rockery in the center of the Central Garden

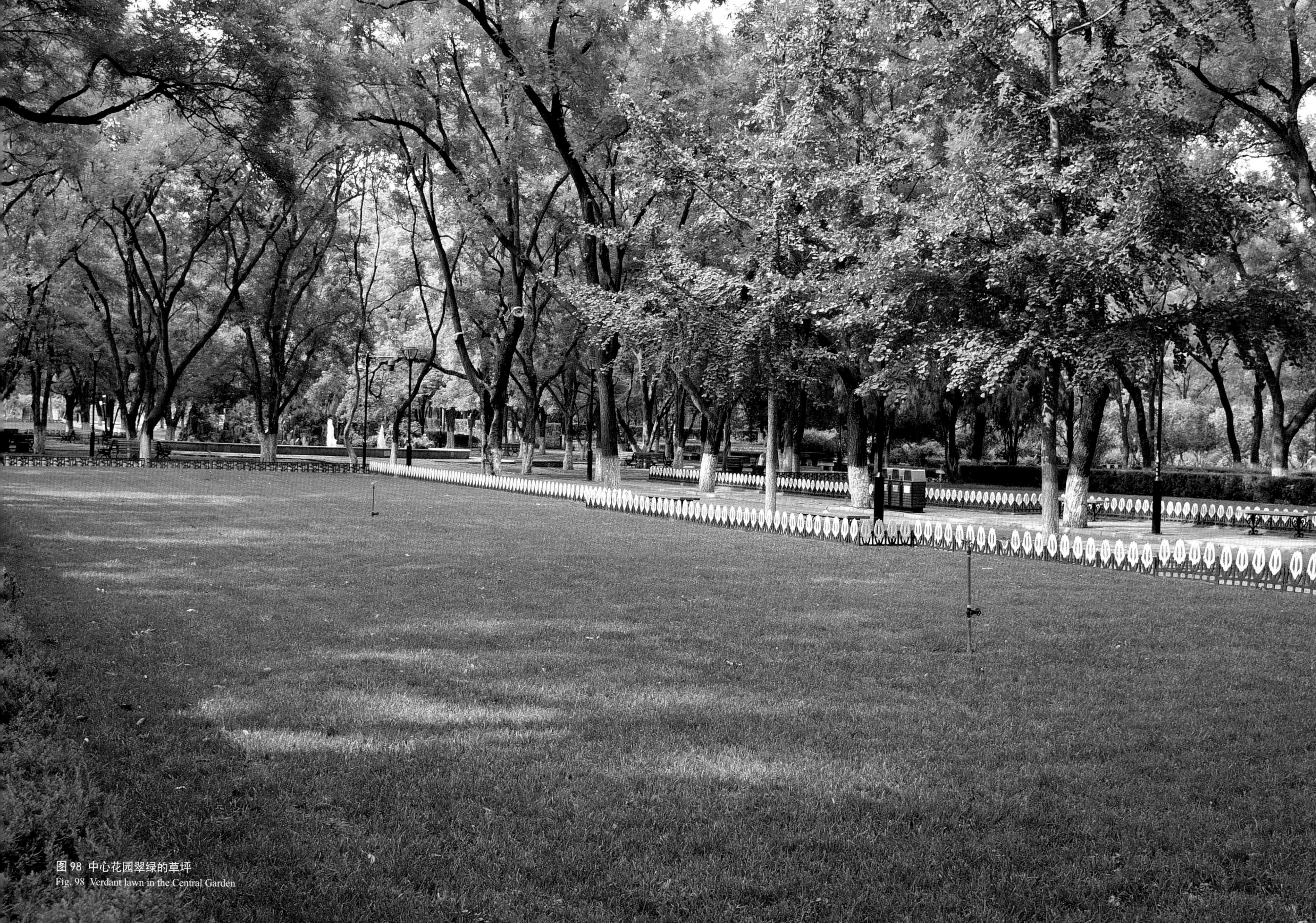

图 98　中心花园翠绿的草坪
Fig. 98　Verdant lawn in the Central Garden

15 中心花园之夏（2）

Summer in the Central Garden (2)

我随航拍器的镜头来到了空中，中心花园恍然变成了绿色的海洋，层层波浪随风翻腾。四周的教学楼就像几艘航船，在绿波中摇荡。假山在花园中央，微微泛黄的枫树环绕四周，构成了一只炯炯有神的“花园之眼”。行人在树下穿梭，时现时隐。即使有千军万马，也会埋伏于这绿帐之下。

虽然夏季绿是主色调，但难掩夏花之绚烂。在十字形伸展的中心花园里，在绿色的背景下，仍盛开着火红的石榴花、白色的槐花和粉红的木槿花。还有很多无名的小花，黄色的、白色的和红色的，它们像天上的星星，镶嵌在如毯的绿茵之上。最令人难忘的夏花莫过于紫薇，有红白两色，花朵图案十分复杂，伸出长长的花蕊犹如金色的龙须。紫薇花期很长，开起来满树繁花似锦，远远望去仿佛绿树披上了轻纱，在微风中长袖起舞。

The view of the aerial camera in the air shows that the Central Garden is like a green ocean with layers of waves billowing with the wind. The teaching buildings around are like a few boats, swaying in the green waves. The rockery is in the center of the garden and it is surrounded by slightly yellow maple trees, forming a bright “eye of the garden”. The pedestrians shuttle through the trees, sometimes hidden. Even if there are thousands of troops, they will become hidden under this green tent.

Although the main color of summer is green, the gorgeous flowers aren’t covered up. In the cross-shaped Central Garden, the fiery-red pomegranate flowers, white sophora flowers and pink hibiscus flowers still bloom against a green background. There are also many nameless flowers of yellow, white and red colors, inlaid in the green carpet like stars. The most memorable flowers of summer are crape myrtle flowers. They have the colors of red and white, and their patterns are very complex, extending long stamens like golden dragon whiskers. The flower phase of the crape myrtle flowers is very long, blooming like brocade. From a distance, it looks as if the green trees put on light gauze and dance with long sleeves in the breeze.

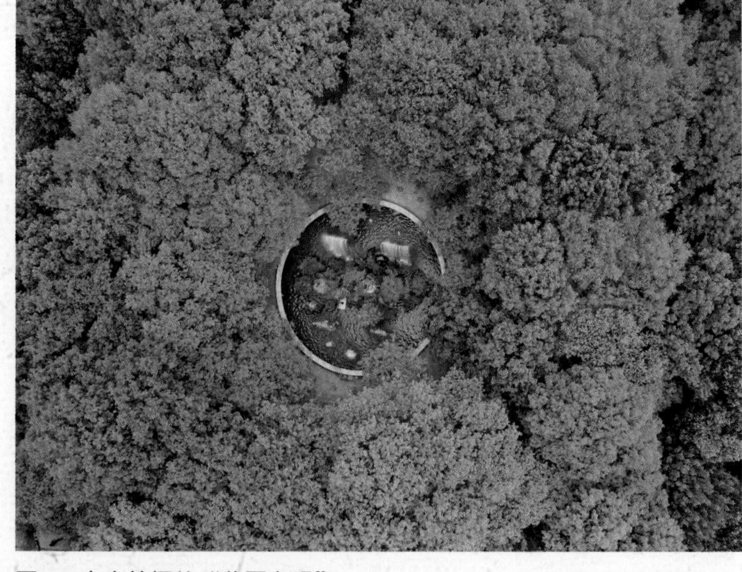

图 99 空中拍摄的“花园之眼”
Fig. 99 Aerial “eye of the garden”

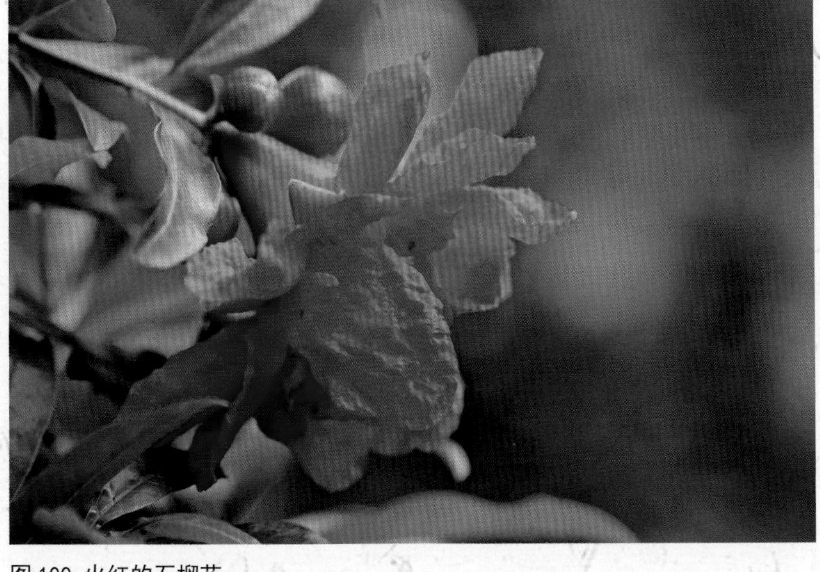

图 100 火红的石榴花
Fig. 100 Fiery-red pomegranate flowers

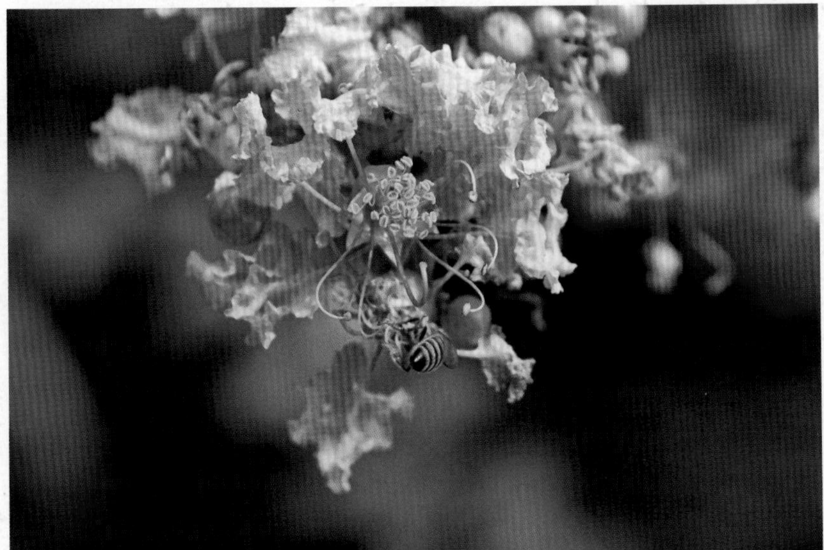

图 101 艳丽的紫薇花
Fig. 101 Gorgeous crape myrtle flowers

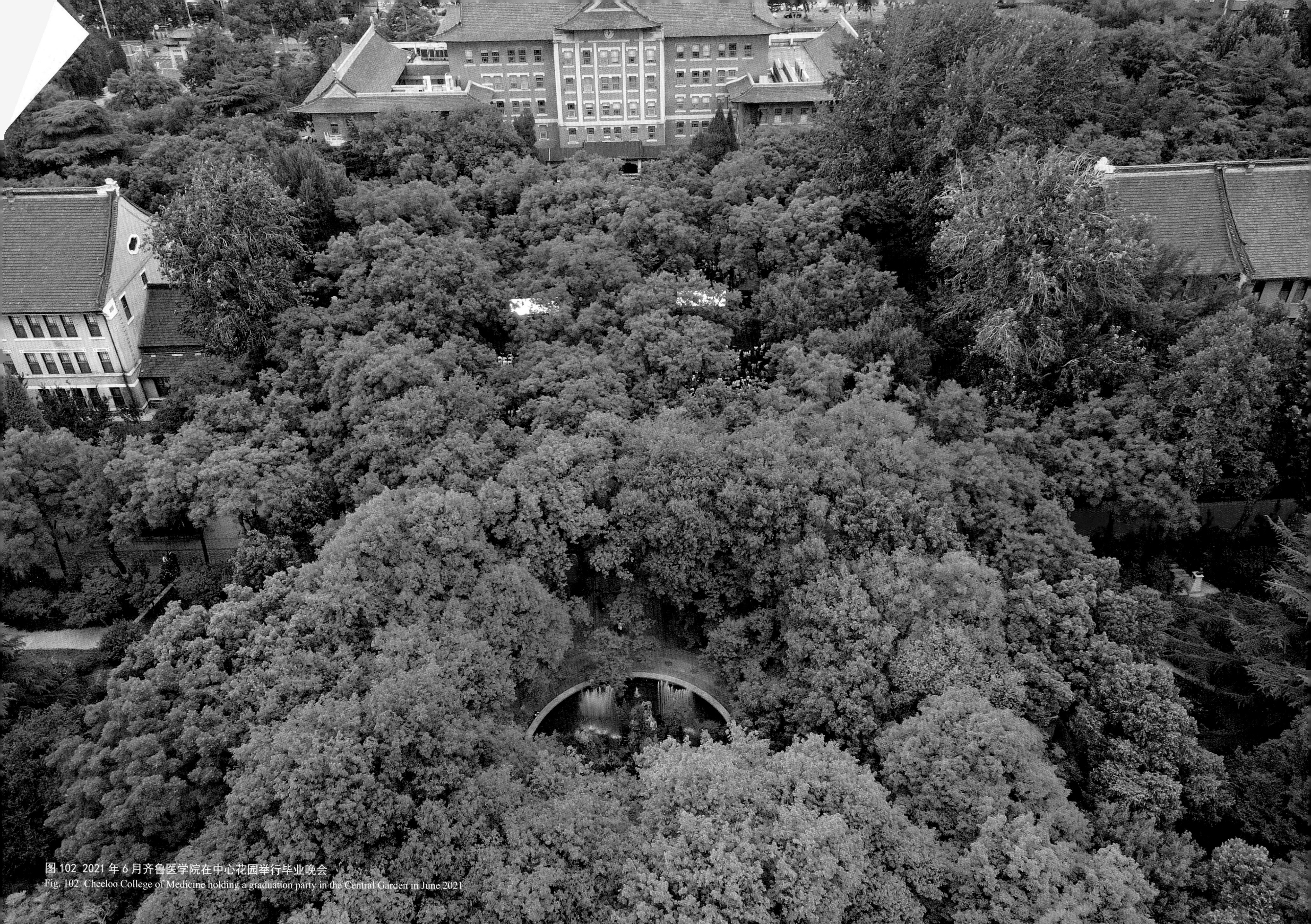

图 102 2021 年 6 月齐鲁医学院在中心花园举行毕业晚会
Fig. 102 Cheeloo College of Medicine holding a graduation party in the Central Garden in June 2021

16 中心花园之秋（1）

Autumn in the Central Garden (1)

“秋风一夜起，满院闪金辉。古瓦红藤照，新思白絮追。乾坤无主次，日月有轮回。谁解春花意？萧萧落叶飞。”这是对秋天校园的最佳写照。秋天的中心花园是五彩缤纷的，但主色调还是金色。中心花园的树主要为枫树，树叶为红色或红黄色，小小巧巧的，精致无比。深秋时节，枫叶落满了地面、石桌、条椅和石凳，令人不忍踩踏和拂去。银杏树最令人惊奇，昨天还是满树金黄，一夜之间，树叶竟然已飘落树下，铺了一层厚厚的金毯，而树上则仅剩下飕飕的枯枝了。每年秋天，赏叶是必备的项目。尽管看到树叶飘落会有瞬间“无边落木萧萧下”的感慨，但随后就会被美景所感染，师生们均仿佛被美景陶醉了，在此嬉戏、照相和高谈阔论，疯狂地在微信朋友圈里发出或转发有关校园落叶的影像，是那样地畅快淋漓，毫无悲秋之感！

The Central Garden in autumn is colorful, but the dominant color is gold. The trees in the Central Garden are mainly maple trees with delicate red or reddish yellow leaves. In late autumn, the maple leaves fall all over the ground, stone tables, chairs and stone benches, and people can not bear to tread and brush away them. The ginkgo trees are the most amazing. The previous golden leaves can fall on the ground overnight, forming a thick golden blanket, and only the dead branches are left on the trees. Enjoying the leaves is a must in autumn. Although there will be an instant feeling of “the boundless forest sheds its leaves shower by shower” when you see the leaves falling, you will then be infected by the beautiful scenery. The teachers and students seem to be intoxicated by the scenery. They play, take photos, talk freely, and send or forward images of fallen leaves on campus on WeChat Moments. They are so happy and feel no sadness with autumn.

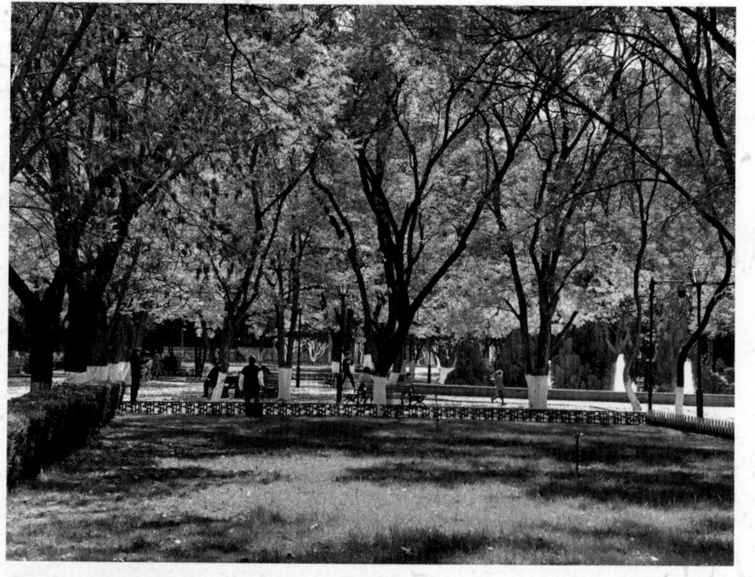

图 103 充满秋色的中心花园
Fig. 103 The Central Garden full of autumn scenery

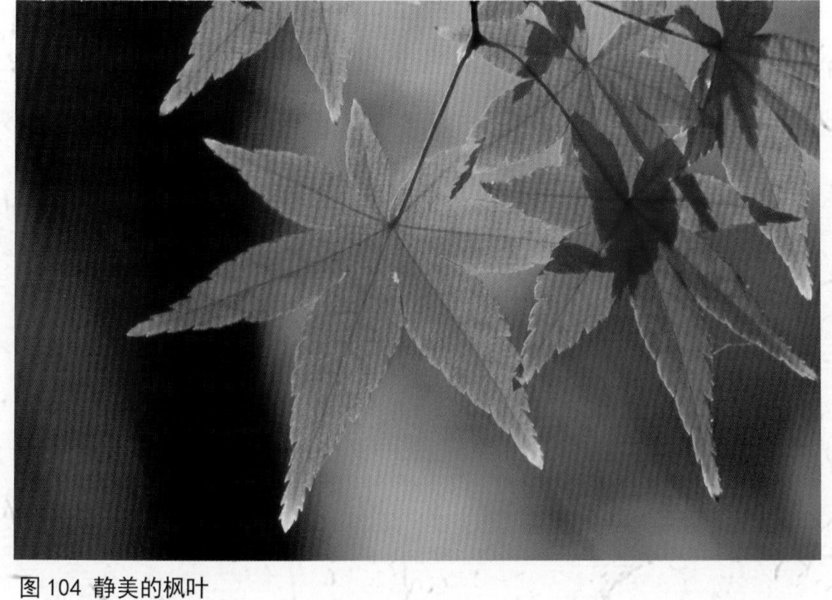

图 104 静美的枫叶
Fig. 104 Quiet and beautiful maple leaves

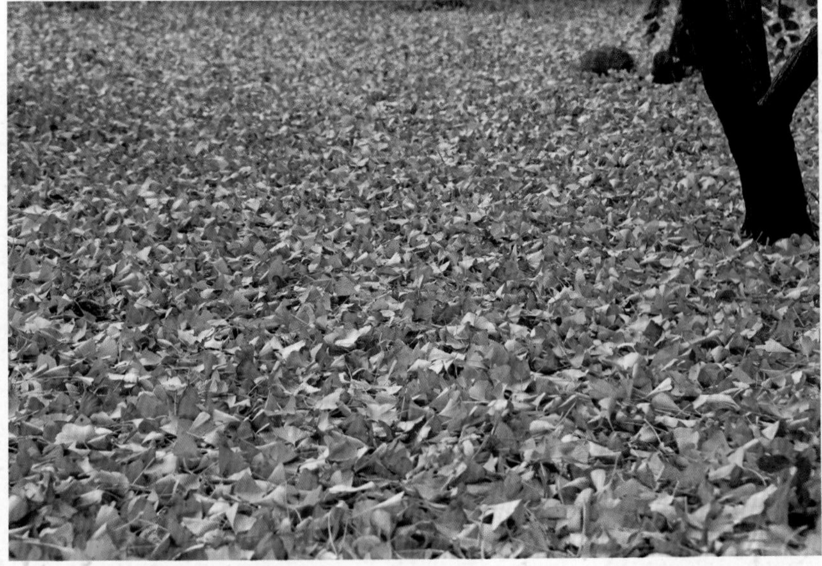

图 105 秋叶织就的金色地毯
Fig. 105 A golden carpet woven by autumn leaves

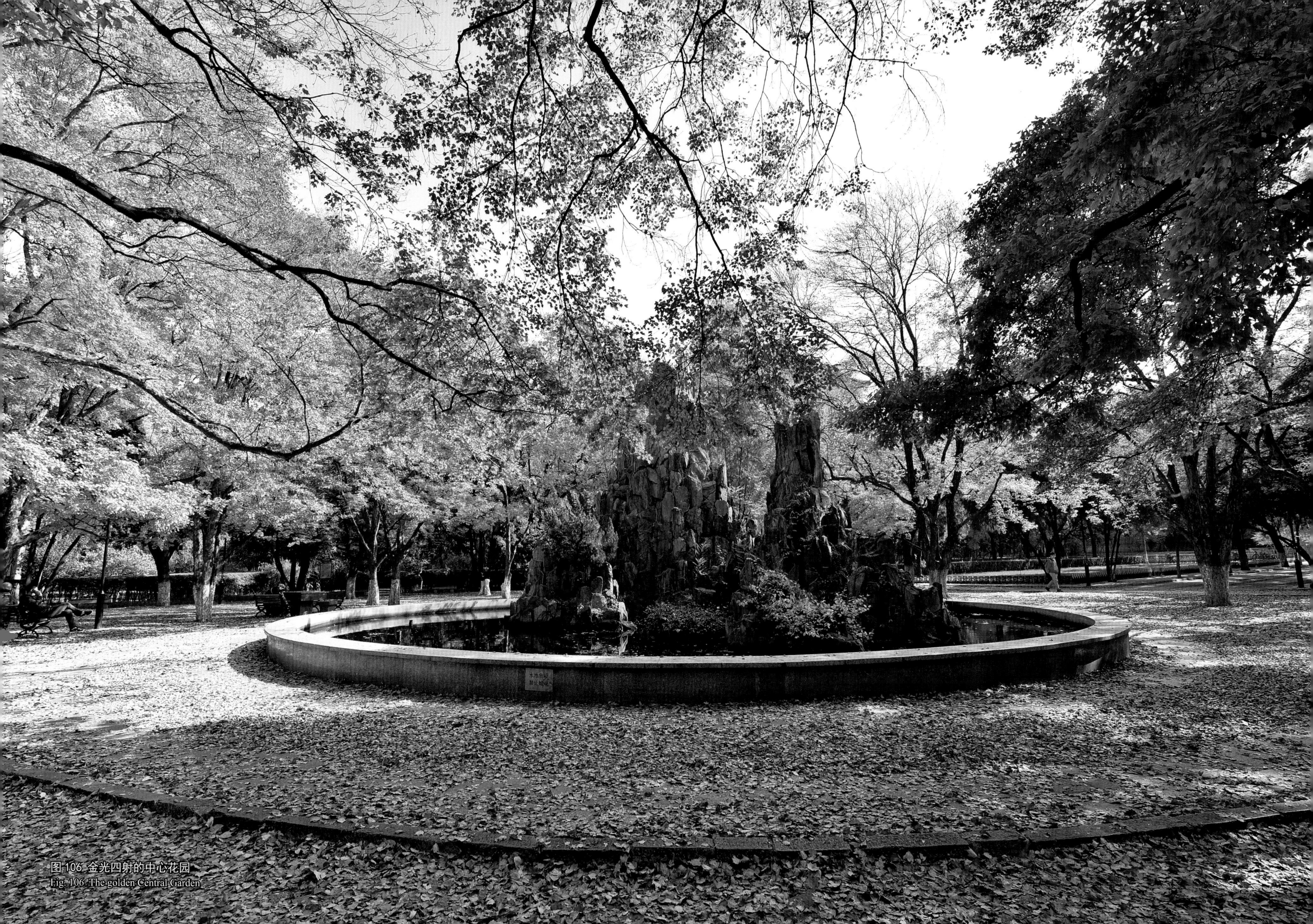

图 106 金光四射的中心花园
Fig. 106 The golden Central Garden

16 中心花园之秋（2）

Autumn in the Central Garden (2)

叶落之后，中心花园呈现出另一番深秋之美。树叶稀疏了，树丛中露出了深秋独有的蓝天。天朗气清之时，站在满地落叶的中心花园林下抬眼望去，树枝间蓝天、白云和枝上残存的几片黄叶和红叶，简直是一幅难以言妙的斑驳画卷。中心花园两侧是笔直的大道，平时路两边树冠交织，形成了两条林荫走廊。秋天树叶成了点缀，现出了树枝编成的木网，网眼中飘动着黄叶、红叶和少许绿叶，昔日的绿色走廊变成了黄金隧道，在阳光的照耀下金碧辉煌，令人流连忘返。

最近我迷上了航拍，那是因为视角不同而致感受迥异。平时我们是仰视，从下往上看。航拍则是俯视，从上往下看。在这个视角下，秋天的中心花园五彩斑斓，就像彩色的森林。枫叶是红的，松枝是绿的，槭树是黄的，还有楼顶红色的飞檐和青色的覆瓦，再加上绿色的草坪，绘制成了一副列维坦式的天然油画。我们天天身处其中，这是何等的幸运！

After the leaves fall, the Central Garden presents another beauty of late autumn. The leaves are sparse, and the blue sky unique to late autumn appears in the trees. On a clear and sunny day, looking up in the trees with fallen leaves in the Central Garden, you can find that the blue sky and white clouds between the branches and the remaining yellow and red leaves on the branches are simply a mottled picture that could not be described. On both sides of the Central Garden are straight avenues, and the crowns on both sides of the avenues are interwoven, forming two tree-lined corridors. The leaves in autumn become embellishments and a wooden net made of branches appears with the floating yellow leaves, red leaves and a few green leaves. The former green corridor has become a golden tunnel, shining brilliantly in the sun and making people forget to return.

Recently, I've become obsessed with aerial photography as different views lead to different feelings. Usually we look up, from bottom to top. Aerial photography is looking down, from top to bottom. In the aerial view, the Central Garden in autumn is colorful like a forest. The red maple leaves, the green pine branches, the yellow maples, the red cornices and grey tiles on the roof, and the green lawn are painted into a natural oil painting of Levitan style. How lucky the students are to be in it every day!

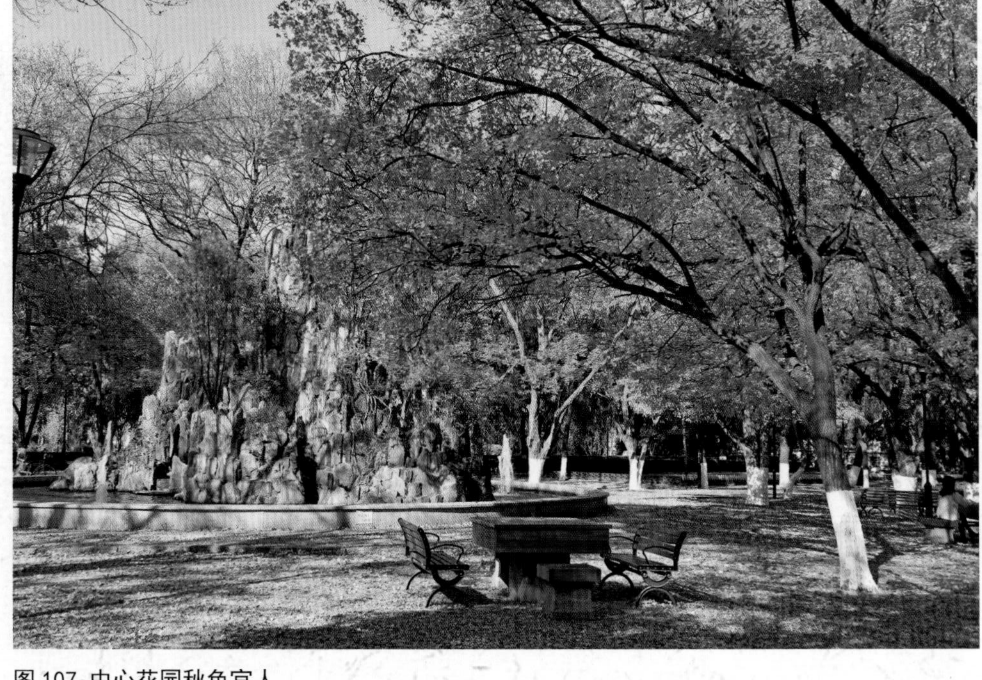

图 107 中心花园秋色宜人

Fig. 107 The pleasant autumn scenery in the Central Garden

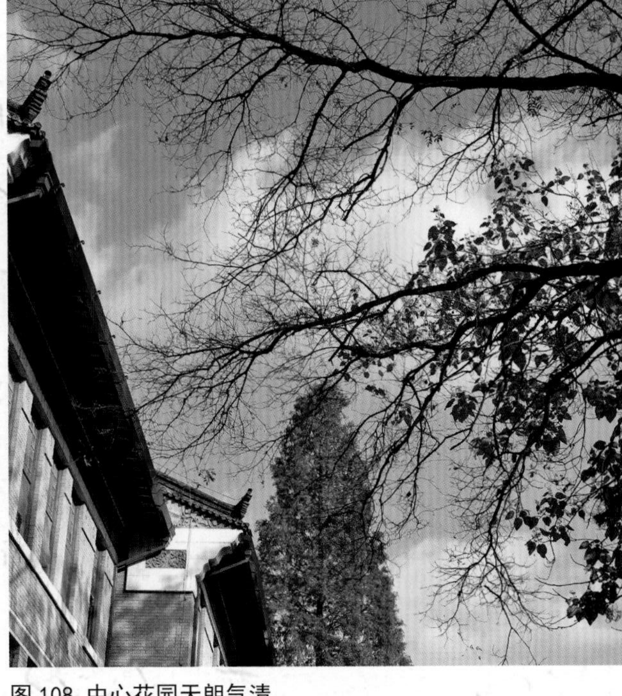

图 108 中心花园天朗气清

Fig. 108 The Central Garden with fine weather

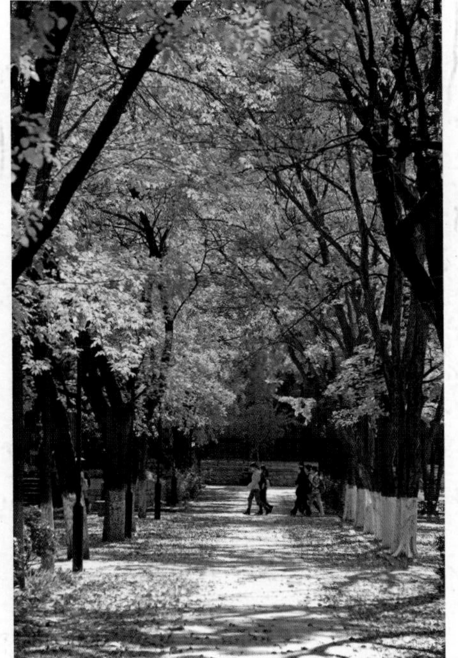

图 109 中心花园两侧的金色隧道

Fig. 109 Golden paths on both sides of the Central Garden

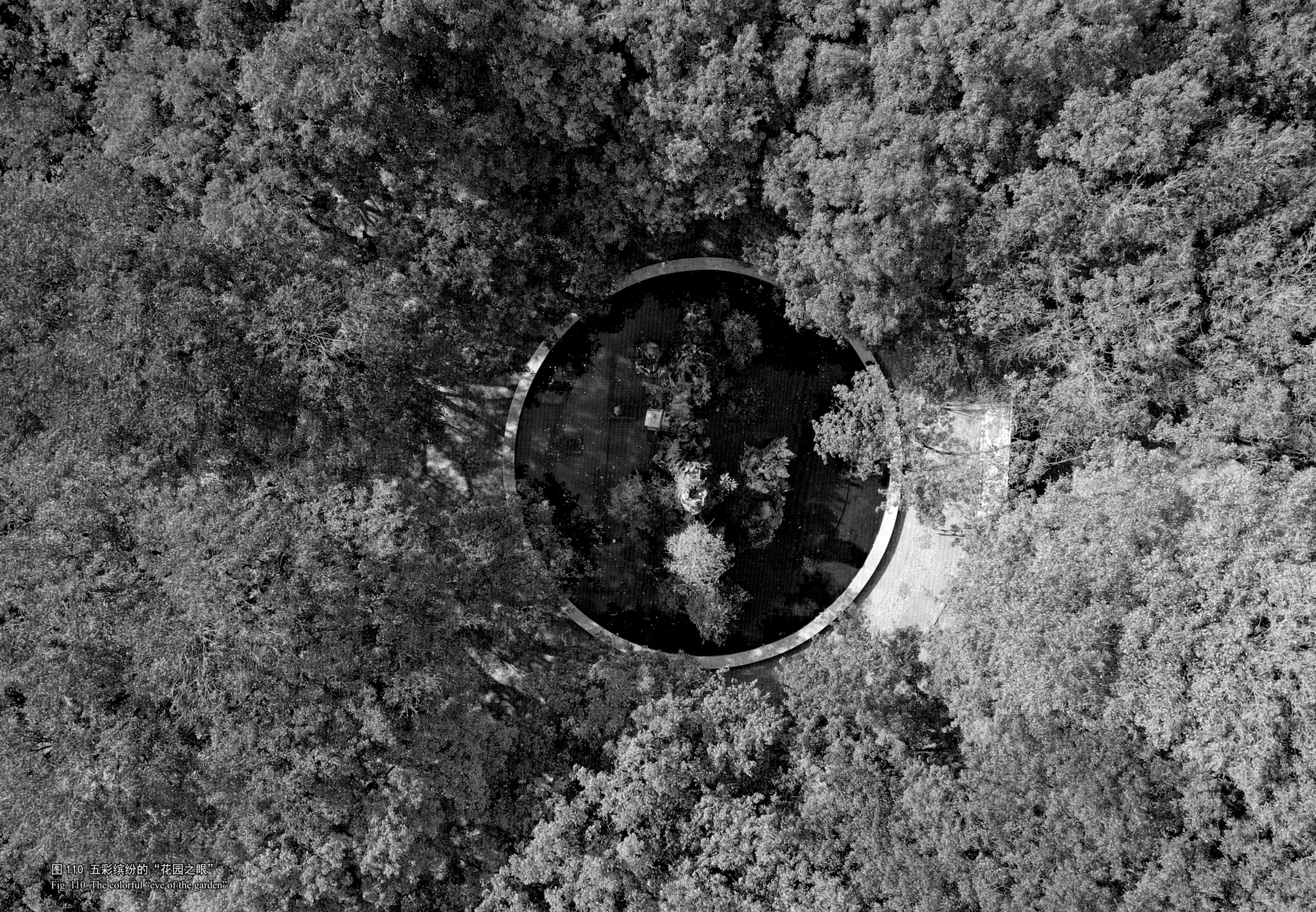

图 110 五彩缤纷的“花园之眼”
Fig. 110 The colorful “eye of the garden”

17 中心花园之冬（1）

Winter in the Central Garden (1)

冬天来了，中心花园的人少了不少，但并不冷清，因为它的主角变了。这时觅食的麻雀多了，草地、树枝都是它们的天地。冬春交接之际，有时会见到成千上万只麻雀飞来，栖息在树上，黑压压一片，很是壮观。长尾的灰喜鹊会在树上跳来跳去，看起来非常优雅。但是，在其繁殖季节，你千万不要得罪它们，否则灰喜鹊会突然从后方撞你的头，吓你一大跳！倒是那种前黑后白的短尾喜鹊比较友好，也不太怕人。路过中心花园时，有时会听到清脆的“哪！哪！哪！”的声音，那是啄木鸟在工作。据说一只啄木鸟每天能吃掉 1500 多只害虫，着实是一种益鸟。啄木鸟十分机灵，见人就飞，所以我从来没有捕捉到它们的图像。树上有很多鸟巢，也是冬天里的一道景观。但也要注意，在林下行走，随时会有天粪降落到你的头上，令人啼笑皆非！

Winter is coming, and the Central Garden has fewer people, but it is not deserted because its protagonist has changed. At this time, there are more sparrows foraging, and the grass and branches are their places of activity. At the turn of winter and spring, sometimes you can see thousands of sparrows flying and perching on trees, dark and spectacular. The long-tailed grey magpies jump around the trees and look very elegant, but you can not offend them during their breeding season, or they will suddenly hit your head from behind and scare you! The short-tailed magpies with black front and white back are friendly and they are not too afraid of people. When you pass the Central Garden, you can sometimes hear the crackling sound of the woodpeckers at work. It is said that a woodpecker can eat more than 1,500 pests a day, and it is really a beneficial bird. The woodpeckers are so alert that they fly away when they see people, so I never catch an image of them. There are many bird's nests in the trees which are also a scenery in winter. When walking under the trees, you must notice that there will be sky dung falling on your head at any time, which is really farcical.

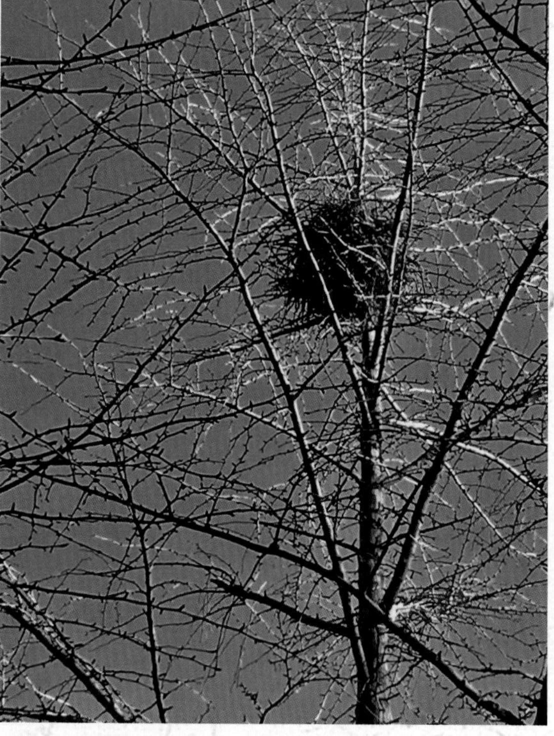

图 111 冬日鸟巢

Fig. 111 A nest in winter

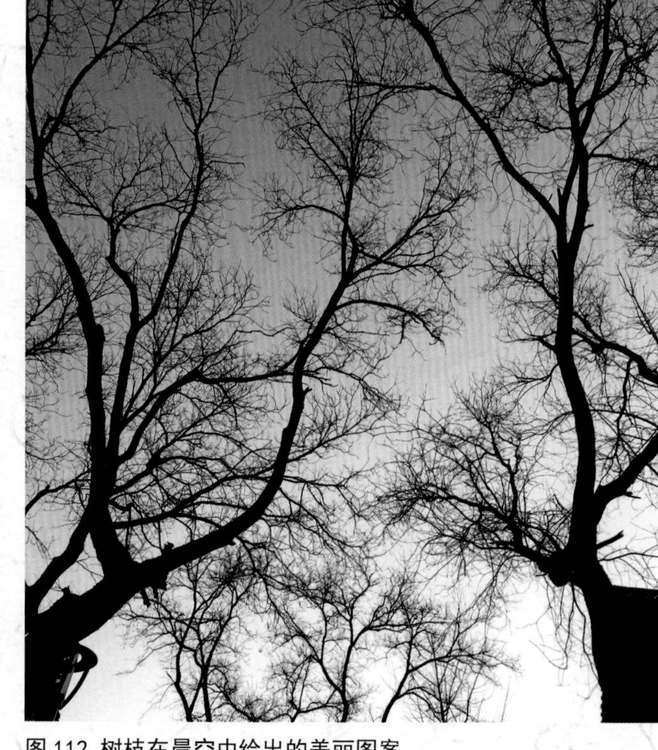

图 112 树枝在晨空中绘出的美丽图案

Fig. 112 Beautiful pattern of branches in the morning sky

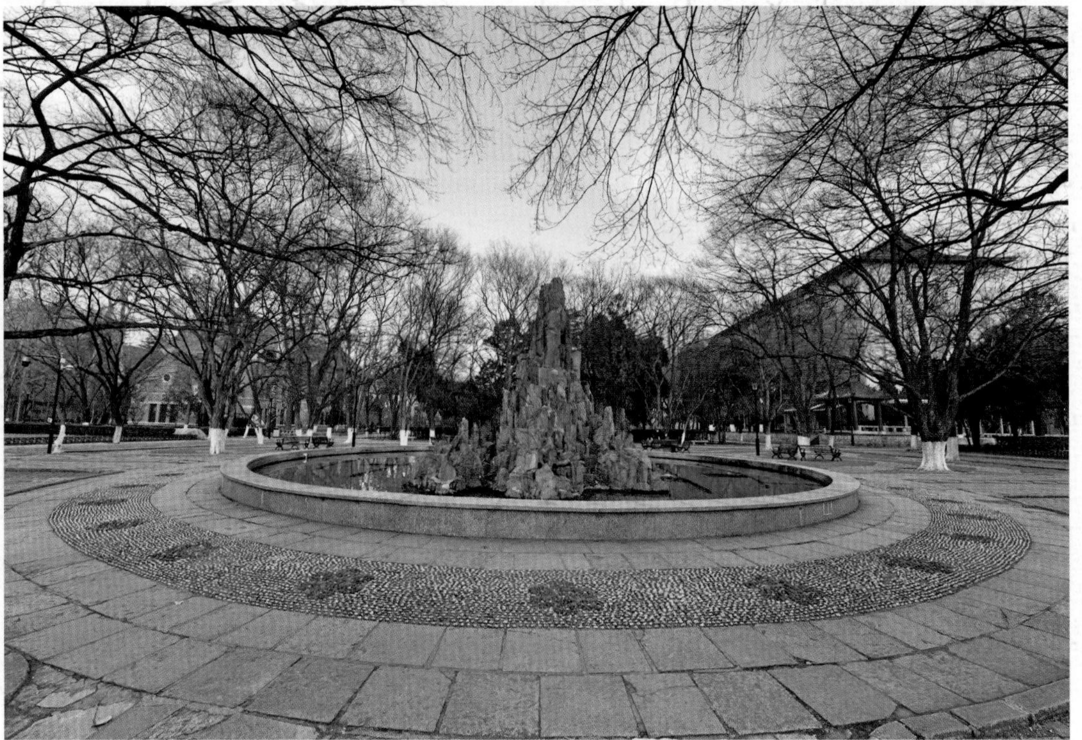

图 113 中心花园冬日晨景

Fig. 113 The morning view of the Central Garden in winter

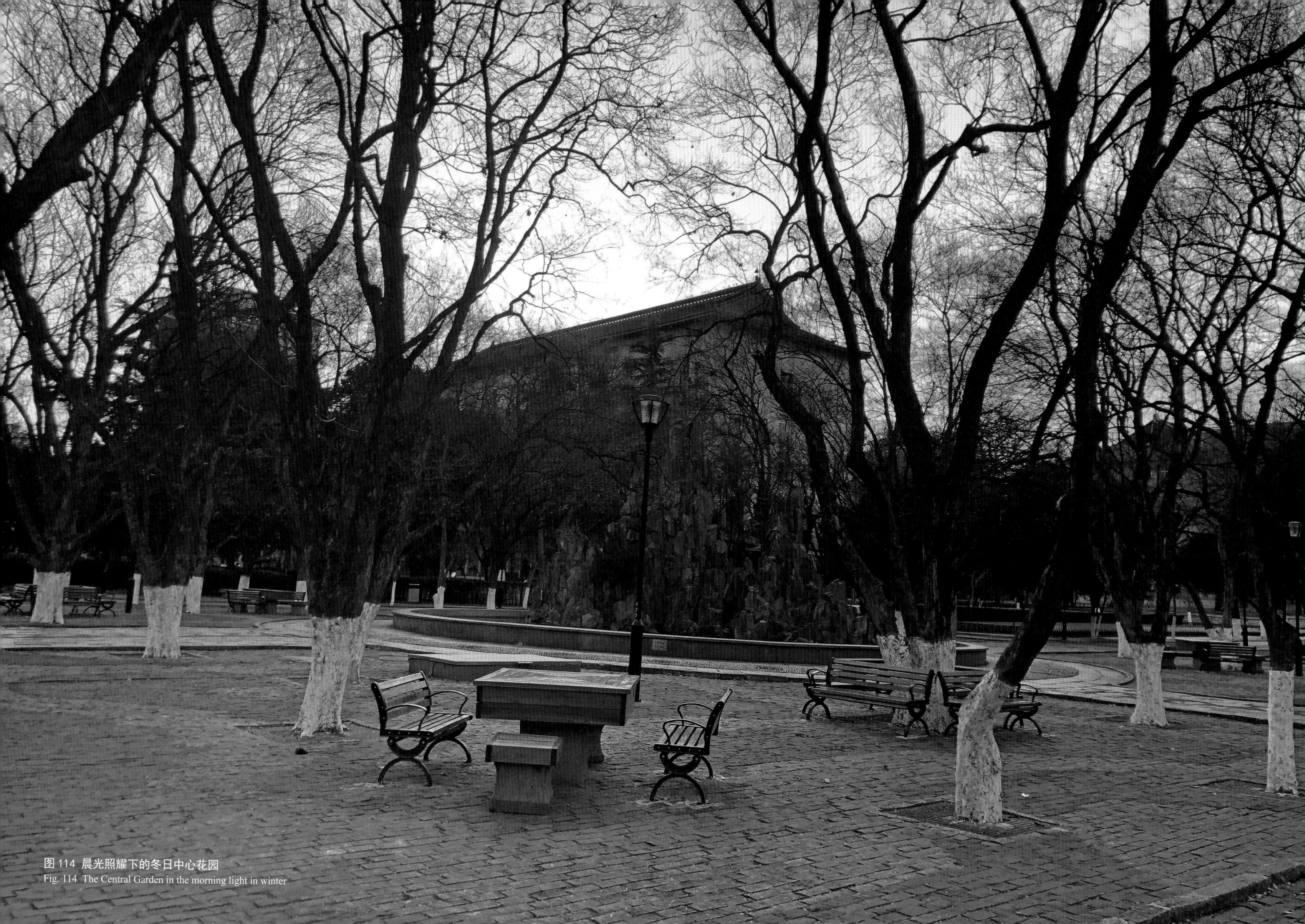

图 114 晨光照耀下的冬日中心花园
Fig. 114 The Central Garden in the morning light in winter

17 中心花园之冬（2）

Winter in the Central Garden (2)

“正气充天地，虽寒万物欣。梅开白雪至，草冒紫风临。格物达晓月，致知越远岑。枝头苞已满，只是待春神。”的确，冬天的中心花园是令人难忘的，即使是寒冷的夜晚。有时一不小心你会踩到刺猬，还以为是块石头。有时你会被猖狂逃跑的黄鼠狼惊得头皮发麻，还以为遇到了什么怪物！下雪前，彤云密布的夜晚，树枝映在空中会出现许多奇妙的图案，有的像毛细血管网，有的像支气管树，有的像墨汁灌注的淋巴管……

雪花飘舞的景象总是令人兴奋的！花园突然冒出了“千树万树梨花开”的琼枝玉树，天地为之一色。此时，我们一定会去花园两侧踏雪寻梅，去呼吸一下蜡梅耐寒的清气，去领略一番“大雪压青松，青松挺且直”的傲骨，去感受一种“长空雪乱飘，改尽江山旧”的气概。南面的千佛山隐约可见，它的悠悠钟声，已传到了不远处它所一脉相连的泰山。

“The healthy trends fill the world; everything is thriving in spite of the cold. The wintersweet flowers bloom with the arrival of the snow; the grass comes out against the wind. To study the nature of things as far as possible; to acquire knowledge as much as possible. The branches are full of buds; the spring is to come.” Indeed, the Central Garden in winter is memorable, even on cold nights. Sometimes you will step on a thorn carelessly and you might think it is a stone. Sometimes you will be shocked by the weasel that suddenly comes out and you might think you have met some monster. Before the snow comes on a cloudy night, there will appear many wonderful patterns of the branches reflected in the sky, some like capillary networks, some like bronchial trees and some like ink-filled lymphatic vessels...

The sight of snowflakes dancing is always exciting! The trees covered with ice and snow present a scene of “thousands of pear trees amazingly in bloom” in the garden and thus the heaven and earth are of the uniform color. At this time, the students will certainly go to both sides of the garden to find plum in the snow and take a breath of the cold-resistant wintersweets. And they can appreciate the lofty and unyielding character of the green pines: “Heavy on the green pine the snow weighs, but the pine remains lofty and straight.” They can also feel the spirit of “the snowflakes floating in the sky changing the old appearance of the country”. The Qianfo Hill in the south is vaguely visible, and its bell tones reach to Mount Tai of the same range not far away.

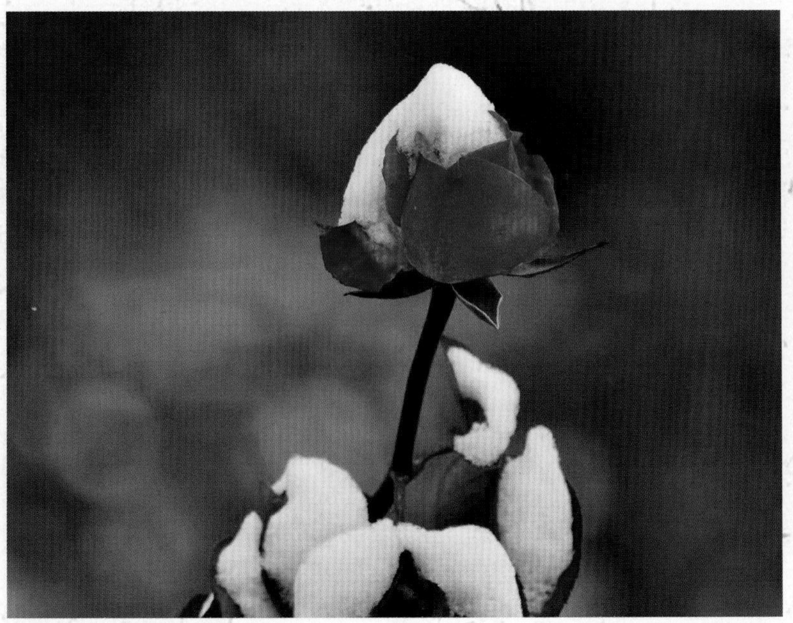

图 115 中心花园的雪中玫瑰
Fig. 115 Roses in the snow in the Central Garden

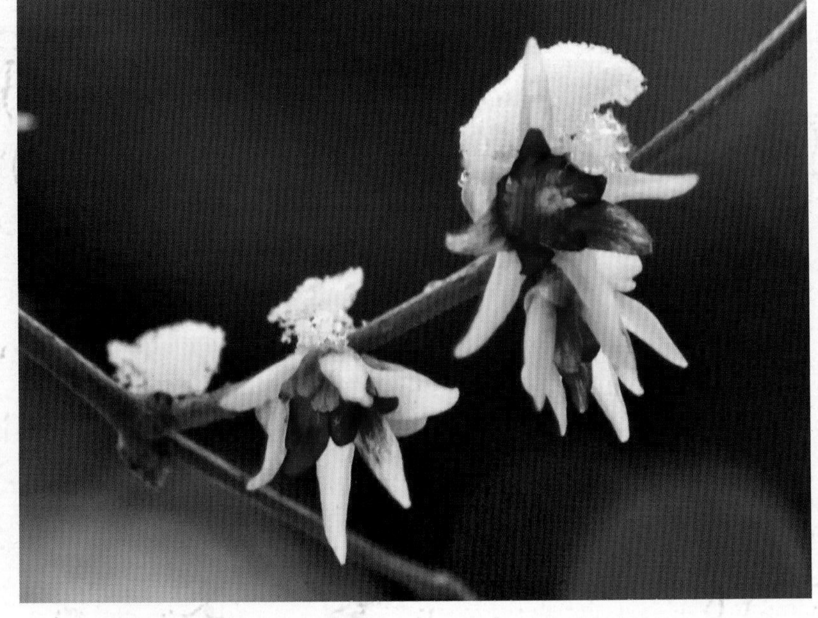

图 116 傲雪的蜡梅
Fig. 116 Wintersweets standing in the snow

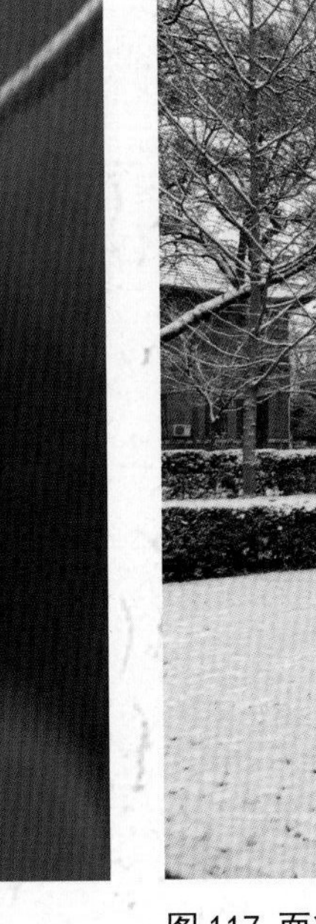

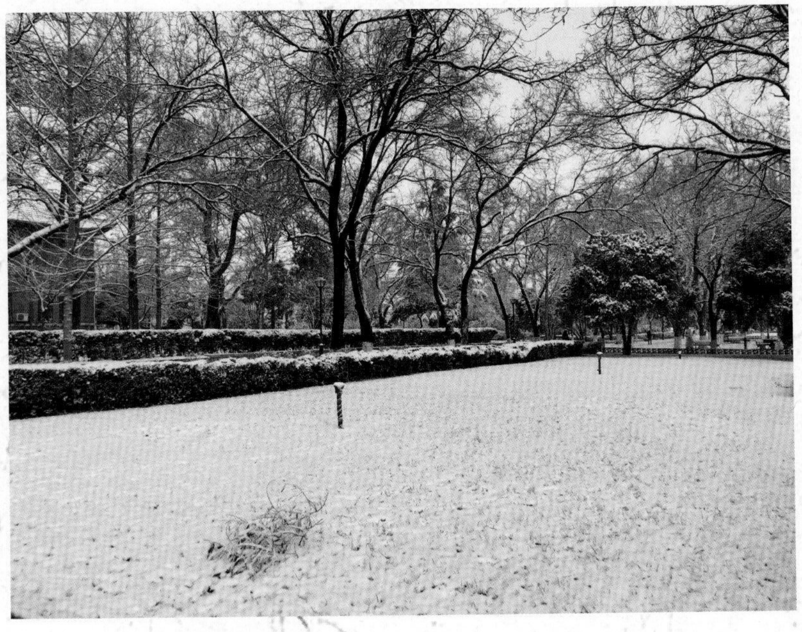

图 117 面貌一新的雪中花园
Fig. 117 The garden with a new look in the snow

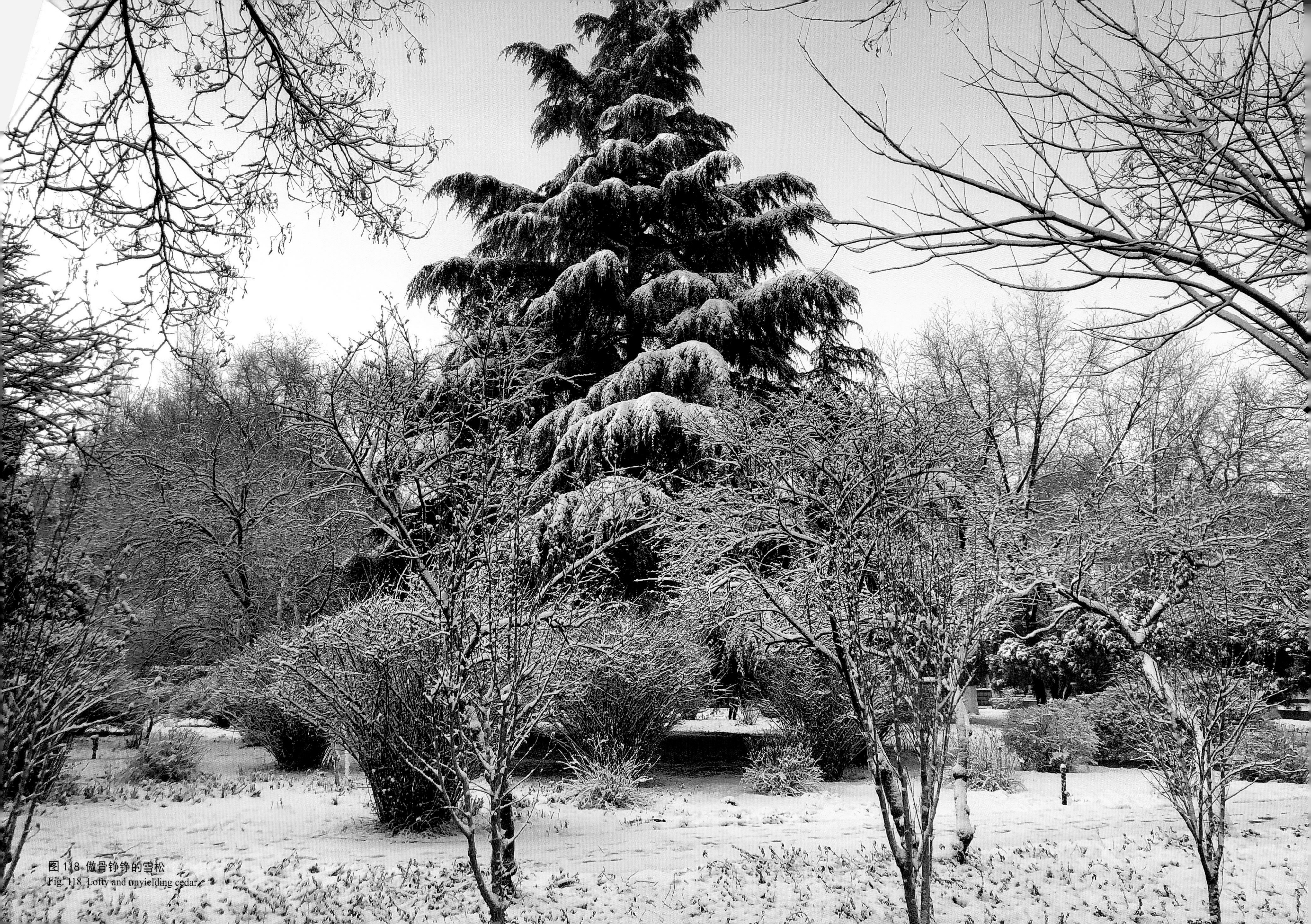

图 118 傲骨铮铮的雪松
Fig. 118 Lofty and unyielding cedar

第五章 Chapter Five

行政楼 Administration Building

18 麦考密可楼（1）

McCormick Hall (1)

麦考密可楼建成于 1923 年，为齐鲁大学行政楼，因纪念为齐鲁大学捐款的美国播种机发明者麦考密可 (Cyrus H. McCormick) 的夫人而命名。该楼位于中心花园中轴线的北端，坐北朝南，两层砖木结构，另有宽大的半地下室。屋顶以中国传统建筑形式和处理手法为主，如交叉脊、花脊和歇山、山墙上精致的砖雕等。建筑的正（南）面横向为三段式的西方古典主义风格，中间一段五开间、略向南突出，东西两翼各六开间，但略有变化。它建筑风格古朴典雅，中西合璧，造型庄重大方，用料上乘，装修考究，比例尺度恰当，细部处理得体，被誉为“中国建筑复兴样式”的代表作。该楼也曾是山东医学院和山东医科大学的行政中心，是学校的标志性建筑。可惜的是 1997 年毁于火灾。

McCormick Hall, built in 1923, is the Administration Building of Cheeloo University named in memory of the wife of Cyrus H. McCormick, the inventor of the mechanical reaper. The building is located at the north end of the Central Garden's central axis, facing south with a two-storey brick-wood structure and a wide semi-basement. The roof is mainly treated in the form of traditional Chinese architecture, such as the cross ridge, the ceramic tile ridge, the gable and hip roof, and the exquisite brick carvings on the gable and so on. The front (south) side of the building is a horizontal three-section style of Western classical technique, with a five-bay section in the middle slightly protruding to the south and six-bay sections in the east and west wings respectively, but with slight changes. With the simple and elegant architectural style of Chinese and Western combination, the nice and solemn shape, the superior materials, the exquisite decoration, the appropriate proportion and the properly handled details, this building is known as the representative of the "Revival Style of the Chinese Architecture". The building was also the administrative center of Shandong Medical College and Shandong Medical University. Unfortunately, as the landmark building of the school, it was destroyed in a fire in 1997.

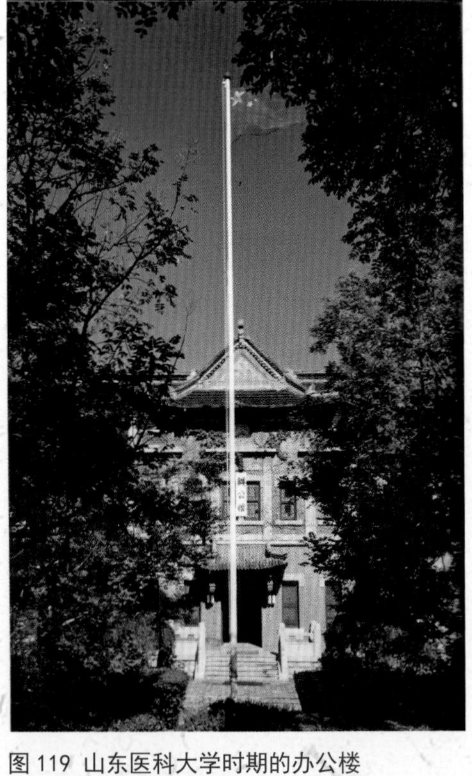

图 119 山东医科大学时期的办公楼
Fig. 119 The Office Building of Shandong Medical University

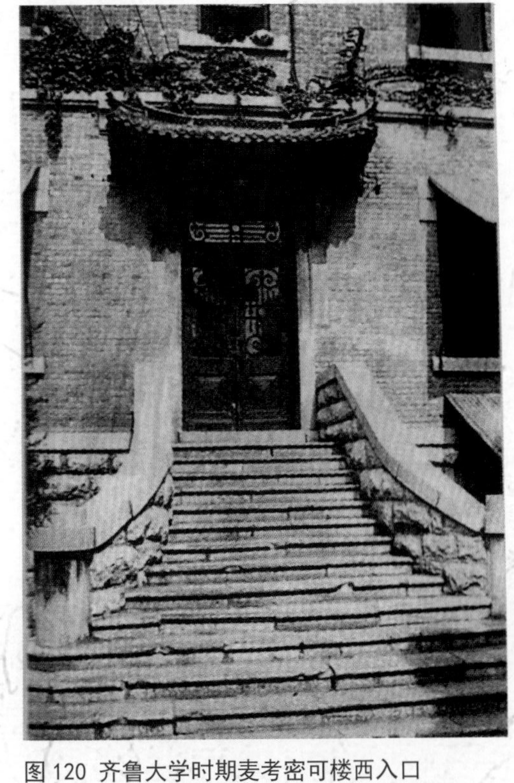

图 120 齐鲁大学时期麦考密可楼西入口
Fig. 120 The west entrance of McCormick Hall at Cheeloo University

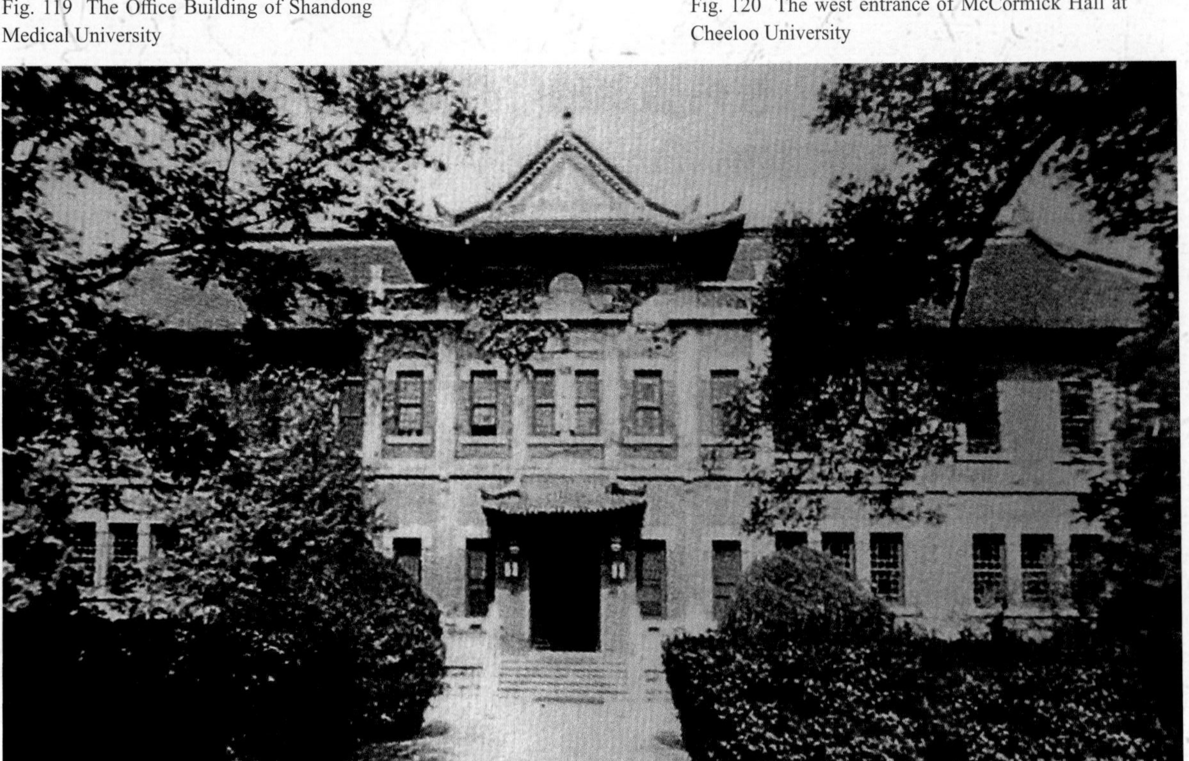

图 121 麦考密可楼南（正）面观
Fig. 121 The south (front) view of McCormick Hall

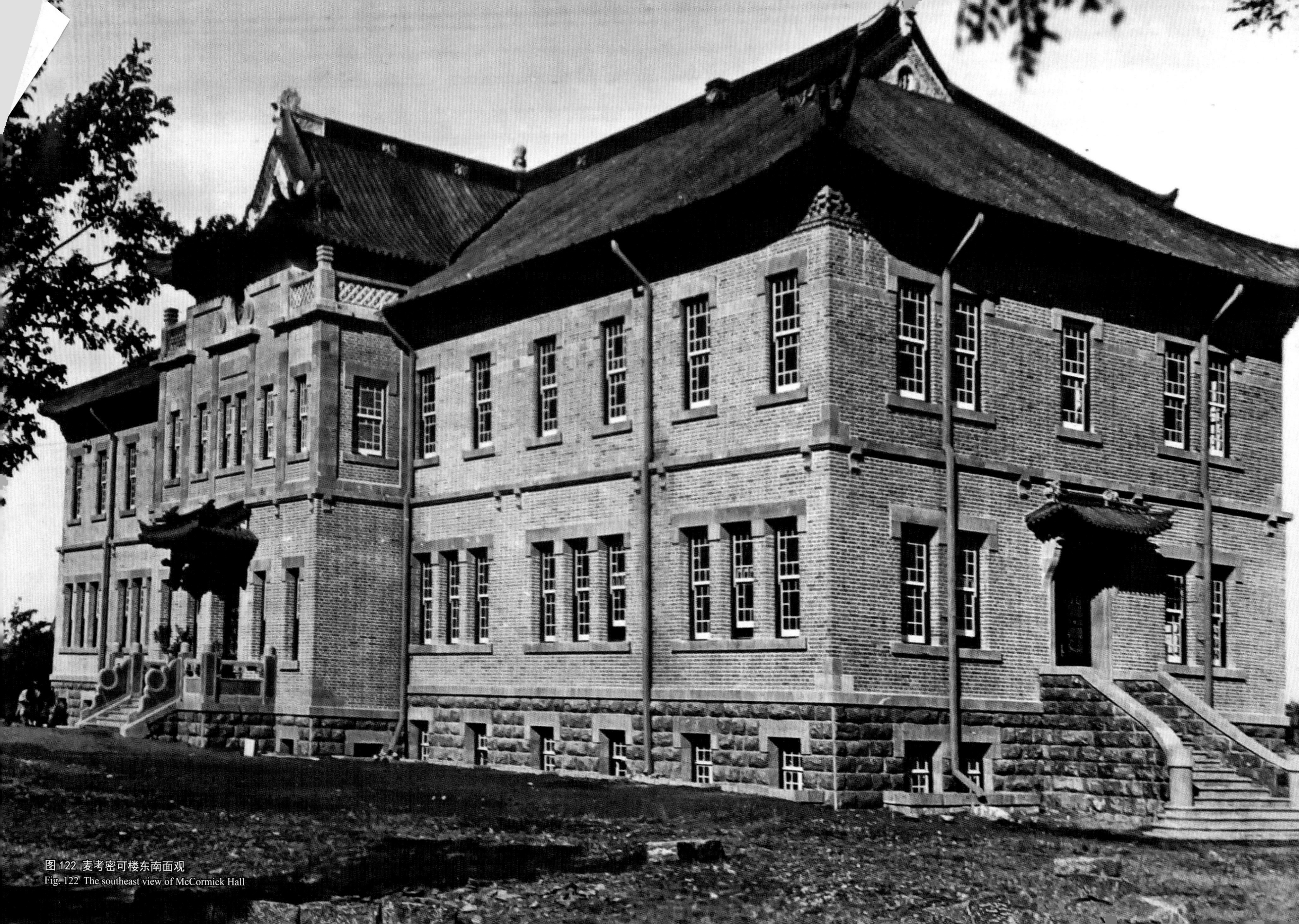
图 122 麦考密可楼东南面观
Fig. 122 The southeast view of McCormick Hall

18 麦考密可楼（2）

McCormick Hall (2)

我国现代著名作家老舍先生（1899 ~ 1966，原名舒庆春，字舍予）曾两度执教于齐鲁大学文学院国文系。第一次为 1930 年 7 月至 1934 年 6 月，第二次为 1937 年 8 月至 11 月，之间在青岛山东大学执教。他第一次执教齐鲁大学期间，先住在麦考密可楼二楼西翼南边的第一个房间里。据其夫人胡絜青后来回忆：“从这间屋子里推窗南望，可以远眺庙宇点点的千佛山；楼下，槐榆夹道，碧草如茵，不远处还有一个圆形喷水池。”1931 年暑假二人结婚，便租住在南新街 54 号（现为 58 号，建有老舍故居）的房子里。在第二次执教齐鲁大学期间，住在位于校内长柏路 2 号（现为 11 号）的一栋小洋楼内。老舍在齐鲁大学担任国学研究所文学主任，除授课外，还创作了大量文学作品，其中有《暑假中的齐鲁大学》和《非正式的公园》两篇散文，专门描写了当时齐鲁大学美丽的校园风光。

Mr. Lao She (1899-1966, his original name is Shu Qingchun and courtesy name is Sheyu) is a famous modern writer in China and once taught in the Department of Chinese Literature, School of Literature of Cheeloo University twice. The first time was from July 1930 to June 1934, and the second time was from August 1937 to November 1937, with a gap teaching at Shandong University, Qingdao. During his first teaching at Cheeloo University, he first lived in the first room south of the west wing on the second floor of McCormick Hall. His wife Hu Jieqing later recalled: “Open the window and look south from this room, you can overlook the Qianfo Hill with many temples. Downstairs, the locust trees and the elms line the road, and the expanse of verdant grass seems like a pleasant carpet. Moreover, there is a round fountain not far away.” In the summer vacation of 1931, the two people married and they rented a house at No. 54 Nanxin Street (now No. 58, the former residence of Lao She). During his second teaching at Cheeloo University, he lived in a small Western-style building located at No. 2 (now No. 11) Changbai Road in the university. Lao She served as the director of literature of the Institute of National Studies at Cheeloo University. In addition to teaching, he also wrote a large number of literary works, including two essays “Cheeloo University in Summer Vacation” and “An Informal Park” which specifically described the beautiful campus scenery of Cheeloo University at that time.

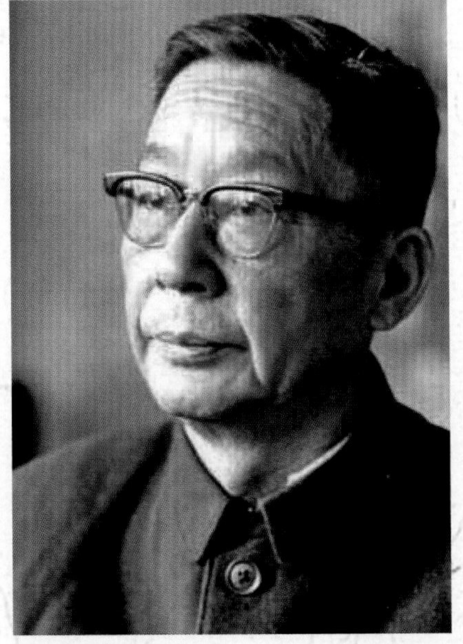

图 123 老舍先生

Fig. 123 Mr. Lao She

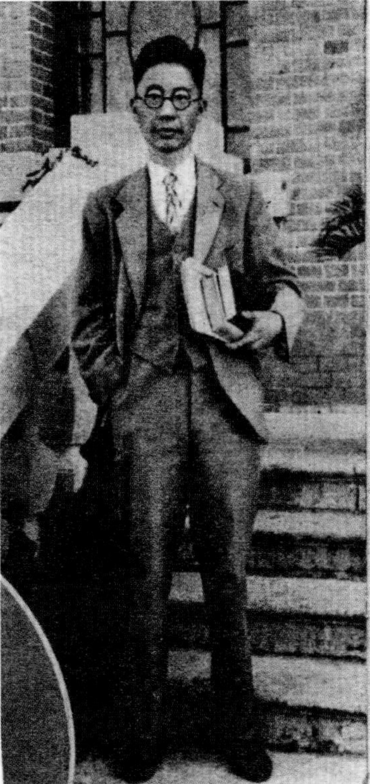

图 124 20 世纪 30 年代老舍在麦考密可楼前留影

Fig. 124 A photo of Lao She in front of McCormick Hall in the 1930s

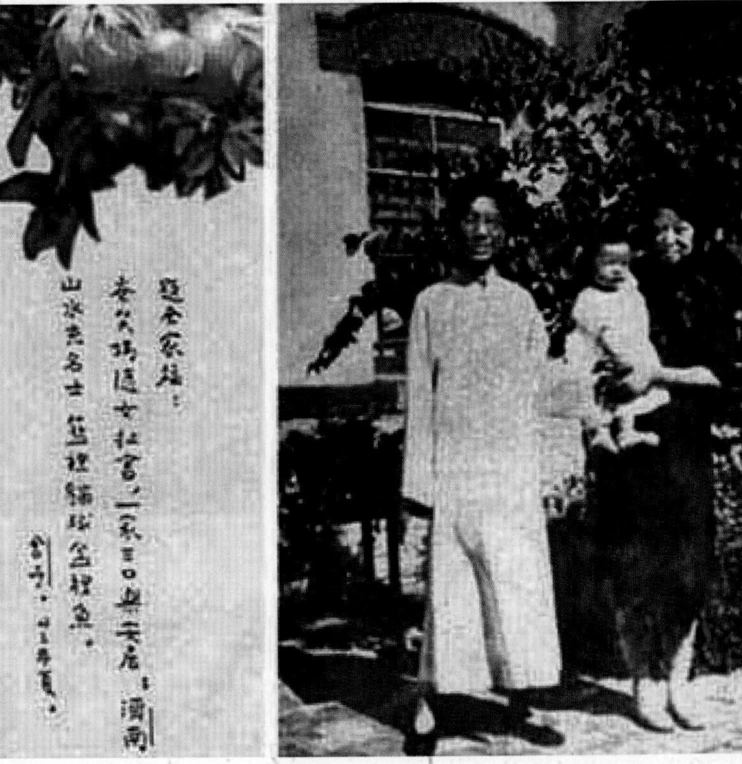

图 125 1934 年夏天，老舍一家在济南南新街 54 号家中

Fig. 125 Lao She’s family staying at home at No. 54 Nanxin Street, Jinan in the summer of 1934

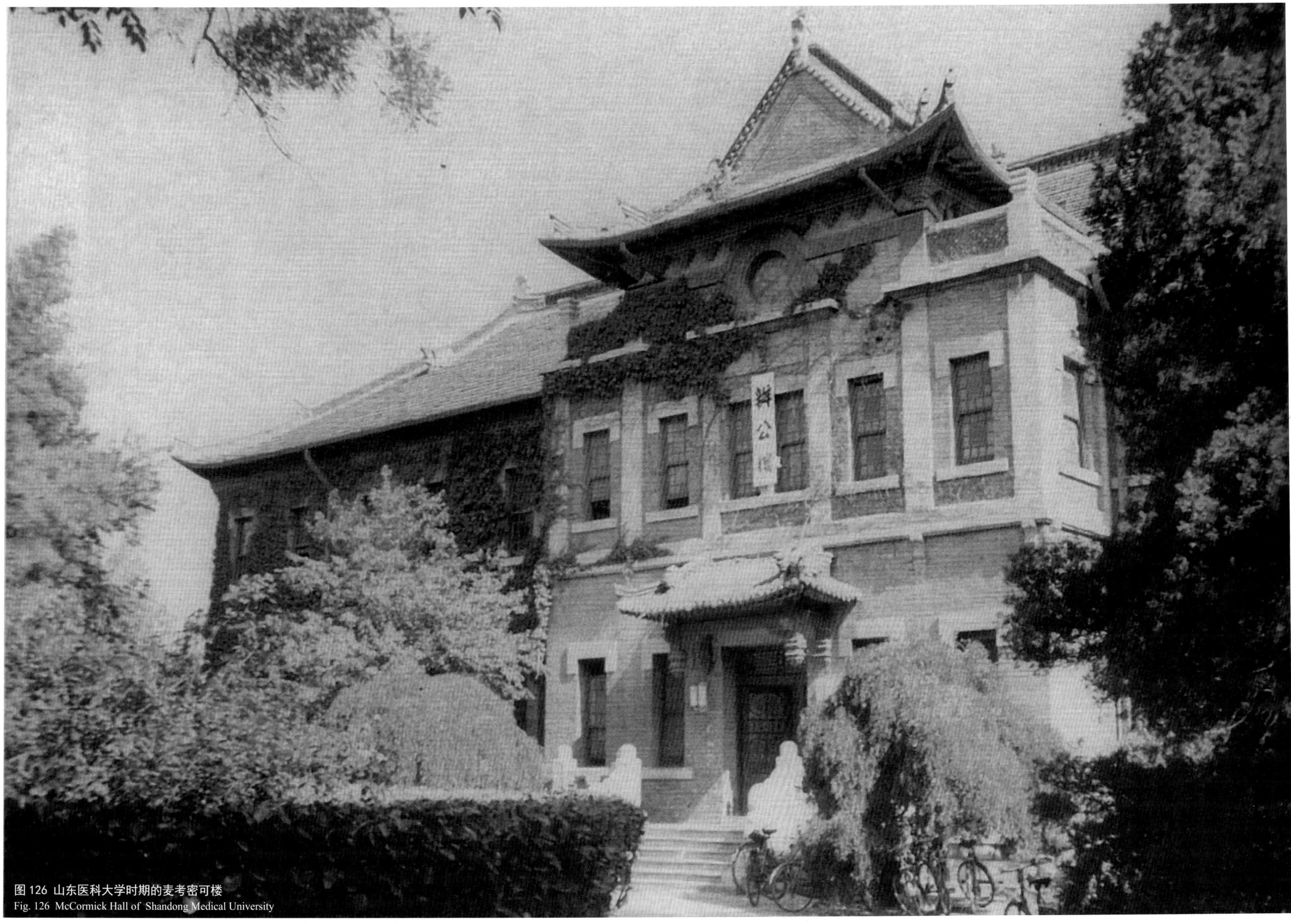

图 126 山东医科大学时期的麦考密可楼
Fig. 126 McCormick Hall of Shandong Medical University

19 新麦考密可楼（1）

New McCormick Hall (1)

新麦考密可楼亦称科研综合楼，建成于 1999 年，在麦考密可楼原址重建，面积大为扩增，建筑风格力图保持原有风貌。新楼为钢筋混凝土结构，主体部分六层，南门为主门，两侧增加了柱廊。建筑的南面横向为五段式，中间部分三段，保持原楼十七开间风貌，两翼为六开间。现为山东大学齐鲁医学院办公楼，以及临床医学院、药学院和公共卫生学院院部，一层建有齐鲁医学院校史馆。山东大学博物馆曾设在此楼，现已迁回中心校区。

The new McCormick Hall, also known as the Comprehensive Building of Scientific Research, was built in 1999 at the original site of McCormick Hall. The area was greatly expanded and the original architectural style was maintained as much as possible. The new building is a reinforced concrete structure, with six floors in the main part. The south gate is the main gate, and colonnades are added on both sides. The south side of the building is horizontal for five sections and the middle part is of three-section style, keeping the original seventeen-bay sections and six-bay sections for two wings. This building now serves as the office building of Cheeloo College of Medicine of Shandong University, as well as the administration office area of School of Medicine, School of Pharmaceutical Sciences and School of Public Health. On the first floor, there is the History Museum of Cheeloo College of Medicine. The Museum of Shandong University, once located in this building, has now moved back to the central campus.

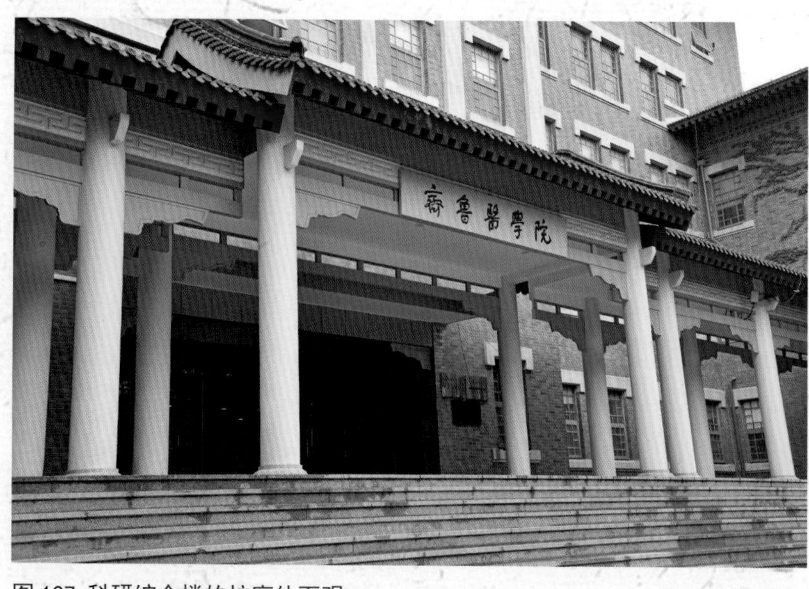

图 127 科研综合楼的柱廊外面观
Fig. 127 Exterior view of the colonnades of the Comprehensive Building of Scientific Research

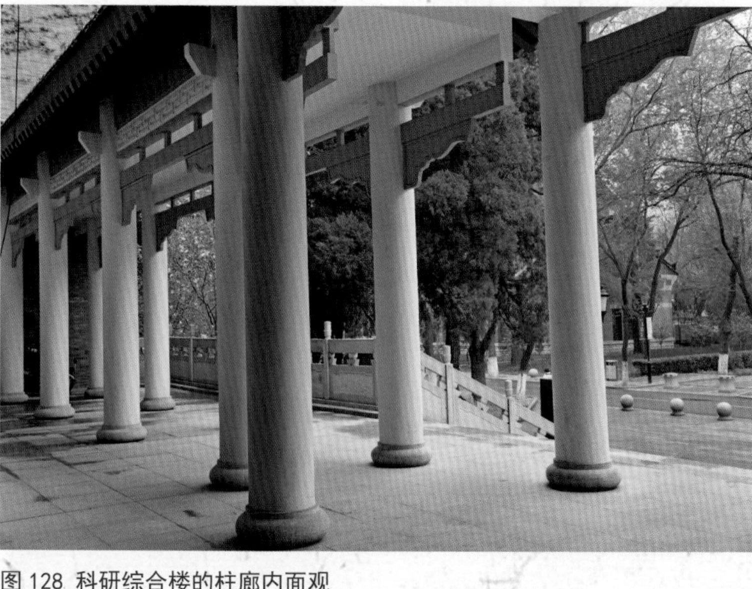

图 128 科研综合楼的柱廊内面观
Fig. 128 The interior view of the colonnades of the Comprehensive Building of Scientific Research

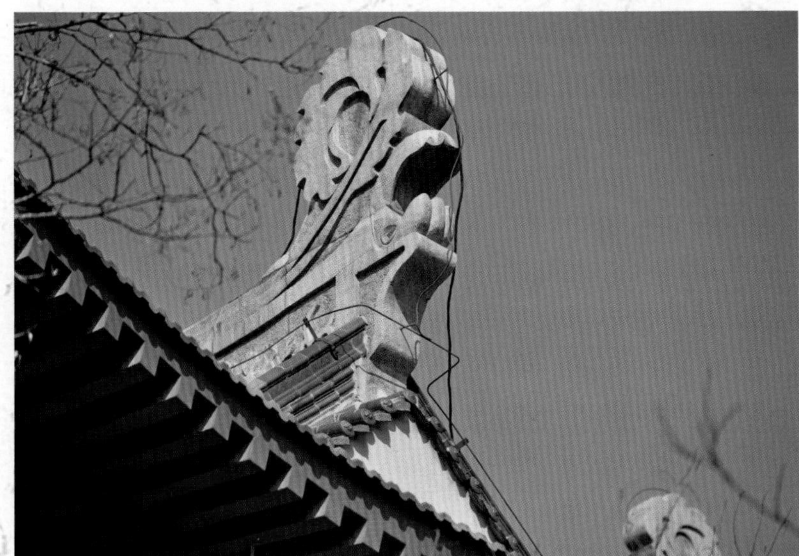

图 129 科研综合楼楼顶的鸱吻
Fig. 129 *Chiwen* (an ornament in the shape of a legendary animal) on the roof of the Comprehensive Building of Scientific Research

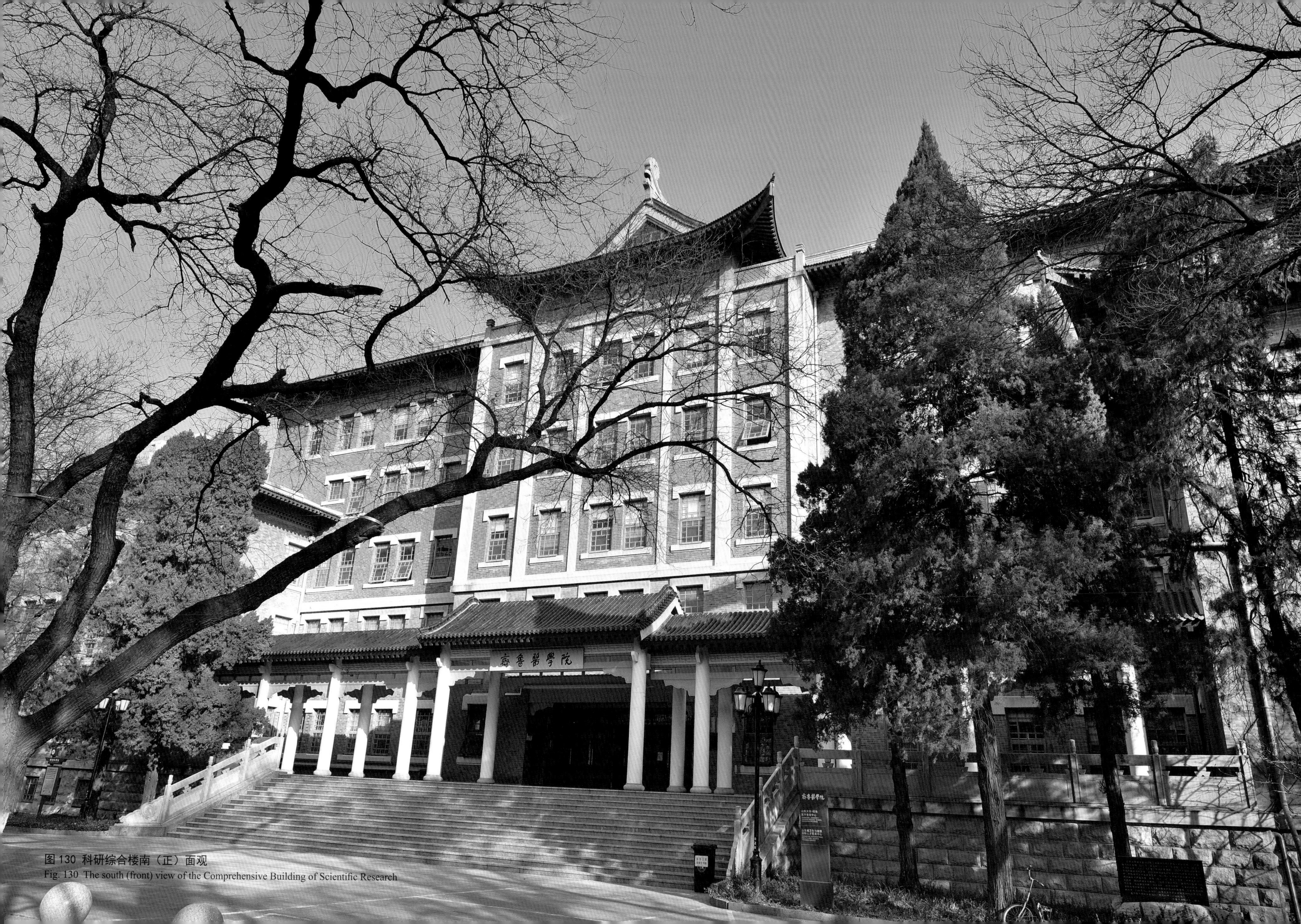

图 130 科研综合楼南（正）面观

Fig. 130 The south (front) view of the Comprehensive Building of Scientific Research

19 新麦考密可楼（2）

New McCormick Hall (2)

齐鲁医学院办公地点位于新麦考密可楼内，承担山东大学医学教育和事业发展的日常管理任务，具有统筹、协调、管理医学教育等职能，协助学校做好医学教学科研单位、附属医院干部队伍建设。齐鲁医学院目前有基础医学院、临床医学院、公共卫生学院、口腔医学院、护理与康复学院和药学院六个学院，高等医学研究院和实验动物中心两个挂靠单位，齐鲁医院、第二医院、口腔医院和生殖医院四所直属附属医院。齐鲁医学院的院训为：博施济众，广智求真；办学宗旨为：培育医学精英，护佑人类健康；办学定位为：创办具有齐鲁特色、国内领先、世界一流的研究型医学院。

The office of Cheeloo College of Medicine is located in the new McCormick Hall, undertaking the daily management tasks of medical education and career development of Shandong University, performing the functions of overall planning, coordination and management of medical education, and assisting the university in constructing the cadres in medical teaching and research units and affiliated hospitals. At present, Cheeloo College of Medicine has six schools, namely School of Basic Medical Sciences, School of Medicine, School of Public Health, School of Stomatology, School of Nursing and Rehabilitation and School of Pharmaceutical Sciences; two attached units, namely the Advanced Medical Research Institute and the Laboratory Animal Center; and four directly affiliated hospitals, namely Qilu Hospital, the Second Hospital, the Stomatological Hospital and the Hospital for Reproductive Medicine. The motto of Cheeloo College of Medicine is "relieving the public by providing extensive medical assistance, and seeking truth via continuing study". The mission is "to cultivate medical elite and protect human health". The orientation is "to establish a Research Medical College, leading in China and world-class with Qilu characteristics".

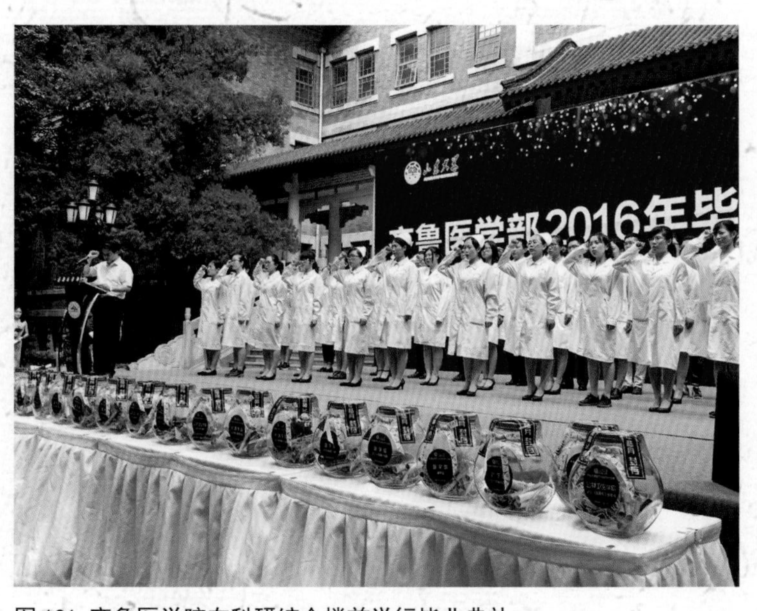

图 131 齐鲁医学院在科研综合楼前举行毕业典礼

Fig. 131 Cheeloo College of Medicine holding graduation ceremony in front of the Comprehensive Building of Scientific Research

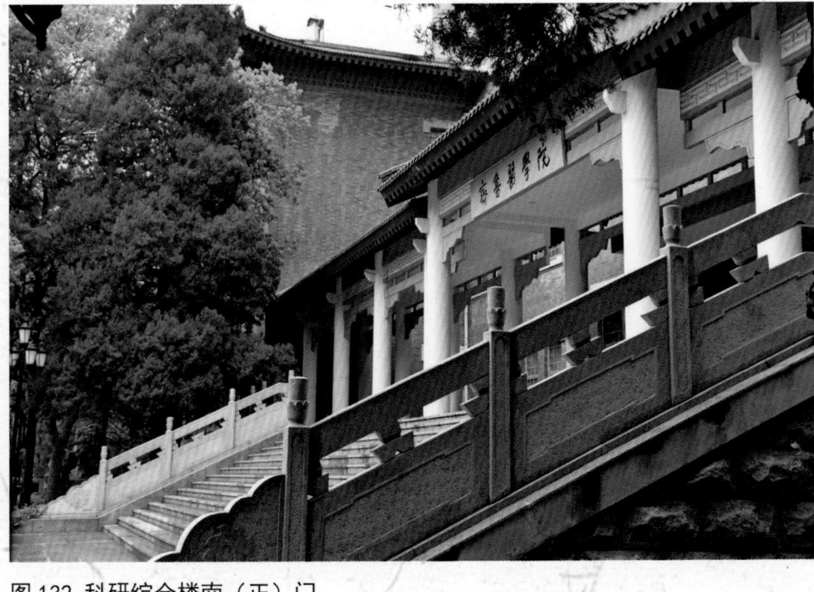

图 132 科研综合楼南（正）门

Fig. 132 The south (front) gate of the Comprehensive Building of Scientific Research

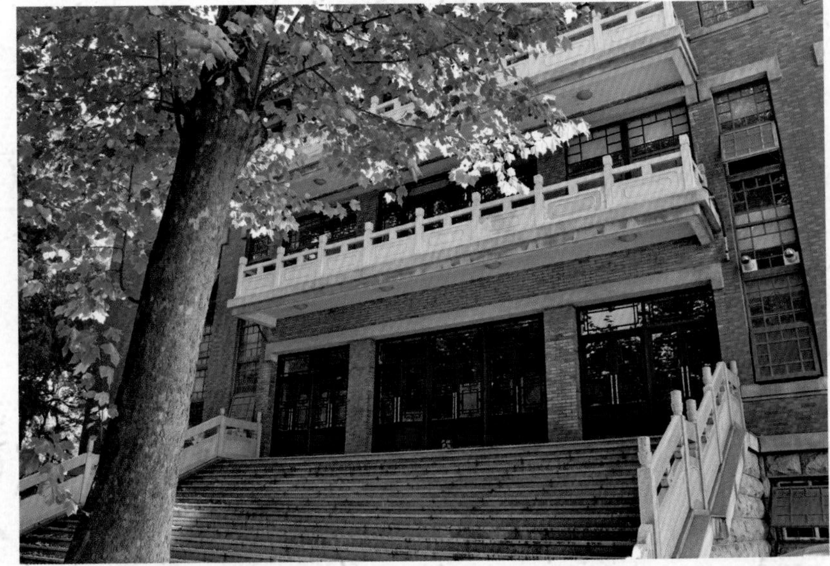

图 133 科研综合楼东门

Fig. 133 The east gate of the Comprehensive Building of Scientific Research

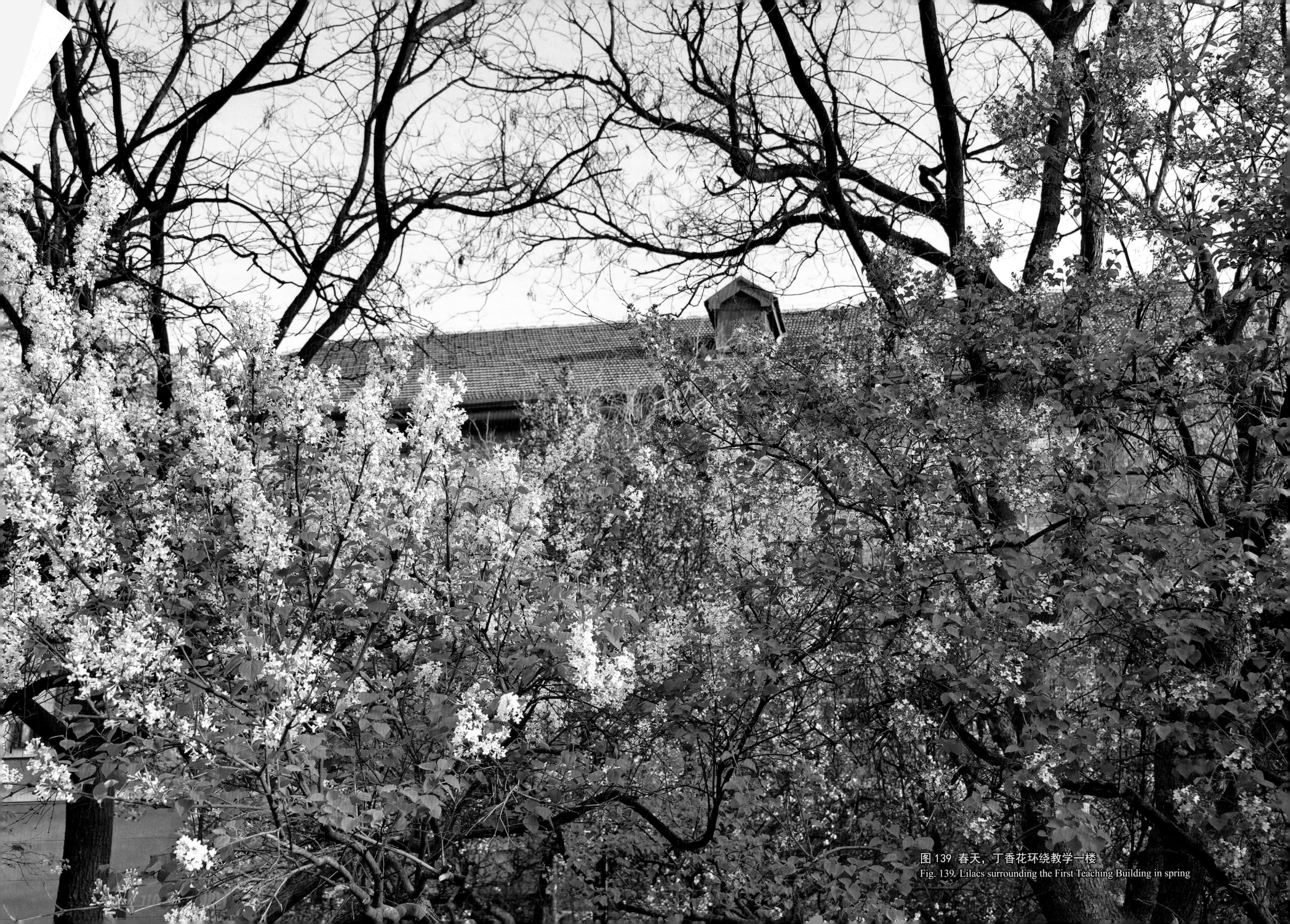

图 139 春天，丁香花环绕教学一楼
Fig. 139. Lilacs surrounding the First Teaching Building in spring

20 第一教学楼（2）

The First Teaching Building (2)

人体解剖学实验教学平台位于第一教学楼二层，共六个教学实验室。伟大导师恩格斯说过：“没有解剖学，就没有医学。”因此，人体解剖学课程受到师生的格外重视，教研成果曾三次获得过国家级教学成果奖。

第一次为教材建设。重点建设了文字教材（教科书、参考书）、直观教材（标本、模型）和电化教材（电影、幻灯）。“‘三材’建设的系列改革，是全面提高教学质量的关键”项目于 1989 年获得国家级优秀教学成果奖。

第二次为课程建设。率先开设断层解剖学课程，探索了新的教学模式。1997 年，“顺应现代影像学发展，创建断层解剖学课程”获得国家级教学成果奖二等奖。

第三次为教学信息化建设。开发了数字解剖学教学软件、虚拟解剖台和应用云平台等。2018 年，“我国数字解剖学教学体系创建与推广”获得国家级教学成果奖二等奖。

The Experimental Teaching Platform of Human Anatomy is located on the second floor of the First Teaching Building, with six teaching laboratories in total. Engels, the great tutor, once said,"Without anatomy, there would be no medicine." Therefore, the teachers and students have paid special attention to the course of Human Anatomy, and their teaching and research achievements have won the National Teaching Achievement Award three times.

The first award is for the construction of teaching materials. The construction of written teaching materials (textbooks and reference books), intuitive teaching materials (specimens and models) and audio-visual teaching materials (films and slides) was treated as a focus. The program with the title of "A Series of Reforms in the Construction of Three Kinds of Materials Is the Key to Improving the Teaching Quality in an All-round Way" won the National Excellent Teaching Achievement Award in 1989.

The second award is for the curriculum construction. The course of Sectional Anatomy was first opened, and a new teaching mode had been explored. In 1997, the subject with the title of "Conforming to the Development of Modern Imaging and Establishing the Course of Sectional Anatomy" won the second prize of the National Teaching Achievement Award.

The third award is for the construction of teaching informatization. The digital anatomy teaching software, the anatomage table and the application cloud platform had been developed. In 2018, the subject with the title of "The Establishment and Promotion of the Teaching System of Digital Anatomy in China" won the second prize of the National Teaching Achievement Award.

一九八九年普通高等学校
优秀教学成果
获奖证书
获奖项目：“三材”建设的系列改革，是全面提高教学质量的关键
获 奖 者：裘法祖 李人光 张光昌
奖励等级：国家级优秀奖
中华人民共和国 国家教育委员会
证书编号(89)Y2201 一九八九年 月 日

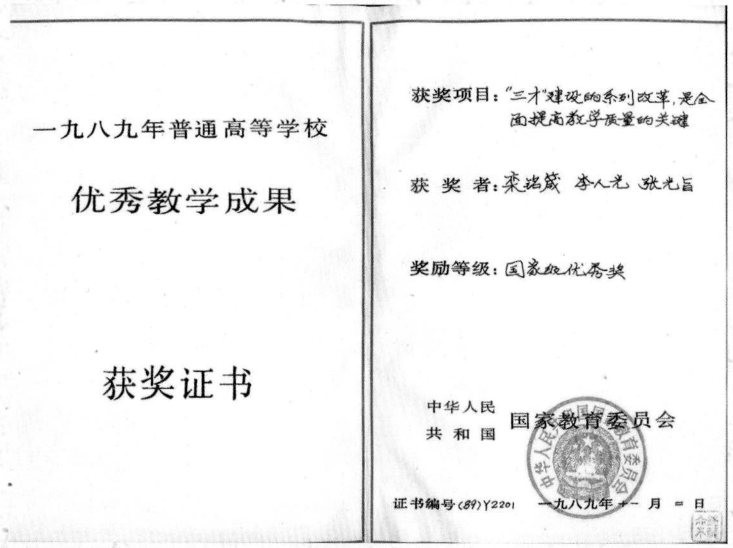

图 140 1989 年的国家级教学成果奖证书
Fig. 140 The certificate of the National Teaching Achievement Award in 1989

国家级教学成果奖
获奖证书
获 奖 成 果：顺应现代影像学发展，创建断层解剖学课程
获 奖 者：刘树伟 刘汉明 李振平 张宪涛 柔铭蔵
获 奖 等 级：二等奖
证 书 号：1997-2-243-5
中华人民共和国 国家教育委员会主任
一九九七年十月二十四日

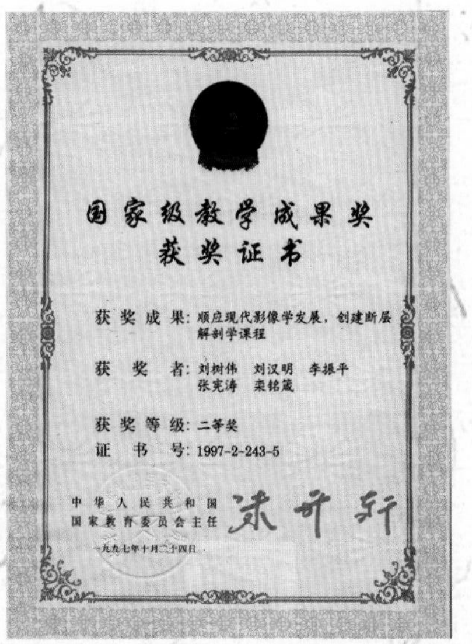

图 141 1997 年的国家级教学成果奖证书
Fig. 141 The certificate of the National Teaching Achievement Award in 1997

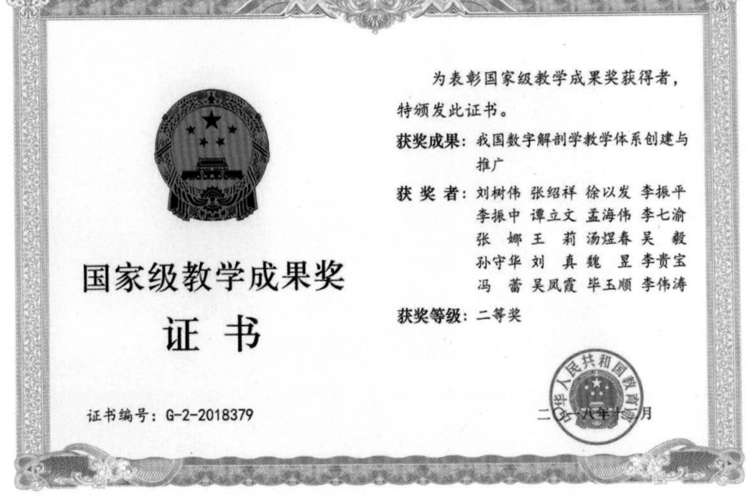

国家级教学成果奖
证 书
为表彰国家级教学成果奖获得者，特颁发此证书。
获奖成果：我国数字解剖学教学体系创建与推广
获 奖 者：刘树伟 张绍祥 徐以发 李振平 李振中 谭立文 孟海伟 李七渝 张 娜 王 莉 汤煜春 吴 毅 孙守华 刘 真 魏 星 李贵宝 冯 蕾 吴凤霞 毕玉顺 李伟涛
获奖等级：二等奖
证书编号：G-2-2018379

图 142 2018 年的国家级教学成果奖证书
Fig. 142 The certificate of the National Teaching Achievement Award in 2018

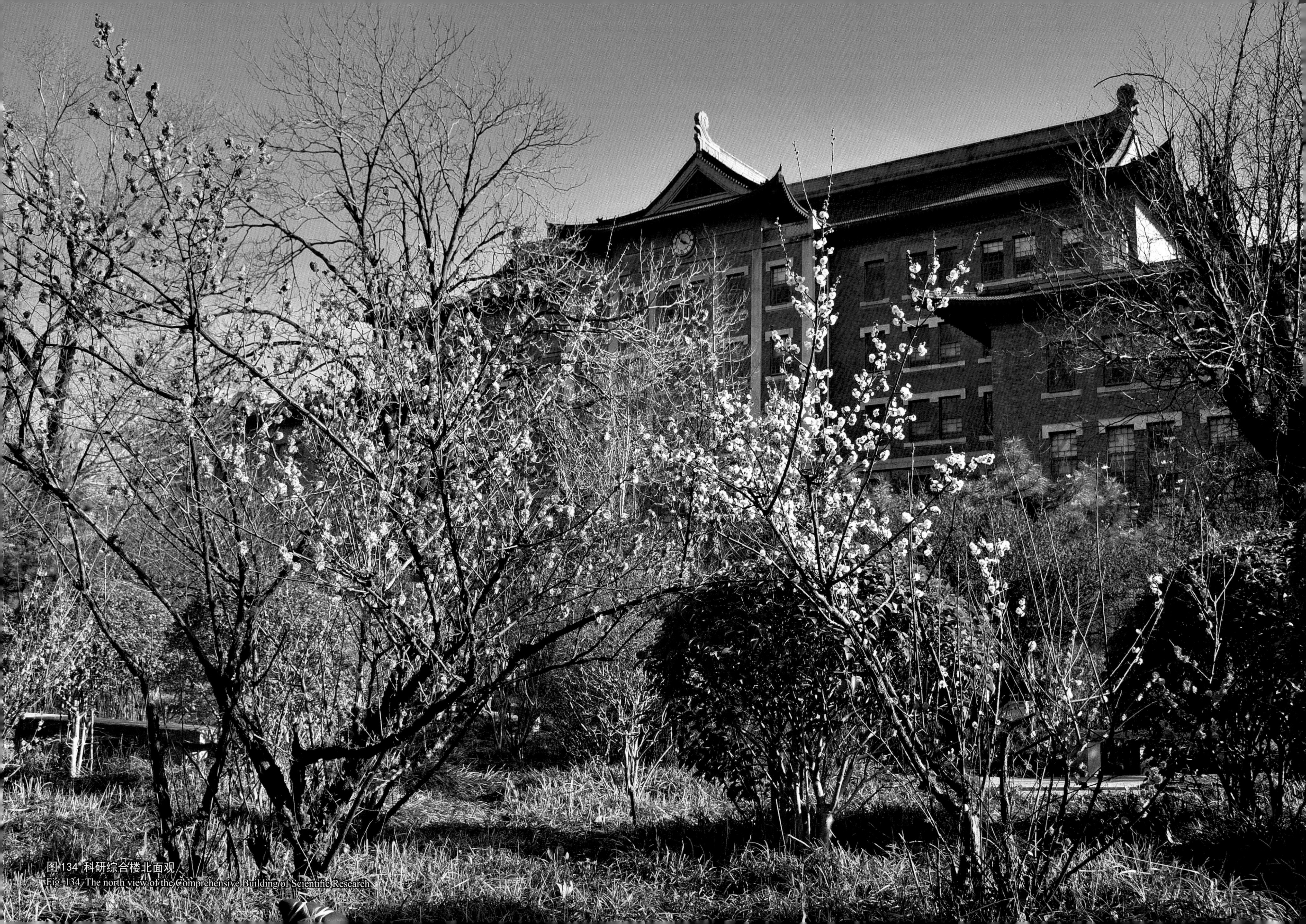
图 134 科研综合楼北面观
Fig. 134 The north view of the Comprehensive Building of Scientific Research

20 第一教学楼（1）

The First Teaching Building (1)

第一教学楼又称解剖楼，建于 1954 年，乃三层仿古建筑，配有地下室，现为解剖学与神经生物学系工作用房。我校的人体解剖学科创建于 20 世纪初，著名解剖学家施尔德、英格尔、叶鹿鸣、苏醒、张季兰、翟允、曹献廷、李人光和栾铭箴等曾在此学科工作过。此学科一直重视科学研究，在神经解剖学、淋巴解剖学和断层影像解剖学等领域研究成绩突出，故 2007 年被教育部评为国家重点学科。早在 1942 年，学校在内迁成都时刚从美国学成归来的叶鹿鸣教授即开展了神经科学研究，并著有《神经解剖学》一书，以后翟允教授、杨琳教授等继续探索于此领域。1959 年，宋景祁教授从苏联获得副博士学位后回国开展了淋巴解剖学研究，此后成为我校的特色研究领域，1991 年王怀经教授开展的脑内淋巴引流研究获得山东省科技进步一等奖。断层影像解剖学研究始于 1989 年，1998 年创建了中国解剖学会断层影像解剖学分会，至今我校依然是主任委员单位。

The First Teaching Building, also known as the Anatomy Building, was built in 1952. It is a three-storey antique building with a basement and is now the working room of the Department of Anatomy and Neurobiology. The Discipline of Human Anatomy of Shandong University was established in the early 20th century. The famous anatomists such as R. T. Shields, Laurence M. Ingle, Ye Luming, Su Xing, Zhang Jilan, Zhai Yun, Cao Xianting, Li Renguang and Luan Mingzhen had once worked here. The researchers of this discipline have attached importance to scientific research and made outstanding achievements in the fields of neuroanatomy, lymphatic anatomy and sectional image anatomy, so this discipline was rated as a National Key Discipline by the Ministry of Education in 2007. As early as 1942 when the university moved to Chengdu, Professor Ye Luming, who had just returned from the United States after finishing school, had carried out neuroscience research and wrote the book *Neuroanatomy*. Later, Professor Zhai Yun and Professor Yang Lin continued to explore in this field. In 1959, Professor Song Jingqi returned home after obtaining an associate doctor's degree from the Soviet Union and carried out the research on lymphatic anatomy, which has become a characteristic research field of our university. In 1991, Professor Wang Huaijing's research on cerebral lymphatic drainage won the first prize of Shandong Provincial Science and Technology Progress Award. The study of sectional image anatomy began in 1989, and the Sectional Image Anatomy Branch of Chinese Society for Anatomical Sciences was established in 1998. Up to now, our university is still the chairman unit.

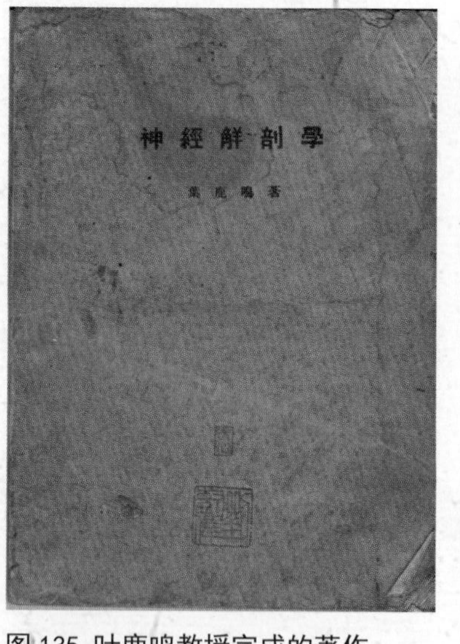

图 135 叶鹿鸣教授完成的著作《神经解剖学》
Fig. 135 *Neuroanatomy* written by Professor Ye Luming

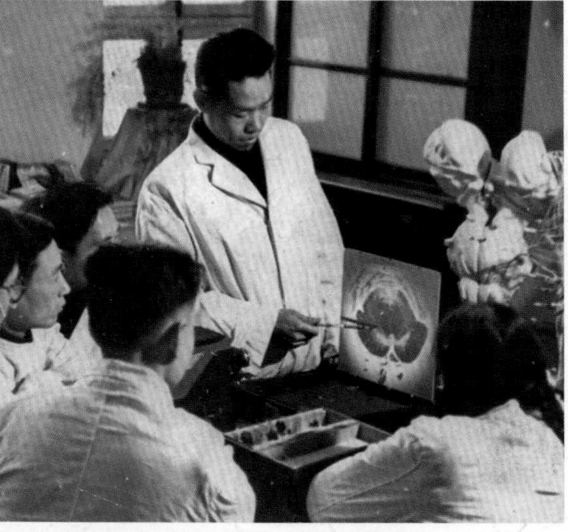

图 136 20 世纪 50 年代翟允教授为学生讲授脑干连片
Fig. 136 Professor Zhai Yun teaching brain stem tablets to students in the 1950s

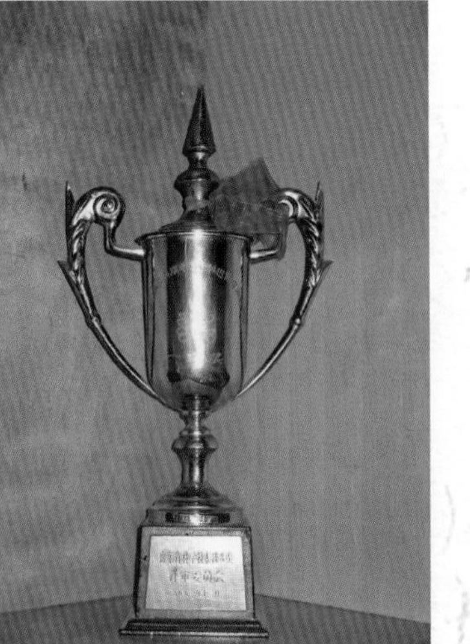

图 137 1991 年王怀经教授获得的山东省科技进步一等奖奖杯
Fig. 137 The first prize trophy of Shandong Provincial Science and Technology Progress Award granted to Professor Wang Huaijing

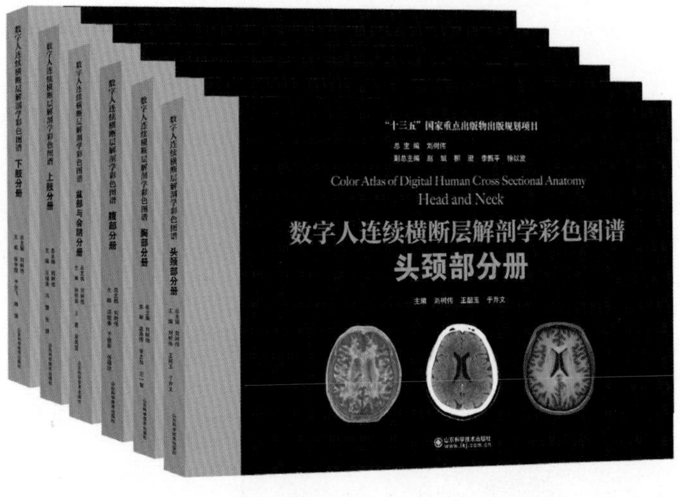

图 138 2020 年刘树伟教授总主编的《数字人连续横断层解剖学彩色图谱》（共 6 个分册）
Fig. 138 *Color Atlas of Digital Human Cross Sectional Anatomy* edited by Professor Liu Shuwei in 2020 (six volumes in total)

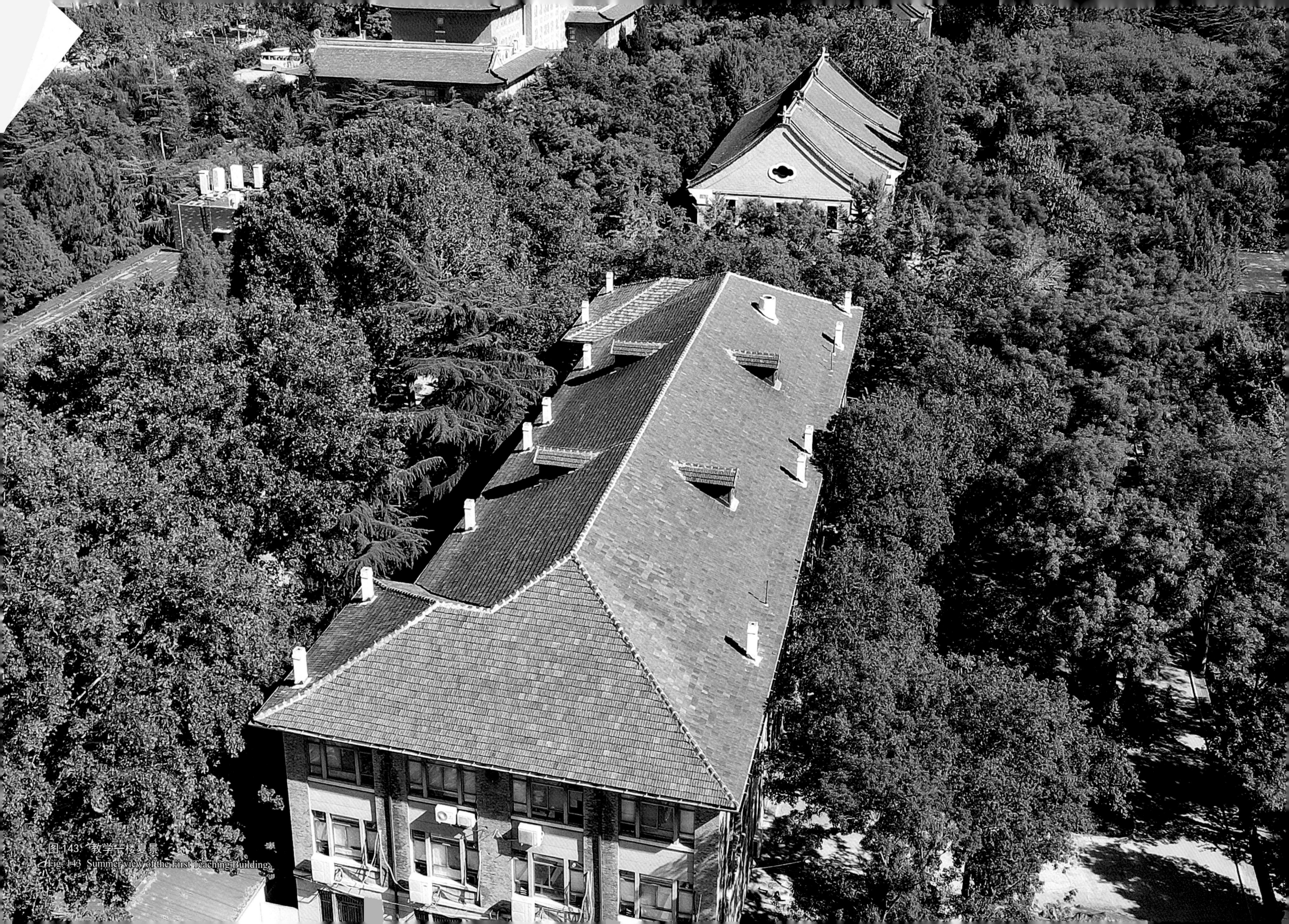

图143　教学一楼夏景

Fig. 143　Summer view of the First Teaching Building

20 第一教学楼（3）

The First Teaching Building (3)

人体标本陈列馆原来也位于第一教学楼，现已迁往第八教学楼。人体解剖学属于形态学范畴，标本多、切片多、图像数据多是其学科特点，因此该学科教师喜欢以图书、影像和展览馆的形式来呈现自己的研究成果。据不完全统计，建校百余年来，我校解剖学教师共主编出版教材、专著和教学课件达 120 余部，尤其在全国规划教材建设中成绩突出。我校教师主编了人民卫生出版社出版的本科全国规划教材《局部解剖学》第 2 版和第 8 版、长学制全国规划教材《局部解剖学》第 1 ~ 2 版，高等教育出版社出版的本科全国规划教材《局部解剖学》第 1 ~ 3 版、《断层解剖学》第 1 ~ 3 版和研究生规划教材《人体断层解剖学》，科学出版社出版的本科全国规划教材《系统解剖学》第 1 ~ 3 版。2021 年，山东大学基础医学院在首届全国教材建设奖评审中荣获“全国教材建设先进集体”称号，解剖学科的贡献巨大。

The Human Specimen Exhibition Hall, which was located in the First Teaching Building, has now moved to the Eighth Teaching Building. Human anatomy belongs to the category of morphology, which is characterized by many specimens, slices and image data. Therefore, teachers of this discipline like to present their research results in the form of books, images and exhibition halls. According to incomplete statistics, the anatomy teachers in our university have edited and published more than 120 textbooks, monographs and teaching courseware since the establishment of the university more than a hundred years ago and have made outstanding achievements in the construction of the National Planning Textbooks. The teachers of our university have edited the second and eighth editions of the National Undergraduate Planning Textbook *Topographic Anatomy* published by the People’s Medical Publishing House; the first and second editions of the National Planning Textbook *Topographic Anatomy* for long-term medical program; the 1-3 editions of the National Undergraduate Planning Textbook *Topographic Anatomy*, the 1-3 editions of *Sectional Anatomy* and the Graduate Planning Textbook *Human Sectional Anatomy* published by the Higher Education Press; the 1-3 editions of the National Undergraduate Planning Textbook *Systematic Anatomy* published by the Science Press. In 2021, School of Basic Medical Sciences of Shandong University won the title of “Advanced Collective of National Textbook Construction” in the evaluation of the First National Textbook Construction Award, and the discipline of anatomy has contributed a lot.

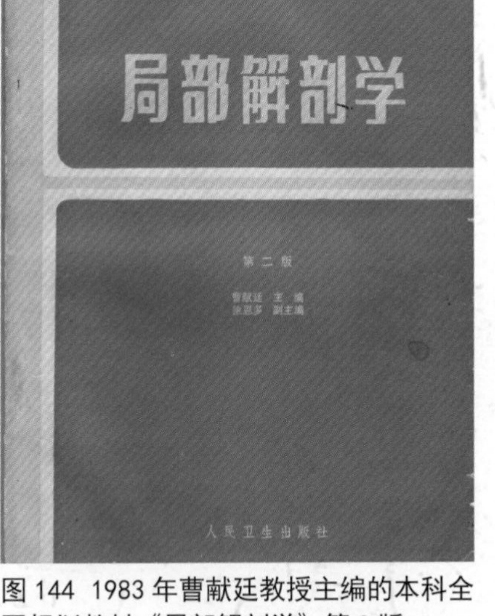

图 144 1983 年曹献廷教授主编的本科全国规划教材《局部解剖学》第 2 版

Fig. 144 The second edition of the National Undergraduate Planning Textbook *Topographic Anatomy* edited by Professor Cao Xianting in 1983

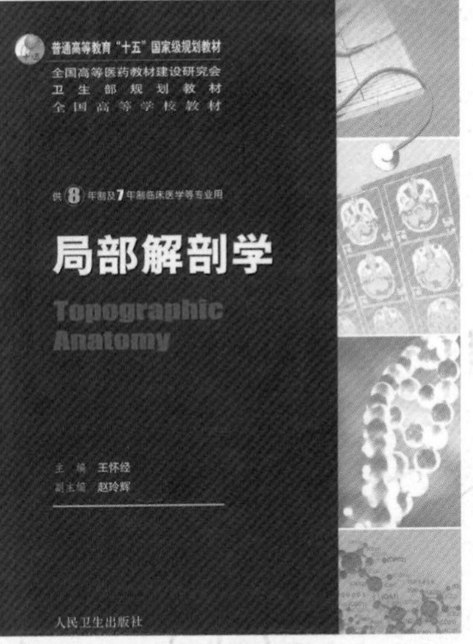

图 145 2005 年王怀经教授主编的长学制全国规划教材《局部解剖学》第 1 版

Fig. 145 The first edition of the National Planning Textbook *Topographic Anatomy* for long-term medical program edited by Professor Wang Huaijing in 2005

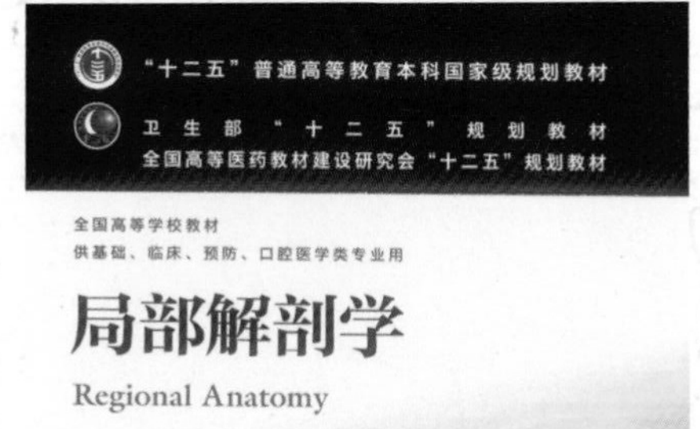
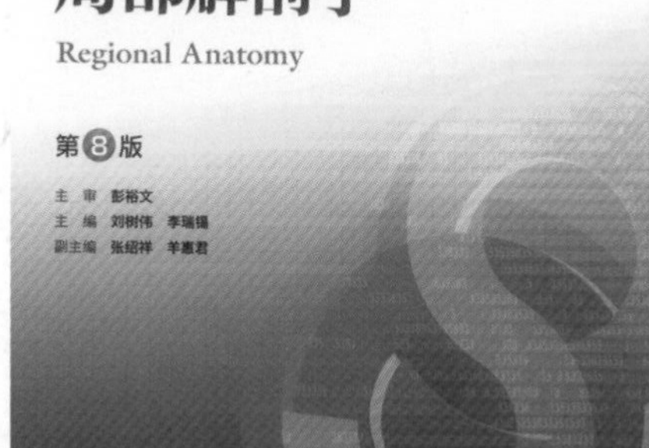

图 146 2013 年刘树伟教授等主编的本科全国规划教材《局部解剖学》第 8 版

Fig. 146 The eighth edition of the National Undergraduate Planning Textbook *Regional Anatomy* edited by Professor Liu Shuwei and others in 2013

图 147 2017 年刘树伟教授主编的本科全国规划教材《断层解剖学》第 3 版

Fig. 147 The third edition of the National Undergraduate Planning Textbook *Sectional Anatomy* edited by Professor Liu Shuwei in 2017

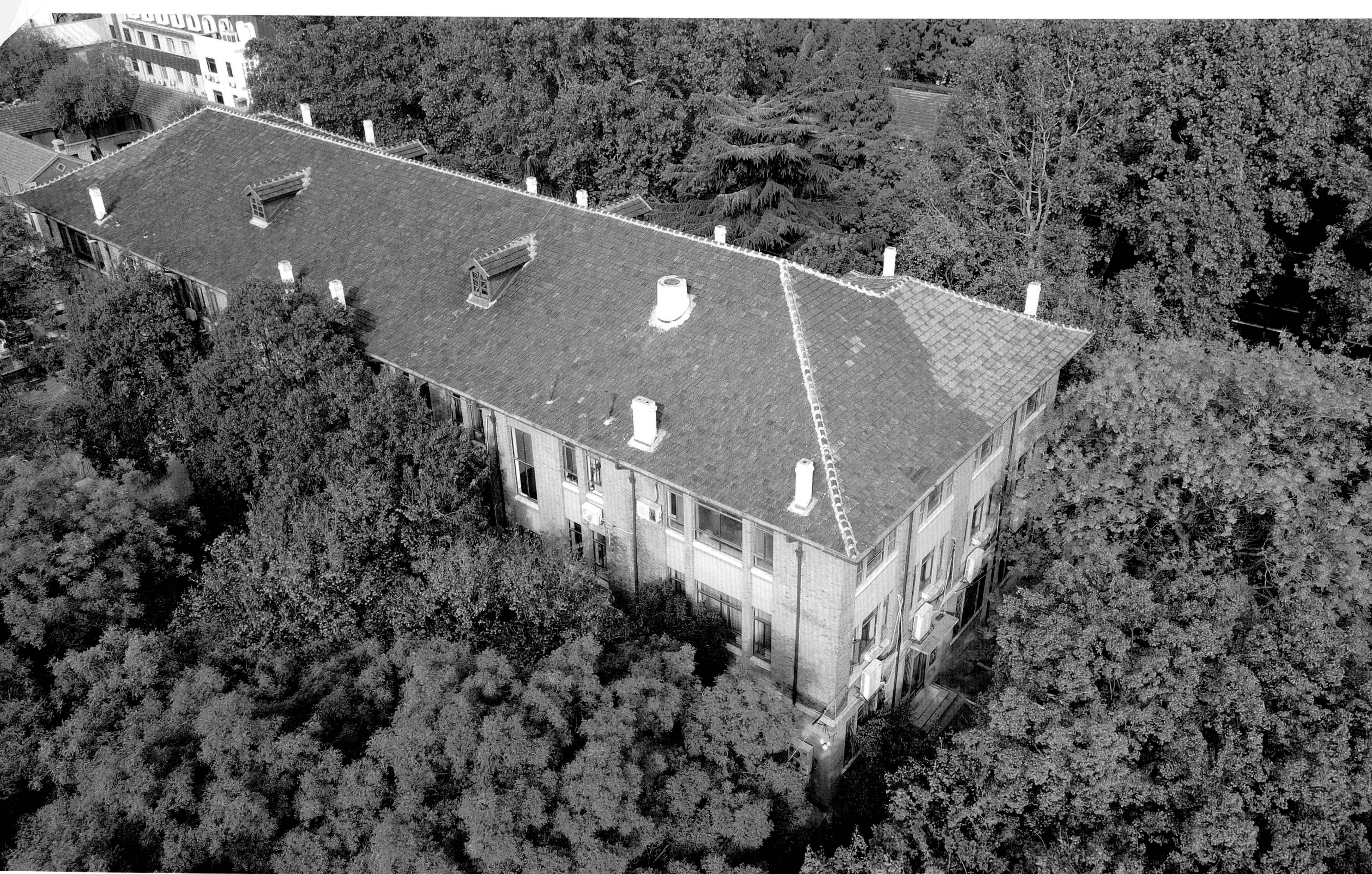

图 148 教学一楼笼罩在一派秋色之中
Fig. 148 The First Teaching Building shrouded in autumn scenery

20 第一教学楼（4）

The First Teaching Building (4)

我校教师四次主译了世界著名的《格氏解剖学》（*Gray's Anatomy*），为我国解剖学的学科建设及解剖学在疾病诊治中的应用做出了重要贡献。

1923 年，齐鲁大学医学院施尔德教授在陈佐庭等的帮助下，翻译了美国版 *Gray's Anatomy of the Human Body* 第 20 版，中文名译为《格氏系统解剖学》，由中国博医会出版、上海美华书馆印刷。

1932 年，齐鲁大学医学院英格尔教授，与陈佐庭合作翻译了英国版 *Gray's Anatomy* 第 23 版，中文名定为《格氏系统解剖学》第 2 版，仍由中国博医会出版发行。

1999 年，山东医科大学杨琳教授与高英茂教授主译了《格氏解剖学》第 38 版，由辽宁教育出版社出版。这是我国自 1932 年以来再次系统翻译《格氏解剖学》，影响巨大。

2017 年，南方医科大学丁自海教授与山东大学刘树伟教授主译了《格氏解剖学》第 41 版，由山东科学技术出版社出版。丁自海与刘树伟的导师分别为曹献廷教授和王永贵教授，两位导师为在齐鲁大学医学院读书时的同班同学。

The teachers of our university have translated the world-famous *Gray's Anatomy* four times, which has made important contributions to the discipline construction of anatomy and the application of anatomy in disease diagnosis and treatment in China.

In 1923, with the help of Chen Zuoting and others, Professor R. T. Shields of the Medical School of Cheeloo University translated the 20th edition of the American edition of *Gray's Anatomy of the Human Body* which was published by the China Medical Missionary Association and printed by the American Presbyterian Mission Press in Shanghai.

In 1932, Professor Ingle of the Medical School of Cheeloo University and Chen Zuoting translated the twenty-third edition of the English edition of *Gray's Anatomy* which was still published by the China Medical Missionary Association.

In 1999, Professor Yang Lin and Professor Gao Yingmao of Shandong Medical University translated the thirty-eighth edition of *Gray's Anatomy* which was published by Liaoning Education Press. This is a systematic translation of *Gray's Anatomy* in China again since 1932, which has produced tremendous impact.

In 2017, Professor Ding Zihai of Southern Medical University and Professor Liu Shuwei of Shandong University translated the forty-first edition of *Gray's Anatomy* which was published by Shandong Science and Technology Press. Ding Zihai and Liu Shuwei's supervisors are Professor Cao Xianting and Professor Wang Yonggui respectively who are classmates at the Medical School of Cheeloo University.

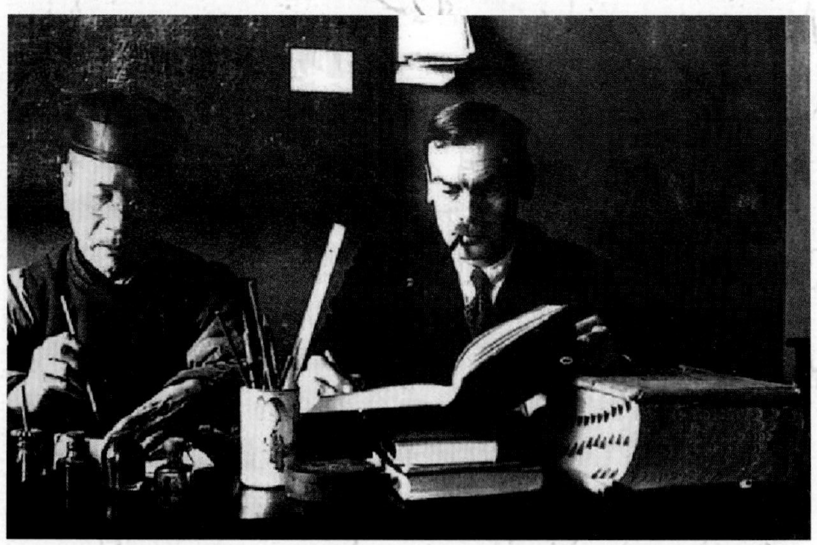

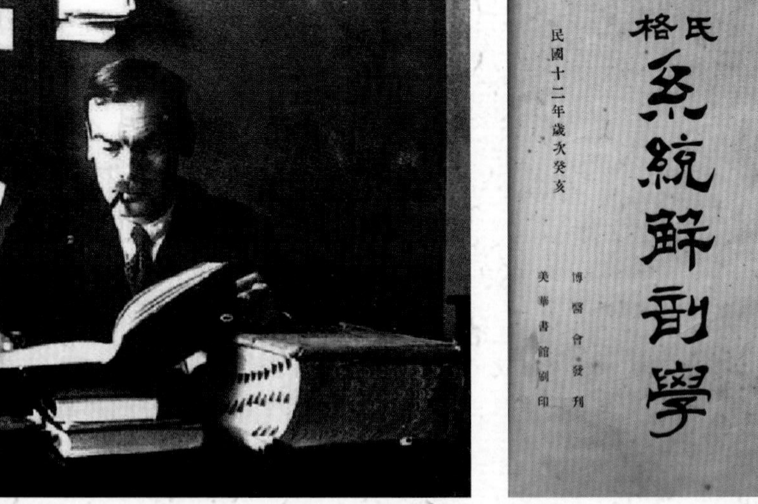

图 149 英格尔在翻译《格氏解剖学》
Fig. 149 Ingle translating *Gray's Anatomy*

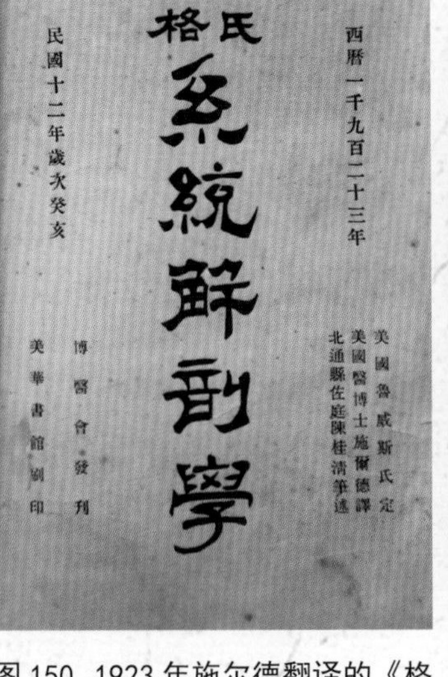

图 150 1923 年施尔德翻译的《格氏系统解剖学》
Fig. 150 *Gray's Anatomy* translated by R. T. Shields in 1923

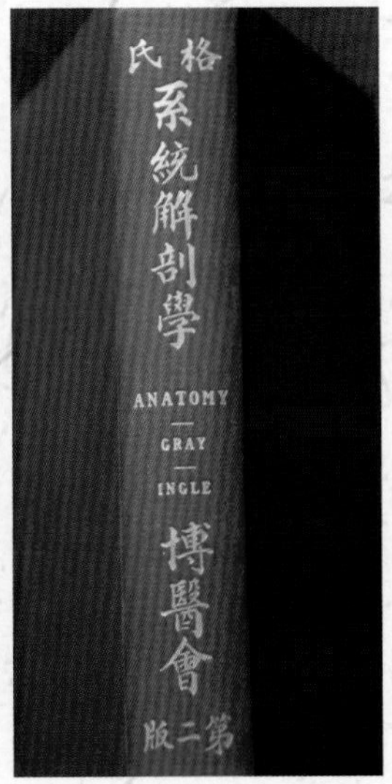

图 151 1932 年，英格尔教授翻译的《格氏系统解剖学》第 2 版
Fig. 151 The second edition of *Gray's Anatomy* translated by Professor Ingle in 1932

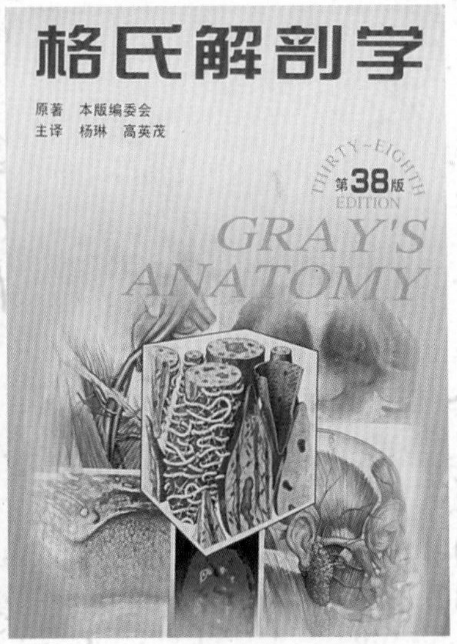

图 152 1999 年，杨琳和高英茂教授主译的《格氏解剖学》第 38 版
Fig. 152 The thirty-eighth edition of *Gray's Anatomy* translated by Professor Yang Lin and Professor Gao Yingmao in 1999

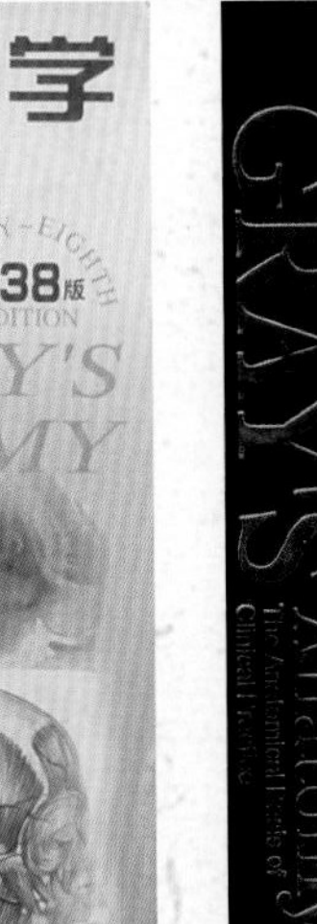

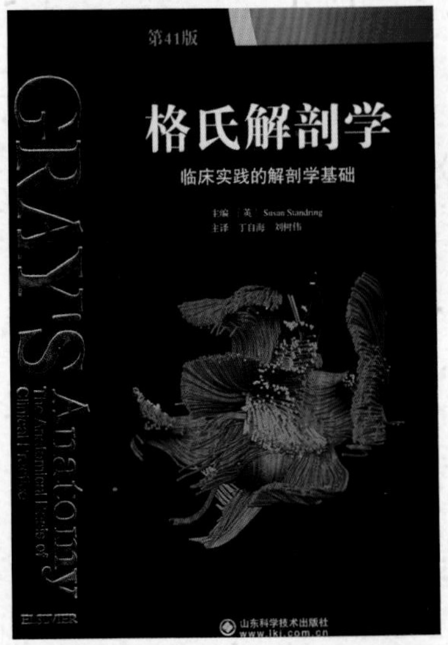

图 153 2017 年，丁自海与刘树伟教授主译的《格氏解剖学》第 41 版
Fig. 153 138 The forty-first edition of *Gray's Anatomy* translated by Professor Ding Zihai and Professor Liu Shuwei in 2017

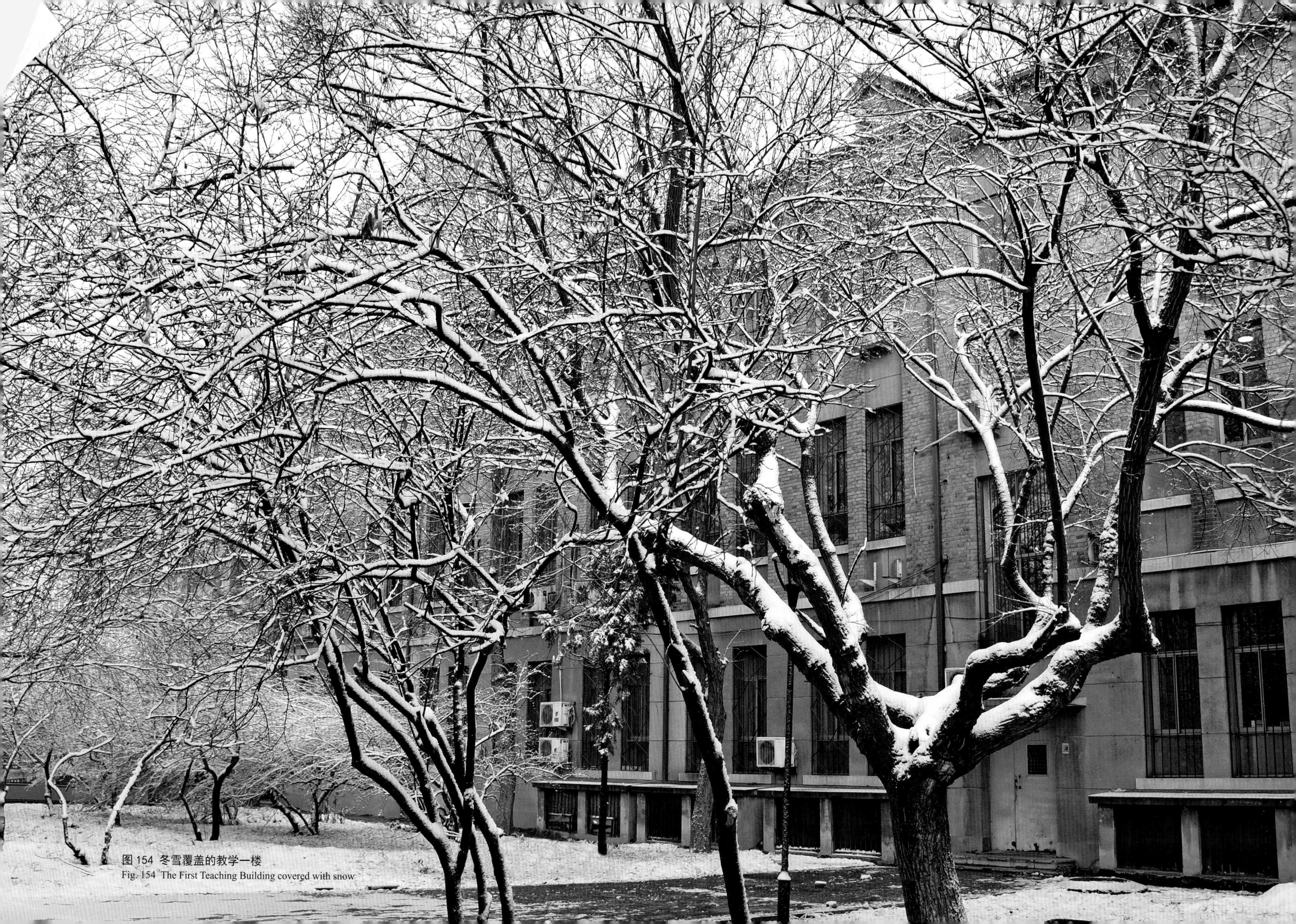

图 154 冬雪覆盖的教学一楼
Fig. 154 The First Teaching Building covered with snow

21 第二教学楼

The Second Teaching Building

第二教学楼建于 1954 年，为三层仿古建筑。为纪念烧伤湿润暴露疗法发明人徐荣祥先生，2018 年冠名“荣祥楼”。第一层长期为公共教室，第二、三层曾为医学微生物教研室和医学免疫学教研室的工作用房，现为分子医学实验教学平台。1950 年 5 月至 1954 年 4 月，著名微生物、免疫及遗传工程专家黄翠芬曾在山东医学院微生物教研室工作，任副教授。

黄翠芬（1921 ~ 2011），广东台山人。1949 年获得美国康奈尔大学理学硕士学位后，与丈夫周廷冲一起回国。1950 年两人到华东白求恩医学院、山东医学院工作，1954 年被调到军事医学科学院。她研制成功四联创伤类毒素，高效甲、乙型肉毒类毒素和“354 装置”，采用分子生物学技术开展细菌毒素的结构与功能研究及基因工程疫苗研究。1996 年当选为中国工程院院士。

The Second Teaching Building, a three-storey antique building, was built in 1954. In memory of Mr. Xu Rongxiang, inventor of the moist exposure therapy of burn, it was named “Rongxiang Building” in 2018. The first floor has been used as public classrooms for a long time; the second and third floors were once used as the working rooms of the Teaching and Research Offices of the Medical Microbiology and the Medical Immunology, and are now used as the experimental teaching platform of Molecular Medicine. Huang Cuifen, a famous expert in microbiology, immunity and genetic engineering, once worked in the Teaching and Research Office of Microbiology of Shandong Medical College as an associate professor from May 1950 to April 1954.

Huang Cuifen (1921-2011) was born in Taishan, Guangdong Province. In 1949, after receiving a degree of Master of Science from Cornell University in the United States, she returned home with his husband Zhou Tingchong. In 1950, they came to work in East China Bethune Medical College and Shandong Medical College, and Huang Cuifen was transferred to Academy of Military Medical Sciences in 1954. She has successfully developed a quadruple wound toxoid, high-efficiency botulinum toxoids A and B and a “354 device”, and has carried out research on the structure and function of bacterial toxins and on genetic engineering vaccines by using technology in molecular biology. She was elected academician of Chinese Academy of Engineering in 1996.

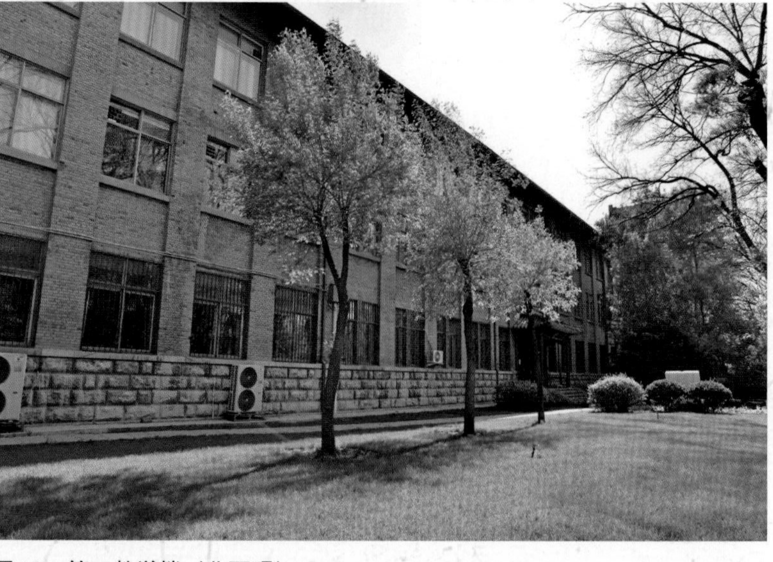

图 155 第二教学楼（北面观）
Fig. 155 The Second Teaching Building (the north view)

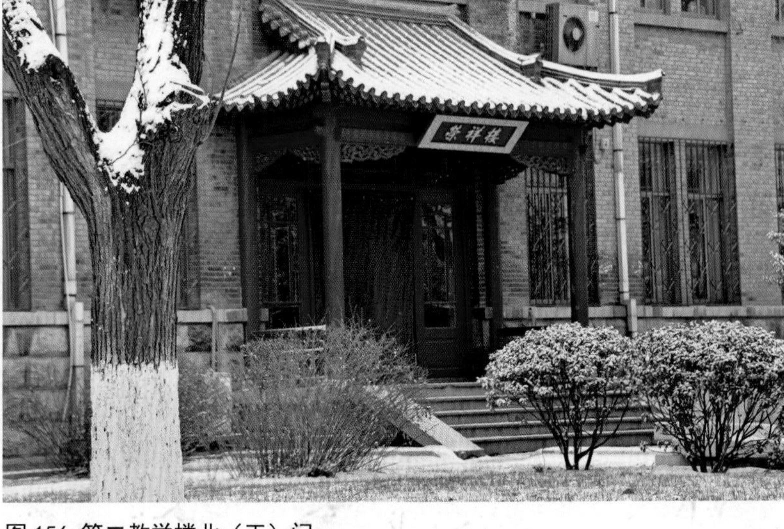

图 156 第二教学楼北（正）门
Fig. 156 The north (front) gate of the Second Teaching Building

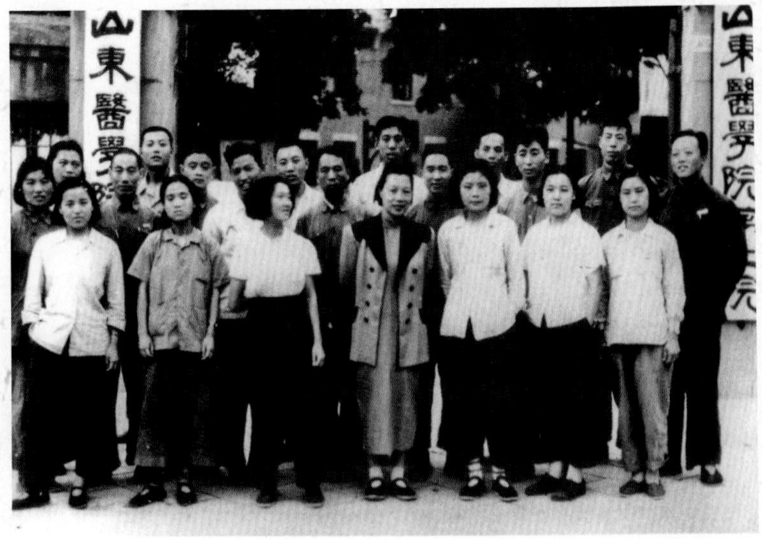

图 157 1951 年，山东医学院微生物教研室全体合影（前排中为黄翠芬）
Fig. 157 Group photo of the Teaching and Research Office of Microbiology of Shandong Medical College (Huang Cuifen in the middle of the front row) in 1951

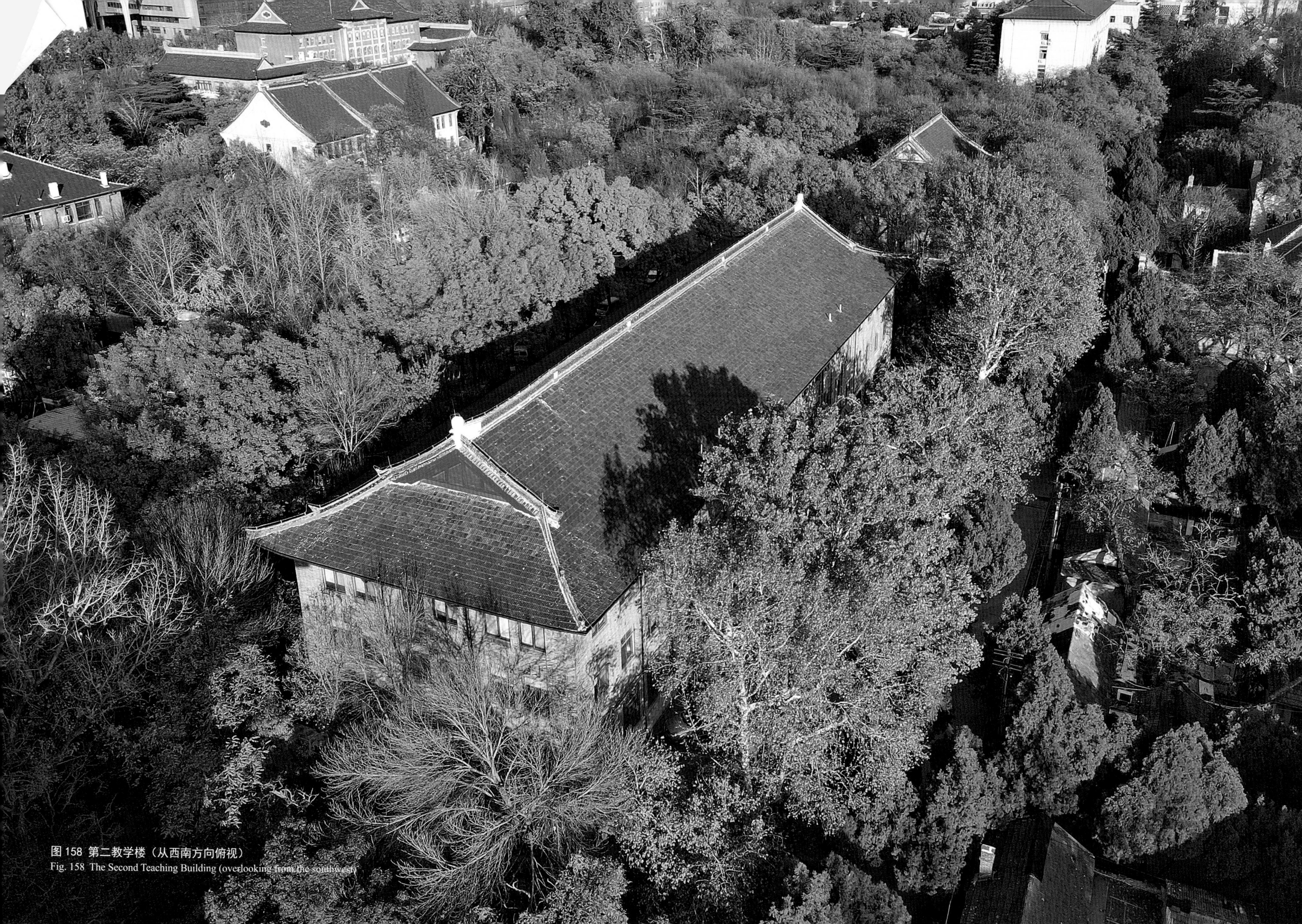

图 158 第二教学楼（从西南方向俯视）
Fig. 158 The Second Teaching Building (overlooking from the southwest)

22 第三教学楼（1）

The Third Teaching Building (1)

第三教学楼又称柏根楼，是为纪念齐鲁大学前身之一广文学堂的首任校长美国北长老会传教士柏根 (Paul D. Bergen) 而命名。此楼建成于 1917 年，是齐鲁大学初期的主要教学建筑之一。柏根楼规模宏伟，中西合璧，呈现出西方古典主义三段式特征与“中国式”大屋顶融于一体的建筑风格。此楼坐南朝北，三层，砖木石结构。楼体北面有两个主入口，南面设两个次入口。入口设计考究，做法精细，两侧装有石制立柱。在门窗装饰上，设计者独具匠心，将中国传统建筑中的“和玺彩画”进行简化、概括，作为此楼所有长条形石窗楣的雕饰纹样。屋檐和窗下墙面上，镶嵌有中国传统的“圆寿”图案。两侧耳房，南北两端较矮的卷棚屋面与中间部分较高的硬山屋面错落有致，呈和谐的组合样式。柏根楼在立面构图、色彩处理与门窗装饰等方面与考文楼、麦考密可楼相互协调一致，共同营造了齐鲁医学院中心地带的浓郁、庄严而古朴的文化氛围。

The Third Teaching Building, also known as Bergen Hall, was named to commemorate Paul D. Bergen, a missionary of the American Presbyterian Missions, North who was the first president of Wei Hsien Arts and Science College, the predecessor of Cheeloo University. This building was built in 1917 and was one of the main teaching buildings in the early days of Cheeloo University. Bergen Hall, of both Chinese and Western styles, is magnificent in scale, showing the integrated architectural style of classical Western three-section style and the large roof of Chinese style. The building faces north, with three-storey structures of brick, wood and stone. There are two main entrances to the north and two secondary entrances to the south of the building. The entrances are exquisite in design and fine in construction, with stone columns on both sides. In the decoration of doors and windows, the designers had unique ingenuity, simplifying and generalizing the “Hexi Color Painting” in the traditional Chinese architecture as the carving pattern of all the long-strip lintels of stone windows in this building. The eaves and walls under the windows are inlaid with the traditional Chinese round pattern of the Chinese character “Shou”. The ear rooms on both sides, the lower rolling shed roof at the north and south ends and the higher flush gable roof in the middle part are well spaced, showing a harmonious combination. In terms of facade composition, color treatment and decoration of doors and windows, Bergen Hall is in harmony with Calvin Mateer Hall and McCormick Hall, which jointly create a strong, solemn and simple cultural atmosphere in the center of Cheeloo College of Medicine.

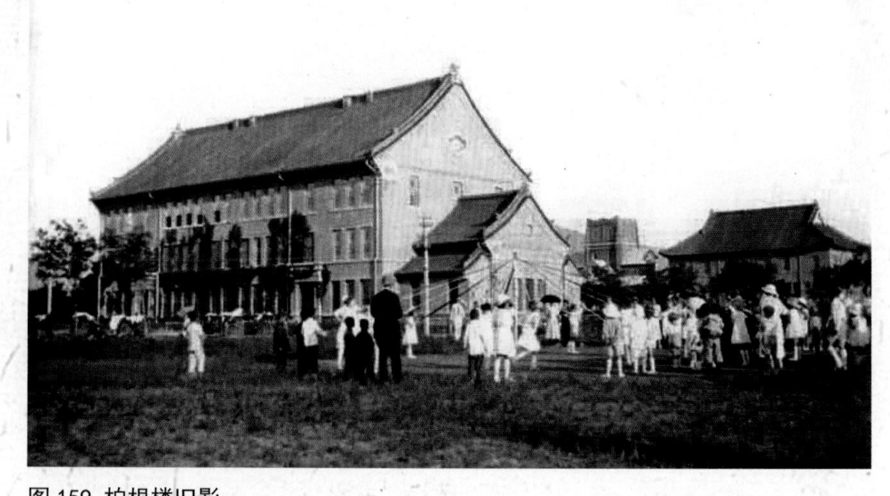

图 159 柏根楼旧影
Fig. 159 An old photo of Bergen Hall

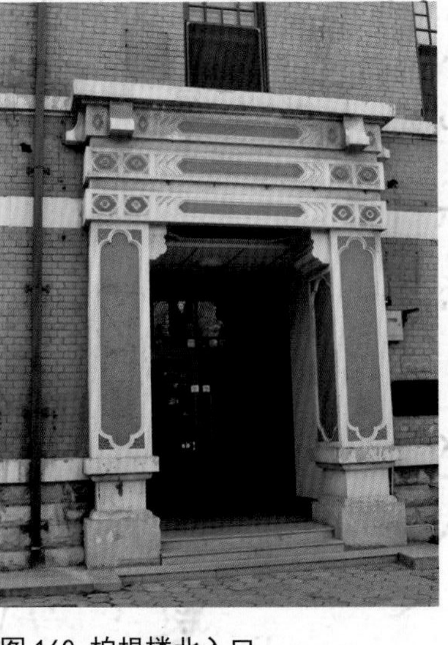

图 160 柏根楼北入口
Fig. 160 The north entrance of Bergen Hall

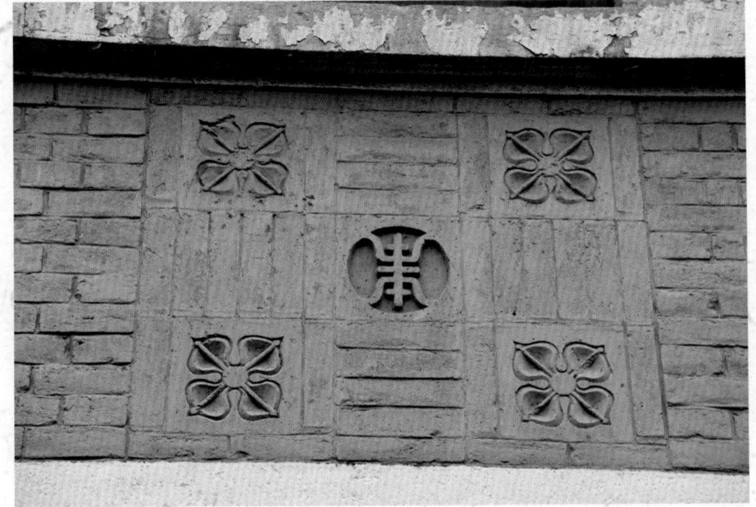

图 161 柏根楼墙面上的“圆寿”图案
Fig. 161 The round pattern of the Chinese character “Shou” on the wall of Bergen Hall

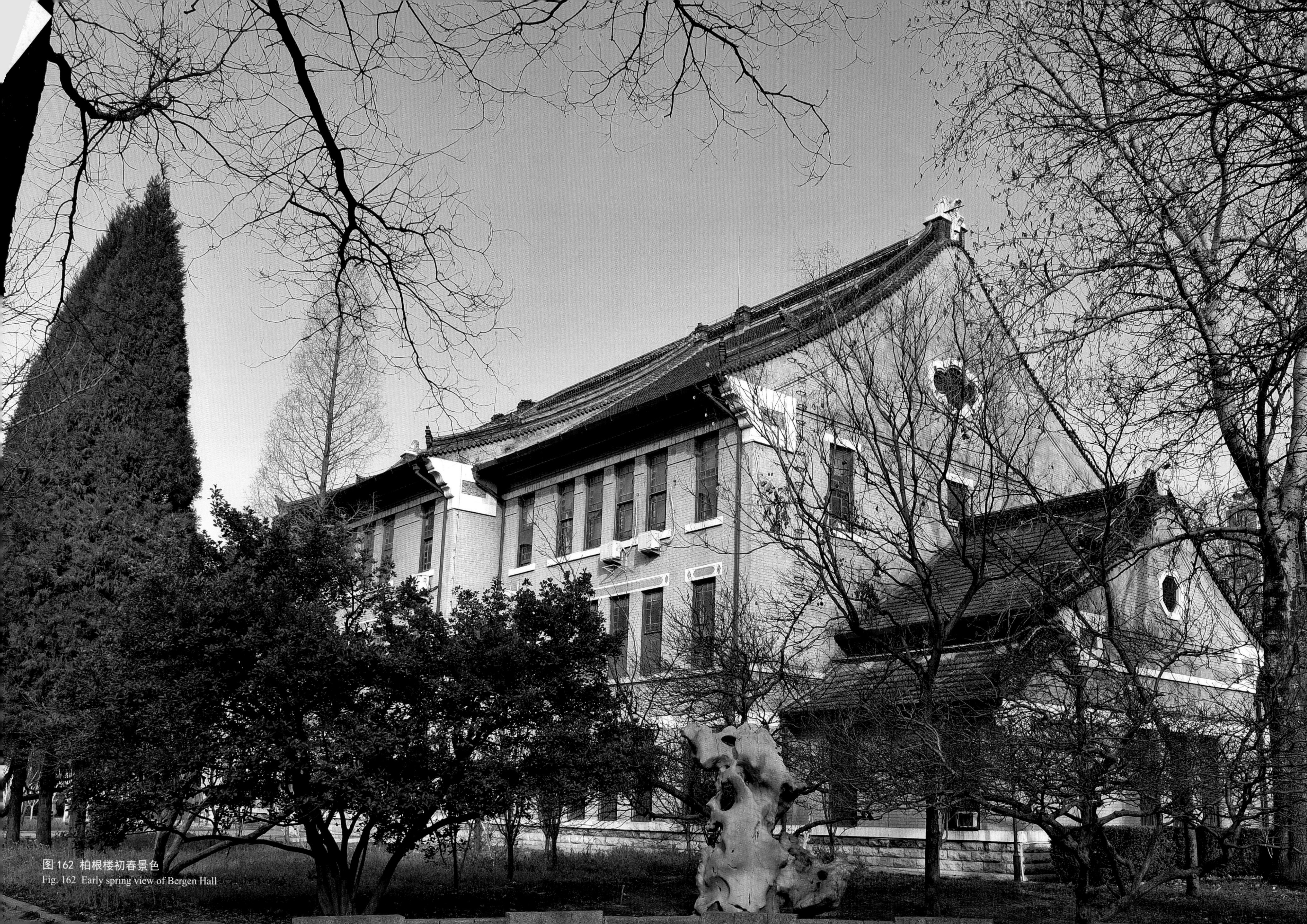

图 162 柏根楼初春景色
Fig. 162 Early spring view of Bergen Hall

22 第三教学楼（2）

The Third Teaching Building (2)

1917年9月，当文理学院和神学院迁来济南时，只有一个教学楼，即柏根楼。直到1919年考文楼建成，文理学院才有了两座教学楼，这种情形一直持续到1952年。此后，柏根楼虽被称为化学、生物学教学楼，但实际上是文理共用。水电及粗重设备、总控制机关均位于地下室；第一层为化学系和生物学系实验室；第二层为教室，文理学院学生均在此上课；第三层供教员使用，还有一个大房间，为学生团体、教员团体的活动地点。

1917年9月，齐鲁大学共有注册学生303人，其中文理学院134人、神学院51人、医学院118人。1924年7月，加拿大政府授予齐鲁大学执照，毕业生授予学士学位，医学院毕业生授予医学博士学位。1931年12月，国民政府批准私立齐鲁大学注册立案，开始同时颁发国民政府教育部统一样式的大学文凭以及原有的加拿大文凭，这也成为齐大毕业生的一大特色。

In September 1917, the College of Arts and Science and the College of Theology moved to Jinan, and there was only one teaching building, Bergen Hall. Calvin Mateer Hall was completed in 1919 and then the College of Arts and Science had two teaching buildings, which continued until 1952. After that, although Bergen Hall was called the Teaching Building of Chemistry and Biology, in fact it is used by the College of Arts and Science. The water and electricity equipment, heavy equipment and the general control switch are all located in the basement. The first floor is used as the laboratories of the Department of Chemistry and the Department of Biology. The second floor is used as the classrooms for students from the College of Arts and Science. The third floor is used by teachers, and there is also a large room for the activities of student groups and teacher groups.

In September 1917, Cheeloo University had a total of 303 registered students, including 134 from the College of Arts and Science, 51 from the College of Theology and 118 from the Medical College. In July 1924, the Government of Canada granted a license to Cheeloo University that graduates were awarded a Bachelor's Degree and graduates of the Medical College were awarded a degree of Doctor of Medicine. In December 1931, the National Government approved the registration of private Cheeloo University, and began to issue the unified university diploma of the Ministry of Education of the National Government and the original Canadian Diploma at the same time, which also became a major feature of the graduates of Cheeloo University.

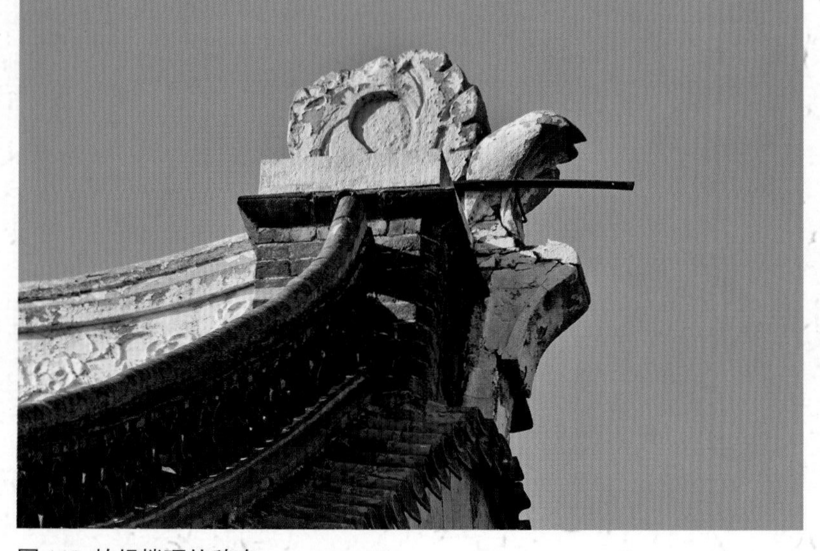

图 163 柏根楼顶的鸱吻

Fig. 163 *Chiwen* on the roof of Bergen Hal

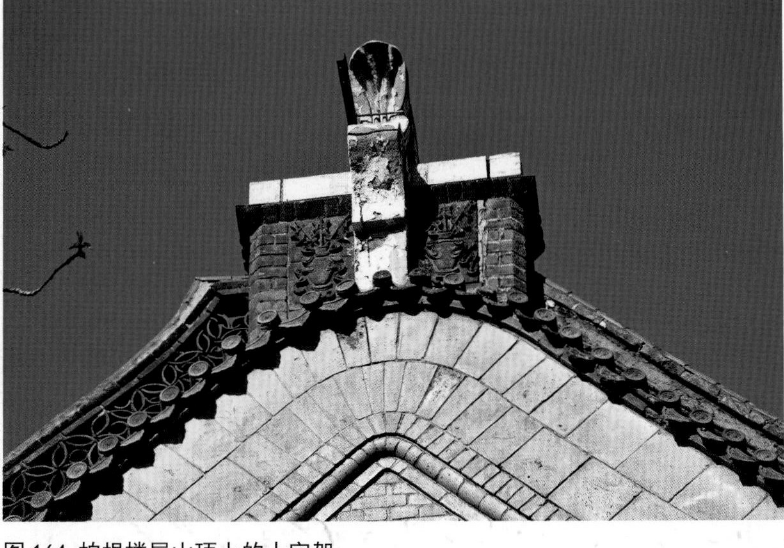

图 164 柏根楼屋山顶上的十字架

Fig. 164 Cross on the roof of Bergen Hall

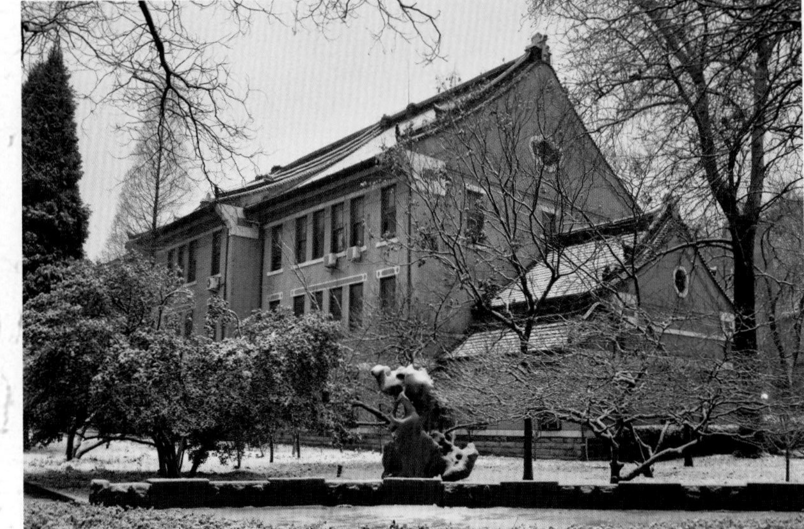

图 165 柏根楼雪景

Fig. 165 Snow view of Bergen Hall

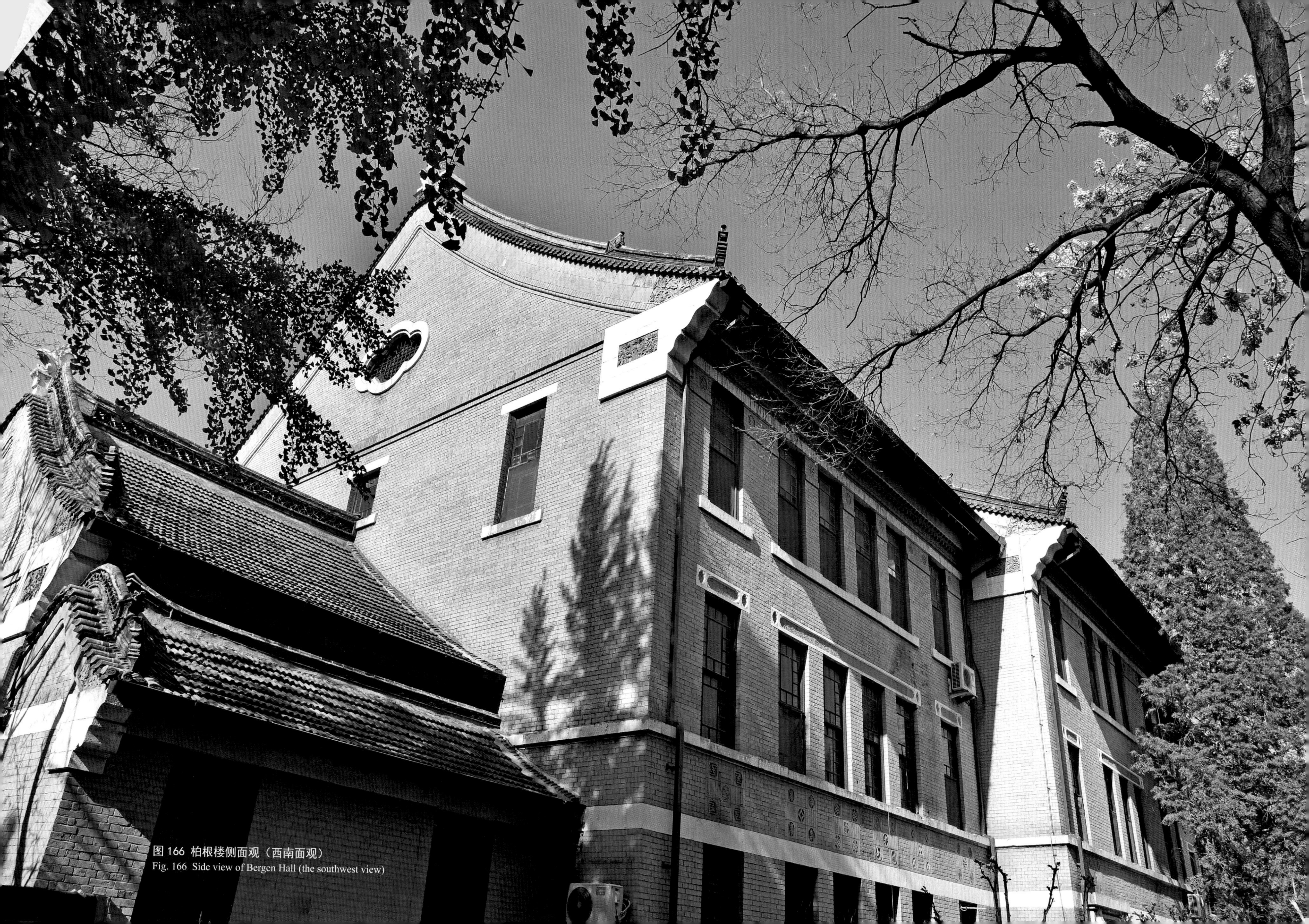

图 166 柏根楼侧面观（西南面观）
Fig. 166 Side view of Bergen Hall (the southwest view)

22 第三教学楼（3）

The Third Teaching Building (3)

1930 年，文理学院分为文学院和理学院。

文学院的鼎盛时期在 1930 年至 1937 年。那时，根据栾调甫教授的倡议，创办了国学研究所，经费来源于哈佛燕京学社。先后有老舍、顾颉刚、钱穆、严耕望、郝立权、余天庥、王敦化、范迪瑞等知名学者在所内做研究，齐鲁大学一时成为全国国学研究的重地。学校除编辑出版学术性校刊《齐大季刊》外，国学研究所还编辑出版了《国学汇编》，在国内外都较有影响。明义士、马彦祥、张维华和孙伏园等一大批文化精英也在此任教。

齐鲁大学的文科学生中，刘谦初是最为出色的一位。1918 年至 1920 年，刘谦初在齐鲁大学预科班学习。因偶然机会，1922 年保送进入北京燕京大学。1927 年 1 月加入中国共产党，1928 年夏任中共福建省委书记。1929 年初，以齐鲁大学助教身份作掩护到山东工作，任山东省委书记兼宣传部长。1929 年 8 月不幸被捕。1931 年 4 月 5 日，与邓恩铭等 22 名党员一起在济南纬八路英勇就义，年仅 34 岁。其妻子为张文秋，女儿是刘思齐（毛岸英妻子）。

In 1930, the College of Arts and Science was divided into the School of Liberal Arts and the School of Science.

The School of Liberal Arts flourished from 1930 to 1937. At that time, according to Professor Luan Diaofu's initiative, the Institute of National Studies was established, with funds from the Harvard-Yenching Institute. Lao She, Gu Jiegang, Qian Mu, Yan Gengwang, Hao Liquan, Yu Tianxiu, Wang Dunhua, Fan Dirui and other well-known scholars did the research in the institute one after another, and Cheeloo University became the focus of the National Studies all over the country for a time. The university also edited the academic journal *Quarterly Journal of Cheeloo University* and the Institute of National Studies edited and published *Compilation of National Studies*, both of which had an influence at home and abroad. A large number of cultural elite such as Ming Yishi, Ma Yanxiang, Zhang Weihua and Sun Fuyuan all once taught here.

Liu Qianchu is the most outstanding student of liberal arts at Cheeloo University. From 1918 to 1920, Liu Qianchu studied in the preparatory class of Cheeloo University. By chance, he was admitted to Yenching University in Beijing in 1922. He joined the Communist Party of China in January 1927 and was appointed Secretary of the Fujian Provincial Committee of the Communist Party of China in the summer of 1928. At the beginning of 1929, he came to work in Shandong under the cover of a teaching assistant of Cheeloo University and served as Secretary of Shandong Provincial Committee of the Communist Party of China and Minister of Publicity. Unfortunately, he was arrested in August 1929. On 5 April 1931, he died bravely at the age of 34 with Deng Enming and other 20 party members on Weiba Road in Jinan. His wife is Zhang Wenqiu and his daughter is Liu Siqi (wife of Mao Anying).

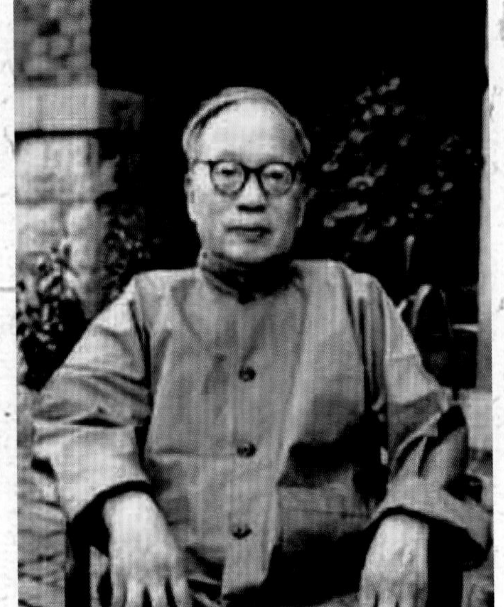

图 167 栾调甫先生

Fig. 167 Mr. Luan Diaofu

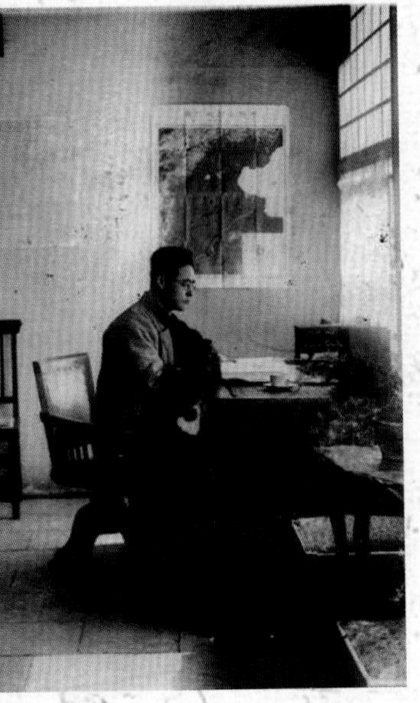

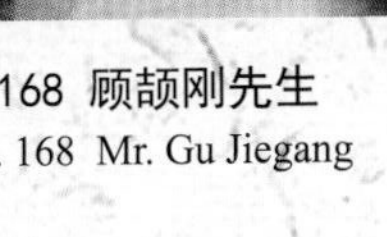

图 168 顾颉刚先生

Fig. 168 Mr. Gu Jiegang

图 169 齐鲁大学校友、原山东省委书记刘谦初

Fig. 169 Liu Qianchu, alumnus of Cheeloo University and former Secretary of Shandong Provincial Committee of the Communist Party of China

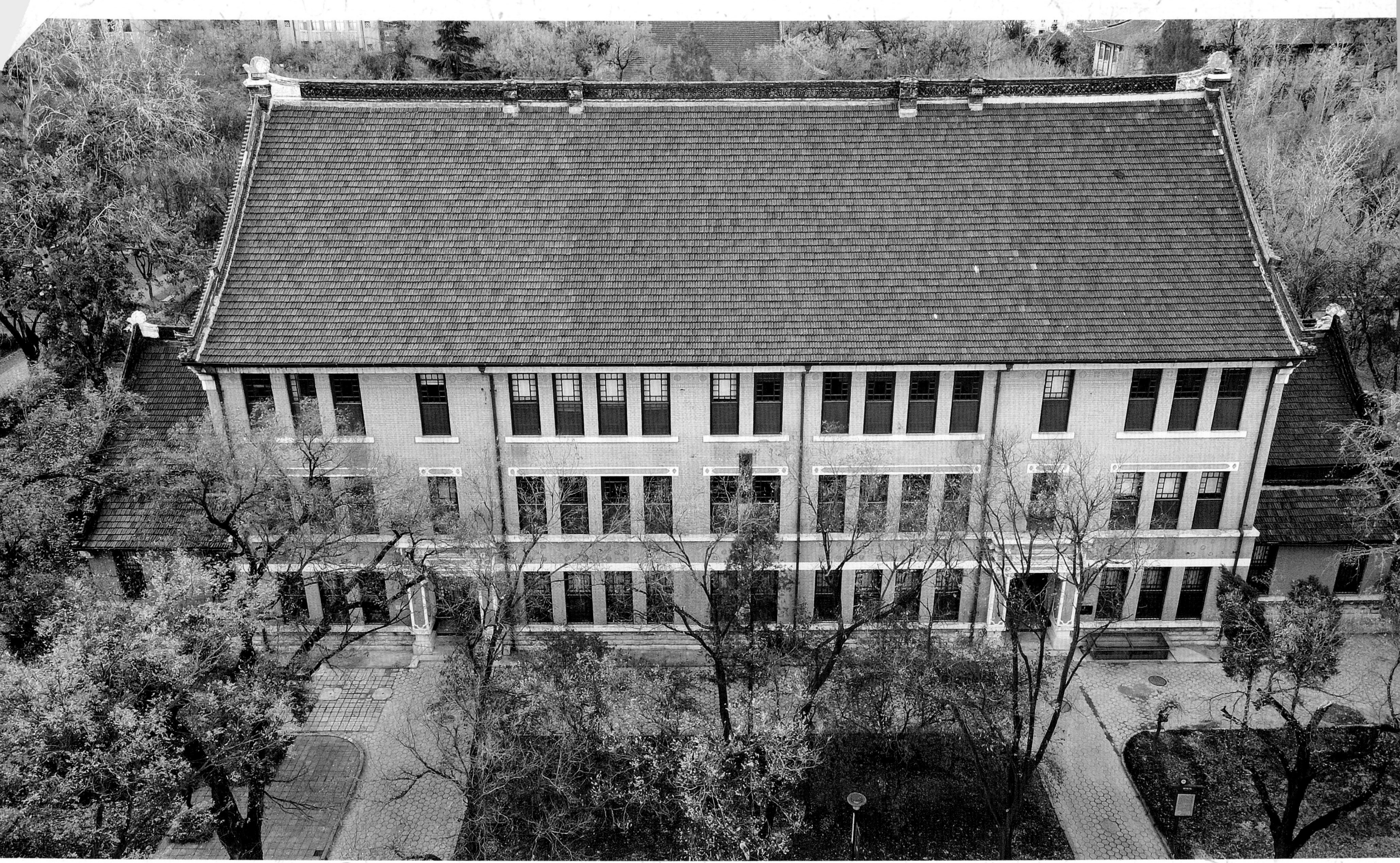

图 170 柏根楼北面观
Fig. 170 The north view of Bergen Hall

22 第三教学楼（4）

The Third Teaching Building (4)

齐鲁大学理学院在教学中除了要求学生准确把握理论知识以外，特别强调实验操作和严谨治学态度的秉持，培养了一大批我国各类学科的奠基人，如化学系毕业生薛愚。

薛愚（1894~1988），药物化学家和药学教育家，湖北襄阳人。1925 年毕业于齐鲁大学化学系，任清华大学讲师。1933 年获巴黎大学理科博士学位，回国任河南大学、暨南大学教授。1939 年至 1944 年任齐鲁大学教授兼化学系、药学系主任及理学院院长。1946 年任国立北京大学医学院药学系教授兼系主任。1949 年出席全国政协第一届全体会议。新中国成立后，任北京医学院药学系主任、教授，北京医科大学药学院名誉院长，中国药学会理事长。编著有《实用有机药物化学》《普通化学定性分析：实验教程》《医用有机化学》《中国药学史料》等。他对中国的药学建设与发展做出了突出贡献，是中国药学教育事业奠基者之一。

In addition to requiring students to accurately grasp the theoretical knowledge, the School of Science of Cheeloo University also emphasized the experimental operation and rigorous scholarship, and it had trained a large number of founders of various disciplines in China, such as Xue Yu, a graduate of the Department of Chemistry.

Xue Yu (1894-1988), a pharmaceutical chemist and educator, was born in Xiangyang, Hubei Province. In 1925, he graduated from the Department of Chemistry of Cheeloo University and then served as a lecturer at Tsinghua University. In 1933, he got a degree of Doctor of Science from the University of Paris and returned home to serve as a professor at Henan University and Jinan University. From 1939 to 1944, he was a professor at Cheeloo University and at the same time served as the director of the Department of Chemistry and the Department of Pharmacy and Dean of the School of Science. In 1946, he served as a professor and director of the Department of Pharmacy of the Medical College of National Peking University. In 1949, he attended the first plenary session of the Chinese People's Political Consultative Conference. After the founding of the People's Republic of China he served as the director and professor of the Department of Pharmacy of Beijing Medical College, honorary dean of the School of Pharmacy of Beijing Medical University, and president of the Chinese Pharmaceutical Association. He had compiled *Practical Organic Pharmaceutical Chemistry*, *Qualitative Analysis of General Chemistry: A Practical Course*, *Medical Organic Chemistry*, *Historical Materials of Chinese Pharmacy* and so on. He has made outstanding contributions to the construction and development of pharmacy in China, and is one of the founders of pharmaceutical education in China.

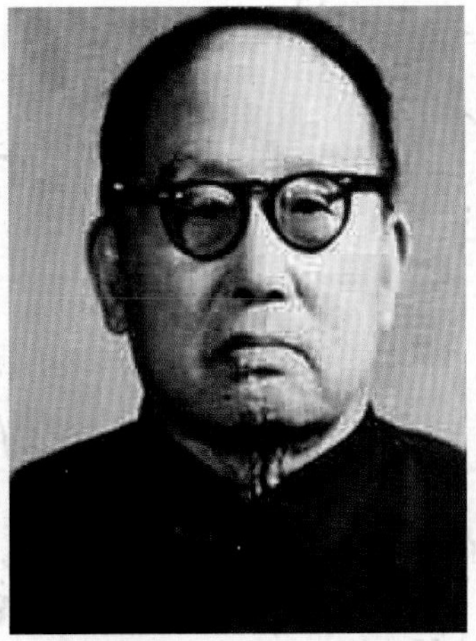

图 171 齐鲁大学化学系毕业生薛愚教授
Fig. 171 Professor Xue Yu, graduate of the Department of Chemistry of Cheeloo University

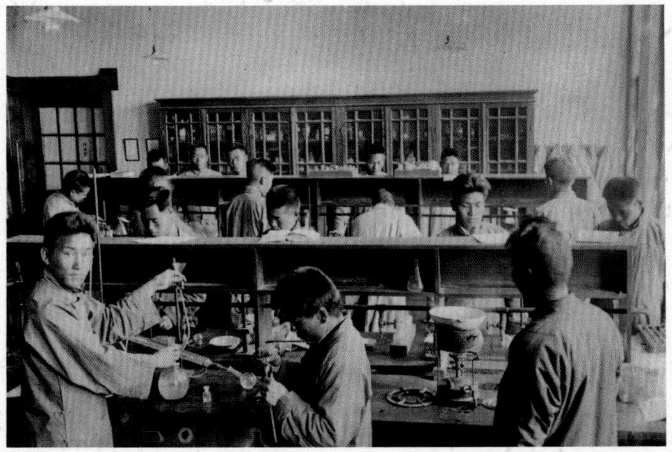

图 172 齐鲁大学学生在做实验
Fig. 172 Students doing experiments at Cheeloo University

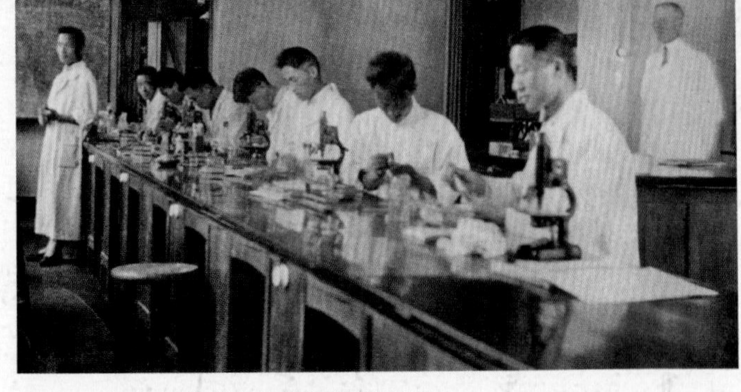

图 173 齐鲁大学学生在做细菌学实验
Fig. 173 Students doing bacteriological experiments at Cheeloo University

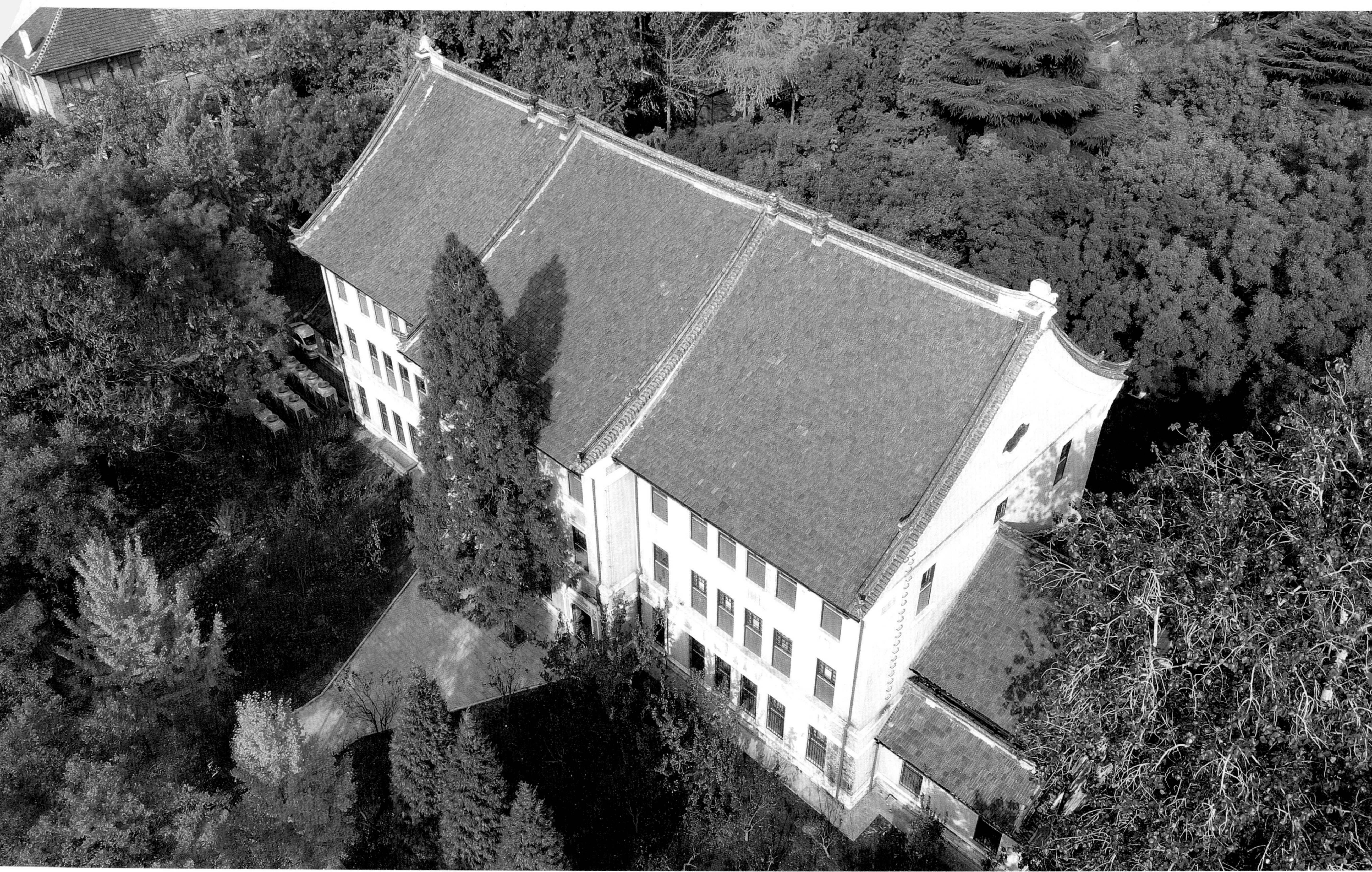

图 174 柏根楼鸟瞰
Fig. 174 A bird's-eye view of Bergen Hall

23 第四教学楼（1）

The Fourth Teaching Building (1)

第四教学楼又称葛罗神学院楼，建成于 1921 年，为齐鲁大学神学院旧址。此楼为齐鲁大学早期的主要建筑之一，与东面的教学七楼（原为奥古斯丁图书馆）隔中心花园相望。

齐鲁大学神学院起源于青州培真书院。1881 年，英国基督教浸礼会传教士仲均安、怀恩光和卜道成于青州最初租用民房创办圣道学堂，培养布道员。1885 年发展成为青州神学院，中文校名“培真书院”。1893 年培真书院得到英国布瑞斯特尔城爱德华 · 罗宾逊夫妇的捐赠，新建校舍。因捐款是为了纪念罗宾逊太太的父亲葛奇博士和罗宾逊先生的父亲伊利沙 · 罗宾逊，故书院改名为“葛罗神学院”（Gotch-Robinson Theological College）。1917 年 9 月葛罗神学院迁来济南，成为齐鲁大学重要的组成部分。

The Fourth Teaching Building, also known as Gotch-Robinson Theological Building, was built in 1921 and is the old site of the Theological College of Cheeloo University. This building is one of the main buildings of Cheeloo University in its early days. It faces the Seventh Teaching Building (former Augustine Library) in the east across the Central Garden.

The Theological College of Cheeloo University originated from Peizhen Academy in Qingzhou. In 1881, the English Baptist missionaries Alfred G. Jones, John Sutherland Whitewright and Joseph Percy Bruce rented private houses to set up Theological Institute in Qingzhou to train preachers. In 1885, the church developed into Tsingchow Theological College, with the Chinese name of “Peizhen Academy”. In 1893, Peizhen Academy was donated by Edward Robinson and his wife in Bristol, the United Kingdom to build new school buildings. The donation was made in memory of Mrs. Robinson’s father, Dr. Gotch, and Mr. Robinson’s father, Elisha Robinson, so the academy was renamed Gotch-Robinson Theological College. In September 1917, Gotch-Robinson Theological College moved to Jinan and became an important part of Cheeloo University.

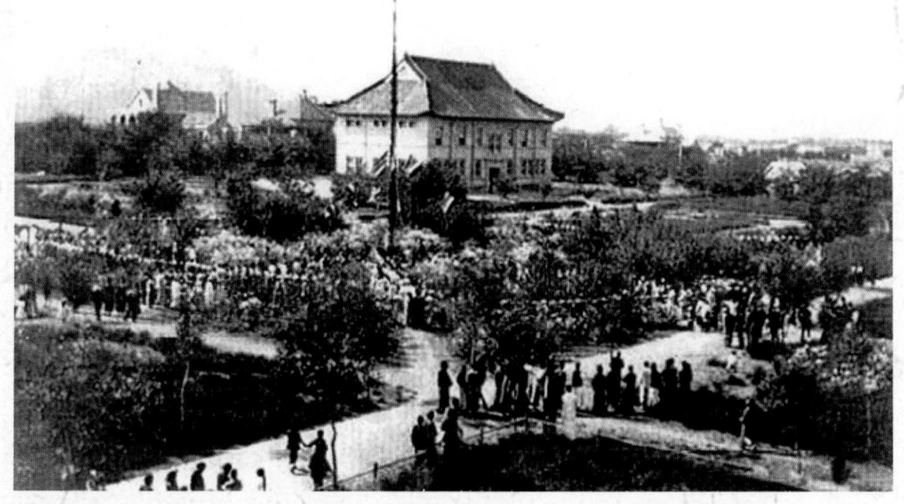

图 175 1921 年 10 月 1 日葛罗神学院楼落成庆典

Fig. 175 The dedication of Gotch-Robinson Theological Building held on 1 October 1921

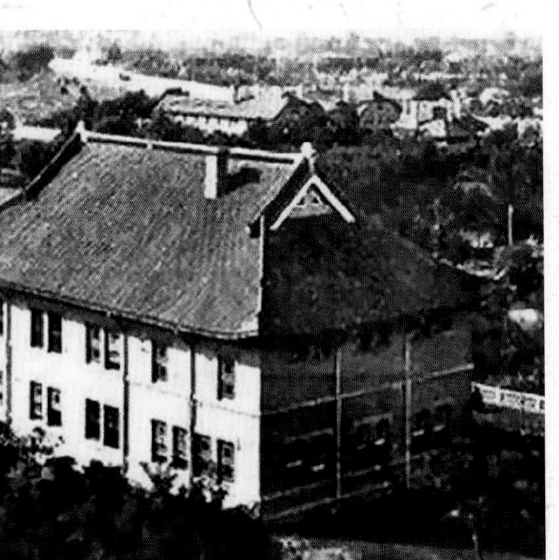

图 176 葛罗神学院楼旧影

Fig. 176 An old photo of Gotch-Robinson Theological Building

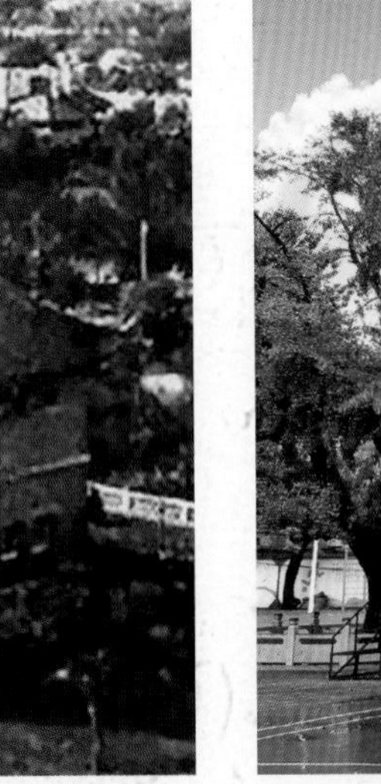

图 177 青州培真书院旧址

Fig. 177 Old site of Peizhen Academy in Qingzhou

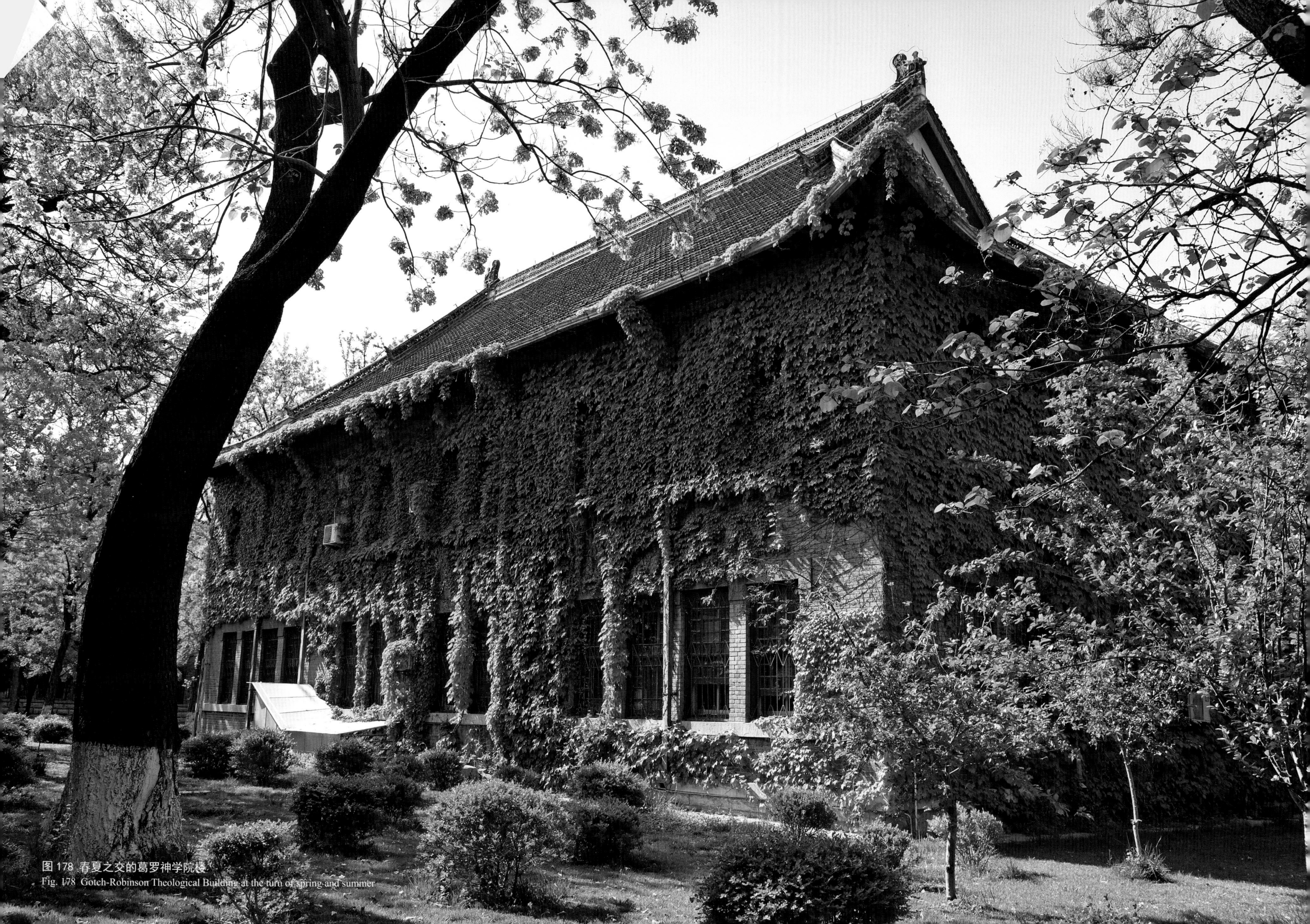

图 178 春夏之交的葛罗神学院楼
Fig. 178 Gotch-Robinson Theological Building at the turn of spring and summer

23 第四教学楼（2）
The Fourth Teaching Building (2)

第四教学楼位于中心花园西南方，中国式大屋顶，二层砖木石结构，带有地下室；歇山灰瓦屋面，内置简易三角形木梁架，翼角具有起翘特征。建筑平面呈规整长方形，由中间东西向长廊串联南北向的房间；主入口位于建筑北侧中央处。此楼布满爬山虎，夏绿秋红，景色怡人。

此楼曾为诊断学教研室用房，现为临床技能培训中心。齐鲁医学院的诊断学在全国具有重要地位，自戚仁铎教授开始，主编了全国规划教材《诊断学》第 1 ~ 9 版。戚仁铎（1921 ~ 2009），山东烟台人，我国著名诊断学和血液病学专家。1947 年考入华东白求恩医学院，毕业后留校任教。1956 年 10 月赴苏联留学，学习血液病，1959 年底获医学副博士学位。曾任山东医科大学诊断学教研室主任、教授，主编全国高等医药院校统编教材《诊断学》第 1 ~ 4 版，一直担任全国高等医药院校诊断学教学咨询委员会主任委员，对我国的诊断学教学影响巨大。

The Fourth Teaching Building is located in the southwest of the Central Garden, with a large Chinese roof, a two-storey structure with brick, wood and stone, and a basement. It has the gable and hip roof of grey tiles and built-in simple triangular frame of wooden beam, and the wing angle with warping characteristics. The building plane is a regular rectangle, and the north-south rooms are connected in series by the east-west corridor in the middle. The main entrance is located in the center of the northern side of the building. This building is full of creepers, green in summer and red in autumn, and the scenery is pleasant.

This building was once used as the Teaching and Research Office of Diagnostics, and is now a training center of clinical skills. The diagnostics of Cheeloo College of Medicine occupies an important position in the whole country. Professor Qi Renduo has edited the National Planning Textbook *Diagnostics* from the first to the ninth editions. Qi Renduo (1921-2009), a native of Yantai, Shandong Province, is a famous expert in diagnostics and hematology in China. In 1947, he was admitted to East China Bethune Medical College and stayed in the university to teach after graduation. In October 1956, he went to the Soviet Union to study blood diseases and obtained an associate doctor's degree in medicine at the end of 1959. He once served as director and professor of the Teaching and Research Office of Diagnostics of Shandong Medical University. He has edited 1-4 editions of the textbook *Diagnostics* of National Higher Medical Colleges and Universities. He has been the chairman of the Teaching Advisory Committee of Diagnostics of National Higher Medical Colleges and Universities, and has a great impact on the teaching of diagnostics in China.

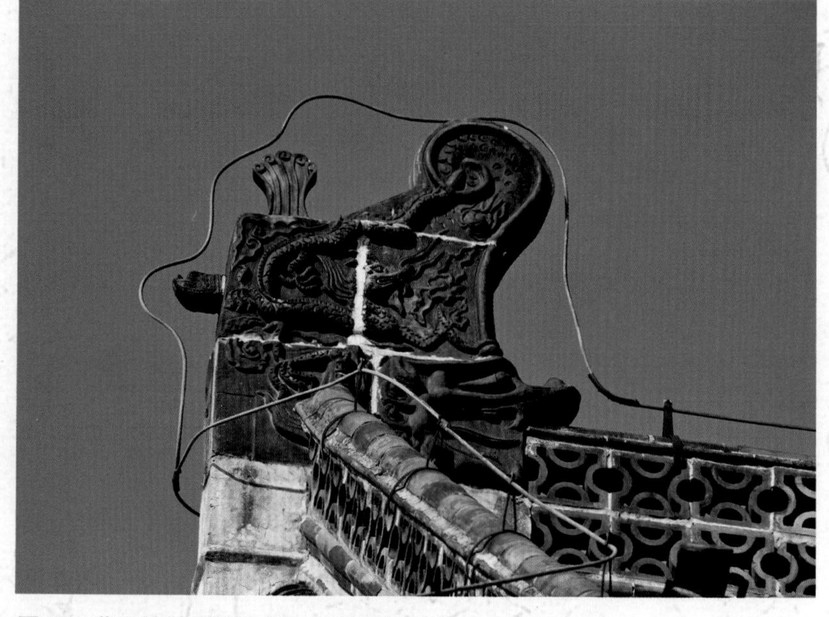

图 179 葛罗神学院楼屋山顶上的鸱吻
Fig. 179 *Chiwen* on the ridge of Gotch-Robinson Theological Building

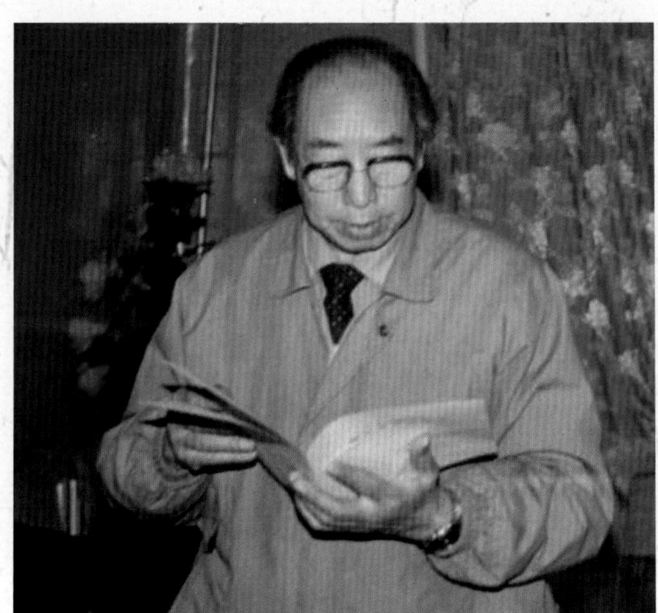

图 180 著名诊断学专家戚仁铎教授
Fig. 180 Professor Qi Renduo, a famous expert in diagnostics

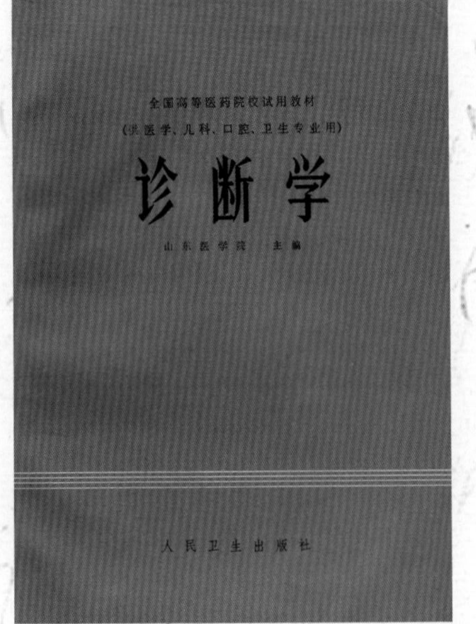

图 181 山东医学院主编的全国统编教材《诊断学》第 1 版
Fig. 181 The first edition of *Diagnosis*, a national textbook edited by Shandong Medical College

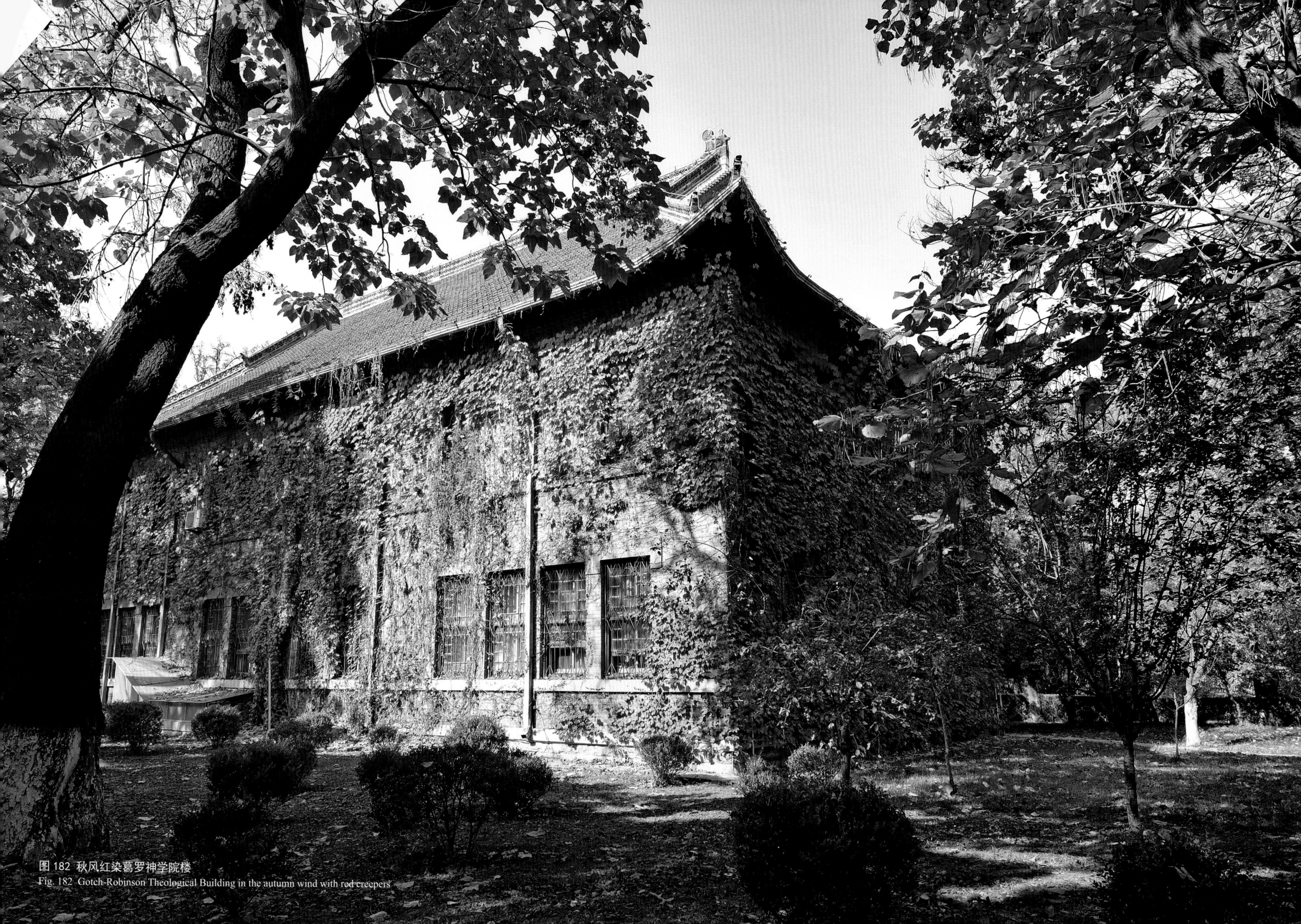

图 182 秋风红染葛罗神学院楼

Fig. 182 Gotch-Robinson Theological Building in the autumn wind with red creepers

24 第五教学楼（1）

The Fifth Teaching Building (1)

第五教学楼建成于 1919 年，又称考文楼，是为了纪念登州文会馆创始人狄考文而命名的。考文楼的设计者为亨利·基拉姆·墨菲，一位崇尚中国传统建筑精神的美国著名建筑设计师。他将中国特别是济南当地的建筑特色与西方古典主义建筑手法融为一体，塑造了考文楼明显的“中国复兴式”建筑风格。整体立面以西方古典主义三段式为主，主楼地上三层、地下一层，两侧设单层耳房。屋顶曲线流畅，舒展大气，正脊两端的鸱吻形态飞扬，暗含“十字架”造形。山墙形式为硬山，有宽大、厚实的挑檐石和墀头。一个大门居北面中间，门楼气质典雅，门外两侧有一对大型抱鼓石，彰显此楼较高的建筑规格。墙面镶嵌着组合有序、变化丰富的万字纹、寿字纹和菊花纹等中国传统图案。总之，考文楼与周围建筑风格相似且富有变化，它们相互呼应，在齐鲁大学校园内共同谱就了一部融会中西、曲调舒缓、和而不同之凝固的华美乐章。

The Fifth Teaching Building was built in 1919, also known as Calvin Mateer Hall in memory of Calvin Wilson Mateer, the founder of Tengchow College. The designer of Calvin Mateer Hall is Henry Killam Murphy, a famous American architect who appreciated the spirit of traditional Chinese architecture. He combined the architectural characteristics of China, especially of Jinan, with Western classical architectural techniques, and shaped the obvious “Chinese architectural style of revival” of Calvin Mateer Hall. The overall facade is mainly of Western classical three-section style, and the main building has three floors above ground and one floor below ground, with single-storey ear rooms on both sides. The curve of the roof is smooth, unfolding and generous, and the shape of *chiwen* at both ends of the main ridge presents a flying posture, implying the “cross” shape. On the flush gable roof are wide and thick cornice stones and *chitou*. A gate is located in the middle of the north. The elegant arch and a pair of large drum stones on both sides outside the gate demonstrate the high architectural specifications of the building. The walls are inlaid with orderly and varied traditional Chinese patterns, such as the swastika pattern, the Chinese character “shou” and chrysanthemums. In a word, the style of Calvin Mateer Hall is similar to that of the surrounding buildings, but full of changes at the same time. They echo each other and jointly compose a beautiful movement on campus of Cheeloo University that is a Chinese and Western fusion with soothing melody, harmonious but different.

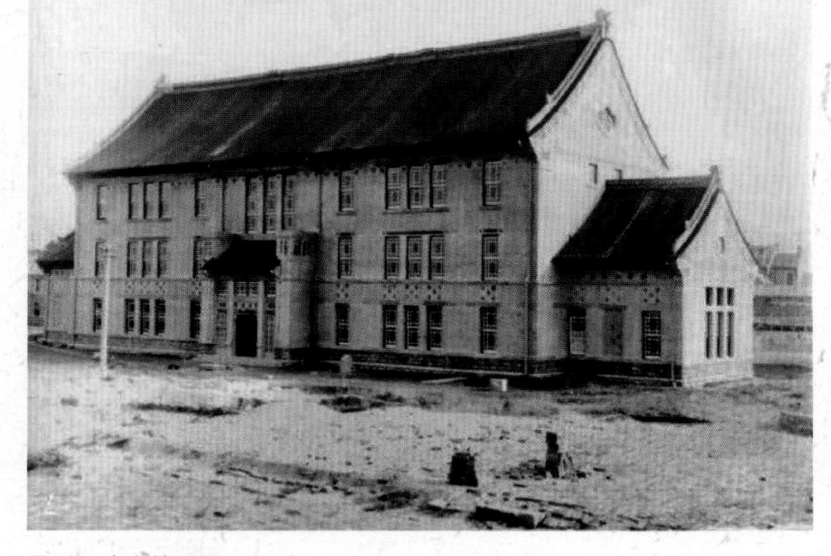

图 183 考文楼旧影
Fig. 183 An old photo of Calvin Mateer Hal

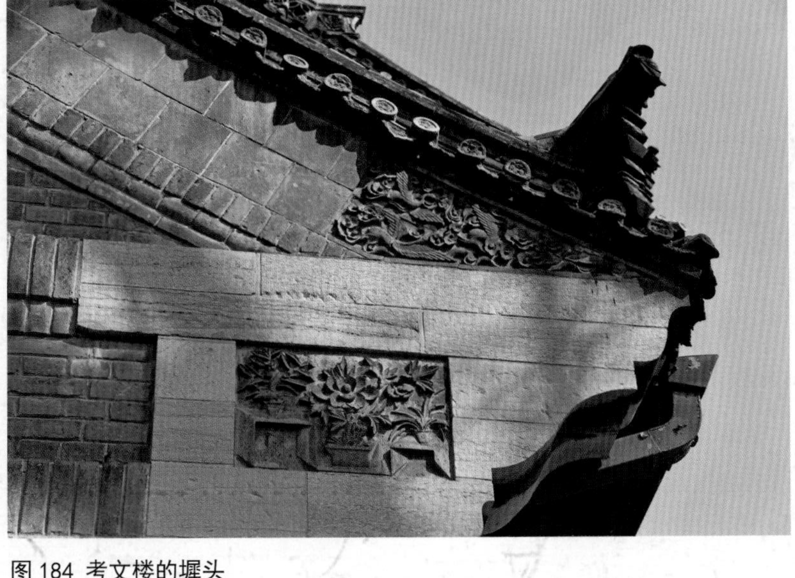

图 184 考文楼的墀头
Fig. 184 *Chitou* of Calvin Mateer Hall

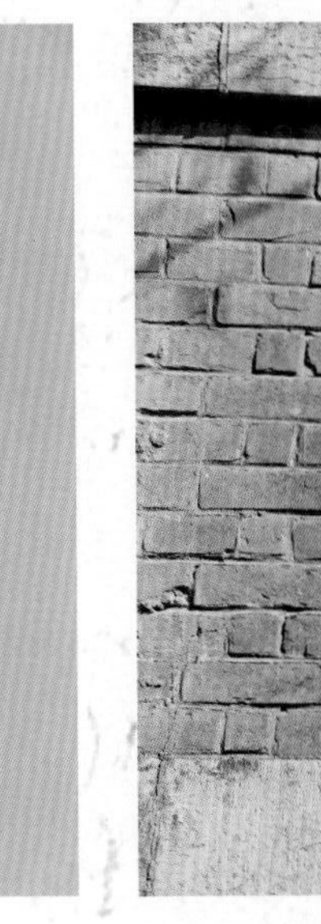

图 185 考文楼墙面上的砖雕
Fig. 185 Brick carvings on the gable of Calvin Mateer Hall

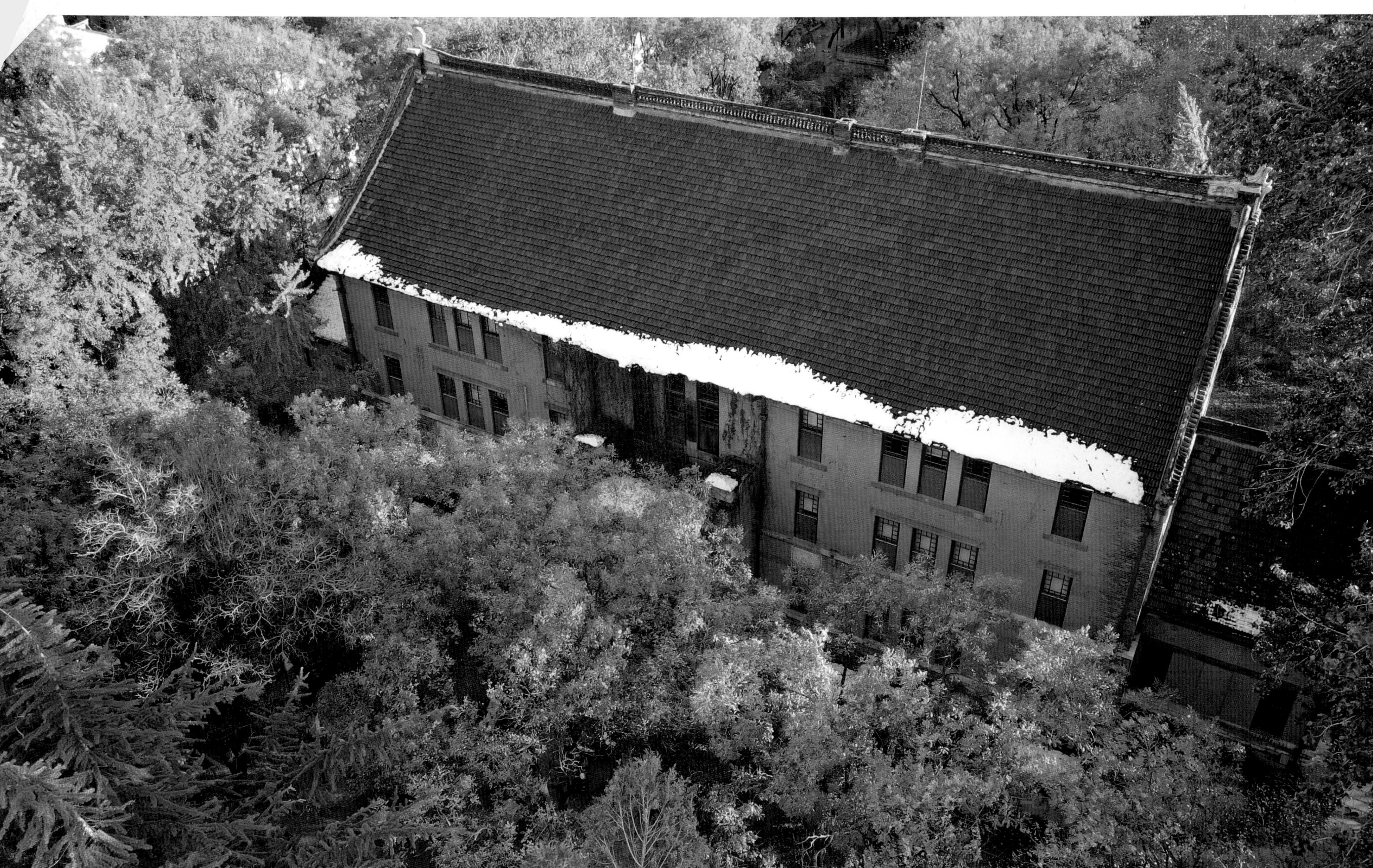

图 186 考文楼北面观
Fig. 186 The north view of Calvin Mateer Hall

24 第五教学楼（2）
The Fifth Teaching Building (2)

考文楼的建筑特色除门楼和抱鼓石外，其内部空间处理吸收了西方建筑理念，在所有的齐鲁大学建筑中是最值得一提的。在入口大厅中轴两侧设有木制楼梯，一层到二层为平行双合楼梯，经过歇步，二层到三层为三跑楼梯，楼梯级数按照中国习俗的“3”“5”“7”为基数而设置。楼梯带有简洁朴素的扶栏，涂以华贵的紫红色。下楼时昂首挺胸，发出咚咚的脚步声，给人一种高傲的满足感。

考文楼是齐鲁大学早期的标志性建筑，为物理学、生理学教学楼，但实际上文理共用。一切水电及粗重设备、总控制机关均位于地下室；第一层为物理学系及其实验室、生理学标本室与实验室；第二层为物理学、生理学、心理学等学科的教室，文理学院学生和医学院预科学生均在此上课；第三层是各社会科学的教室以及教员用房。

In addition to the arch and drum stones, the architectural features of Calvin Mateer Hall absorb the Western architectural concept in the internal space treatment, which is the most worthy of mention in all buildings at Cheeloo University. Wooden stairs are arranged on both sides of the central axis of the entrance hall. The first floor to the second floor are parallel double stairs, and after a rest is the second floor to the third floor with three-run stairs. The number of stairs is set according to the Chinese custom of “3”, “5” and “7” as the base. The stairs have simple handrails, painted with luxurious purple color. When you go downstairs, hold the head high, and you will have a feel of proud satisfaction with a knock of footsteps.

Calvin Mateer Hall is a landmark building in the early days of Cheeloo University. Although it was called the Teaching Building of Physics and Physiology, in fact it is used by the College of Arts and Science. The water and electricity equipment, heavy equipment and the general control switch are all located in the basement. The first floor is for the Department of Physics and its laboratories, and specimen rooms and laboratories of physiology. The second floor is used as the classrooms of physics, physiology, psychology and other disciplines, where students from the College of Arts and Science and preparatory students from the Medical School attend classes. The third floor is used as the classrooms of social sciences and the rooms for teachers.

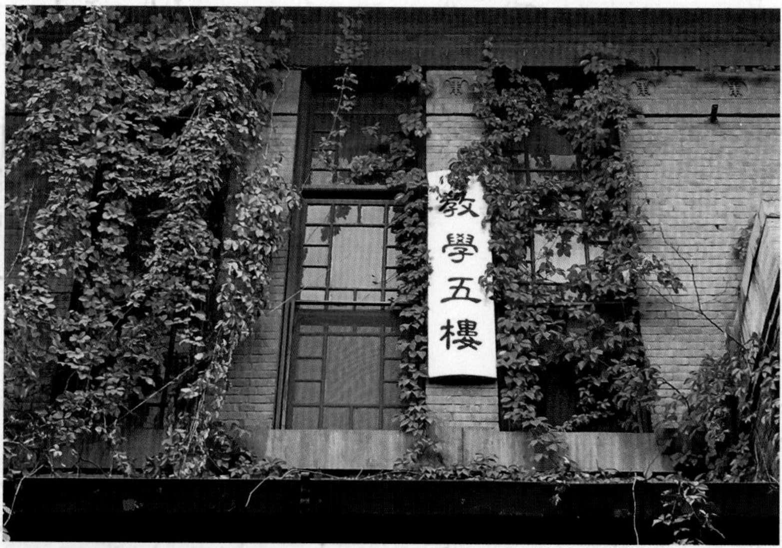

图 187 考文楼大门秋色宜人
Fig. 187 The charming autumn scenery of the gate of Calvin Mateer Hall

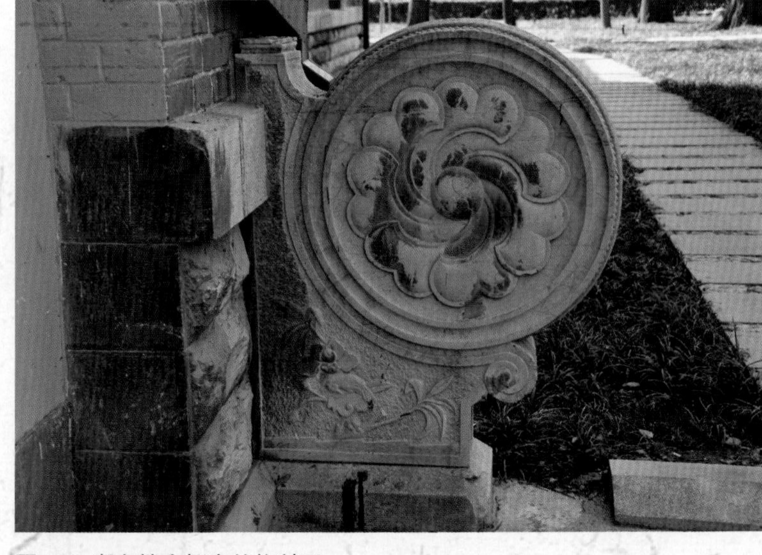
图 188 考文楼大门旁的抱鼓石
Fig. 188 Drum stone by the gate of Calvin Mateer Hall

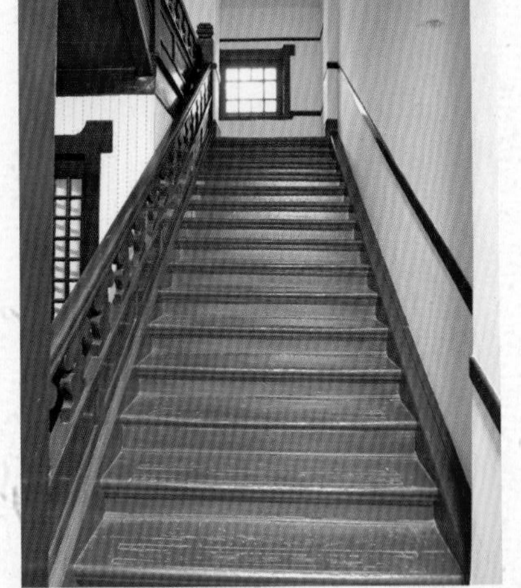
图 189 考文楼内部楼梯
Fig. 189 Interior staircase of Calvin Mateer Hall

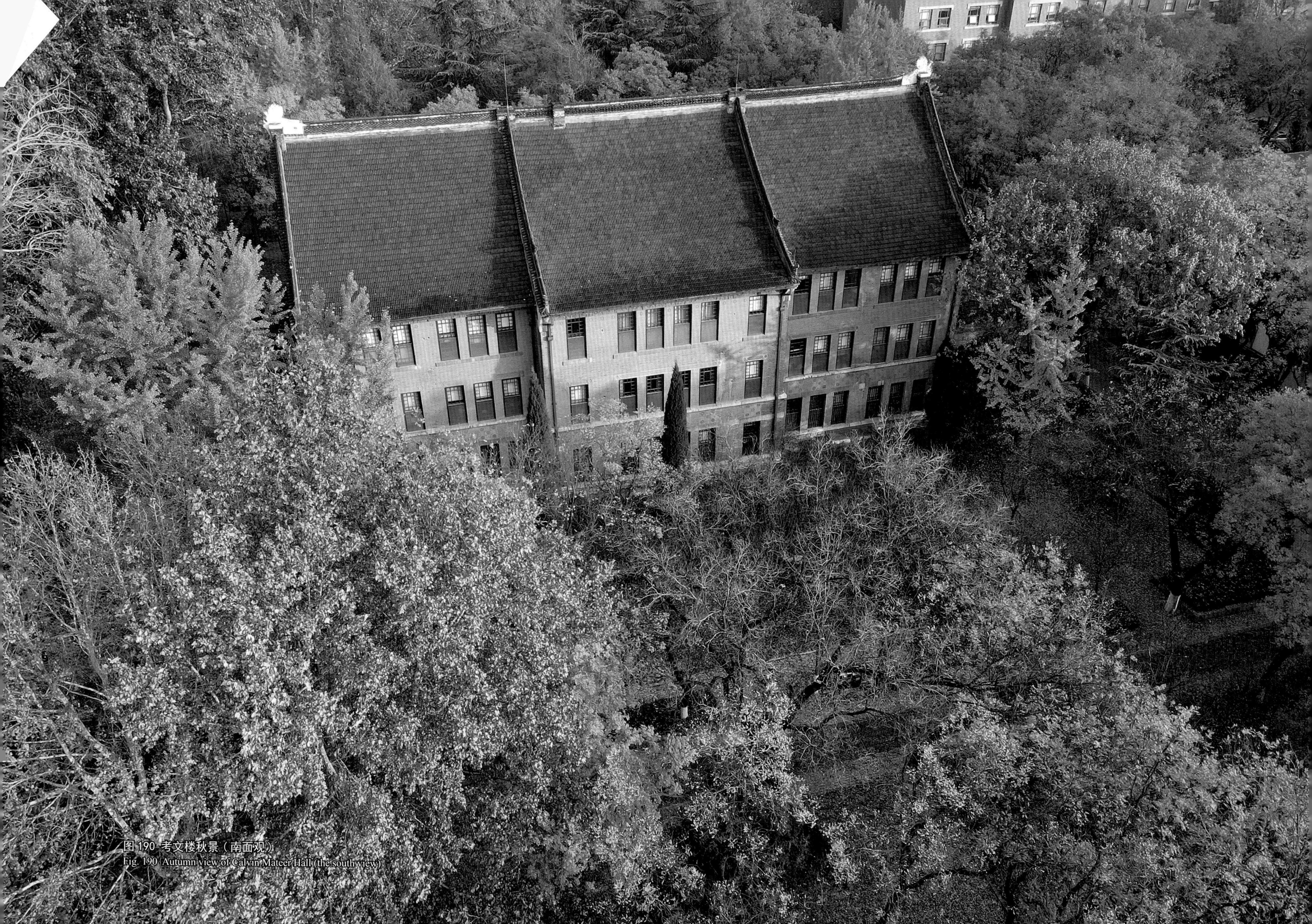

图 190 考文楼秋景（南面观）
Fig. 190 Autumn view of Calvin Mateer Hall (the south view)

24 第五教学楼（3）

The Fifth Teaching Building (3)

考文楼与柏根楼为齐鲁大学文学院和理学院的两个主要教学楼。文学院设有中国文学系、历史社会系、政治经济系与教育系。理学院包括天文系、数学系、物理学系、化学系、生物学系与制药系，附设无线电专修科。

齐鲁大学物理学系有一位天才学子，被称为“中国的爱因斯坦”和“中国雷达之父”，他就是著名的理论物理学家束星北。束星北（1907 ~ 1983），江苏南通人，1925 年 9 月至 1926 年 4 月在齐鲁大学物理学系学习，后至欧洲和美国留学。1927 年在柏林大学威廉皇家物理研究所给爱因斯坦当了一段时间研究助手，开始研究相对论。1931 年回国，赴浙江大学任教。1948 年齐鲁大学理学院暂迁杭州，束星北偕同苏步青、陈建功和王淦昌等一流名师被邀请到齐鲁大学兼课。1952 年，因院系调整，到山东大学物理系任教，并转向大气动力学研究。束星北是诺贝尔物理学奖获得者李政道和中国科学院院士程开甲等的物理学启蒙老师。

Calvin Mateer Hall and Bergen Hall are the two main teaching buildings of the School of Literature and the School of Science of Cheeloo University. The School of Literature has the Department of Chinese Literature, the Department of Historical Sociology, the Department of Political Economy and the Department of Education. The School of Science includes the Department of Astronomy, the Department of Mathematics, the Department of Physics, the Department of Chemistry, the Department of Biology and the Department of Pharmacy, with a specialty in radio.

There was a talented student in the Department of Physics of Cheeloo University, known as “China’s Einstein” and “the Father of Radar in China”. He is the famous theoretical physicist Shu Xingbei. Shu Xingbei (1907-1983), born in Nantong, Jiangsu Province, studied in the Department of Physics of Cheeloo University from September 1925 to April 1926, and then went to study in Europe and the United States. In 1927, he worked as a research assistant for Einstein at the Kaiser Wilhelm Institute for Physics of Berlin University for a period of time and began to study relativity. In 1931, he returned home and taught at Zhejiang University. In 1948, the School of Science of Cheeloo University temporarily moved to Hangzhou. Shu Xingbei, along with Su Buqing, Chen Jiangong, Wang Ganchang and other first-class teachers, was invited to teach part-time at Cheeloo University. In 1952, due to the adjustment of school and department, he came to teach in the Department of Physics of Shandong University and turned to the study of atmospheric dynamics. Shu Xingbei is the first physics teacher of Nobel Prize winner Li Zhengdao and academician Cheng Kaijia of Chinese Academy of Sciences.

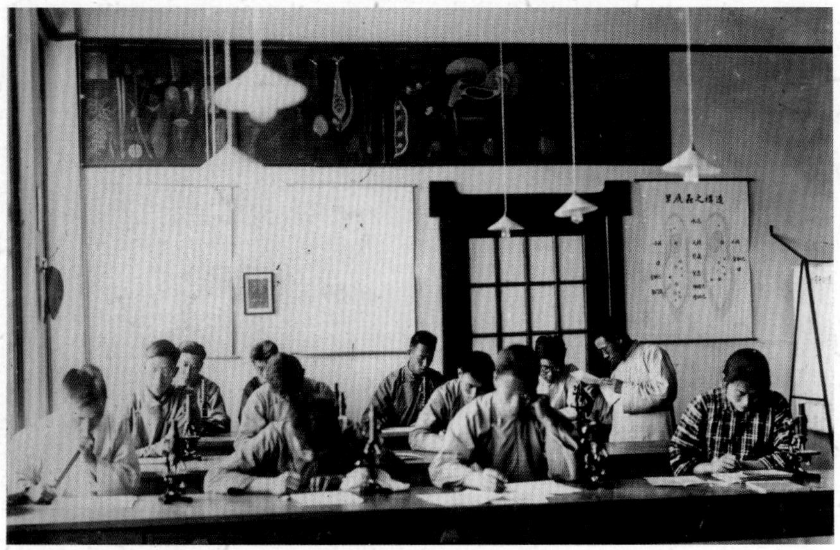

图 191 齐鲁大学学生在做生物学实验
Fig. 191 Students doing biology experiments at Cheeloo University

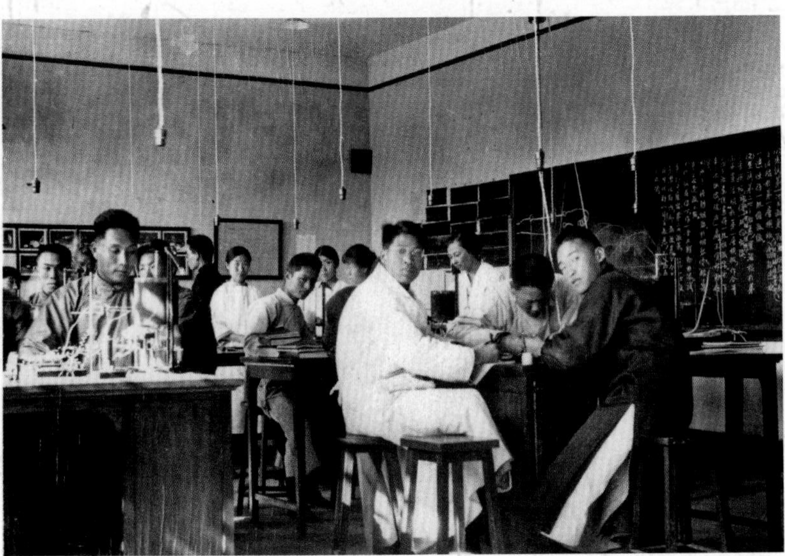
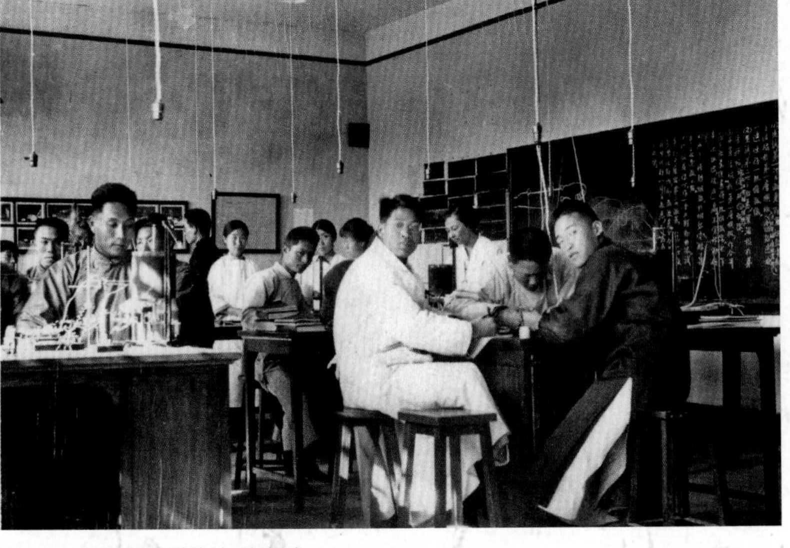

图 192 齐鲁大学学生在做实验
Fig. 192 Students doing experiments at Cheeloo University

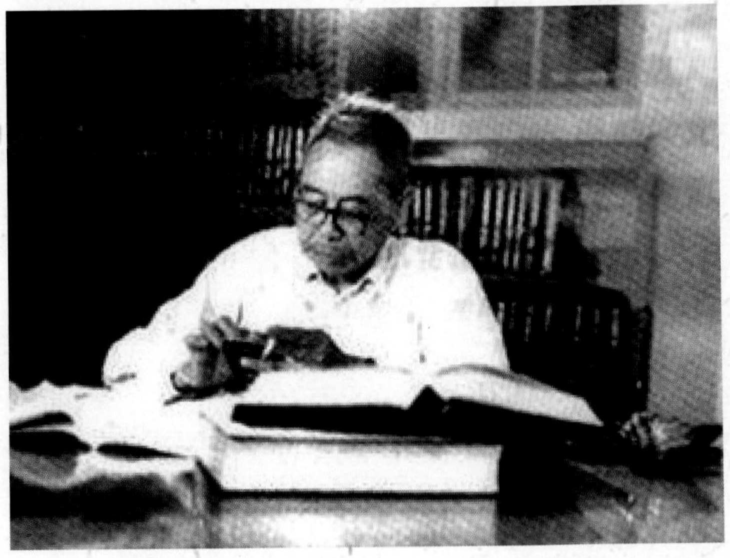

图 193 齐鲁大学校友束星北教授
Fig. 193 Professor Shu Xingbei, an alumnus of Cheeloo University

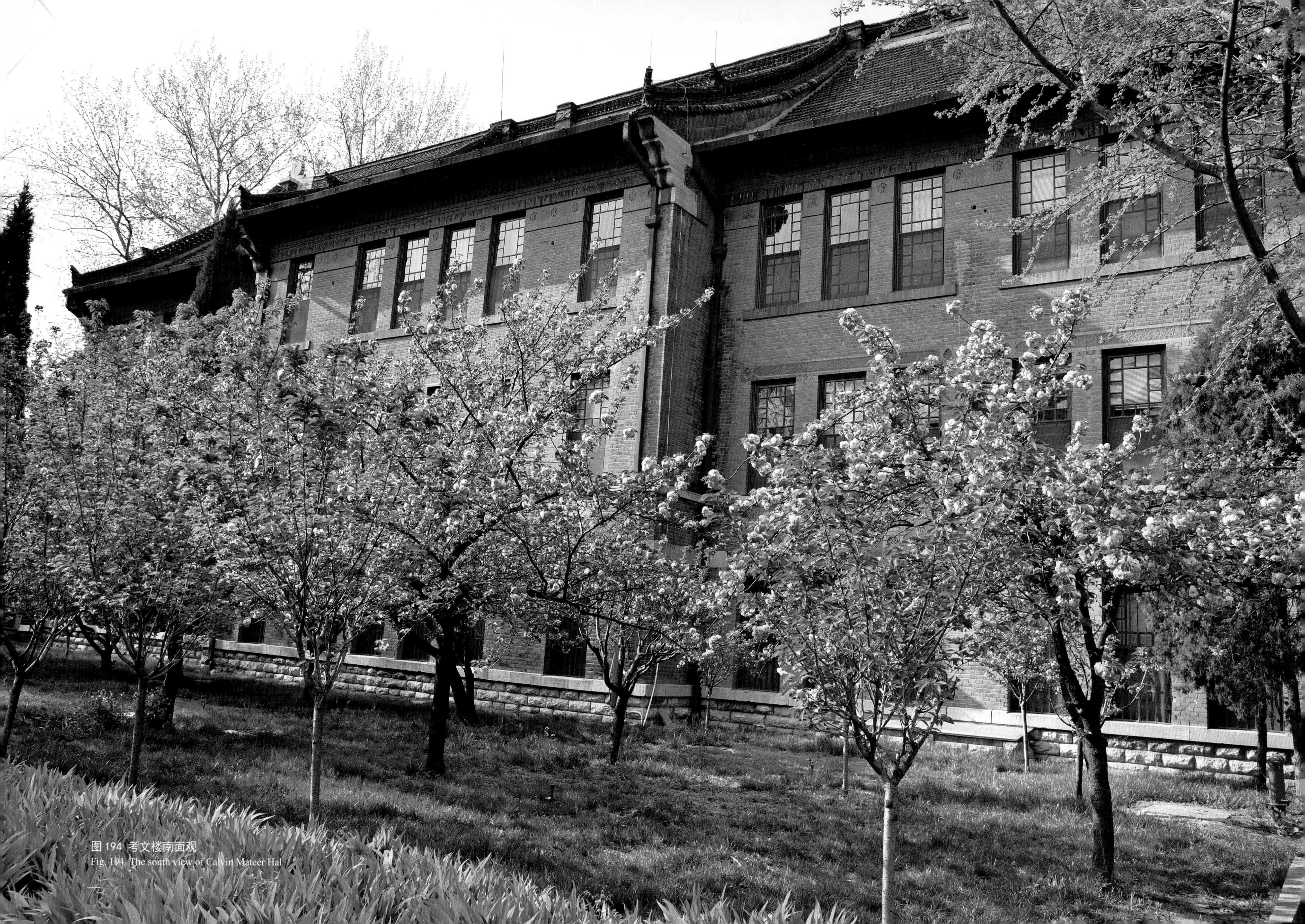

图 194 考文楼南面观
Fig. 194 The south view of Calvin Mateer Hal

24 第五教学楼（4）

The Fifth Teaching Building (4)

齐鲁医学院的人体寄生虫学教学和研究机构一直在考文楼。寄生虫严重危害人类健康，齐鲁大学生物学系和医学院对此进行了长期专门研究。20 世纪 20 年代施尔德医生将《斯氏实验诊断寄生动物学部》译成中文教授学生，培养了我国第一批寄生虫学人才。1933 年开展对华北寄生虫的调查与研究。1937 年，张奎博士回国并到内迁成都的齐鲁大学任教，担任生物学系教授、理学院院长，并于 1942 年创建了齐鲁大学寄生虫研究所，深入研究了四川人体肠寄生虫之防治。

说起寄生虫学，不能不提到齐鲁大学校友冯兰洲。他 1920 年考入齐鲁大学医学院，因学费太高曾两次辍学，1929 年毕业后至中国医学科学院工作，曾任寄生虫病研究所教授、所长。他确定了我国疟疾和丝虫病的主要蚊虫媒介，并对媒介白蛉传播黑热病的作用进行了深入研究。因其对消灭丝虫病做出了重大贡献，1957 年当选中国科学院学部委员（院士）。

The Teaching and Research Institute of Human Parasitology at Cheeloo College of Medicine had been in Calvin Mateer Hall. Parasites pose a serious threat to human health, and the Department of Biology and Medical School of Cheeloo University had conducted long-term specialized research on this. In the 1920s, Dr. Shields translated *Practical Bacteriology, Blood Work and Animal Parasitology* into Chinese to teach students, and trained the first batch of talents of Parasitology in China. The investigation and study of parasites in North China were carried out in 1933. In 1937, Dr. Zhang Kui returned to China and taught at Cheeloo University which moved to Chengdu. He served as a professor in the Department of Biology and dean of the School of Science. In 1942, he established the Institute of Parasitology of Cheeloo University and carried out in-depth research on the prevention and treatment of human intestinal parasites in Sichuan.

Speaking of Parasitology, we can not but mention Feng Lanzhou, an alumnus of Cheeloo University. He was admitted to the Medical School of Cheeloo University in 1920 but dropped out of school twice because of the high tuition fee. After graduating in 1929, he worked in Chinese Academy of Medical Sciences and served as a professor and director of the Institute of Parasitology. He identified the main mosquito vectors of malaria and filariasis in China, and conducted in-depth research on the role of the vector sandflies in transmitting kala-azar. In 1957, he was elected member of Chinese Academy of Sciences (academician) because of his great contribution to the elimination of filariasis.

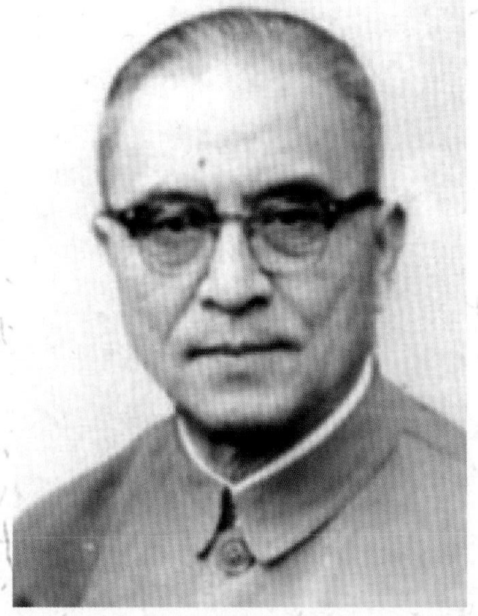

图 195 齐鲁大学校友张奎教授
Fig. 195 Professor Zhang Kui, an alumnus of Cheeloo University

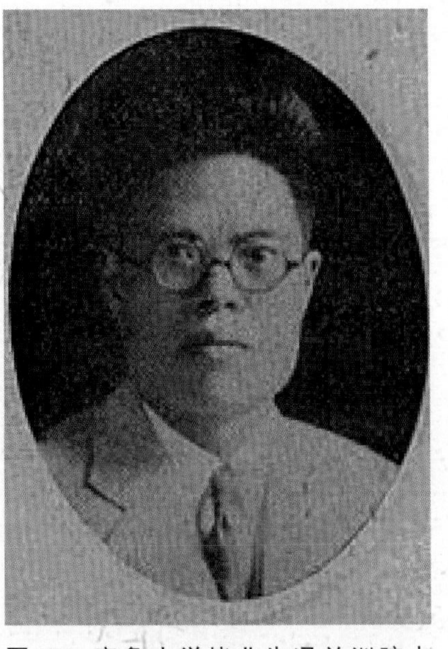

图 196 齐鲁大学毕业生冯兰洲院士（1903 ～ 1972）
Fig. 196 Academician Feng Lanzhou, graduate of Cheeloo University (1903-1972)

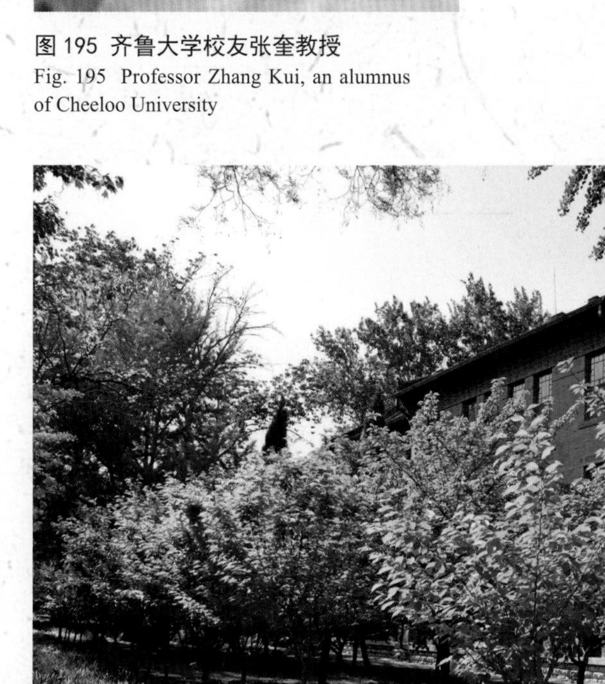

图 197 考文楼夏景
Fig. 197 Summer view of Calvin Mateer Hall

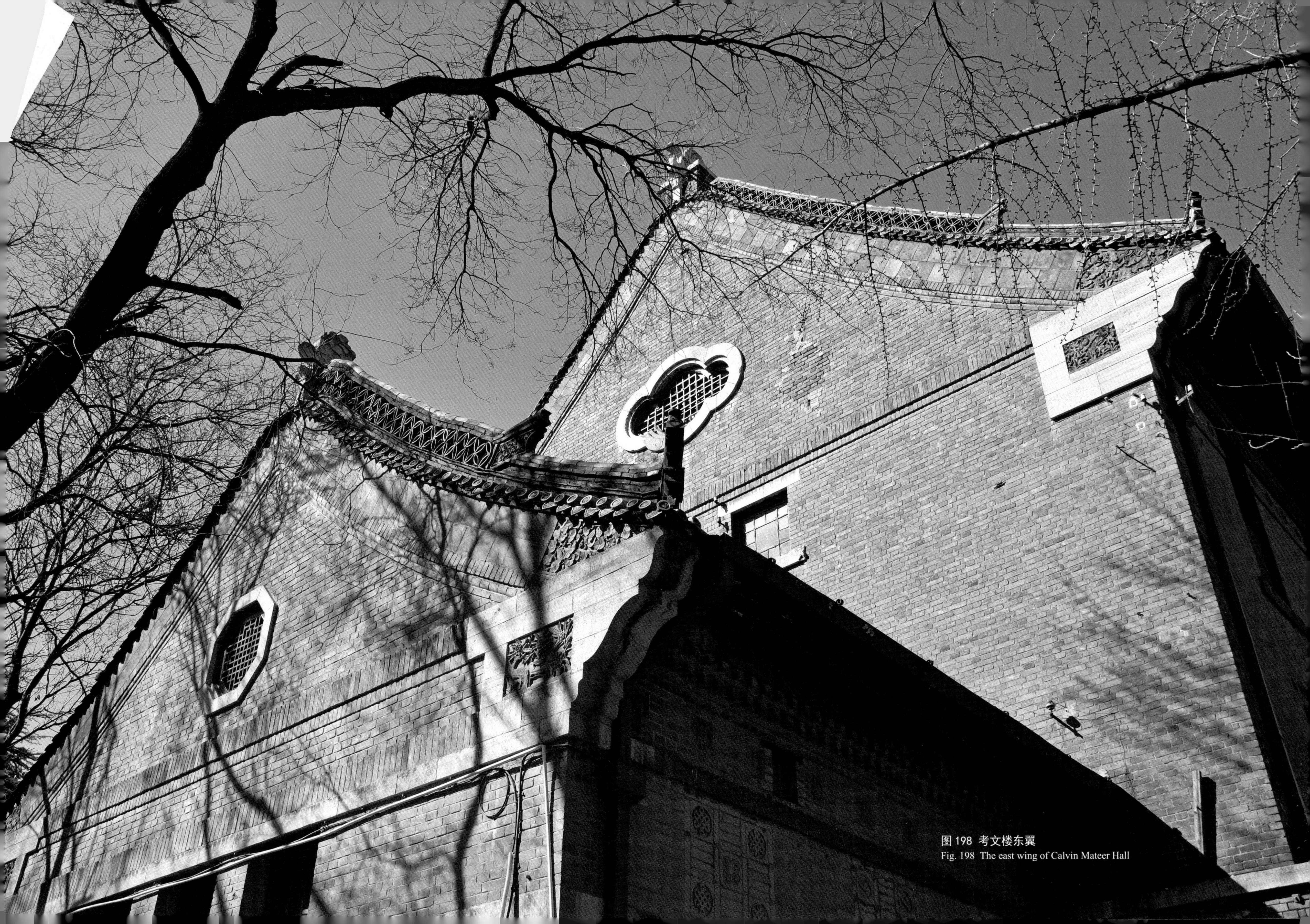

图 198 考文楼东翼
Fig. 198 The east wing of Calvin Mateer Hall

25 第六教学楼（1）

The Sixth Teaching Building (1)

第六教学楼是在拆除老教学六楼后于 2007 年建成的，典型的“中国式”大屋顶与西方楼体相结合的中西合璧式建筑。建筑南面横向分为五段，中轴部分七层带凌空欲飞的大屋顶，稍外为六层，最外侧的两翼为五层，错落有致，层次分明。整个大楼坐落于花草林木之中，远远望去，规模宏大，气势雄伟。因建设年代较晚，此楼屋脊与墙面装饰明显简化。屋顶的飞檐较大，给人以乘风腾飞之感。屋山平滑高耸，迎面而立，墀头装饰有花草图案。大门位于南面，其外侧东西方向上廊式排列以头戴镂空方帽的四棱立柱，也是此楼明显的建筑特色之一。第六教学楼的设计有模仿麦考密可楼的痕迹，但为适应不同的功能而有明显变化。第六教学楼为基础医学院主体建筑，集合了九个二级学科和三个省部级重点实验室。

The Sixth Teaching Building was built in 2007 after the demolition of the the old one. It is a typical building of Chinese and Western fusion with a large roof of Chinese style and the building body of Western style. The south side of the building is divided into five sections horizontally. The centraxonial part has seven floors with a large roof in the air. The outer side has six floors, and the outermost two wings have five floors. They are scattered orderly and have distinct layers. The whole building is located among the flowers and trees and looks grand and magnificent from a distance. Due to the later years of construction, the ridge and gable of this building are obviously decorated simply. The cornices of the roof are large, giving people the feeling of taking off in the wind. The smooth and towering gable stands head-on, and *chitou* is decorated with flowers and plants. The gate is located in the south, and its outer side is arranged in an east-west corridor manner with quadrangular colonnades wearing hollowed-out square hats, which is also one of the obvious architectural features of this building. The design of the Sixth Teaching Building has traces of imitating McCormick Hall, but with obvious changes to adapt to different functions. The Sixth Teaching Building is the main building of the School of Basic Medical Sciences, which integrates nine secondary disciplines and three key laboratories at the provincial and ministerial levels.

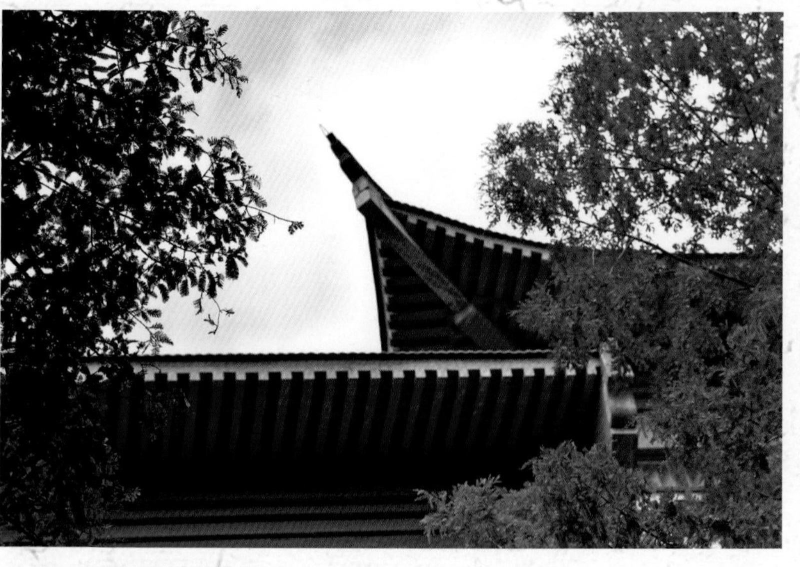

图 199 凌空欲飞的大屋顶

Fig. 199 Large roof in the sky

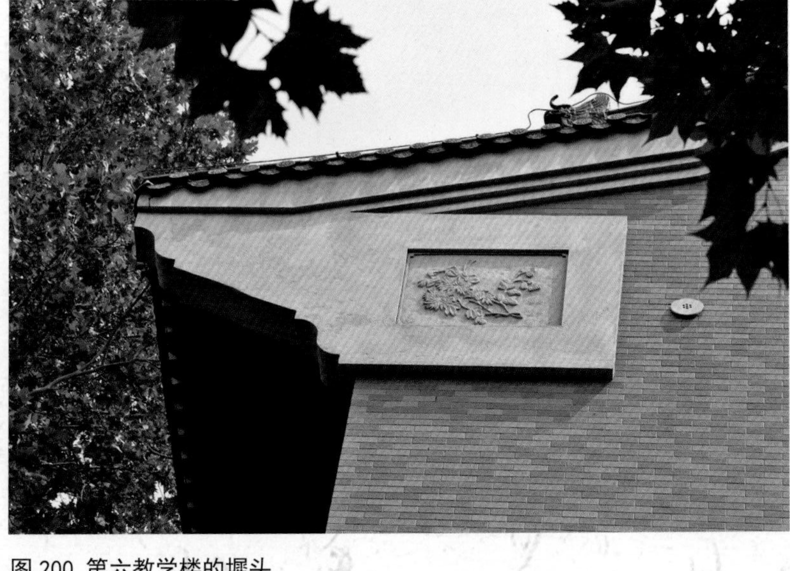

图 200 第六教学楼的墀头

Fig. 200 *Chitou* of the Sixth Teaching Building

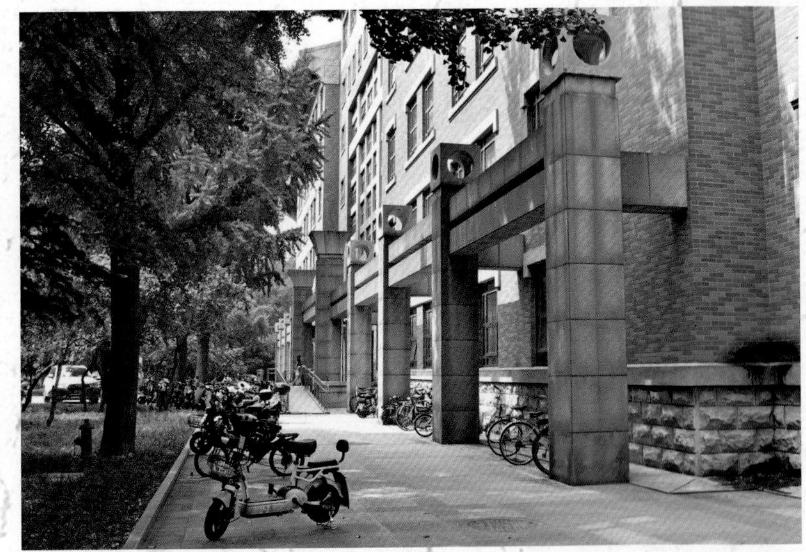

图 201 第六教学楼南面的四棱廊柱

Fig. 201 Quadrangular colonnades in the south of the Sixth Teaching Building

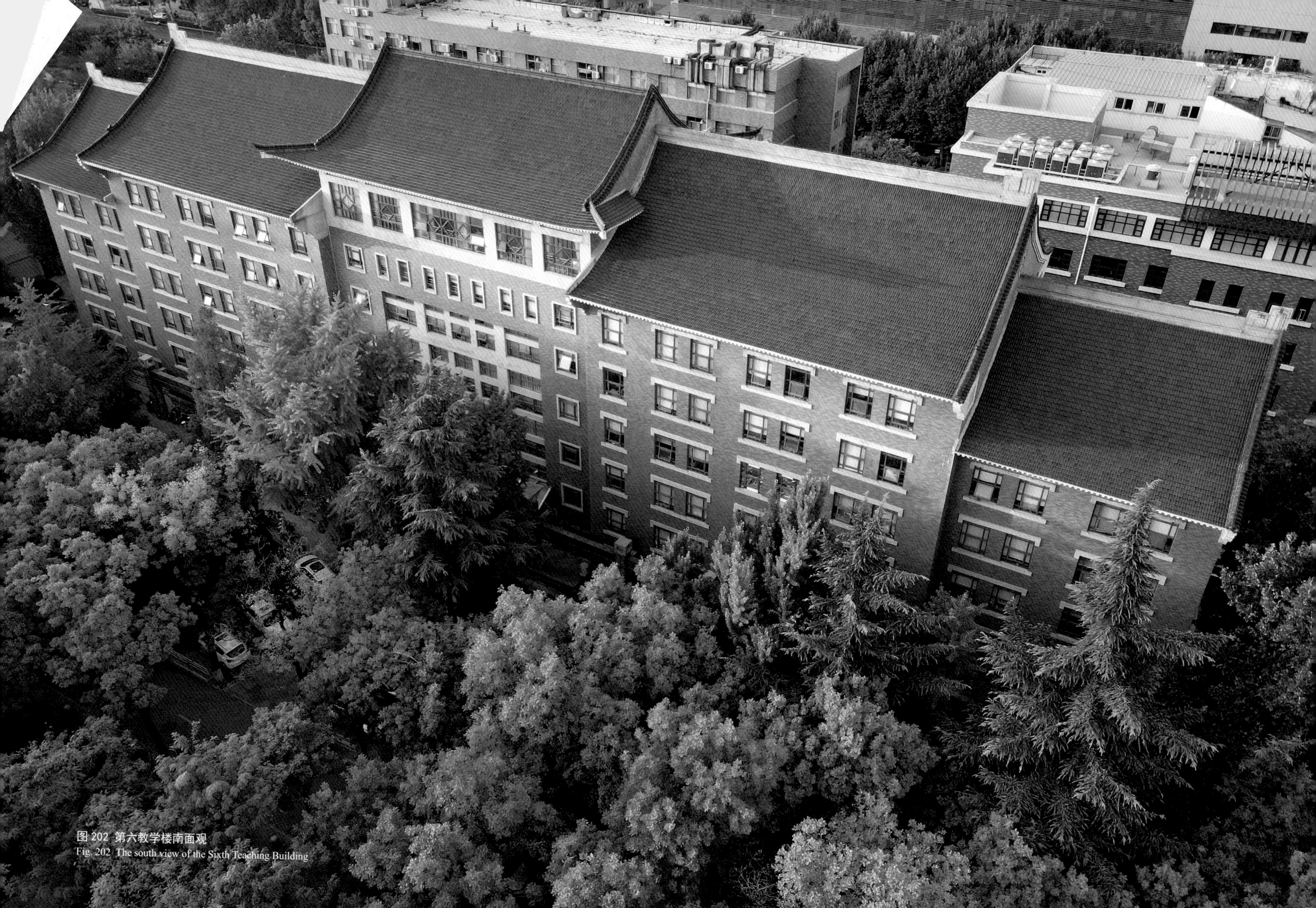

图 202 第六教学楼南面观
Fig. 202 The south view of the Sixth Teaching Building

25 第六教学楼（2）

The Sixth Teaching Building (2)

第六教学楼第一层东侧为齐鲁医学院显微表征平台，西侧为病理学系。病理学系为国家级临床重点专科，不但承担全校的病理学教学、科研任务，而且还要在齐鲁医院做病理诊断工作。我国著名病理学家侯宝璋教授为该学科的发展做出了重大贡献。

侯宝璋（1893~1967），安徽凤台人，中国病理学先驱，医学教育家。1920 年毕业于齐鲁大学医学院并留校工作，后任病理学系教授、主任。抗日战争爆发后，他随校到成都，任华西齐鲁大学联合医院病理系教授及主任，并代理齐鲁大学医学院院长。1948 年任香港大学医学院病理系主任、教授，代理院长。因国家病理学研究之需，受周恩来总理之邀，1962 年任北京中国医科大学（现北京协和医学院）副校长，兼病理教研室主任。他编写了我国第一部《实用病理组织学》。第一次提出并证明了寄生虫在人体肝内寄生可以引起恶性肿瘤的现象。1967 年 3 月 12 日病逝，骨灰存放于北京八宝山革命公墓。

The east side of the first floor of the Sixth Teaching Building is the Center for Microscopic Imaging and Analysis of Cheeloo College of Medicine, and the west side is the Department of Pathology. The Department of Pathology is a national key clinical specialty. It not only undertakes the teaching and scientific research tasks of pathology in the university, but also does pathological diagnosis in Qilu Hospital. Professor Hou Baozhang, a famous pathologist in China, has made great contributions to the development of this discipline.

Hou Baozhang (1893-1967), a native of Fengtai, Anhui Province, is a pioneer of Chinese pathology and a medical educator. In 1920, he graduated from the Medical School of Cheeloo University and then stayed there to work. Later, he served as professor and director of the Department of Pathology. After the outbreak of the War of Resistance Against Japanese Aggression, he went to Chengdu with the university and served as a professor and director of the Department of Pathology of West China and Cheeloo University Union Hospital, and as dean of the Medical School of Cheeloo University at the same time. In 1948, he served as the director and professor of the Department of Pathology of the Medical School, University of Hong Kong, and as the acting dean of the school. Due to the need of national pathology research, he was appointed vice president of Chinese Medical University in Beijing(now Peking Union Medical College) and director of the Teaching and Research Office of Pathology in 1962 at the invitation of Premier Zhou Enlai. He compiled *Practical Pathological Histology* in China. He is the first to put forward and prove that parasites in human liver can cause malignant tumors. He died of illness on 12 March 1967 and his ashes were stored in Babaoshan Revolutionary Cemetery in Beijing.

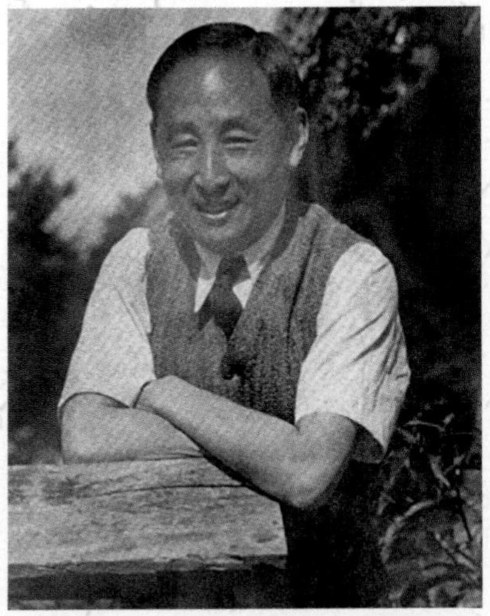

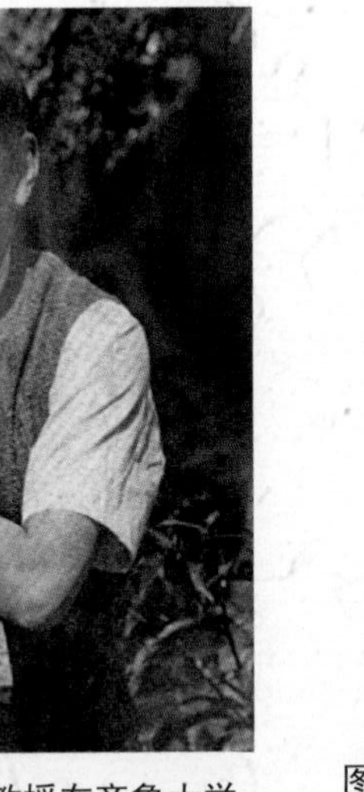

图 203 1932 年侯宝璋教授在齐鲁大学
Fig. 203 Professor Hou Baozhang at Cheeloo University in 1932

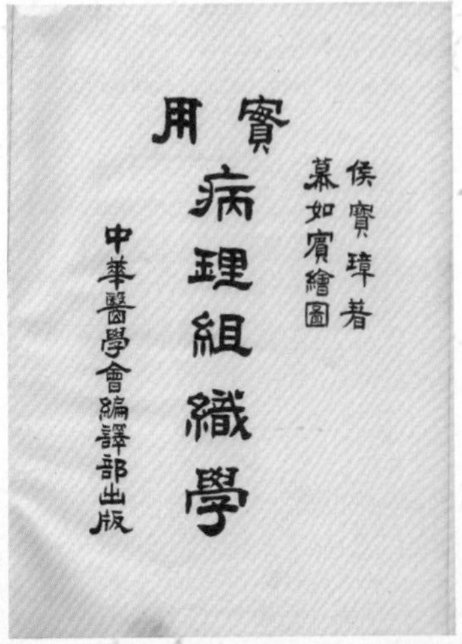

图 204 1934 年侯宝璋编写的《实用病理组织学》
Fig. 204 *Practical Pathological Histology* edited by Hou Baozhang in 1934

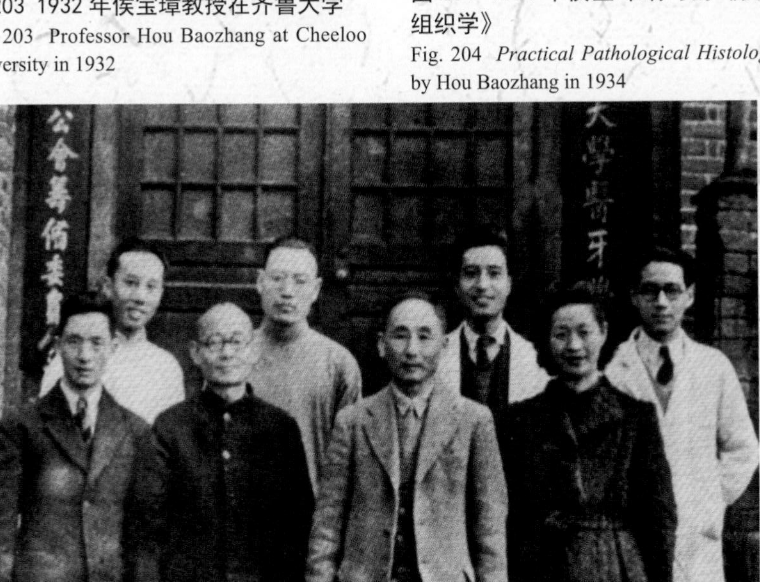

图 205 抗日战争期间侯宝璋教授与同事在成都华西协和大学医牙学院门前合影
Fig. 205 Professor Hou Baozhang and his colleagues taking a photo in front of the School of Dentistry of West China Union University in Chengdu during the War of Resistance Against Japanese Aggression

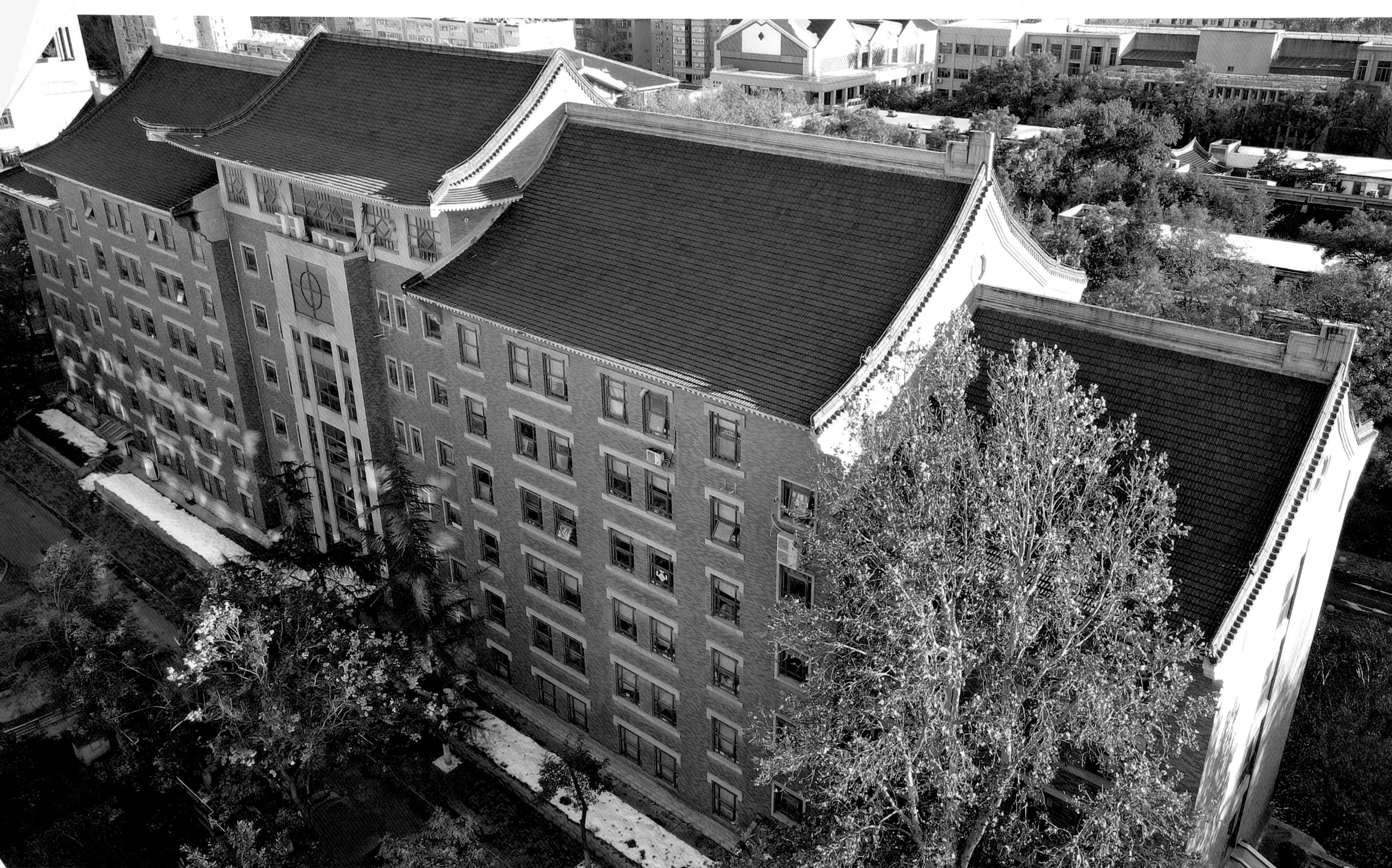

图 206 第六教学楼北面观
Fig. 206 The north view of the Sixth Teaching Building

25 第六教学楼（3）

The Sixth Teaching Building (3)

第六教学楼二层西侧由组织学与胚胎学系使用。山东大学的人体解剖与组织胚胎学为国家重点学科，在百余年的发展历程中，有三位人物不能不提及。第一位是施尔德（Randolph T. Shields），美国人，医学博士，长期担任齐鲁大学医学院组织学与胚胎学教授，1919 年编译了《路氏组织学》，1920 年与丁立成一起翻译了《胎生学引阶》，1923 年翻译了美国版 Gray's Anatomy 第 20 版，中文译名为《格氏系统解剖学》。第二位是张汇泉，1926 年毕业于齐鲁大学医学院，留校主讲组织学与胚胎学，1921 年他亲自送邓恩铭去上海参加中共一大会议，先后撰写了《胚胎图谱》《组织胚胎学》《胚胎学》和《人体畸形学》等著作，是我国组织学与胚胎学的主要奠基人之一。第三位是高英茂，国家级教学名师，1962 年毕业于山东医学院，创建了我国第一个实验畸形学实验室，先后主编了 30 多部教材、专著和译著。

The west side of the second floor of the Sixth Teaching Building is the Department of Histology and Embryology. Human Anatomy and Histoembryology of Shandong University is a national key discipline. In the development process of more than 100 years, three people have to be mentioned. The first one is Randolph T. Shields, an American doctor of medicine and long-term professor of Histology and Embryology of the School of Medicine of Cheeloo University. In 1919, he compiled and translated *A Text-Book of Histology: Arranged upon an Embryological Basis*. In 1920, he translated An Introduction to Vertebrate Embryology: Based on the Study of the Frog, Chick, and Mammal with Ding Licheng. In 1923, he translated the 20th edition of the American edition of *Gray's Anatomy*, which was translated into Chinese as *Geshi Xitong Jiepouxue*. The second one is Zhang Huiquan, who graduated from the School of Medicine of Cheeloo University in 1926 and then stayed there to teach histology and embryology. In 1921, he personally sent Deng Enming to Shanghai to attend the First National Congress of the Communist Party of China. He had written such works as *Atlas of Embryo Atlas, Histoembryology*, *Embryology* and *Teratology of the Human Body*, and is one of the main founders of histology and embryology in China. The third one is Gao Yingmao, a famous state-level teacher. He graduated from Shandong Medical College in 1962 and established the first laboratory of Experimental Teratology in China. He had edited more than 30 textbooks, monographs and translated works.

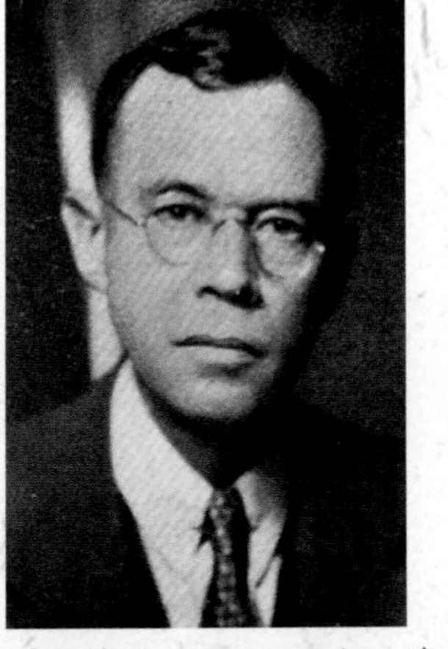

图 207 施尔德（1877 ～ 1958），齐鲁大学医学院组织学与胚胎学教授，曾任齐鲁大学医科科长、医学院院长、齐鲁医院院长。

Fig. 207 Randolph T. Shields(1877-1958),a professor of Histology and Embryology of the School of Medicine of Cheeloo University, once served as chief of Medicine and dean of the School of Medicine of Cheeloo University and president of Cheeloo Hospital.

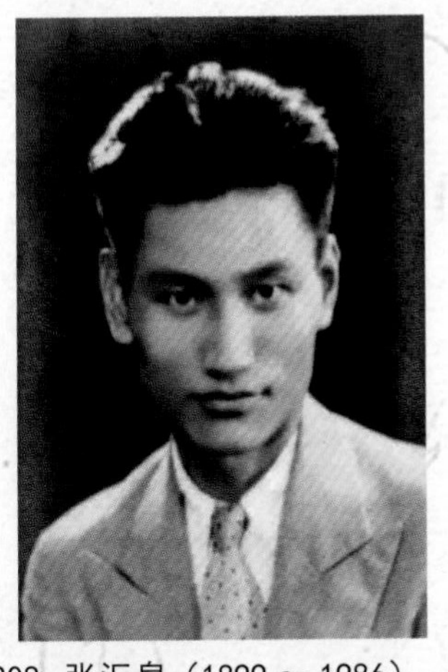

图 208 张汇泉（1899 ～ 1986），我国组织胚胎学奠基人之一，曾任齐鲁大学医学院院长、山东医学院副院长等职。

Fig. 208 Zhang Huiquan (1899-1986), one of the founders of histoembryology in China, served as dean of Cheeloo College of Medicine of Cheeloo University and vice president of Shandong Medical College.

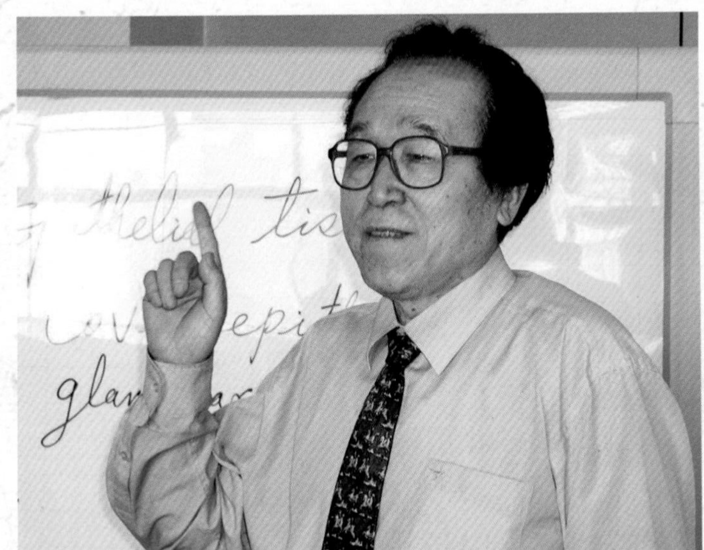

图 209 国家级教学名师、高英茂教授

Fig. 209 Professor Gao Yingmao, a famous state-level teacher

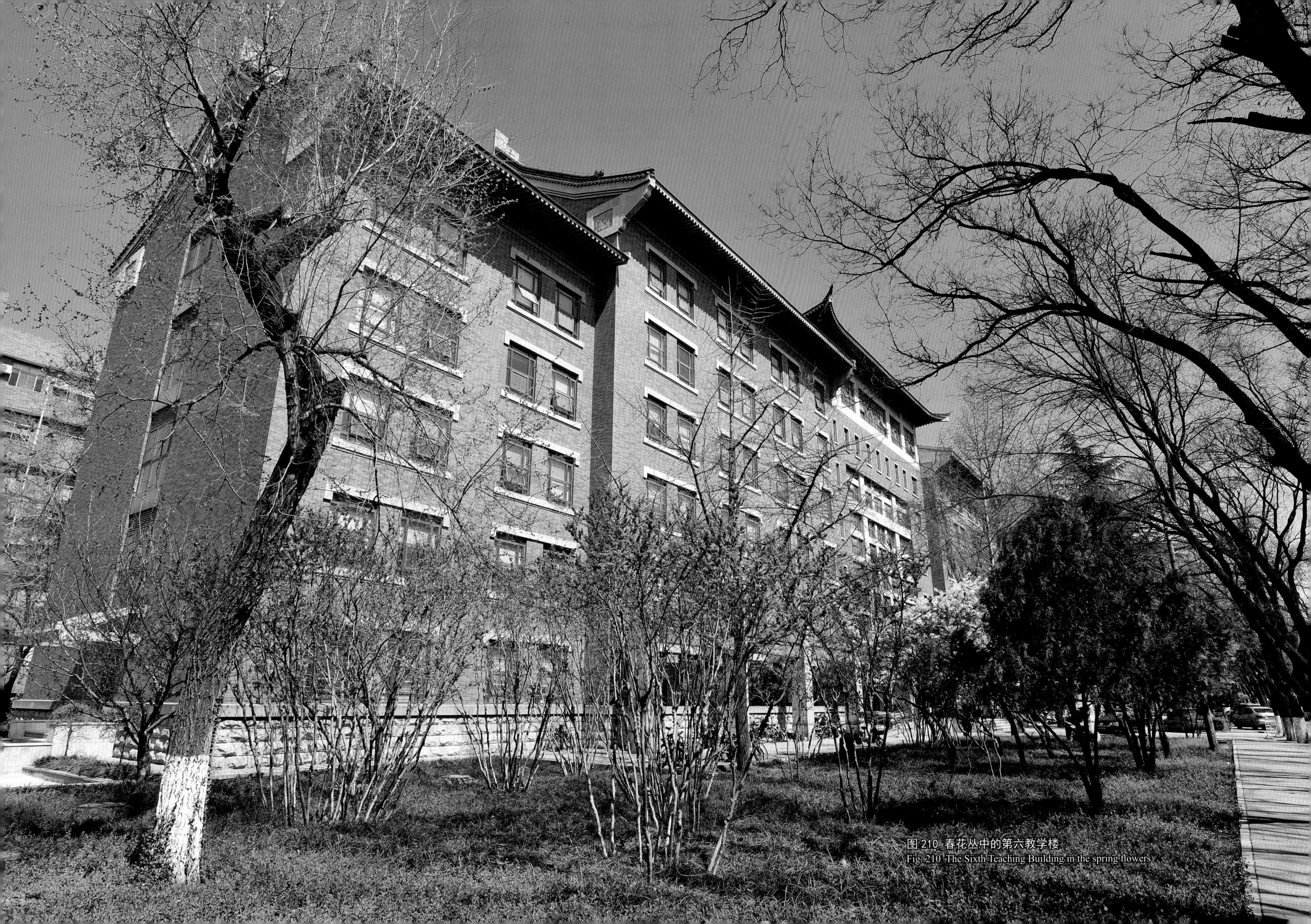

图 210 春花丛中的第六教学楼

Fig. 210 The Sixth Teaching Building in the spring flowers

25 第六教学楼（4）

The Sixth Teaching Building (4)

第六教学楼二层东侧由药理学系使用。此系传统上主要研究心、脑血管药理学，近期在国家杰出青年科学基金获得者易凡教授带领下，在肾病与免疫药理学等研究方向上取得了较大成绩。著名药理学家周廷冲和吴葆杰等曾在此工作过。

周廷冲（1917 ~ 1996），浙江新登人，著名生化药理学家。1941 年从上海医学院医学系毕业后进入中央卫生实验院药理室工作，1945 年赴英国牛津大学贝利奥学院进修，1947 年获得牛津大学药理学博士学位，1948 年赴美国康奈尔大学酶化学实验室进行博士后研究，1950 年与夫人黄翠芬一起回国，并到华东白求恩医学院、山东医学院工作，1953 年调到军事医学科学院。一直从事生物活性因子的分子生物学研究，首次阐明梭曼膦酰化乙酰胆碱酯酶的老化机制，证明梭曼膦酰化酶老化的实质是毒剂残基上特己氧基的去烷基反应，从而为毒剂防治中的药物设计指明了方向。1980 年当选为中国科学院院士。

The east side of the second floor of the Sixth Teaching Building is used by the Department of Pharmacy. Traditionally, the department mainly studies cardiovascular and cerebrovascular pharmacology. Recently, under the leadership of Professor Yi Fan, winner of the National Science Fund for Distinguished Young Scholars, it has made great achievements in nephrology and immunopharmacology. The famous pharmacologists Zhou Tingchong and Wu Baojie had once worked in the department.

Zhou Tingchong (1917-1996), born in Xindeng, Zhejiang Province, is a famous biochemical pharmacologist. In 1941, after graduating from the Department of Medicine of Shanghai Medical College, he entered the Department of Pharmacy of the Central Health Experimental Institute to work. In 1945, he went to Balliol College of the University of Oxford to study, and in 1947, he received a doctor's degree in pharmacology from Oxford University. In 1948, he went to the Laboratory of Zymochemistry of Cornell University to carry out postdoctoral research. In 1950, he returned home with his wife Huang Cuifen, and worked in East China Bethune Medical College and Shandong Medical College. In 1953, he was transferred to the Academy of Military Medical Sciences. He had been engaged in the molecular biology research of bioactive factors, explained the aging mechanism of Soman phosphoryl acetylcholinesterase for the first time, and proved that the essence of Soman phosphoryl acetylcholinesterase aging is the dealkylation reaction of the special hexyloxy group on the poison residue, thus pointing out the direction for the drug design in the prevention and treatment of poison. He was elected academician of Chinese Academy of Sciences in 1980.

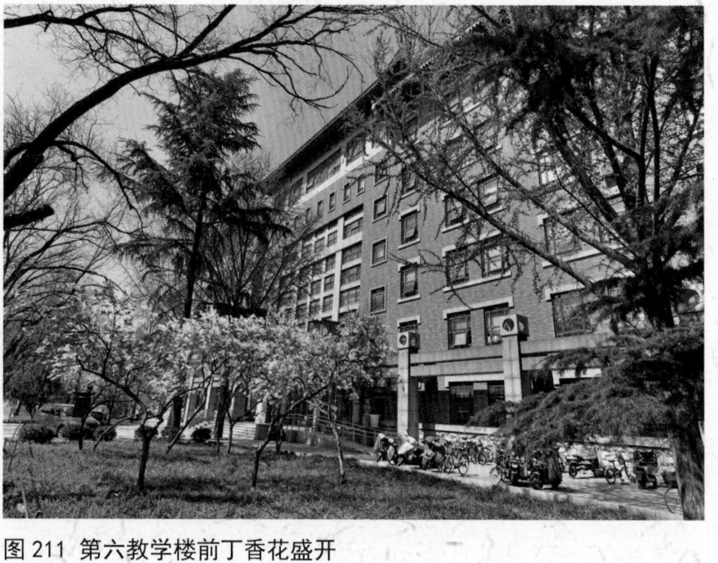

图 211 第六教学楼前丁香花盛开
Fig. 211 Lilacs blooming in front of the Sixth Teaching Building

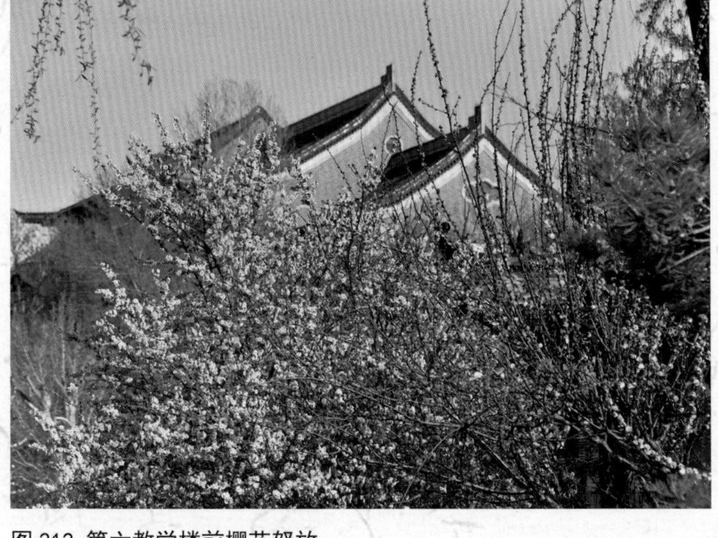

图 212 第六教学楼前樱花怒放
Fig. 212 Cherry blossoms blooming in front of the Sixth Teaching Building

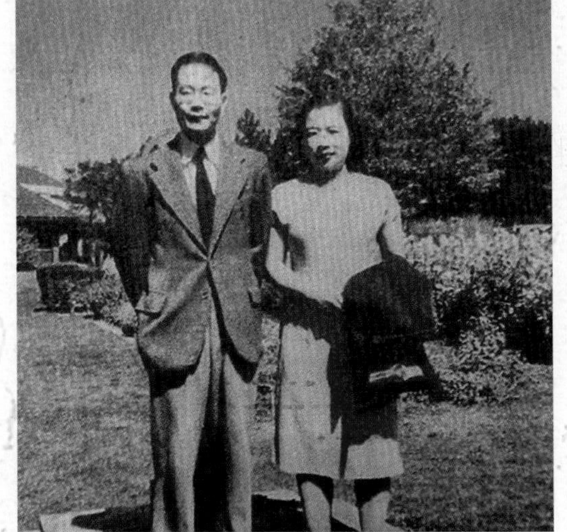

图 213 1948 年周廷冲、黄翠芬夫妇在美国康奈尔大学
Fig. 213 Zhou Tingchong and Huang Cuifen at Cornell University in the United States in 1948

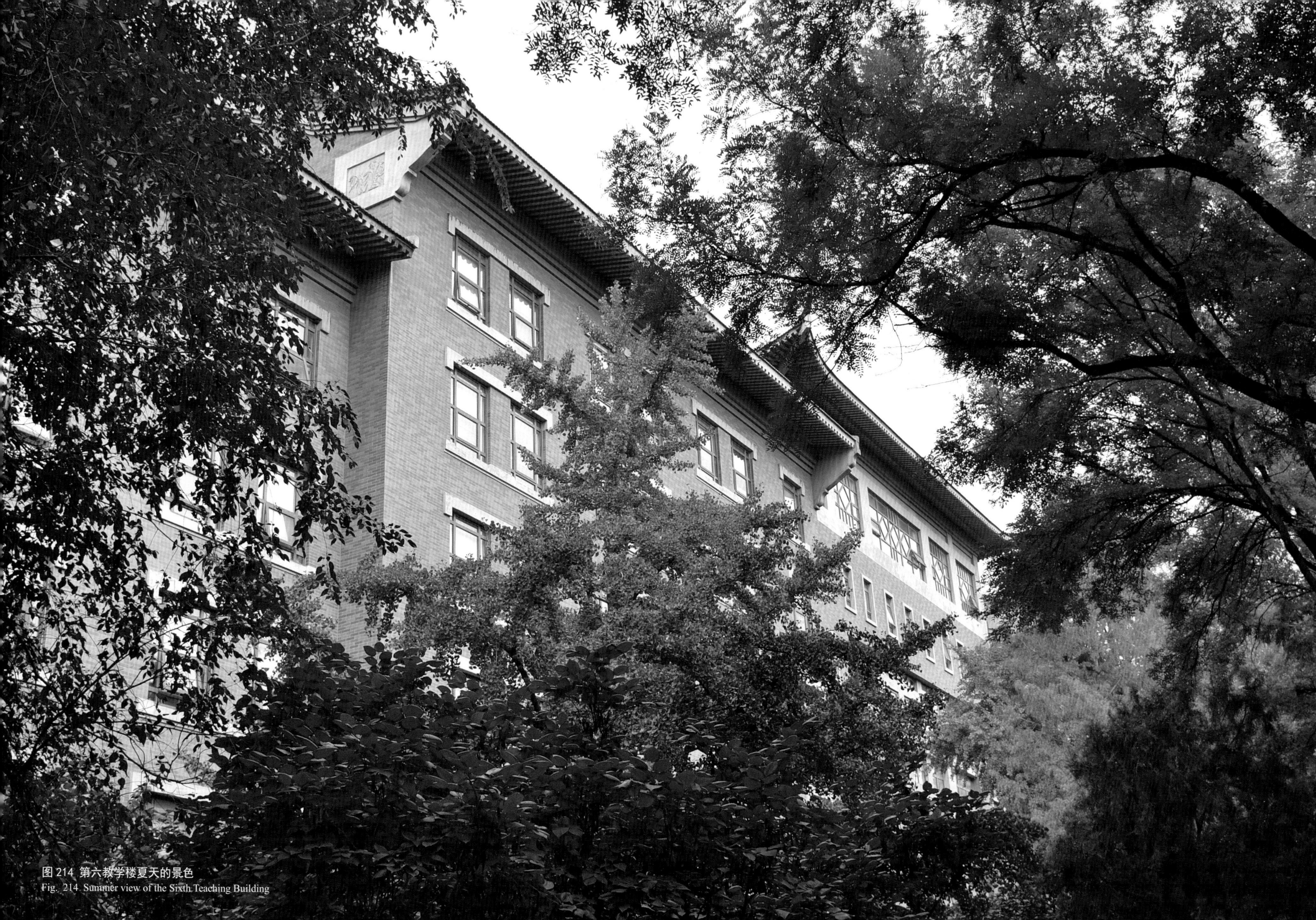

图 214 第六教学楼夏天的景色
Fig. 214 Summer view of the Sixth Teaching Building

25 第六教学楼（5）

The Sixth Teaching Building (5)

第六教学楼三层属生理学与病理生理学系，四层属生物化学与分子生物学系。

1911 年美国人聂会东和英国人易文士在齐鲁大学讲授生理学。1948 年在山东省立医学院创建的华东生理学研究所，由沈霁春教授任首任所长。于秉振教授主持的“针麻原理研究——穴位与针感专题”和刘磊教授主持的“穴位与针感”项目 1978 年双双获得全国科学大会奖。2021 年 2 月于晓教授团队在国际著名杂志 *Cell* 上发表了题为“Ligand recognition and allosteric regulation of DRD1-Gs signaling complexes”的论文，首次揭示快乐荷尔蒙受体 DRD1 的配体识别和别构调节机制。

江清教授为我国生物化学先驱，早在 20 世纪 20 年代，就与李缵文、鲁德馨等合作翻译了我国第一部中文生物化学教科书《良氏 (Conant) 生物化学教科书》。李缵文教授等于 1952 年创建了生物化学教研室，发展到今天，在国家杰出青年科学基金获得者孙金鹏带领下 2021 年 1 月在 *Nature* 发表了题为“Structures of the glucocorticoid-bound adhesion receptor GPR97-Go complex”的论文，首次鉴定并解析了糖皮质激素与其膜受体 GPR97 结合的复合物电镜结构。

In 1911, James Boyd Neal from the United States and P. S. Evans from the United Kingdom taught physiology at Cheeloo University. In 1948, East China Institute of Physiology was established in Shandong Provincial Medical College, with Professor Shen Jichun as the first director. In 1978, the project “Research on Acupuncture and Anesthesia—Acupuncture Points and Acupuncture Sensation” hosted by Professor Yu Bingzhen and the project “Acupuncture Points and Acupuncture Sensation” hosted by Professor Liu Lei both won the National Science Conference Award. In February 2021, Professor Yu Xiao’s team published a paper entitled “Ligand recognition and allosteric regulation of DRD1-Gs signaling complexes” in the internationally famous journal *Cell*, which revealed the ligand recognition and allosteric regulation mechanism of feel good hormone receptor DRD1 for the first time.

As a pioneer of biochemistry in China, Professor Jiang Qing translated *Conant Biochemistry* in cooperation with Li Zuanwen and Lu Dexin as early as the 1920s and it became the first Chinese biochemistry textbook in China. Professor Li Zuanwen led the establishment of the Teaching and Research Office of Biochemistry in 1952. Today, under the leadership of Sun Jinpeng, winner of the National Science Fund for Distinguished Young Scholars, the office published a paper entitled “Structures of the glucocorticoid-bound adhesion receptor GPR97-Go complex” in *Nature* in January 2021, identifying and analyzing the electron microscope structure of the complex of the glucocorticoid-bound adhesion receptor GPR97 for the first time.

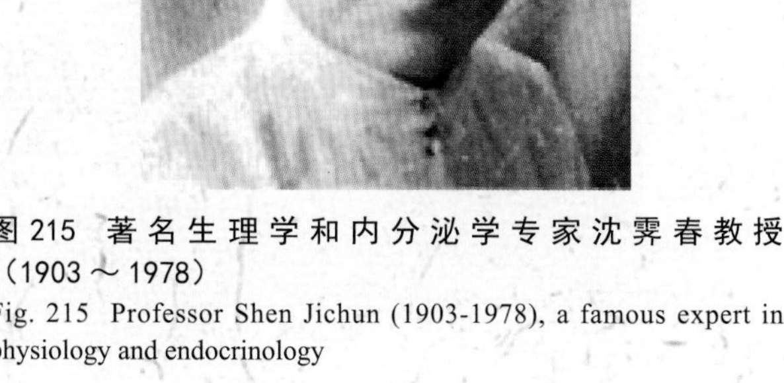

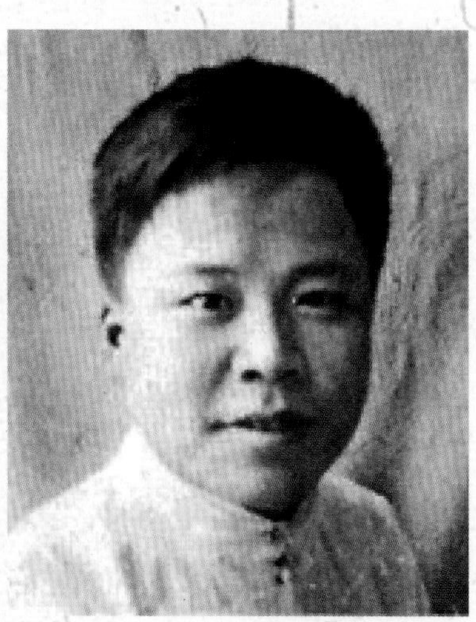

图 215　著名生理学和内分泌学专家沈霁春教授（1903 ～ 1978）

Fig. 215　Professor Shen Jichun (1903-1978), a famous expert in physiology and endocrinology

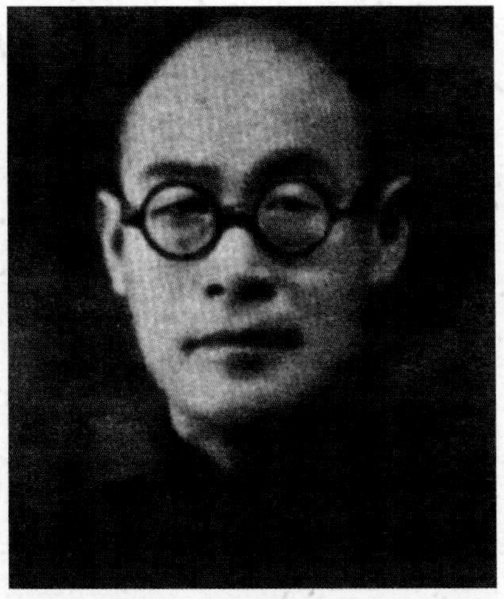

图 216　江清（1886 ～ 1939）教授，著名生物化学家，历任齐鲁大学医学院生理学系生物化学教授、医学院院长等职。

Fig. 216　Professor Jiang Qing (1886-1939), a famous biochemist, served as professor of biochemistry in the Department of Physiology and dean of the School of Medicine of Cheeloo University.

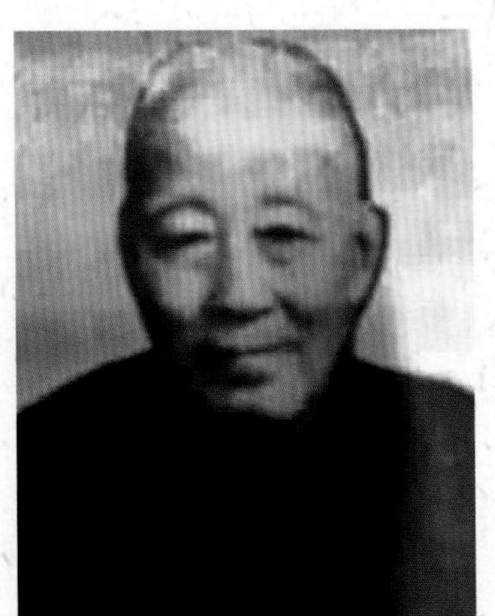

图 217　李缵文（1900 ～ 1977），生物化学家，曾任齐鲁大学医学院教授、代理院长。新中国成立后，历任山东医学院教授、生物化学教研室主任。

Fig. 217　Li Zuanwen (1900-1977), a biochemist, was a professor and acting dean of the School of Medicine of Cheeloo University. After the founding of the People’s Republic of China, he served as a professor and director of the Teaching and Research Office of Biochemistry of Shandong Medical College.

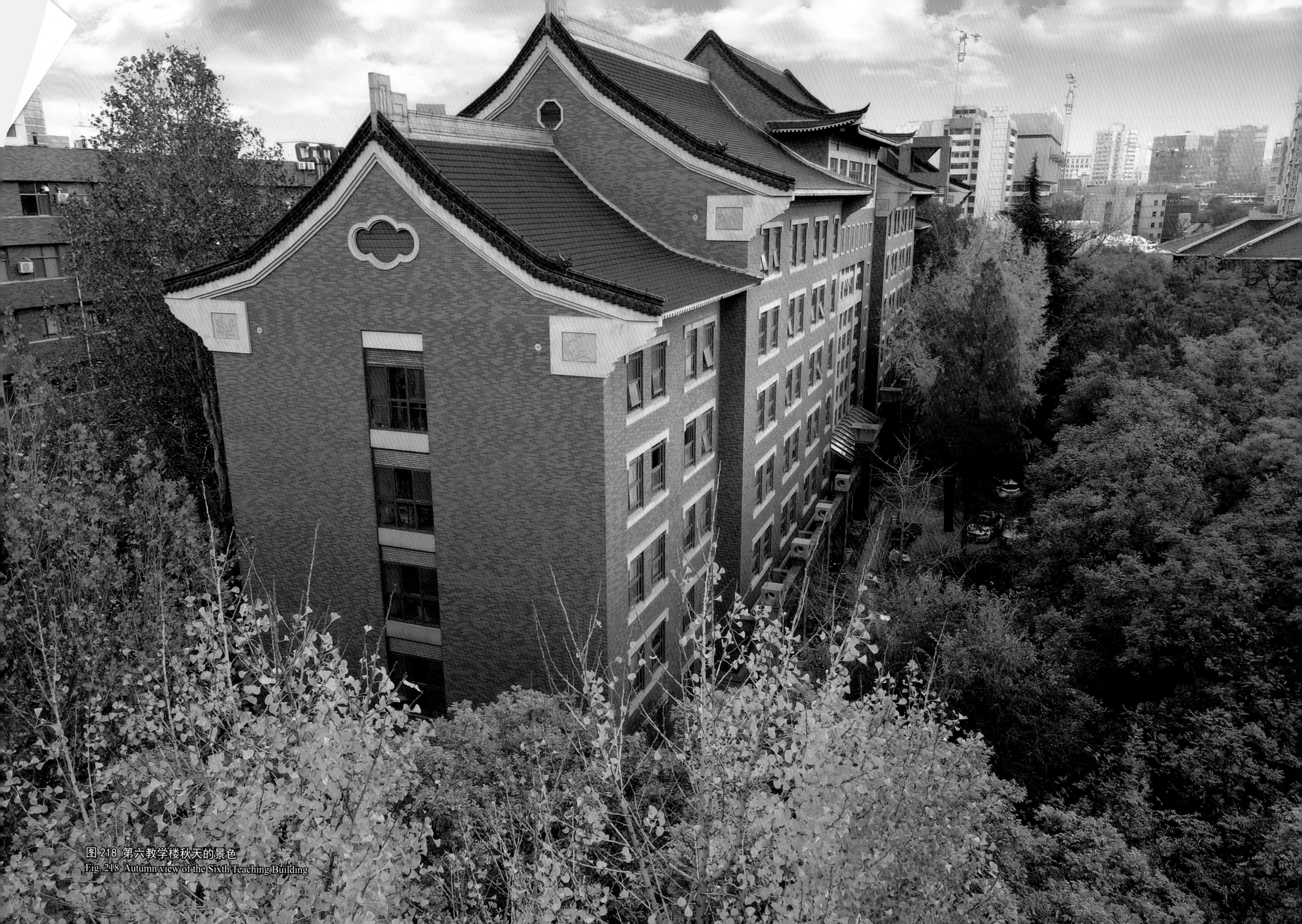

图 218 第六教学楼秋天的景色
Fig. 218 Autumn view of the Sixth Teaching Building

25 第六教学楼（6）

The Sixth Teaching Building (6)

第六教学楼五层东侧属病原生物学系，西侧属医学免疫学系，亦合称感染与免疫山东省重点实验室。中国工程院黄翠芬院士曾在病原生物学系工作过。国家级教学名师于修平教授主持的“基础医学融合性实验教学课程体系改革”项目 2005 年获国家级教学成果奖二等奖。著名医学超微结构和病毒学专家洪涛教授 1955 年于山东医学院毕业后至中国疾病预防控制中心工作，1996 年当选中国工程院院士。医学免疫学系近期成果丰硕，特别是长江学者和国家杰出青年科学基金获得者高成江教授、国家杰出青年科学基金获得者马春红教授和国家优秀青年基金获得者赵伟教授，在 *Nature* 系列杂志上发表了多篇论文。

此楼六层东侧为细胞生物学系，西侧为山东省精神疾病基础与临床重点实验室。此重点实验室由长江学者和国家杰出青年科学基金获得者陈哲宇教授创建，他于 2006 年 10 月在 *Science* 杂志上发表了题为“Genetic variant BDNF (Val66Met) polymorphism alters anxiety-related behavior”的论文，揭示脑源性神经营养因子基因突变的转基因小鼠能产生人类大脑带有此等位基因突变的表型特征。

The east side of the fifth floor of the Sixth Teaching Building is the Department of Pathogen Biology, and the west side is the Department of Medical Immunology. They are also jointly called Shandong Provincial Key Laboratory of Infection and Immunization. Huang Cuifen, the academician of Chinese Academy of Engineering, once worked in the Department of Pathogen Biology. The project “Curriculum System Reform of Integrated Experimental Teaching of Basic Medical Sciences” hosted by Professor Yu Xiuping, a famous state-level teacher, won the second prize of National Teaching Achievement Award in 2005. Professor Hong Tao, a famous expert in medical ultrastructure and virology, worked in the Chinese Center for Disease Control and Prevention after graduating from Shandong Medical College in 1955 and was elected academician of Chinese Academy of Engineering in 1996. Recently, the Department of Medical Immunology has achieved fruitful results. Professor Gao Chengjiang, winner of Chang Jiang Scholars Program and the National Science Fund for Distinguished Young Scholars, and Professor Ma Chunhong, winner of the National Science Fund for Distinguished Young Scholars, and Professor Zhao Wei, winner of the Excellent Young Scientists Fund, have published many papers in *Nature* and its journal series.

The east side of the sixth floor of the building is the Department of Cell Biology, and the west side is Shandong Provincial Key Laboratory of Basic and Clinical Psychiatric Disorders. This key laboratory was established by Professor Chen Zheyu, a winner of Chang Jiang Scholars Program and the National Science Fund for Distinguished Young Scholars. In October 2006, he published a paper entitled “Genetic variant BDNF (Val66Met) polymorphism alters anxiety-related behavior” in the journal *Science* which revealed that transgenic mice with brain-derived gene mutations of neurotrophic factor can show phenotypic characteristics of human brain with this allele mutation.

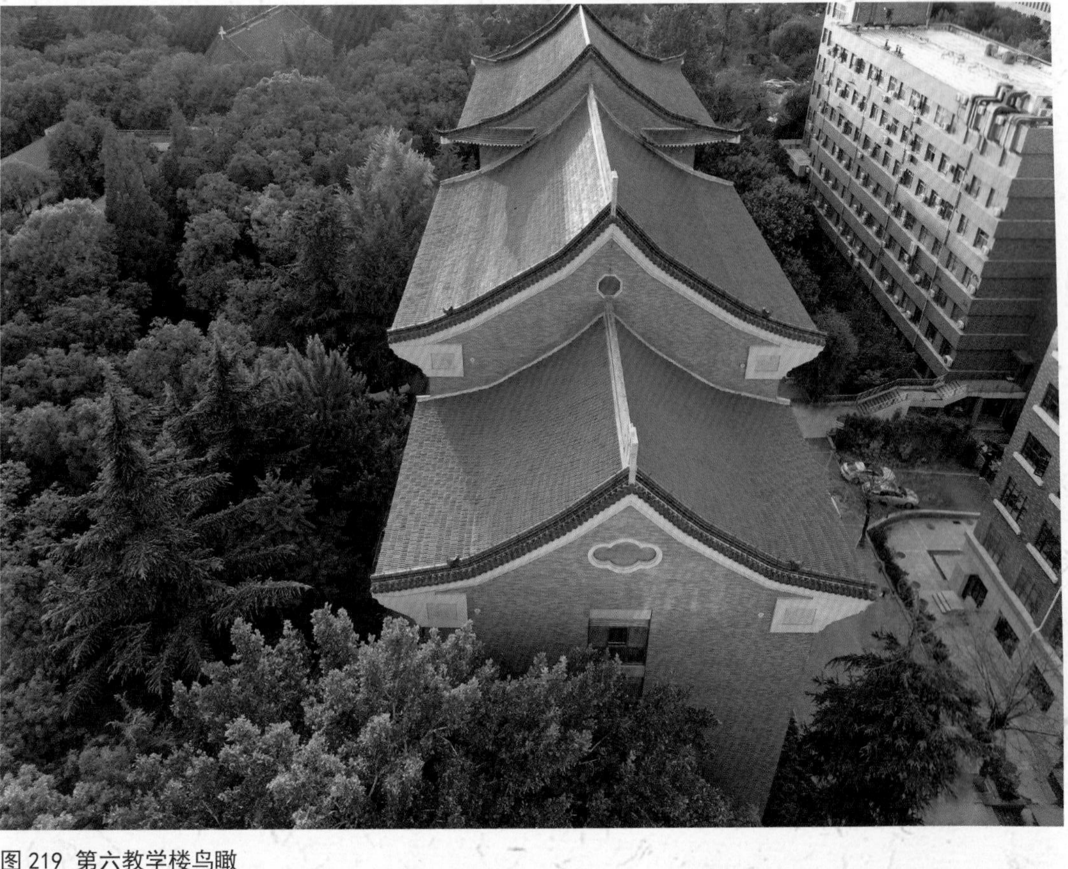

图 219 第六教学楼鸟瞰

Fig. 219 A bird’s eye-view of the Sixth Teaching Building

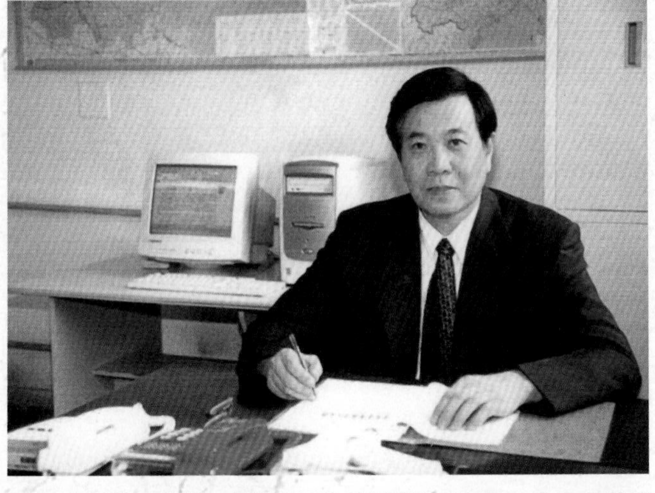

图 220 于修平教授，曾任病原生物学研究所所长、山东大学副校长兼医学院院长。

Fig. 220 Professor Yu Xiuping, former director of the Institute of Pathogen Biology, vice president of Shandong University and dean of the Medical School.

图 221 中国工程院洪涛院士，20 世纪 40 年代末和 50 年代初曾在山东医学院工作和学习。

Fig. 221 Hong Tao, the academician of Chinese Academy of Engineering, worked and studied in Shandong Medical College in the late 1940s and early 1950s.

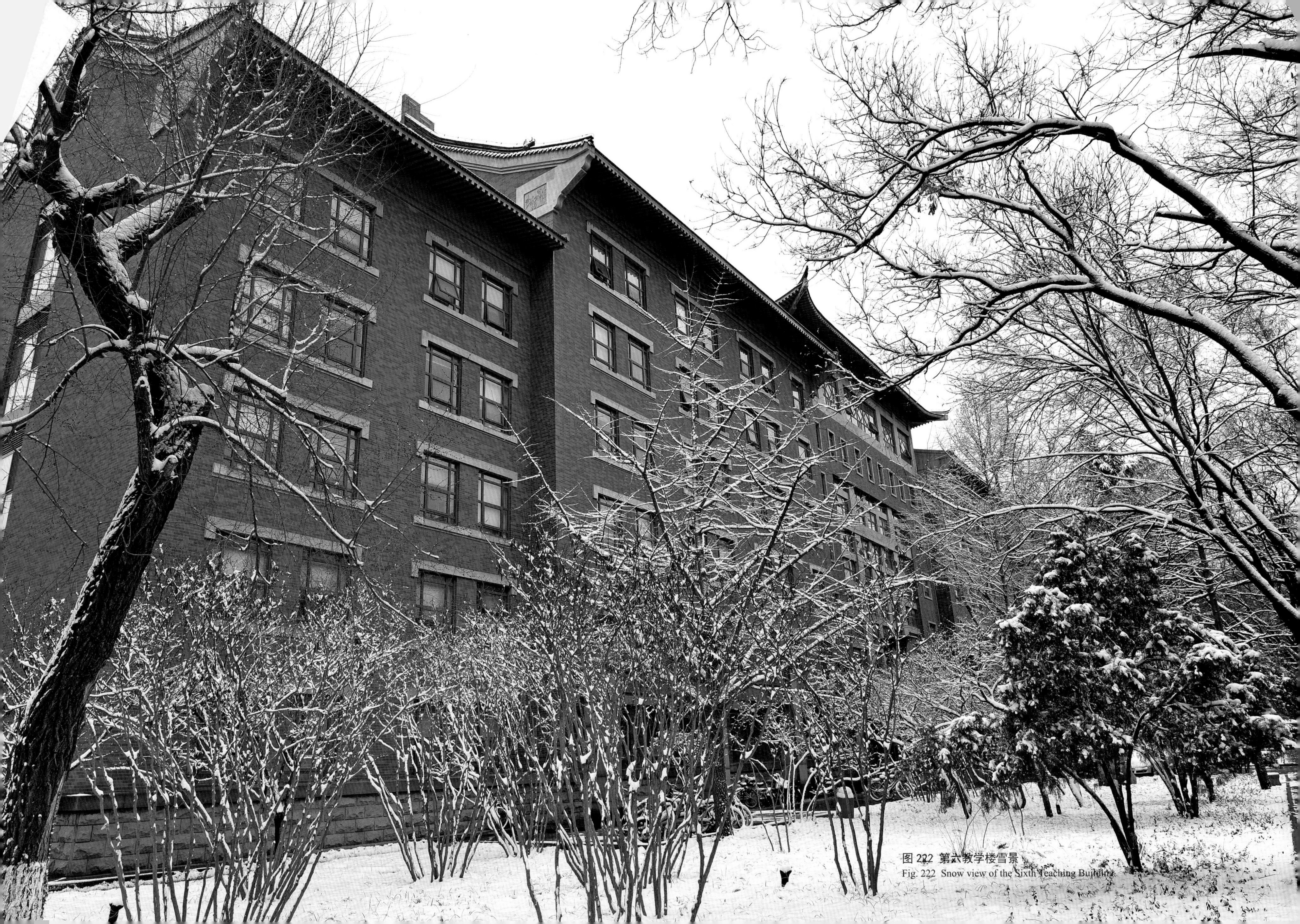

图 222 第六教学楼雪景

Fig. 222 Snow view of the Sixth Teaching Building

26 第七教学楼（1）

The Seventh Teaching Building (1)

第七教学楼是在 1983 年拆除奥古斯丁图书馆后，于 1985 年建成的。在中心花园周围的六座建筑中，这座楼的建筑风格和精神气韵有些卓尔不群。如果说中轴线上的综合楼和教学八楼给人以凝重、庄严和典雅的气质，东西相望的柏根楼与考文楼显得高贵精致、仪态万方的话，那么拔地而起、直插云霄的第七教学楼就令人产生一种“山从人面起，云傍马头生”的感觉。

在艺术设计上，可将中心花园周围的六座楼分为南、北两个“品”字形。南“品”字形的三个建筑在墙体装饰上比北“品”字形的明显简化，而且都坐落于一个高坛之上，需要登上台阶才能到达一层。第七教学楼通体雪白，头戴红沿大屋顶，在碧绿的草坪和浓密的树林衬托下，显得格外光彩照人，潇洒从容。特别是其南北两个大门，门楼被粗壮的廊柱撑起，上覆黄色琉璃瓦，檐下装饰以各种草药图案，楼角飞翅，飘飘欲仙，气派十足。

The Seventh Teaching Building was built in 1985 after the demolition of the Augustine Library in 1983. Of the six buildings around the Central Garden, this building’s architectural style and artistic conception are eminent above all others. If the Comprehensive Building and the Eighth Teaching Building on the central axis manifest a dignified, solemn and elegant temperament, and Bergen Hall and Calvin Mateer Hall facing each other in the east and west sides appear noble, exquisite and graceful, then the Seventh Teaching Building which rises straight from the ground and climbs straight into the sky gives people a feeling of “the cliff suddenly rises from the face side of people walking on the plank road, and the clouds rise and billow beside the horse’s head”.

In terms of the artistic design, the six buildings around the Central Garden are in the shape of the Chinese character “pin” in the south and north respectively. The three buildings in the shape of “pin” in the south are obviously simpler in wall decoration than those in the shape of “pin” in the north, and they all are located on a high altar, which requires to walk up the steps to reach the first floor. The Seventh Teaching Building is snow-white, with a large red roof, shining and calm against the green lawn and dense woods. In particular, the gatehouses of its two gates in the north and south look ethereal and imposing which are supported by strong colonnades, covered with yellow glazed tiles and decorated with a variety of herbal patterns under the eaves.

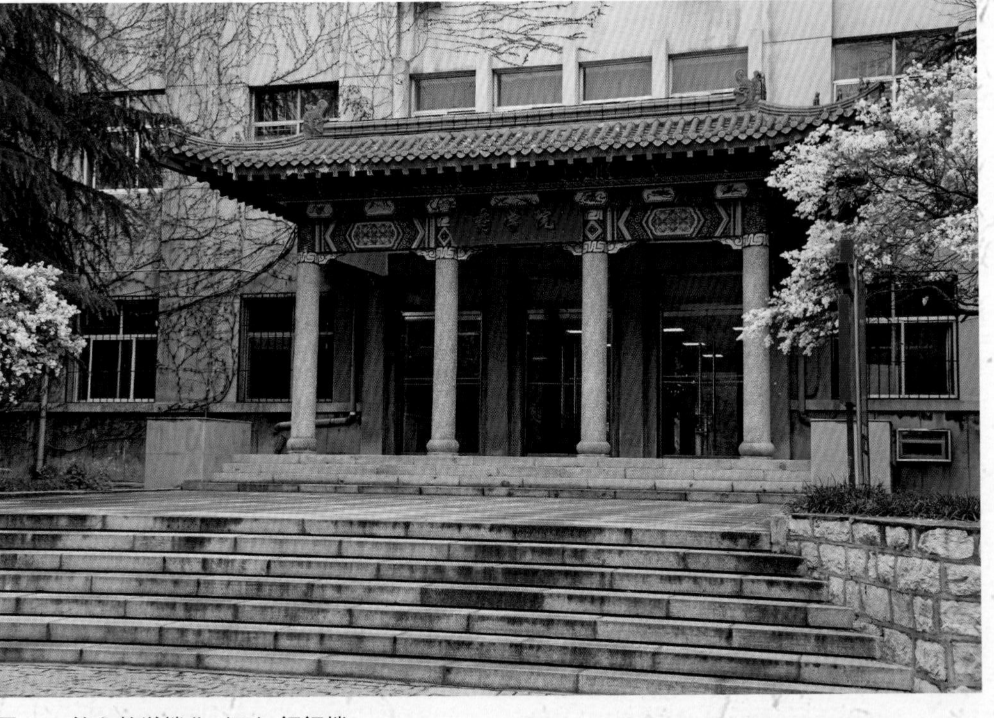

图 223 第七教学楼北（正）门门楼

Fig. 223 Gatehouse of the north (front) gate of the Seventh Teaching Building

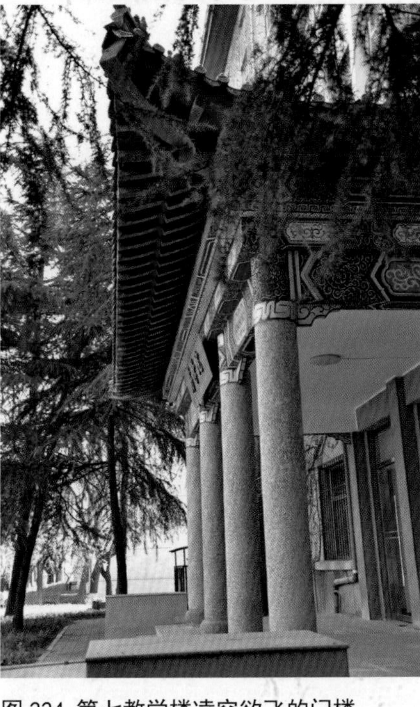

图 224 第七教学楼凌空欲飞的门楼

Fig. 224 Gatehouse of the Seventh Teaching Building in the sky

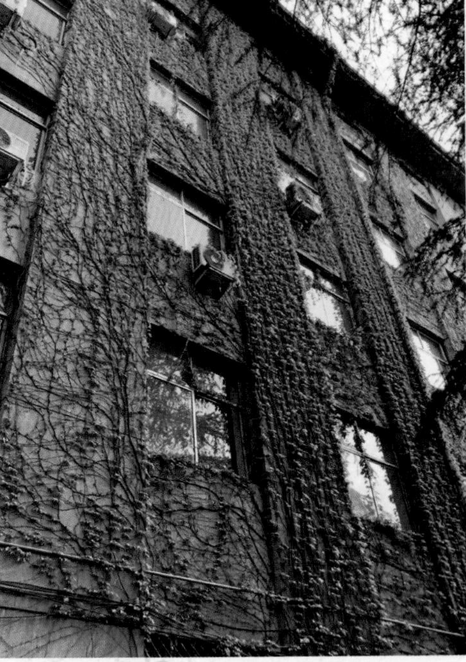

图 225 第七教学楼北立面的爬山虎

Fig. 225 Creepers on the north wall of the Seventh Teaching Building

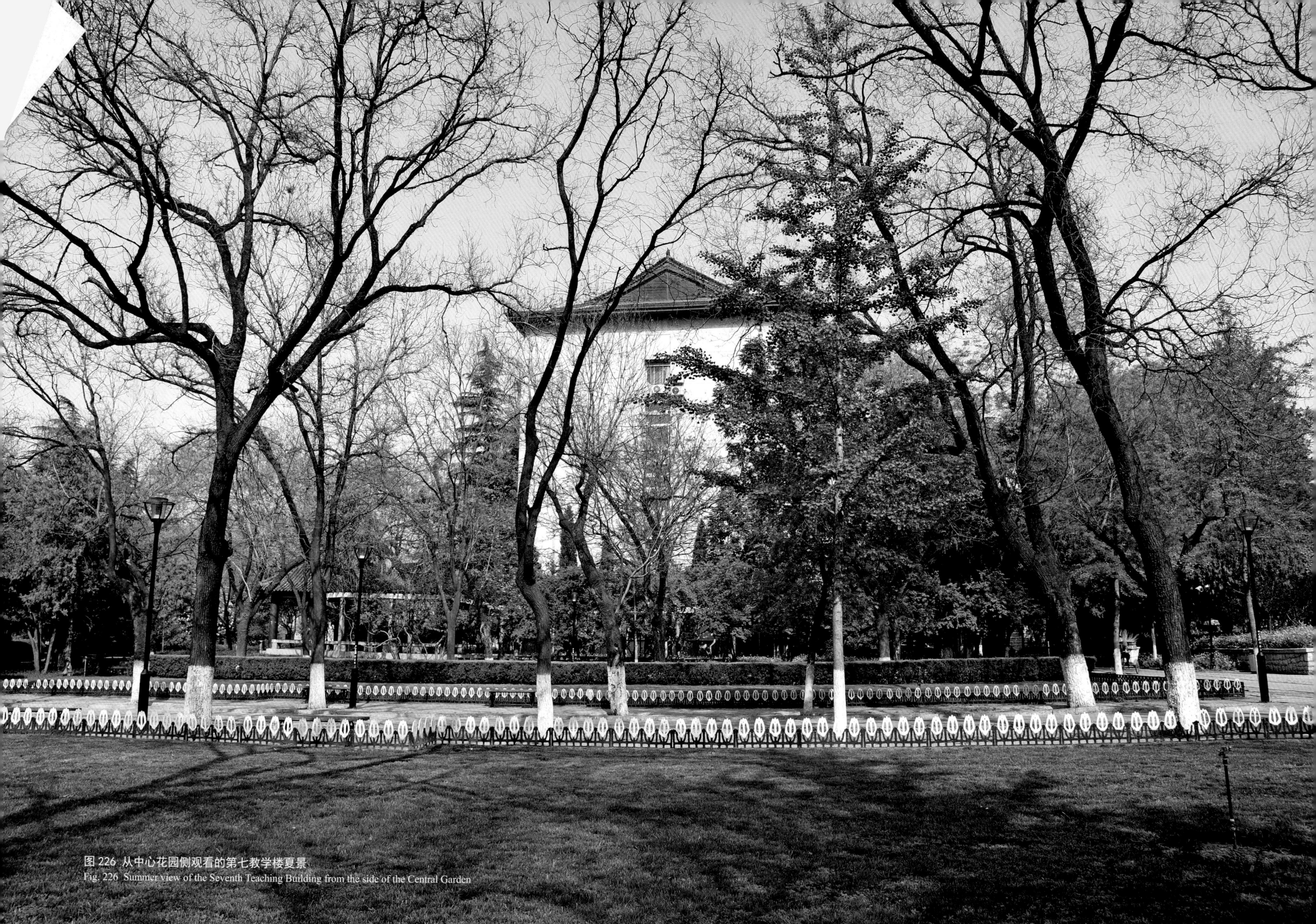

图 226 从中心花园侧观看的第七教学楼夏景
Fig. 226 Summer view of the Seventh Teaching Building from the side of the Central Garden

26 | 第七教学楼（2）

The Seventh Teaching Building (2)

第七教学楼为药学院主体建筑，见证了山东大学药学专业三十余年来的快速发展。山东大学药学院的前身是齐鲁大学药科，由英国传教士裴维廉博士（Willim P.Pailing）于1920 年创办，隶属医学系，是我国第三所现代高等药学教育院校。1941 年，内迁成都的齐鲁大学设立药学系，隶属理学院，薛愚教授担任首任药学系主任。历经几度调整和变迁，1971 年山东医学院药学系恢复招生，1997 年改称山东医科大学药学院，2000 年成为山东大学药学院。20 世纪 70 年代，张天民教授等率先开展微生物与生化药物研究，1978 年获得两项全国科学大会奖。1992 年，王慧才教授等研制的抗癌新药卡铂获国家科技进步奖三等奖。特别是进入 21 世纪以来，在娄红祥、王凤山和刘新泳三任院长领导下，经过全院职工的努力和拚搏，实现了药物研发从仿制到创新的重大转变，综合实力已跻身于国内同类院校的先进行列。

The Seventh Teaching Building is the main building of the School of Pharmaceutical Sciences which has witnessed the rapid development of pharmacy in Shandong University in the past thirty-odd years. The predecessor of the School of Pharmaceutical Sciences of Shandong University is the Department of Pharmacy of Cheeloo University, which was founded in 1920 by the English missionary Dr. William P. Pailing and affiliated to the Department of Medicine. It is the third modern high academy of pharmaceutical education in China. In 1941, Cheeloo University which moved to Chengdu set up the Department of Pharmacy affiliated to the School of Science and Professor Xue Yu served as the first director of the department. After several adjustments and transitions, the Department of Pharmacy of Shandong Medical College resumed enrollment in 1971. It changed its name to the School of Pharmaceutical Sciences of Shandong Medical University in 1997 and became the School of Pharmaceutical Sciences of Shandong University in 2000. In the 1970s, Professor Zhang Tianmin and others took the lead in carrying out research on microorganisms and biochemical drugs, and won two awards of the National Conference on Science in 1978. In 1992, the new anti-cancer drug carboplatin developed by Professor Wang Huicai and others won the third prize of National Science and Technology Progress Award. Since the beginning of the 21st century, under the leadership of the three deans of Lou Hongxiang, Wang Fengshan and Liu Xinyong, and through the efforts and hard work of the faculty, the major transformation of drug research and development from imitation to innovation has been realized, and the comprehensive strength of the School of Pharmaceutical Sciences has been among the advanced ranks of similar colleges and universities in China.

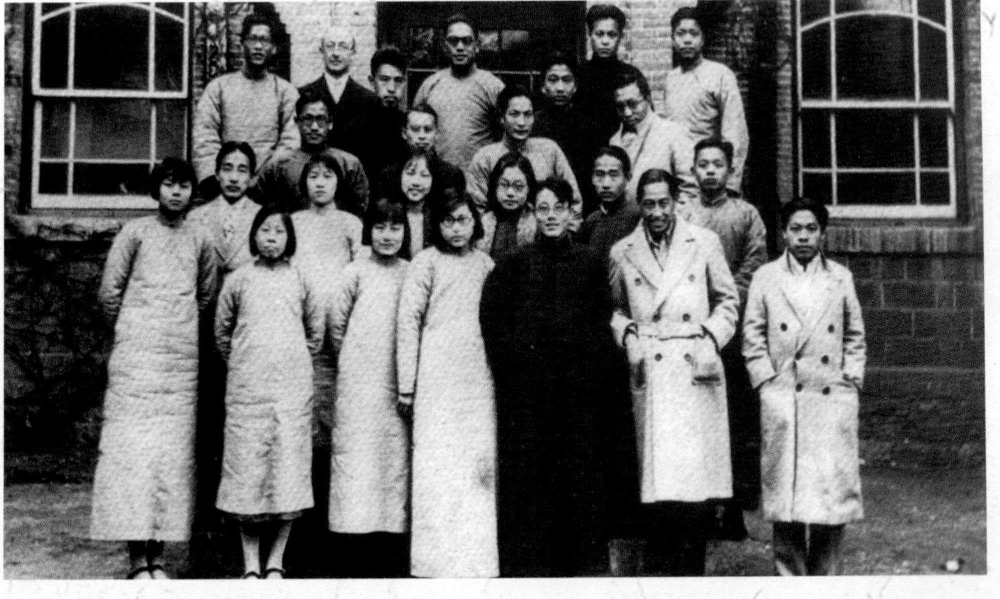

图 227 1934 年齐鲁大学药专班师生合影，后排左二为创办人裴维廉博士

Fig. 227 Teachers and students of the pharmaceutical class of Cheeloo University taking a photo in 1934, with the founder Doctor Willim P. Pailing, the second from the left in the back row.

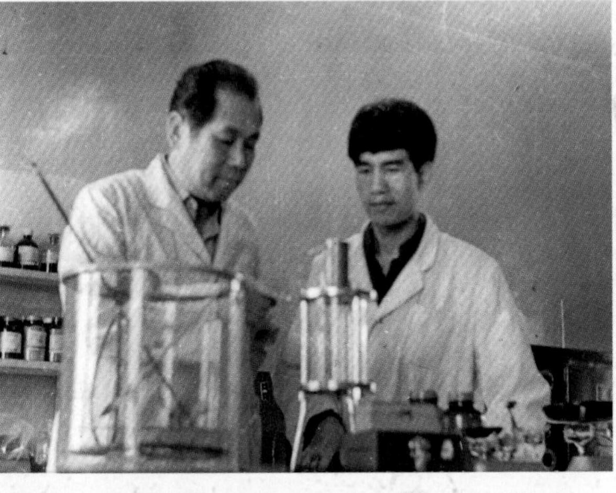

图 228 张天民教授（1928 ～ 2014，左），中国生化药学创始人之一

Fig. 228 Professor Zhang Tianmin (1928-2014,left), one of the founders of biochemical pharmacy in China

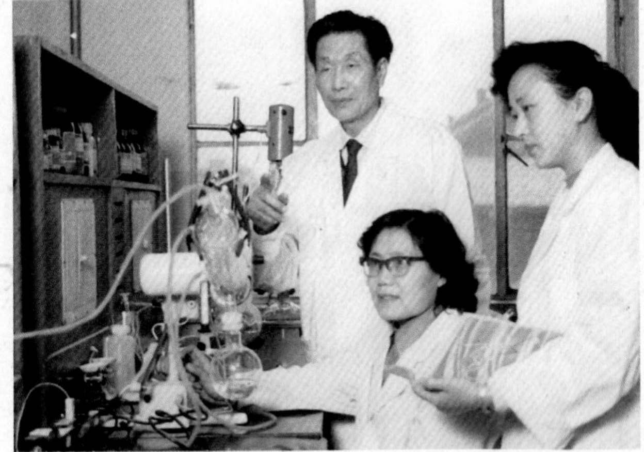

图 229 王慧才教授（1930 ～ 2019，左一）等研制的抗癌新药卡铂，获得国家科技进步奖三等奖

Fig. 229 The new anti-cancer drug carboplatin developed by Professor Wang Huicai (1930-2019,first from left) and others won the third prize of National Science and Technology Progress Award

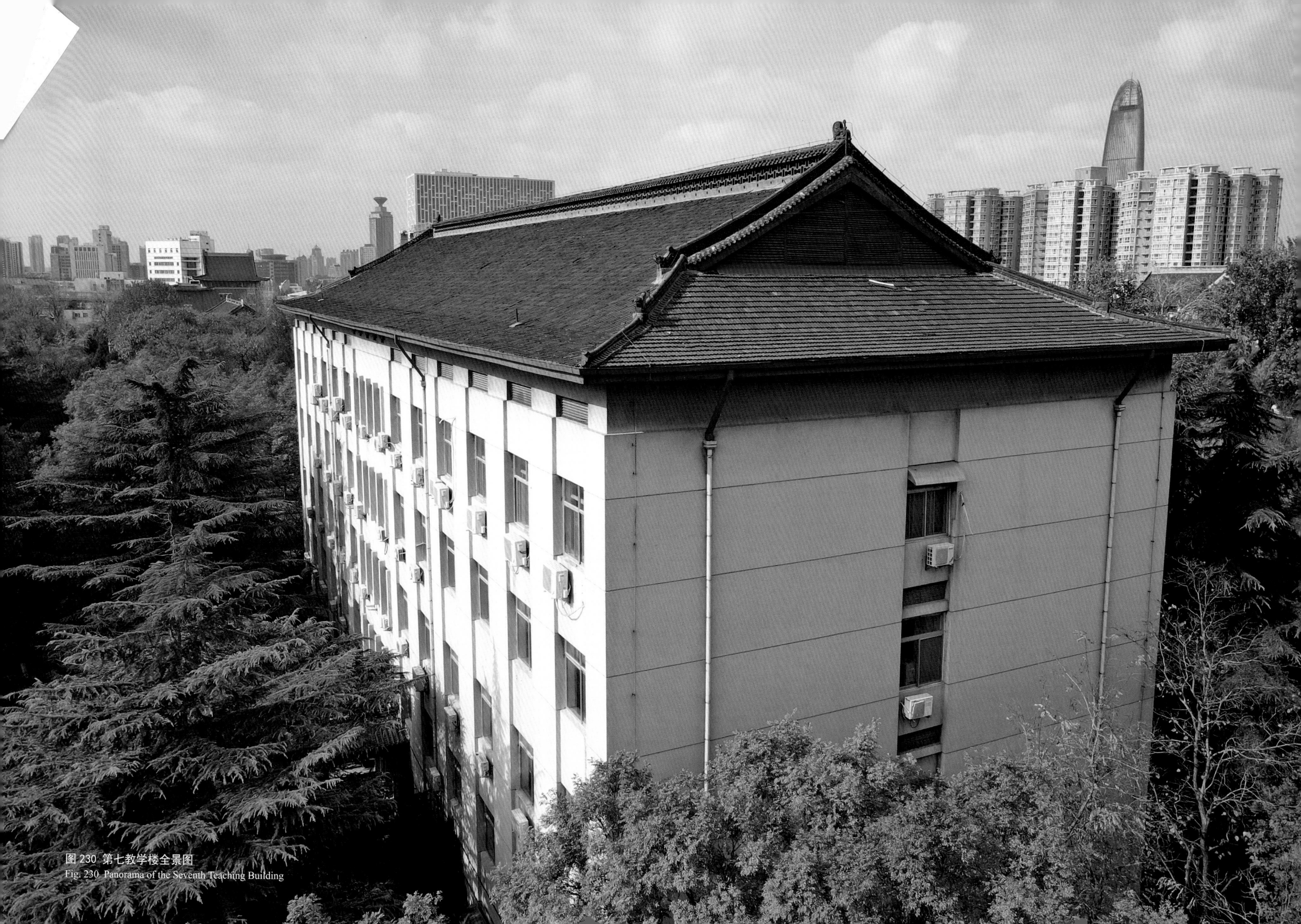

图 230 第七教学楼全景图
Fig. 230 Panorama of the Seventh Teaching Building

27 第八教学楼（1）

The Eighth Teaching Building (1)

第八教学楼是在 1958 年拆除康穆堂后，于 1963 年建成并投入使用的，是齐鲁医学院的主体建筑之一。此楼规模宏大，位于中心花园中轴线的南端，为观赏校园四季变化的最佳去处。若登临此楼高处，南可眺望千佛山连绵之翠峰，北能静听趵突泉喷涌之波涛，东允尽赏春花与旭日齐辉，西许饱览秋菊共晚霞一色。当晚风吹拂，皓月当空，若能于此楼北侧高台之上，设坛慷慨演讲，或轻歌曼舞，或围坐畅谈，定能尽释平日案牍之劳神，岂不快哉！

由于建设的时代背景，第八教学楼的建筑风格颇受苏联的影响。作为中轴线上的压轴之作，此楼舒展扩张，稳重大方，有独领风骚之气魄。楼体正中部分五层，前后稍凸出，上方冠以中国式大屋顶；两翼四层，向东西伸展，至两端时转向南北延伸。鸟瞰全楼，平面十分规整，呈现“王”字外形，蔚为壮观。南北面正中各开一门，设有门楼，均有廊柱支撑，倍感庄严威武。楼体正中部墙面和门楼飞檐下装饰以如意、星星和祥云图案，显得中华文化氛围十足。

The Eighth Teaching Building, which was completed and put into use in 1963 after the demolition of Kumler Chapel in 1958, is one of the main buildings of Cheeloo College of Medicine. Located at the south end of the central axis of the Central Garden, the grand building is the best place to watch the changes of the campus in the four seasons. If you climb to the height of this building, you can see the continuous lush peaks of Qianfo Hill in the south, listen to the flowing waves of Baotu Spring in the north, enjoy the spring flowers and the rising sun in the east, and feast your eyes on the chrysanthemums and sunset of the same color in the west. With the night breeze and bright moon, if you could present your views vehemently on the high platform on the north side of this building, sing and dance lightly, or sit around and talk freely, you would definitely be able to release the daily cares! Wouldn't you be happy!

Due to the background of the construction, the architectural style of the Eighth Teaching Building was greatly influenced by the former Soviet Union. As an important building on the central axis, this unfolding and generous building has the spirit of taking the lead. The middle part of the building has five floors, slightly protruding from the front and back, with a large Chinese roof. The two wings have four floors, extending to the east and west respectively and turning to the south and north respectively when reaching both ends. A bird's-eye view of the whole building shows that the plane is very regular and presents the shape of the Chinese character "wang" , looking very spectacular. A door is opened in the middle of the north and south respectively with the gatehouse supported by the colonnades, feeling solemn and powerful. The wall in the middle of the building and the cornices of the archway are decorated with patterns of ruyi, stars and auspicious clouds, full of Chinese cultural atmosphere.

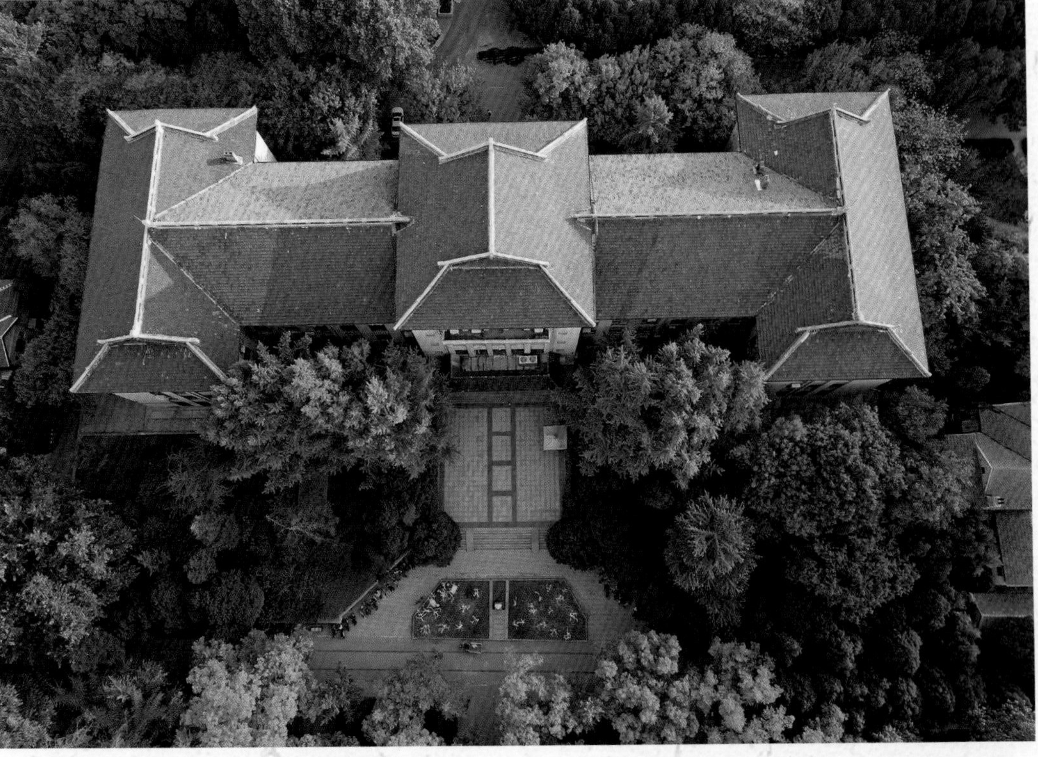

图 231 呈“王”字外形的第八教学楼
Fig. 231 The Eighth Teaching Building in the shape of the Chinese character "wang"

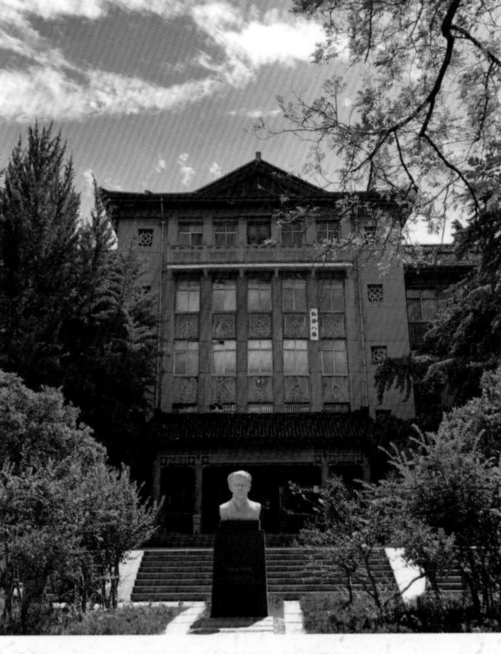

图 232 第八教学楼北（正）面观
Fig. 232 The north (front) view of the Eighth Teaching Building

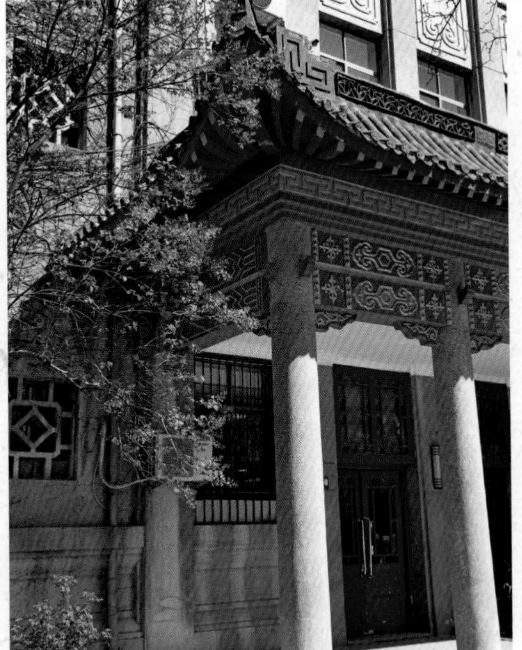

图 233 第八教学楼南门
Fig. 233 The south gate of the Eighth Teaching Building

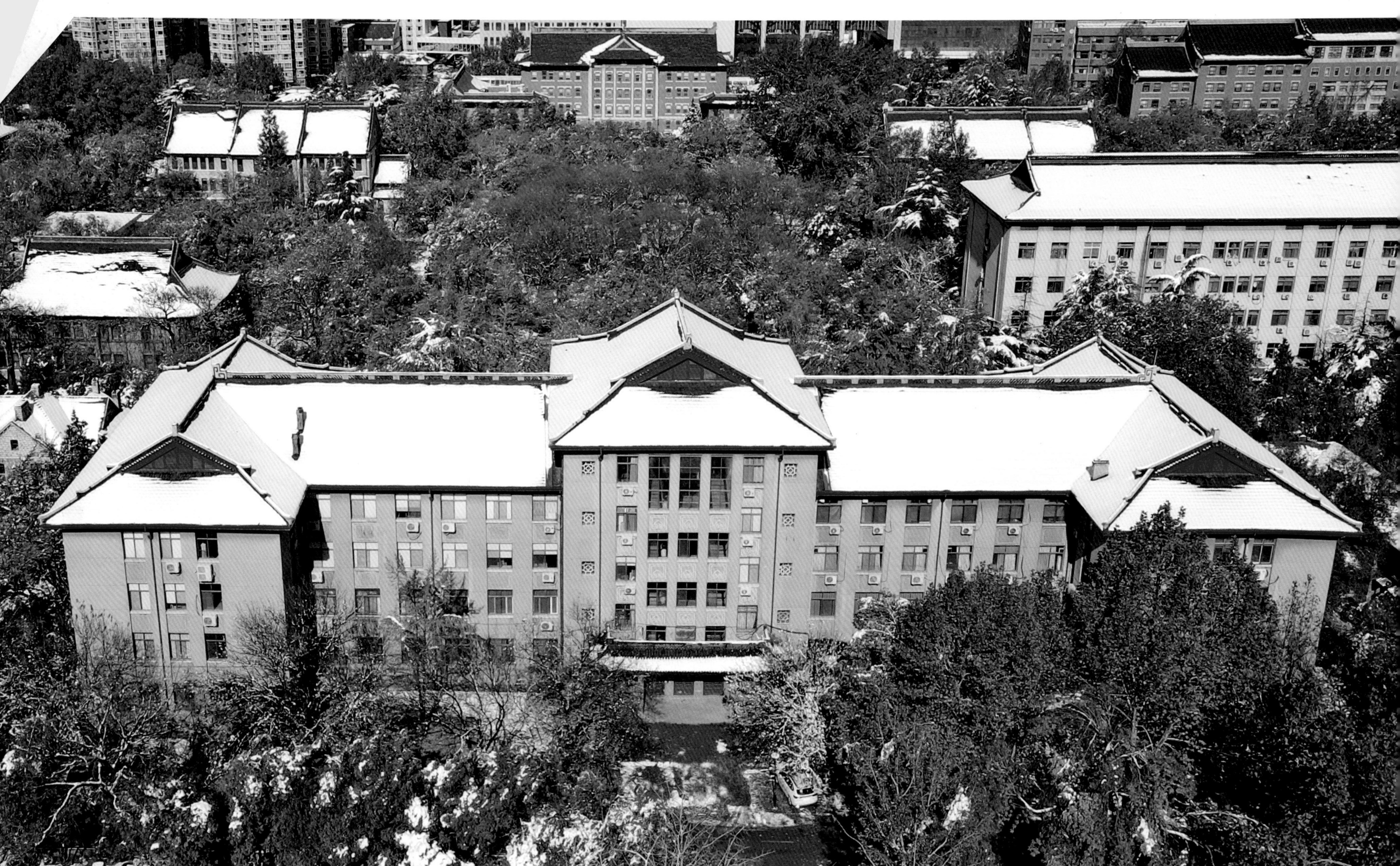

图 234 第八教学楼位于中心花园中轴线的南端
Fig. 234 The Eighth Teaching Building located at the south end of the central axis of the Central Garden

27 | 第八教学楼（2）

The Eighth Teaching Building (2)

除公共教室外，第八教学楼主要有人体科学馆、手术学教研室、信息化教学研究中心、现代教育技术研究中心、形态学实验教学平台、机能学实验教学平台、计算机教学中心和大学外语教学部等机构。

山东大学人体科学馆主要依托国家重点学科人体解剖与组织胚胎学和首批国家临床重点专科病理学的学科力量建设而成，收藏本校师生制作的人体标本逾千件，共分为人体胚胎学、人体解剖学、病理学和学科发展史四个展区，充分展示了人体发生与演变过程、形态结构和常见疾病病理特征，也反映了我校人体解剖与组织胚胎学和病理学一代代师生的科学探索精神和卓越成就。

形态学实验教学平台和机能学实验教学平台成立于 1999 年，完成的“基础医学融合性实验教学课程体系改革”项目于 2005 年获国家级教学成果奖二等奖。手术学教学实验室最近完成了升级改造，以满足现代外科学发展的需要。

Apart from the public classrooms, the Eighth Teaching Building mainly has the Museum of Human Sciences, the Teaching and Research Department of Surgery, the Informationized Teaching and Research Center, the Research Center for Modern Educational Technology, the Experimental Teaching Platform of Morphology, the Functional Experimental Teaching Platform, the Computer Teaching Center and the School of Foreign Languages Teaching.

The Museum of Human Sciences of Shandong University is mainly built on the strength of the national key discipline of Human Anatomy and Histoembryology and the first batch of national key clinical specialty of Pathology. It has collected more than 1,000 human specimens made by teachers and students of the university. It is divided into four exhibition areas: Human Embryology, Human Anatomy, Pathology and the Development History of Disciplines, fully demonstrating the process of anthropogenesis and evolution, the morphological structure and pathological characteristics of common diseases, and also reflecting the scientific exploration spirit and outstanding achievements of generations of teachers and students in human anatomy and histoembryology and pathology in our school.

The Experimental Teaching Platform of Morphology and the Functional Experimental Teaching Platform were established in 1999, and their project of "Curriculum System Reform of Integrated Experimental Teaching of Basic Medical Sciences" won the second prize of National Teaching Achievement Award in 2005. The Teaching and Research Department of Surgery has recently been upgraded to meet the needs of the development of modern surgery.

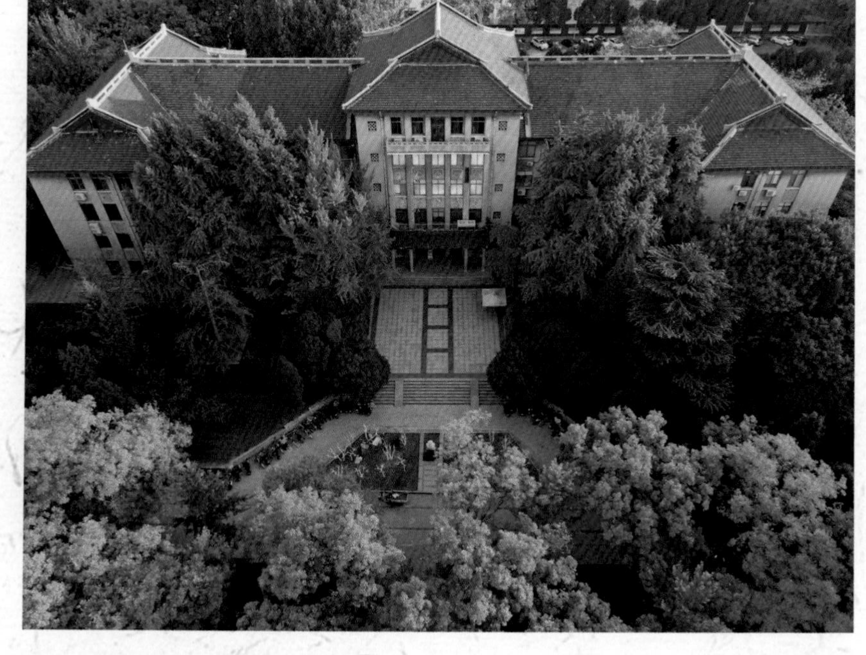

图 235 初秋的第八教学楼（正面观）

Fig. 235 The Eighth Teaching Building in early autumn (front view)

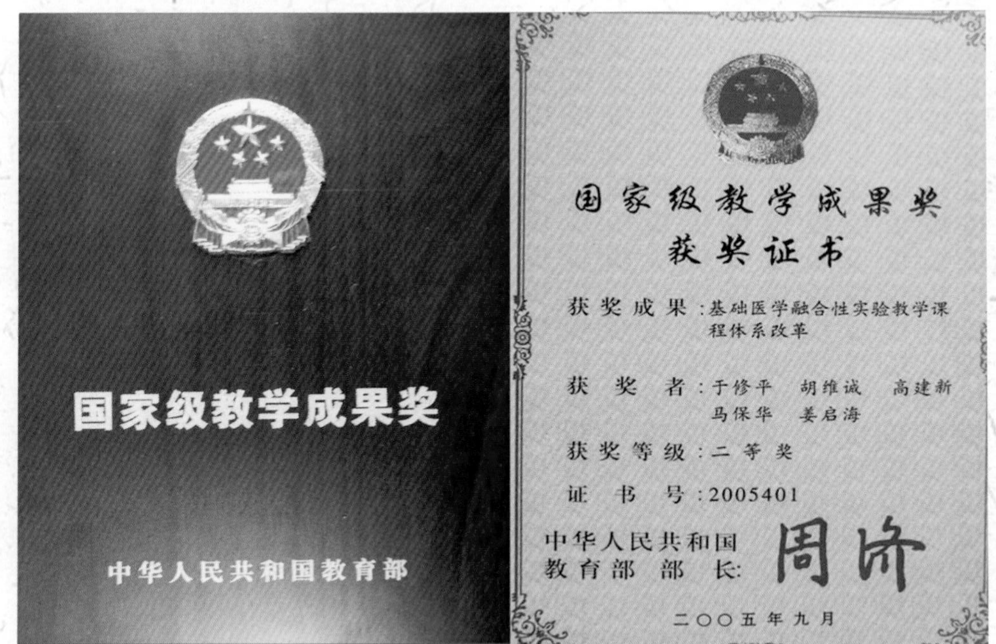

图 236 “基础医学融合性实验教学课程体系改革”项目于 2005 年获国家级教学成果奖

Fig. 236 The project "Curriculum System Reform of Integrated Experimental Teaching of Basic Medical Sciences" winning the second prize of National Teaching Achievement Award in 2005

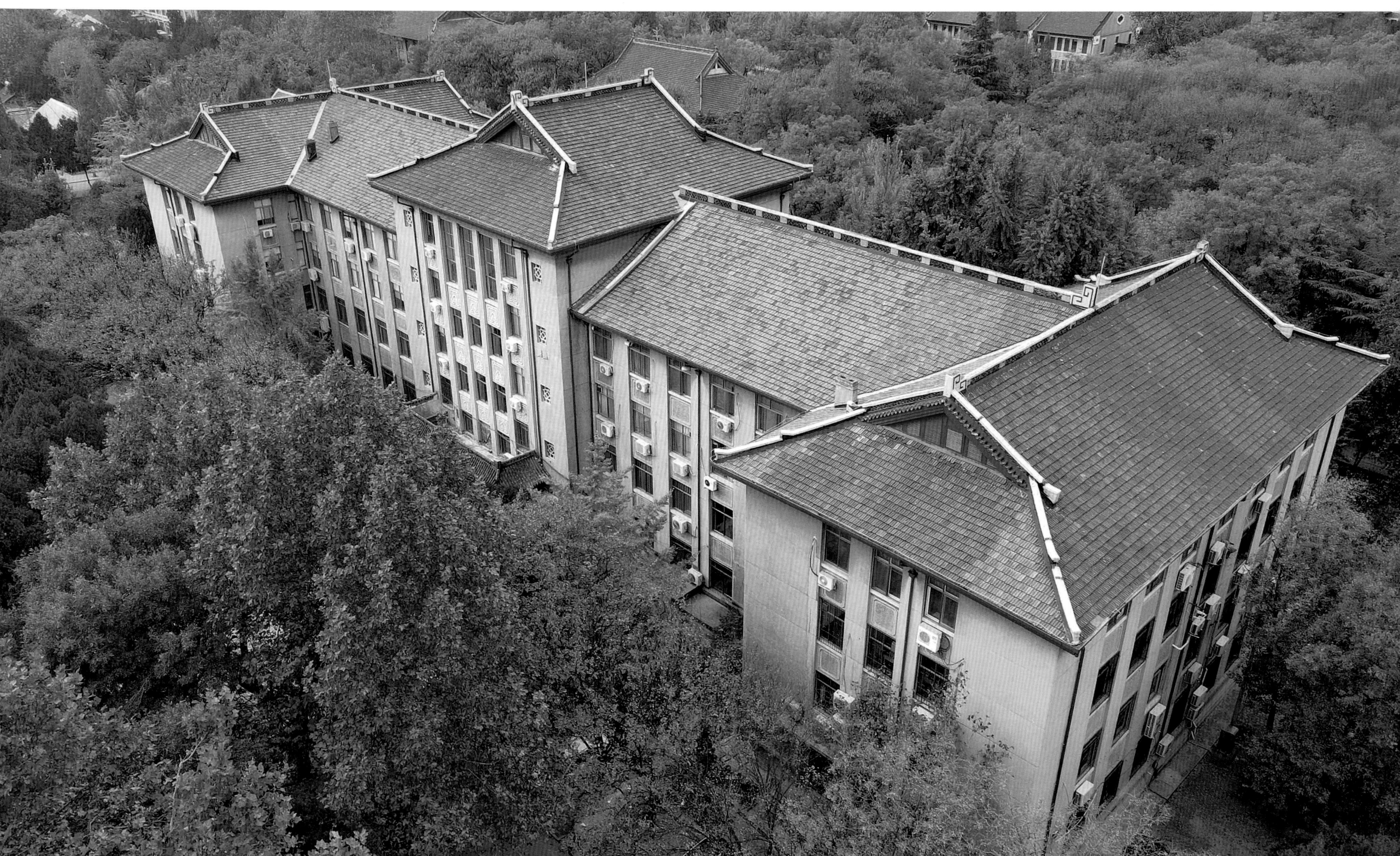

图 237 第八教学楼笼罩在盎然秋色之中
Fig. 237 The Eighth Teaching Building shrouded in the exuberant autumn scenery

28 第九教学楼

The Ninth Teaching Building

第九教学楼兴建于 20 世纪 80 年代初期，钢筋混凝土结构，共七层，一层为公共教室，其余由公共卫生学院使用。

山东大学公共卫生学院悠久的历史可追溯至 1926 年创建的齐鲁大学医学院公共卫生科，1952 年建立山东医学院卫生系，其后历经两次建撤，1977 年恢复建制，1996 年升格为山东医科大学公共卫生学院，2000 年更名为山东大学公共卫生学院。学院底蕴深厚，流行病与卫生统计学为国家重点学科，建有国家卫健委卫生经济与政策研究重点实验室、山东大学健康医疗大数据研究院、山东大学生态健康研究院等研究机构。2020 年与山东省、济南市共建“国家健康医疗大数据研究院”。历史上的知名专家有王福溢、方春望、王均乐和束怀符等。

方春望（1915~1995），原名聂崇铭，浙江常山人，著名传染病学专家。1943 年毕业于上海医学院。曾任山东医学院院长、山东医科大学校长等职。主编有《实用传染病学》《传染病与流行病学》和《实用临床流行病学》等著作。

The Ninth Teaching Building was built in the 1980s, with reinforced concrete structure and seven floors. The first floor is for public classrooms and the rest is used by the School of Public Health.

The long history of the School of Public Health of Shandong University can be traced back to the Discipline of Public Health of the Medical School of Cheeloo University established in 1926. In 1952, the Department of Public Health of Shandong Medical College was established. In 1977, the department was restored after two times of establishment and cancellation. In 1996, It was upgraded to the School of Public Health of Shandong Medical University. In 2000, it changed its name to School of Public Health of Shandong University. With profound foundation, the school has the national key discipline of epidemiology and health statistics and has established some research institutions such as the key Laboratory of Health Economy and Policy Research of the National Health Commission, the Health and Medical Research Institute of Shandong University, the Research Institute of Ecological Health of Shandong University and so on. In 2020, the school has jointly built the National Institute of Health Data Science with Shandong Province and Jinan City. The famous experts of this school include Wang Fuyi, Fang Chunwang, Wang Junle, Shu Huaifu and so on.

Fang Chunwang (1915-1995), the original name as Nie Chongming, was born in Changshan, Zhejiang Province, and is a famous expert in infectious diseases. He graduated from Shanghai Medical College in 1943 and once served as president of Shandong Medical College and president of Shandong Medical University. He once edited *Practical Infectious Diseases*, *Infectious Diseases and Epidemiology*, *Practical Clinical Epidemiology* and so on.

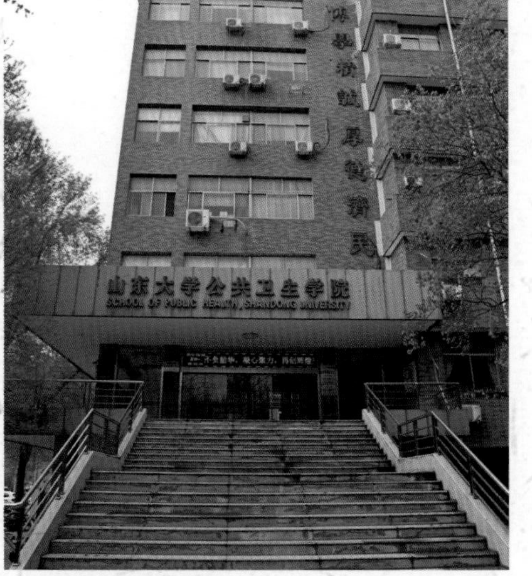

图 238 第九教学楼大门
Fig. 238 Gate of the Ninth Teaching Building

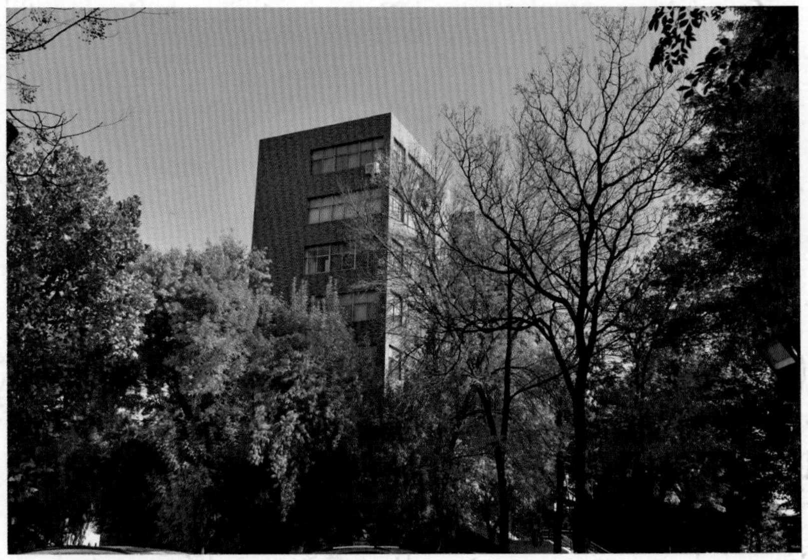

图 239 第九教学楼西面观
Fig. 239 The west view of the Ninth Teaching Building

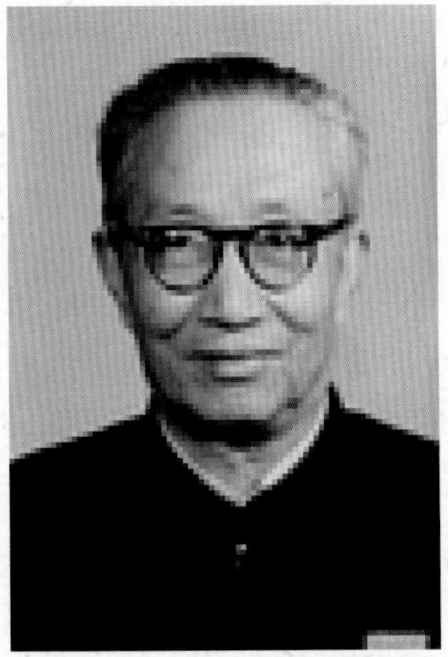

图 240 著名传染病学专家、医学教育家方春望教授
Fig. 240 Professor Fang Chunwang, a famous expert in infectious diseases and medical educator

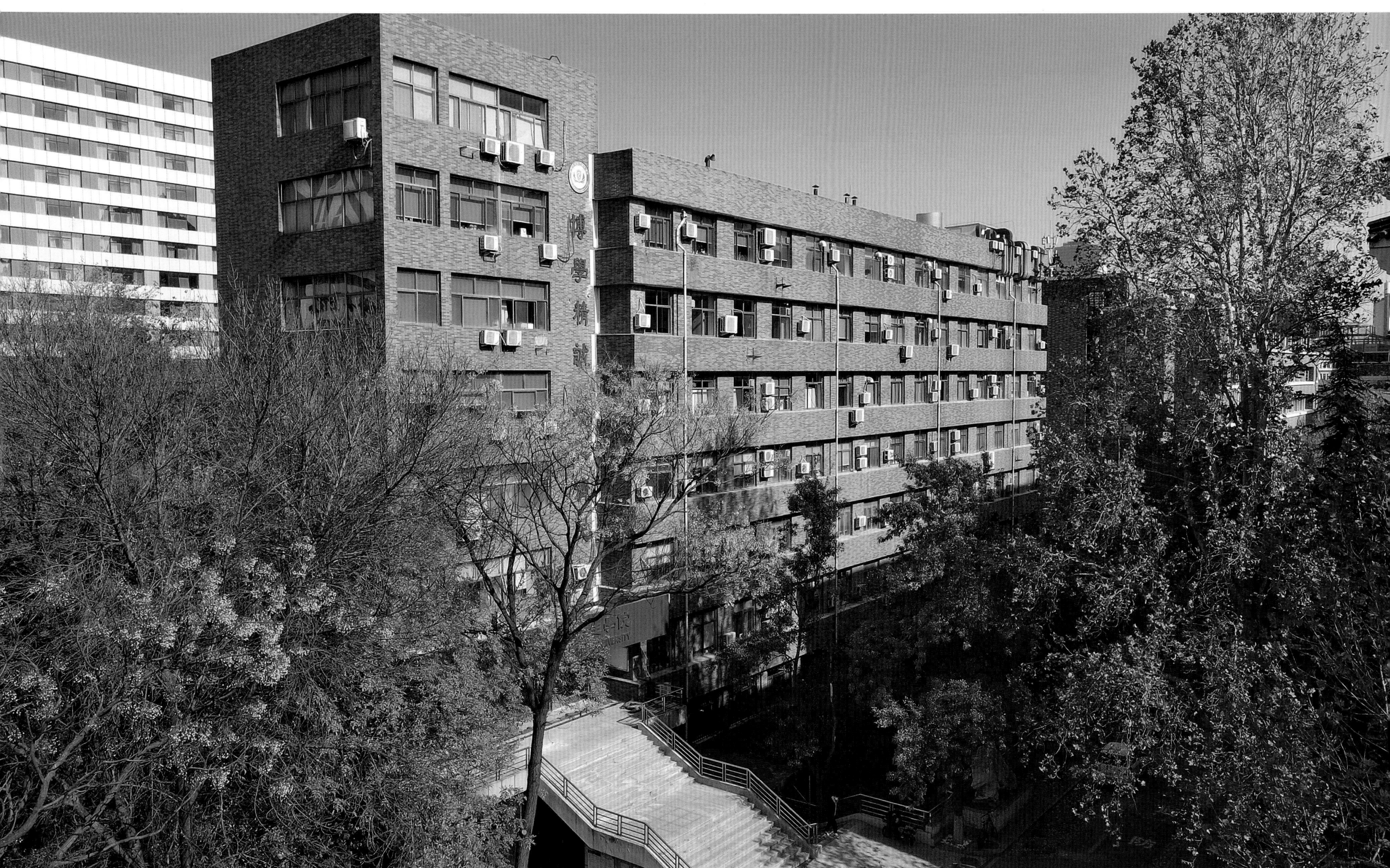

图 241 秋叶映照第九教学楼

Fig. 241 The autumn leaves shining on the Ninth Teaching Building

29 口腔医学大楼（1）

Building of Stomatology（1）

口腔医学大楼共六层，包括南北两部分，北楼 20 世纪 80 年代兴建，南楼落成于 2018 年，均为钢筋混凝土结构，现由口腔医学院（口腔医院）使用。

山东大学口腔医学院（口腔医院）的前身为山东医学院口腔系，始建于 1977 年。1985 年更名为山东医科大学口腔系，1992 年附属口腔医院开诊，2000 年改称山东大学口腔学院（口腔医院），2006 年增名山东省口腔医院。山东大学口腔医学院、山东大学口腔医院、山东省口腔医院实行三院合一管理体制，集教育教学、科学研究、医疗服务和预防保健等功能于一体，是山东省口腔医学教学、科研、医疗和预防保健中心。学院（医院）综合实力雄厚，第四轮学科评估位居全国第八位。作为我国重要的口腔医学研究平台，学院（医院）拥有山东省口腔组织再生重点实验室和山东省口腔生物材料与组织再生工程实验室，并完成了国家临床药物试验机构口腔医疗器械试验备案，获得了口腔器械临床试验的资质。

The Building of Stomatology has six floors, including the North Building and the South Building. The North Building was built in the 1980s and the South Building was completed in 2018. Both buildings are of reinforced concrete structures and are now used by the School of Stomatology (The Stomatological Hospital).

The School of Stomatology of Shandong University (The Stomatological Hospital) was founded in 1977, formerly known as the Department of Stomatology of Shandong Medical College. In 1985, it was renamed the Department of Stomatology of Shandong Medical University. In 1992, the Affiliated Stomatological Hospital opened. In 2000, it was renamed the School of Stomatology of Shandong University (The Stomatological Hospital), and in 2006, it got another name of Shandong Stomatological Hospital. The School of Stomatology of Shandong University, the Stomatological Hospital of Shandong University and Shandong Stomatological Hospital implement a three-in-one management system, which integrates the functions of education and teaching, scientific research, medical service and prevention and healthcare, and serves as the center for teaching, scientific research, medical treatment and prevention and healthcare of stomatology in Shandong Province. With strong comprehensive strength, the School (Hospital) ranked the eighth in the fourth round of China Discipline Ranking. As an important research platform of stomatology in China, the School (Hospital) has Shandong Provincial Key Laboratory of Oral Tissue Regeneration and Shandong Provincial Engineering Laboratory for Dental Materials and Oral Tissue Regeneration, and it has completed the trial filing of oral medical devices of the national clinical drug trial institution and obtained the qualification of clinical trial of oral devices.

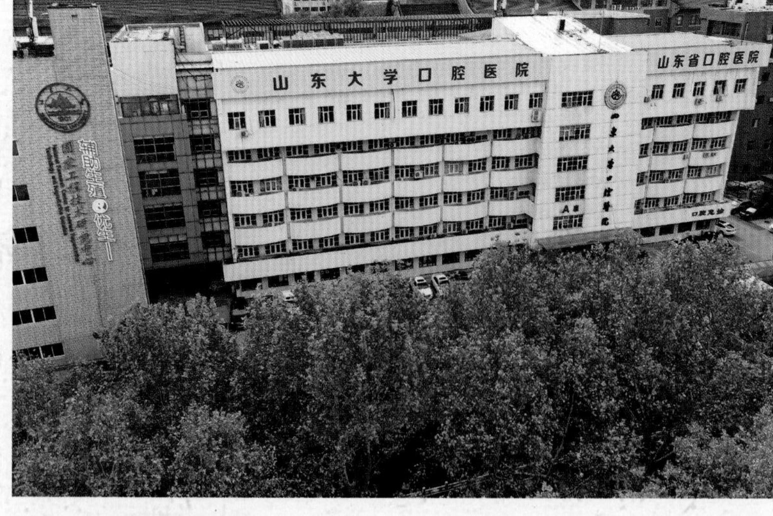

图 242 口腔医学院北楼
Fig. 242 The North Building of the School of Stomatology

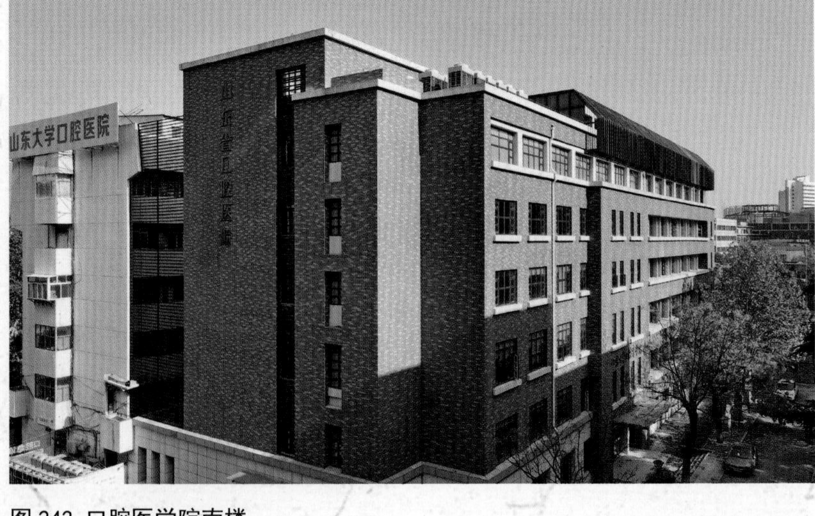

图 243 口腔医学院南楼
Fig. 243 The South Building of the School of Stomatology

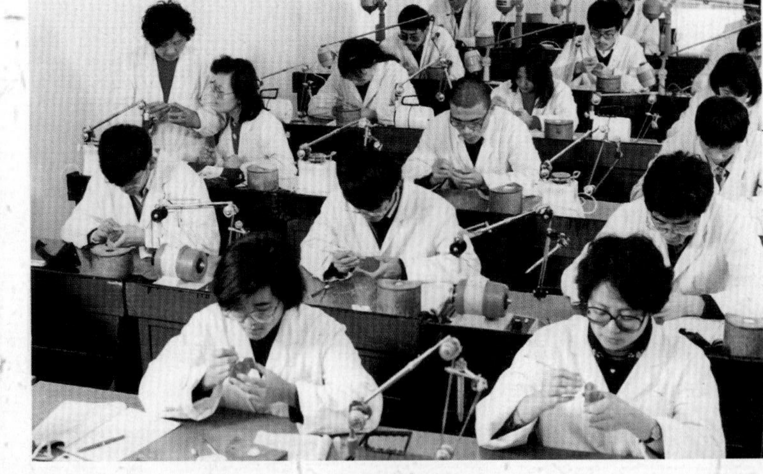
图 244 20 世纪 90 年代初的口腔医学实验教学
Fig. 244 Experimental teaching of stomatology in the early 1990s

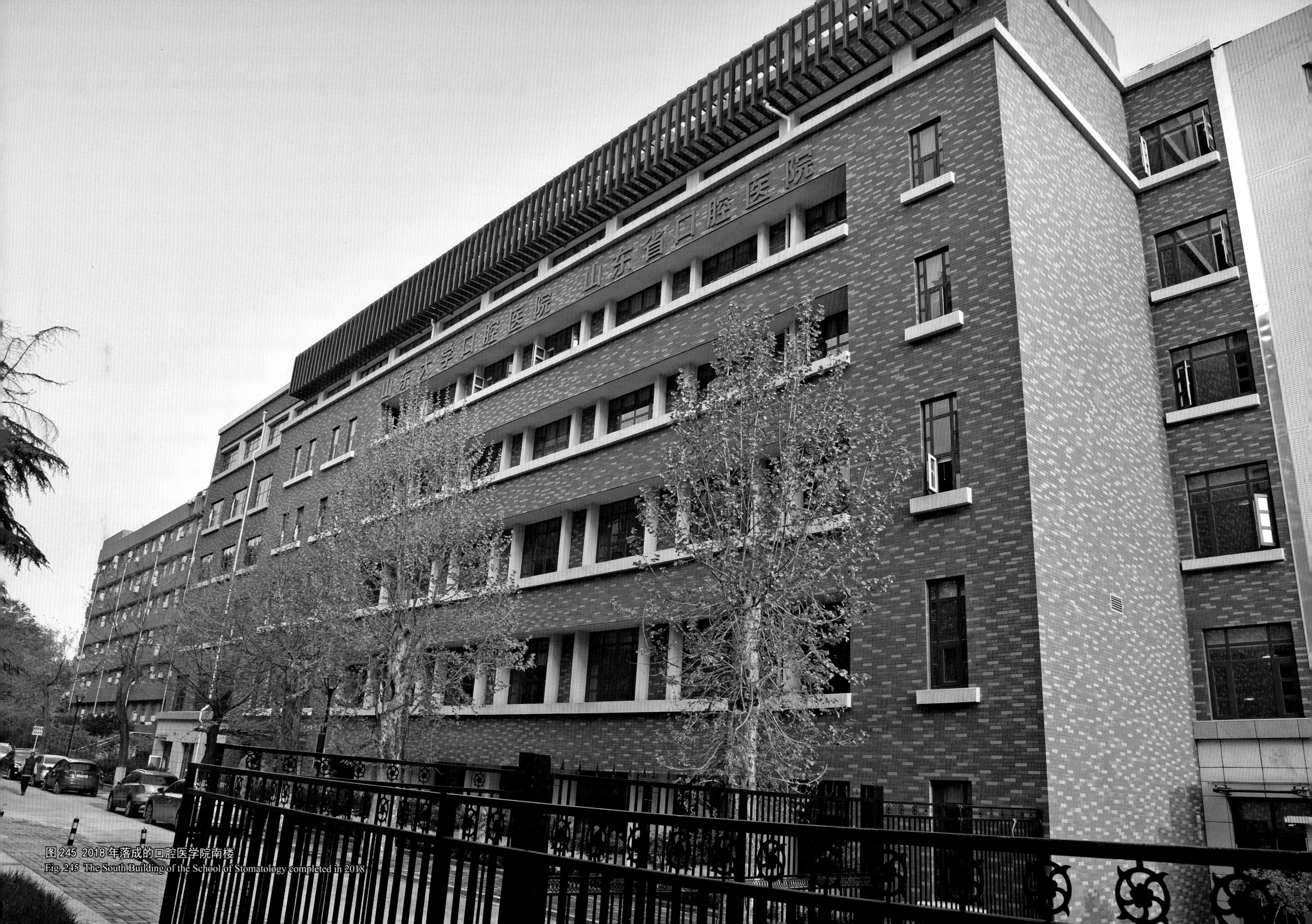

图 245　2018 年落成的口腔医学院南楼

Fig. 245　The South Building of the School of Stomatology completed in 2018

29 口腔医学大楼（2）

Building of Stomatology（2）

在我校口腔医学的发展中，张光溥教授和孙涌泉教授发挥了重要作用。

张光溥（1914 ~ 1989），山东高密人，著名牙科专家，山东医科大学教授，山东省口腔医学奠基人。1940 年毕业于华西协和大学牙医学院，获美国纽约州立大学口腔医学博士学位。毕业后任华西协和大学牙科助教兼住院医师。1950 年到齐鲁医院工作，历任副教授、教授、学校口腔教研室主任、附属医院口腔科主任，1952 ~ 1956 年兼任山东省立第一医院口腔科主任。1977 年山东医科大学建立口腔系，他为首任主任。

孙涌泉 (1918 ~ 1993)，山东博兴人，著名口腔颌面外科专家，山东医科大学教授。1948 年毕业于华西协和大学口腔学院，获美国纽约州立大学口腔医学博士学位。历任我校口腔颌面外科教研室主任、教授，口腔系副主任和附院口腔科副主任，培养的 15 名口腔医学硕士现今已成为我省口腔颌面外科界的学术带头人和骨干力量。他开展的腭裂整复改良手术“腭咽环扎术”，一直沿用至今。

Professor Zhang Guangpu and Professor Sun Yongquan have played an important role in the development of stomatology in our university.

Zhang Guangpu (1914-1989), a native of Gaomi, Shandong Province, is a famous dental expert. He is a professor of Shandong Medical University and founder of stomatology in Shandong Province. He graduated from the School of Dentistry of West China Union University in 1940 and obtained his doctorate in stomatology from the State University of New York in the United States. After graduation, he served as a dental assistant and resident of West China Union University. He came to work in Qilu Hospital in 1950 and successively served as associate professor, professor, director of Dental Teaching and Research Office and director of Dental Department of the Affiliated Hospital. From 1952 to 1956, he concurrently served as director of Dental Department of Shandong Provincial First Hospital. In 1977, Shandong Medical University established the Department of Stomatology, and Zhang Guangpu served as the first director.

Sun Yongquan (1918-1993), a native of Boxing, Shandong Province, is a famous expert in oral and maxillofacial surgery and a professor at Shandong Medical University. He graduated from the School of Stomatology of West China Union University in 1948 and obtained his doctorate in stomatology from the State University of New York in the United States. He successively served as the director and professor of the Teaching and Research Office of Oral and Maxillofacial Surgery, the deputy director of the Department of Stomatology and the deputy director of the Dental Department of the Affiliated Hospital. The fifteen masters of stomatology trained by him have become the academic leaders and backbone in the field of the Oral and Maxillofacial Surgery in our province. He developed the “velopharyngeal ring ligation” in the palatopharyngeal repair surgery which is still in use today.

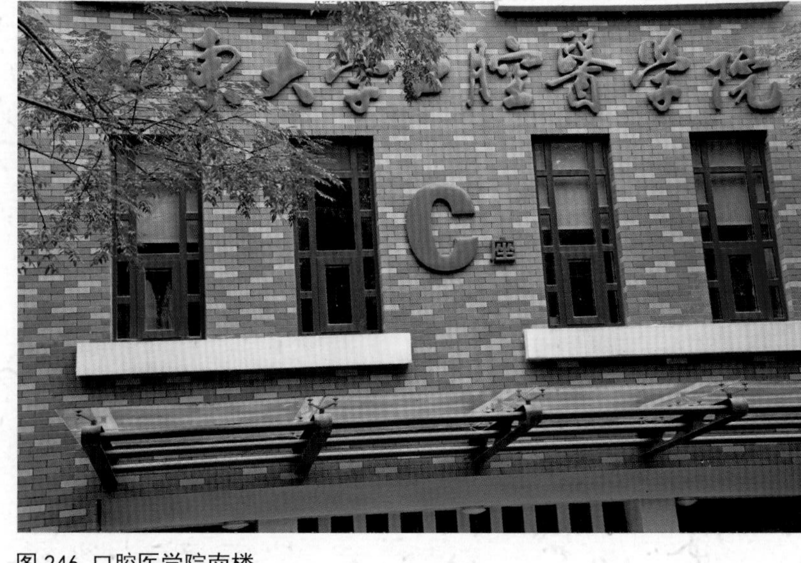

图 246 口腔医学院南楼
Fig. 246 The South Building of the School of Stomatology

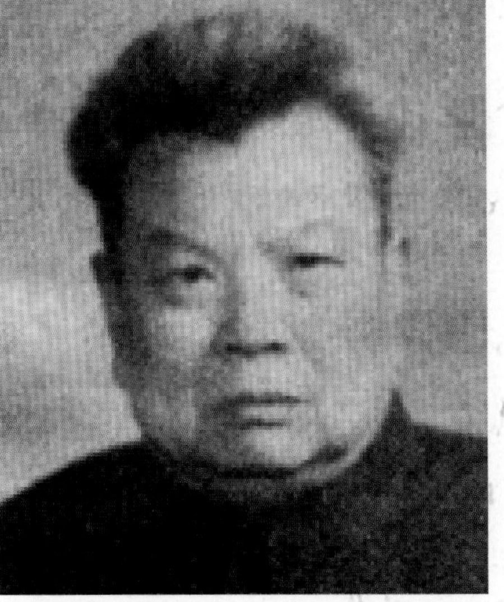
图 247 张光溥教授
Fig. 247 Professor Zhang Guangpu

图 248 孙涌泉教授
Fig. 248 Professor Sun Yongquan

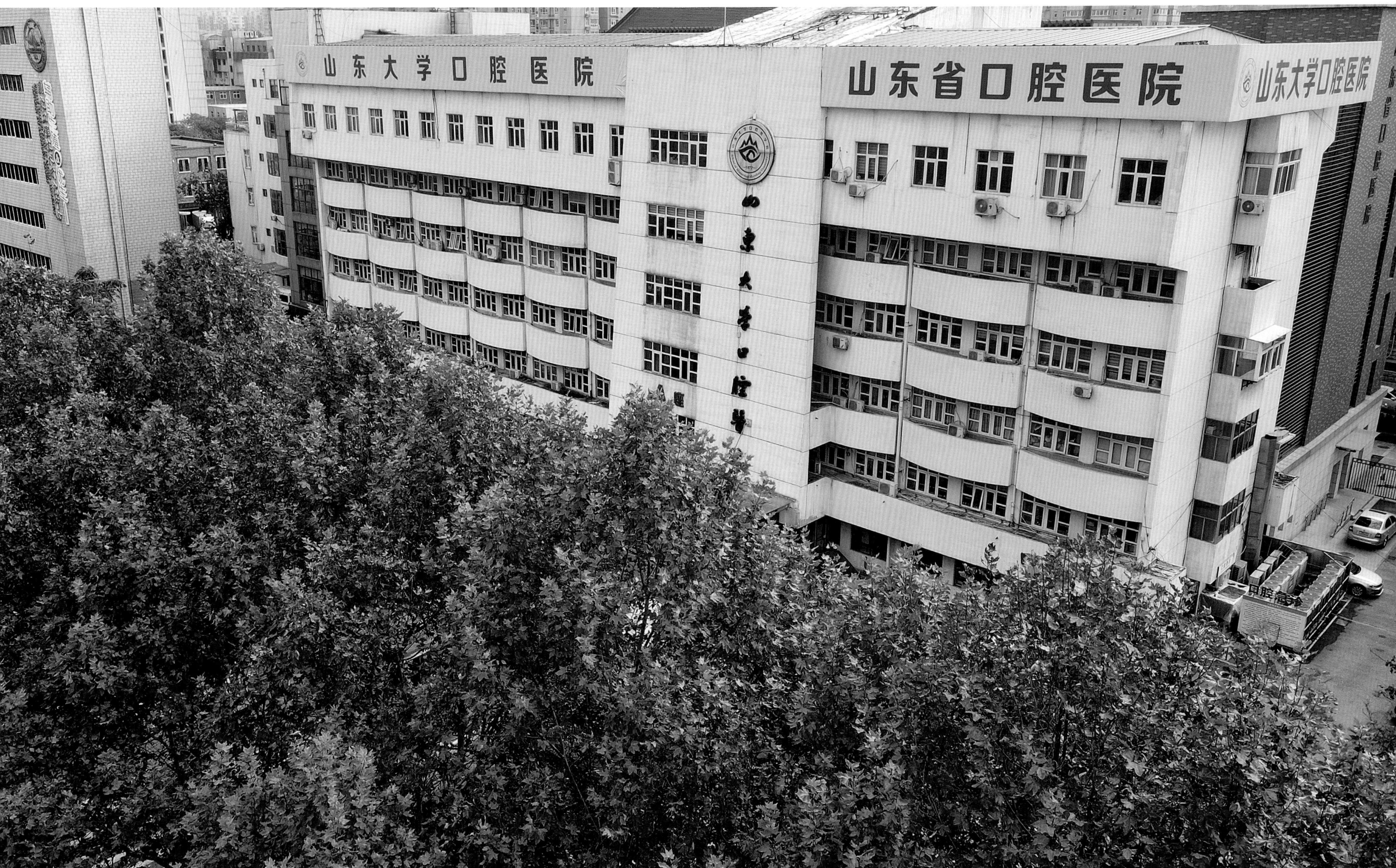

图 249 口腔医学院北楼
Fig. 249 The North Building of the School of Stomatology

30 护理大楼

Nursing Building

护理大楼是拆除原游泳池于 2009 年建成使用的，仿古风格，共六层，由山东大学护理与康复学院及高等医学研究院共同使用。

山东大学的护理教育始于 1914 年，当时山东共合医道学堂（齐鲁大学医学院前身）附设护士养成学校开设有四年制护士班。1985 年开始护理本科教育，是全国首批恢复高等护理教育的院校之一。2000 年升格为山东大学护理学院。2020 年 10 月 20 日，成立山东大学护理与康复学院。学院是国家首批护理学专业一级学科博士授权点、首批专业硕士授权点，2012 年获批设立国家首批护理学博士后科研流动站，目前已形成本科、硕士、博士、博士后在内的护理人才培养体系。学院国际合作成绩突出，已与美国、日本、澳大利亚和瑞典等 10 余个国家的高水平大学建立了实质性合作关系，是世界卫生组织在中国大陆设有合作发展中心的两个护理院校之一。

The Nursing Building was completed and put into use in 2009 after the original swimming pool was demolished. It has six floors in antique style and is jointly used by the School of Nursing and Rehabilitation and the Advanced Medical Research Institute of Shandong University.

The nursing education in Shandong University began in 1914 when a four-year nursing class was set up in the Nurse Training School attached to Shandong Union Medical College (the predecessor of the School of Medicine of Cheeloo University). Shandong University started undergraduate nursing education in 1985, and is one of the first universities to resume higher nursing education in China. In 2000, it was upgraded to the Nursing School of Shandong University. On 20 October 2020, the School of Nursing and Rehabilitation of Shandong University was established. The school is among the first batch to have the authorized discipline of the first-level doctoral programs of nursing and the professional master programs in the country. In 2012, it was approved to be among the first batch of setting up post-doctoral research mobile stations in nursing in the country, thus forming a training system of nursing talents including undergraduate, master, doctor and post-doctor. The school has made outstanding achievements in international cooperation. It has established substantive cooperation relations with high-level universities in more than 10 countries, including the United States, Japan, Australia, Sweden and so on. It is one of the two nursing schools with a cooperative development center set up by the World Health Organization in mainland China.

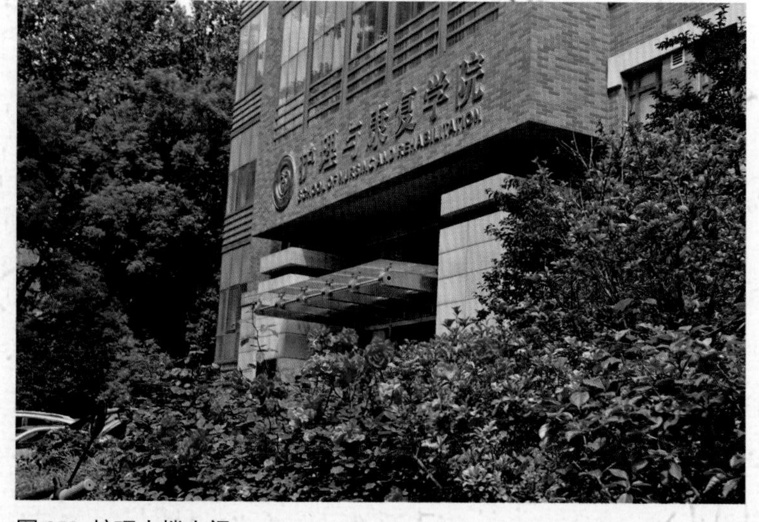

图 250 护理大楼大门
Fig. 250 Gate of the Nursing Building

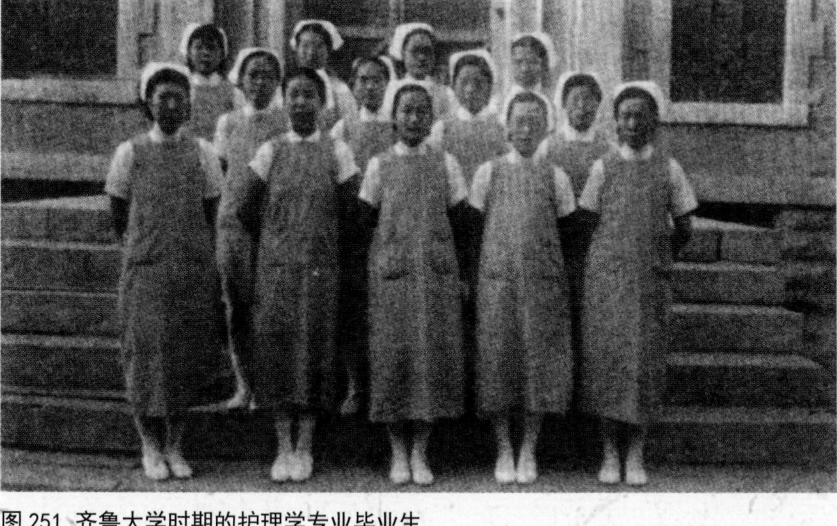

图 251 齐鲁大学时期的护理学专业毕业生
Fig. 251 Nursing graduates of Cheeloo University

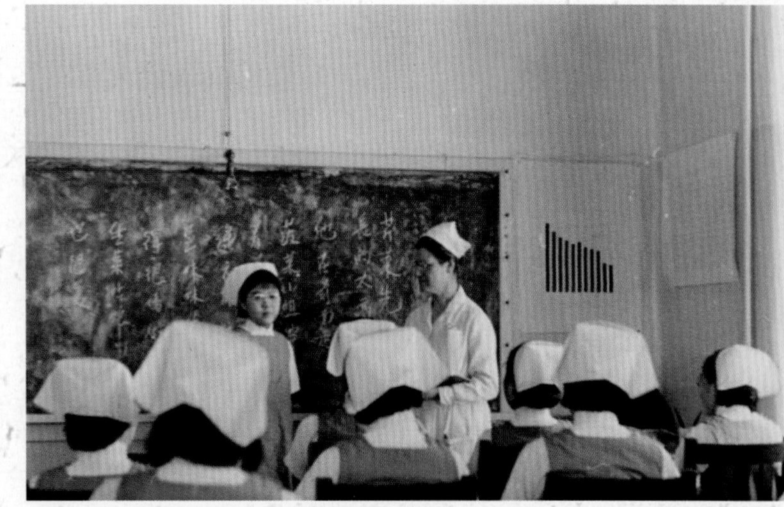

图 252 1941 年，齐鲁大学护校的营养课堂
Fig. 252 Nutrition class at the Nursing School of Cheeloo University in 1941

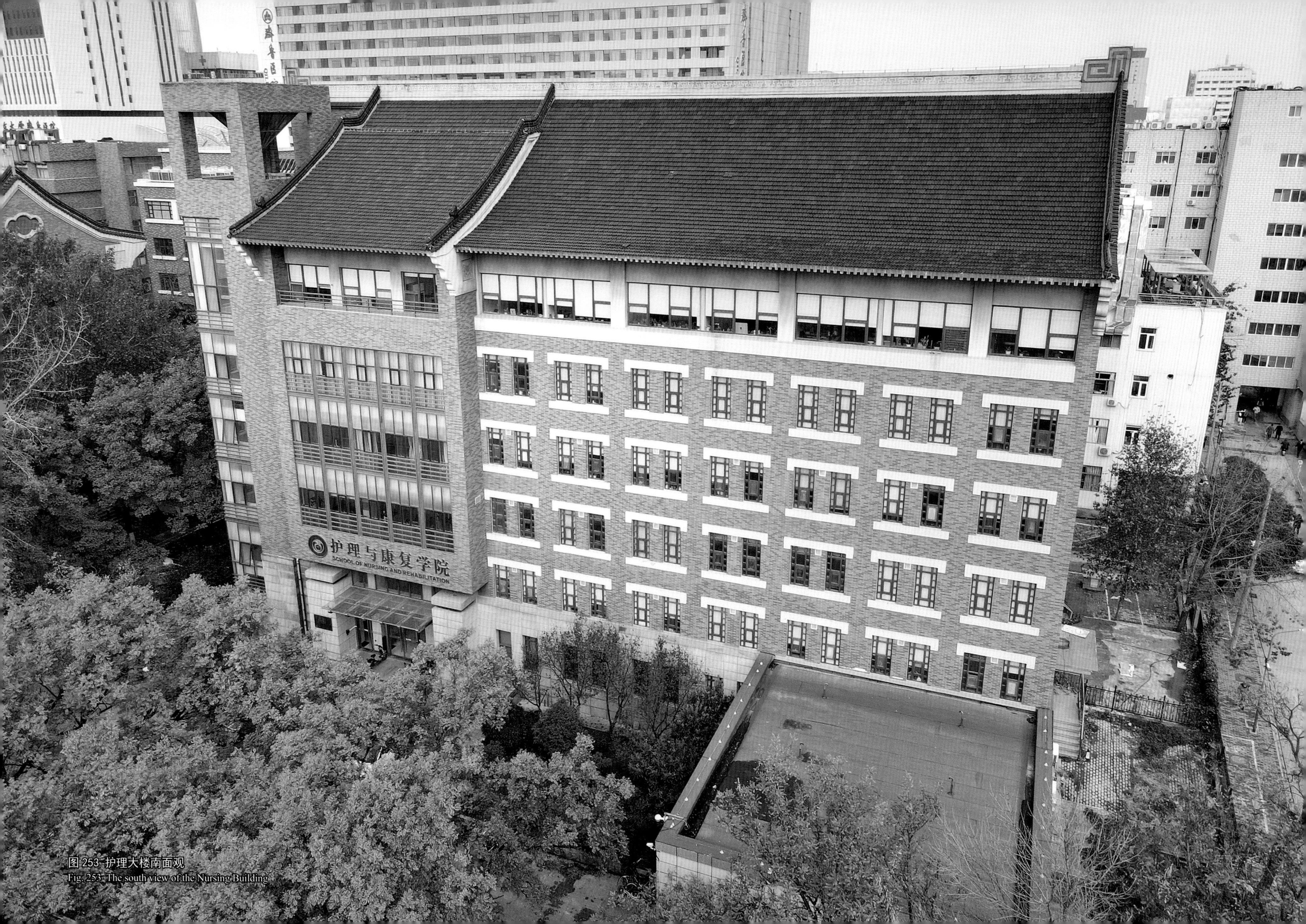

图 253 护理大楼南面观
Fig. 253 The south view of the Nursing Building

31 电镜楼

Building of Electron Microscopy

电镜楼建于 1974 年，钢筋混凝土结构，主体建筑共三层。一层建有电子显微镜实验室，二、三层为医学遗传学系所在地。

山东大学医学遗传学系起源于 1950 年成立的山东医学院生物学教研组，1989 年山东医科大学医学遗传学教研室成立，郭亦寿教授担任主任。2001 年更名为山东大学医学院医学遗传学研究所，由长江学者和国家杰出青年科学基金获得者龚瑶琴教授担任所长。2014 年改称医学遗传学系。此系拥有山东省遗传病重点实验室，也是实验畸形学教育部重点实验室的主要组成部分。实验畸形学教育部重点实验室由国家级教学名师高英茂教授于 2001 年创建，主要围绕遗传病、出生缺陷、基因组病及其他发育异常相关疾病的病因、发病机制、预防和干预策略开展基础和应用基础研究，已鉴定分离了多个具有自主知识产权的致病基因，文章发表于 *Cell* 和 *Nature Genetics* 等杂志。

The Building of Electron Microscopy was built in 1974, with reinforced concrete structure. The main building has a total of three floors. The first floor is equipped with an Electron Microscope Laboratory, and the second and third floors are the locations of the Department of Medical Genetics.

The Department of Medical Genetics of Shandong University originated from the Teaching and Research Group of Biology of Shandong Medical College established in 1950. In 1989, The Teaching and Research Department of Medical Genetics of Shandong Medical University was established, with Professor Guo Yishou as the director. In 2001, it was renamed the Institute of Medical Genetics of School of Medicine of Shandong University, with Professor Gong Yaoqin, winner of Chang Jiang Scholars Program and the National Science Fund for Distinguished Young Scholars, as the director. In 2014, it was renamed the Department of Medical Genetics. This department has the Key Laboratory of Genetic Diseases of Shandong Province, the main part of the Key Laboratory of Experimental Teratology of the Ministry of Education. The Key Laboratory of Experimental Teratology of the Ministry of Education was established in 2001 by Professor Gao Yingmao, a famous state-level teacher. It mainly carries out basic research and applied basic research on the etiology, pathogenesis, and prevention and intervention strategies of genetic diseases, birth defects, genomic diseases and other dysplasia-related diseases. It has identified and isolated a number of pathogenic genes with independent intellectual property rights, and the research papers have been published in the journals such as *Cell* and *Nature Genetics*.

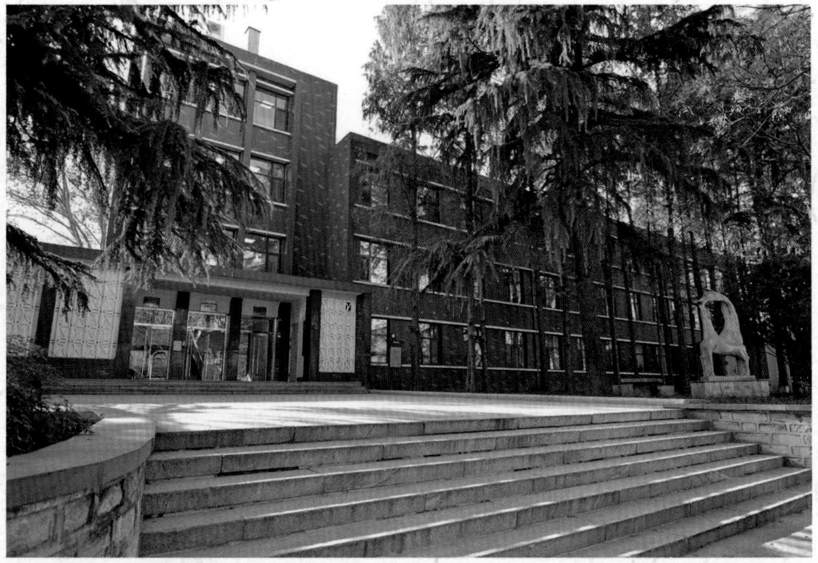

图 254 电镜楼北面观
Fig. 254 The north view of the Building of Electron Microscopy

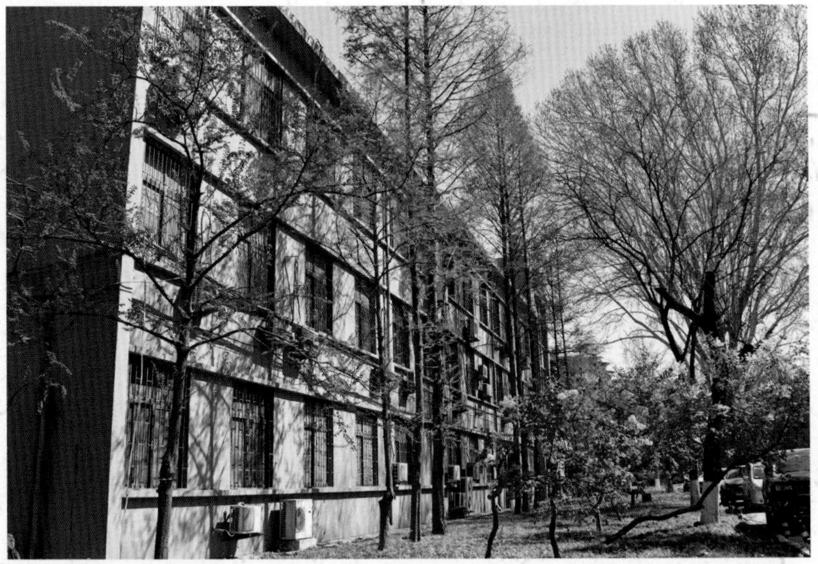

图 255 电镜楼南面观
Fig. 255 The south view of the Building of Electron Microscopy

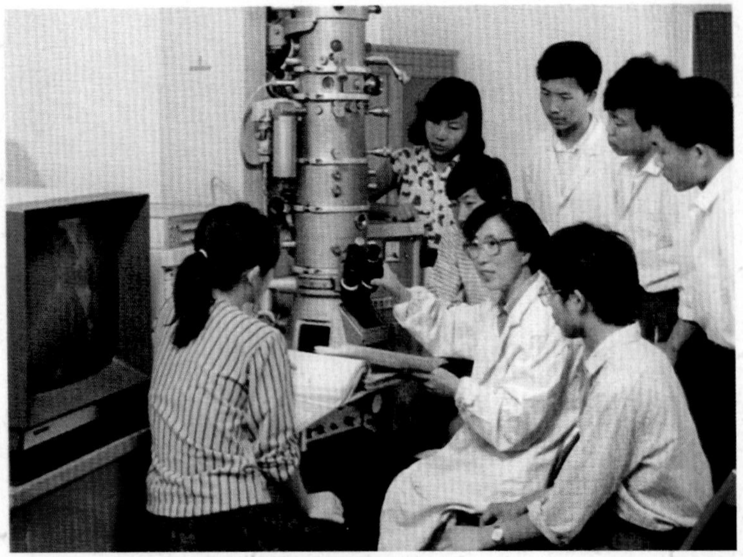

图 256 20 世纪 90 年代初的电子显微镜教学
Fig. 256 Teaching of electron microscope in the early 1990s

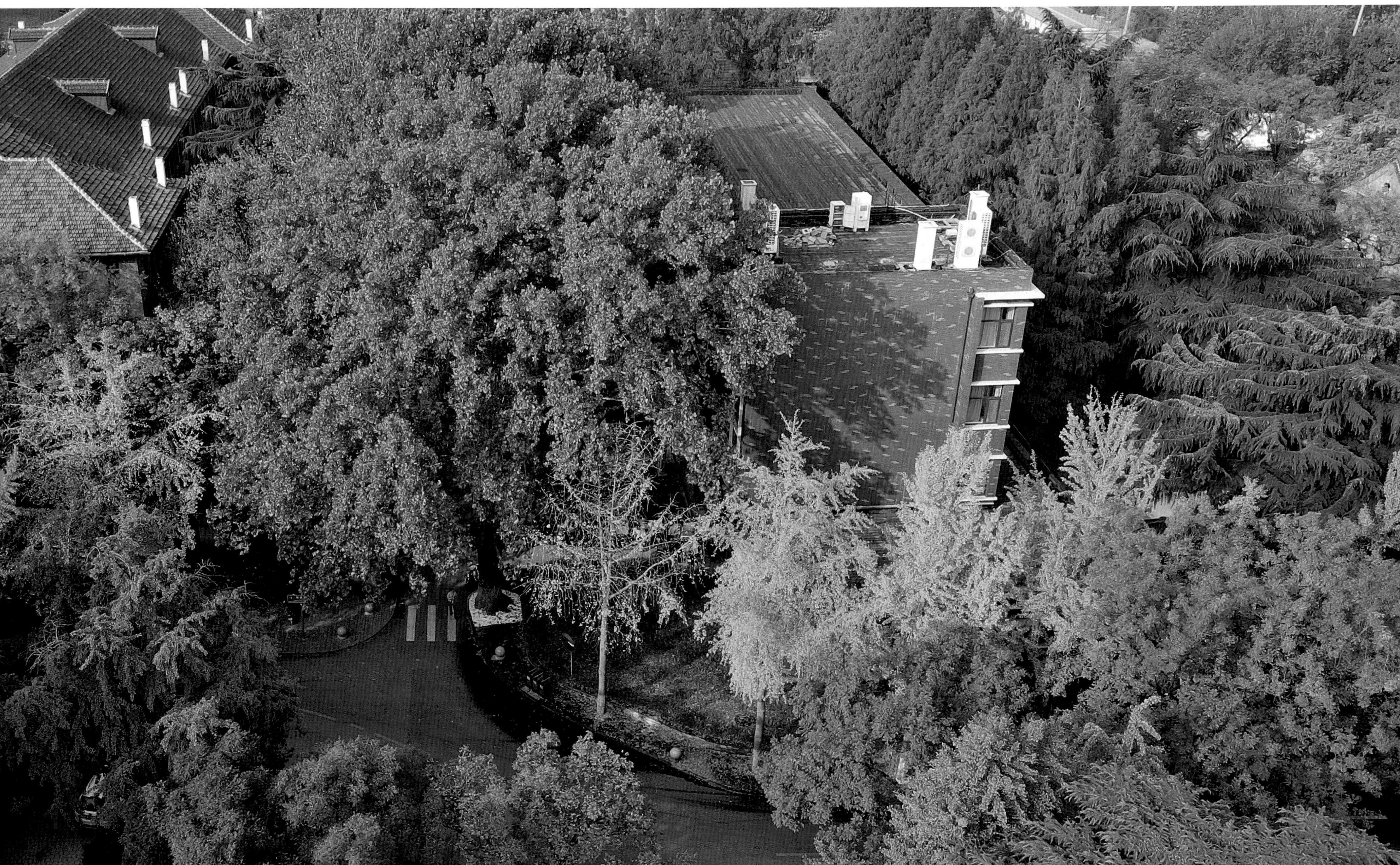

图 257 电镜楼鸟瞰

Fig. 257 A bird's-eye view of the Building of Electron Microscopy

32 桐荫阁与核医学楼

Tongyin Pavilion and the Nuclear Medicine Building

桐荫阁原为教授别墅，建于 20 世纪 20 年代初，内为木质楼梯及楼板，设计及装潢别致，西方风格，曾供蓝娜德博士及其他女教师居住，一度为核医学教研室办公及科研用房。

核医学楼兴建于 1962 年，现为山东大学实验核医学研究所（原同位素中心实验室）所在地。研究所作为山东大学利用放射性核素进行科研、教学的基地，同时还承担血清超微量物质放射免疫检测的临床科技服务工作。建所以来，主编过《核医学》国家级规划教材第 1 ~ 4 版、《实验核医学与核药学》研究生教材、《生物医学标记示踪技术》等专著。2021 年为进一步加强学科建设，学校购置了先进的小动物 PET/CT，还将电子显微镜实验室并入实验核医学研究所，成立了实验核医学与电镜中心。

Tongyin Pavilion, built in the early 1920s, was originally a villa for professors. The interior is equipped with wooden stairs and floors, unique in design and decoration of western style. It was once the residence of Dr. Leonard and other female teachers and also used as the office and scientific research room for the Teaching and Research Department of Nuclear Medicine.

Built in 1962, the Nuclear Medicine Building is now the site of the Institute of Experimental Nuclear Medicine of Shandong University (former Central Laboratory of Isotope). As the base for scientific research and teaching of Shandong University by using radionuclides, the institute also undertakes clinical scientific and technological services for radioimmunoassay of ultramicro substances of the serum. Since establishment, it has edited the 1-4 editions of the National Planning Textbook *Nuclear Medicine*, the postgraduate textbook *Experimental Nuclear Medicine and Nuclear Pharmacy*, *The Marker and Tracer Technique of Biomedicine* and so on. In 2021, in order to further strengthen the discipline construction, the university purchased advanced PET/CT for small animals, and merged the Electron Microscope Laboratory into the Institute of Experimental Nuclear Medicine to establish the Center for Experimental Nuclear Medicine and Electron Microscope.

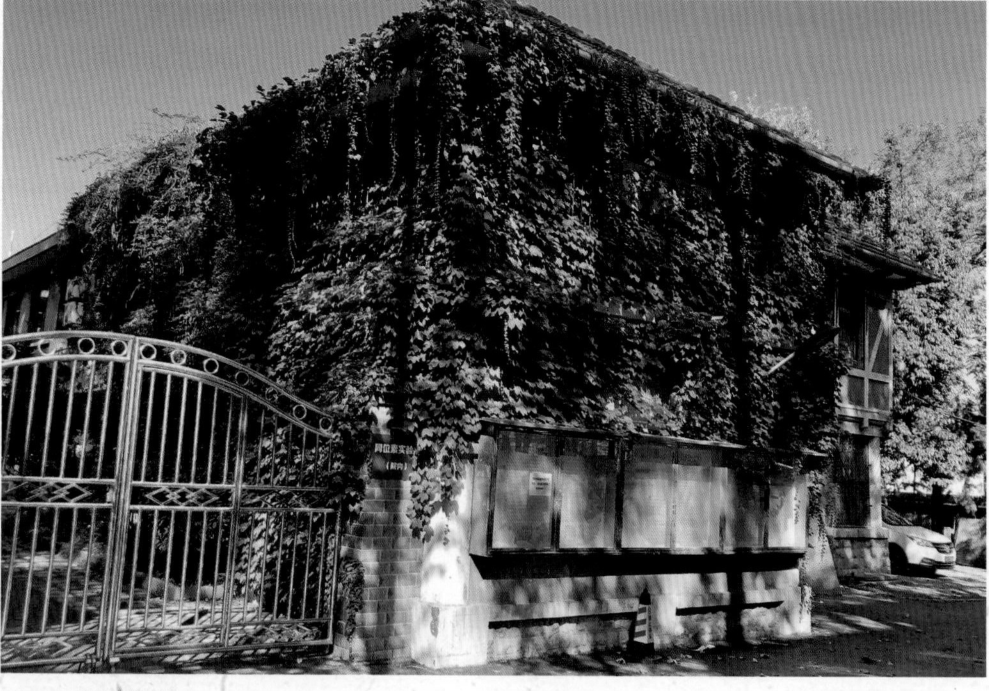

图 258 桐荫阁夏景

Fig. 258 Summer view of Tongyin Pavilion

图 259 桐荫阁秋色

Fig. 259 Autumn color of Tongyin Pavilion

图 260 著名核医学专家周申教授主编的全国统编教材《核医学》

Fig. 260 *Nuclear Medicine*, a national textbook edited by Professor Zhou Shen, a famous expert in nuclear medicine

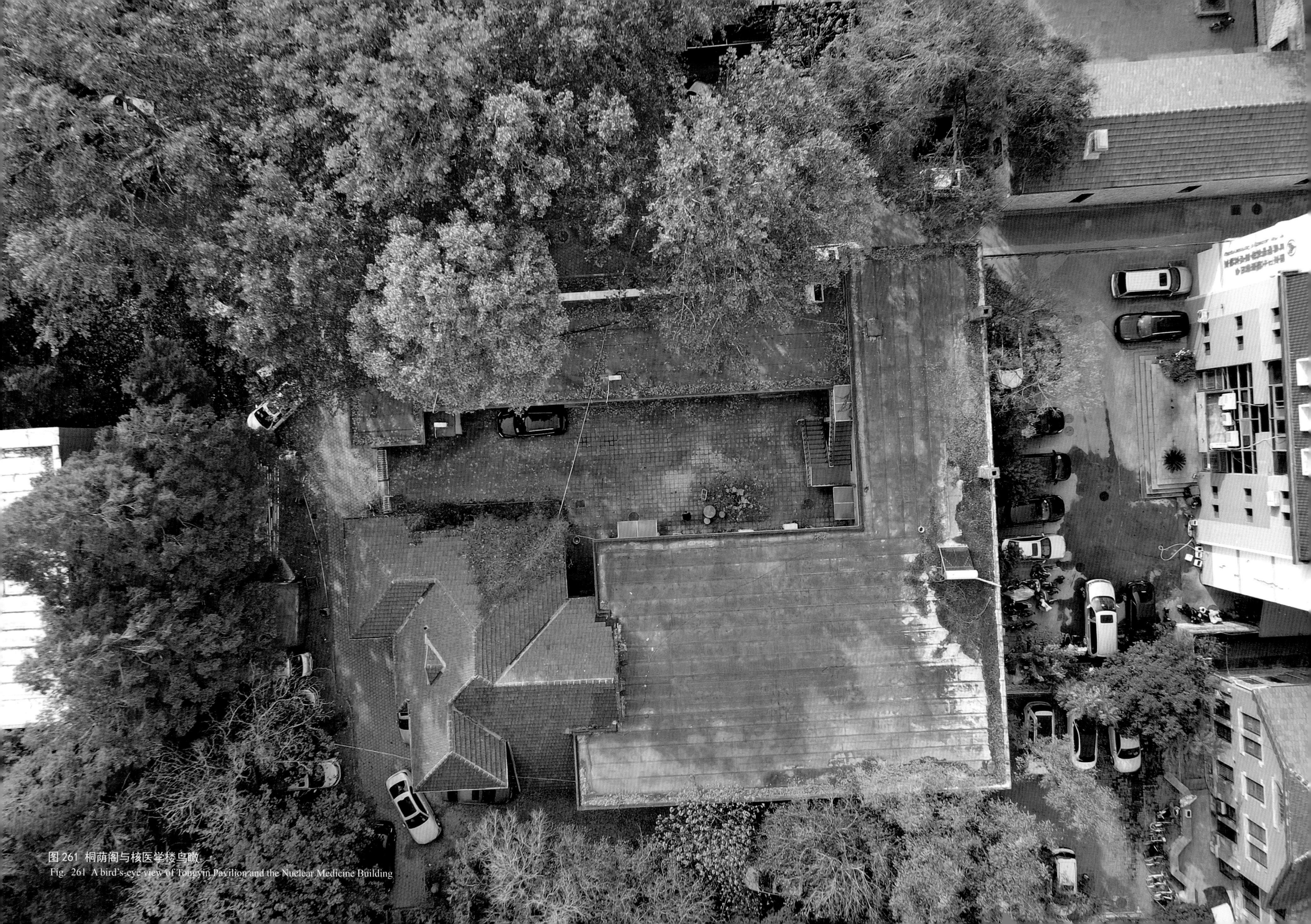

图 261 桐荫阁与核医学楼鸟瞰
Fig. 261 A bird's-eye view of Tongyin Pavilion and the Nuclear Medicine Building

33 耳鼻咽喉科学重点实验室楼

Building of the Key Laboratory of Otorhinolaryngology

国家卫生健康委员会（原卫生部）耳鼻咽喉科学重点实验室成立于 1989 年，其实验楼于 1994 年建成开放，实验室首任主任为著名耳鼻喉专家王廷础教授。齐鲁医学院的耳鼻咽喉科始建于 1924 年，学科创建者孙鸿泉教授是我国耳鼻咽喉科学的奠基人之一。他在国内率先开展了全喉切除术、内耳开窗术、喉移植术、喉再造术等。杨仁中教授创造了世界首例“中国人工喉”，曾获 1978 年全国科学大会奖。王天铎教授率先在国内开展了保留喉功能的喉癌和下咽癌手术，曾获国家科技进步奖。王廷础教授研制成功的“喉癌切除（后）硅橡胶喉成形术”荣获国家技术发明奖三等奖。此学科在继续保持头颈肿瘤手术治疗传统优势的基础上，在保留喉功能的喉癌和下咽癌的手术治疗领域一直保持国内领先水平，是目前国内外喉功能保留率最高的研究和治疗中心。

The Key Laboratory of Otorhinolaryngology of the National Health Commission (former Ministry of Health) was established in 1989. Its experimental building was completed and opened in 1994, with Professor Wang Tingchu, a famous expert in otolaryngology, as the first director of the laboratory. The Discipline of Otolaryngology of Cheeloo College of Medicine was founded in 1924 and the founder Professor Sun Hongquan is one of the founders of otolaryngology in China. He took the lead in carrying out total laryngectomy, fenestration of inner ear, laryngeal transplantation, laryngeal reconstruction and so on in China. Professor Yang Renzhong created the first “Chinese artificial larynx” in the world and won the award of the National Science Conference in 1978. Professor Wang Tianduo took the lead in carrying out the surgery of laryngeal cancer and hypopharyngeal cancer with laryngeal function preservation in China, and won the National Science and Technology Progress Award. The “silicone rubber laryngoplasty after laryngectomy” successfully developed by Professor Wang Tingchu won the third prize of National Technology Invention Awards. On the basis of maintaining the traditional advantages of surgical treatment of head and neck neoplasm, this discipline has always been maintaining the leading level in China in the surgical treatment of laryngeal cancer and hypopharyngeal cancer with laryngeal function preservation, and the laboratory is the research and treatment center with the highest rate of laryngeal function preservation at home and abroad.

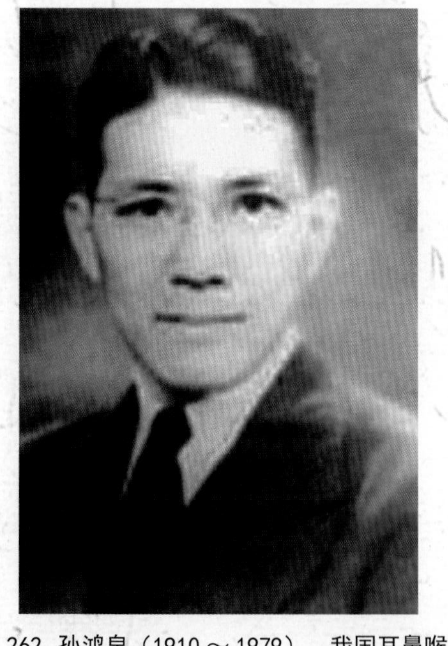

图 262 孙鸿泉（1910 ～ 1979），我国耳鼻喉科奠基人之一，一级教授

Fig. 262 Sun Hongquan (1910-1979), a first-level professor and one of the founders of otolaryngology in China

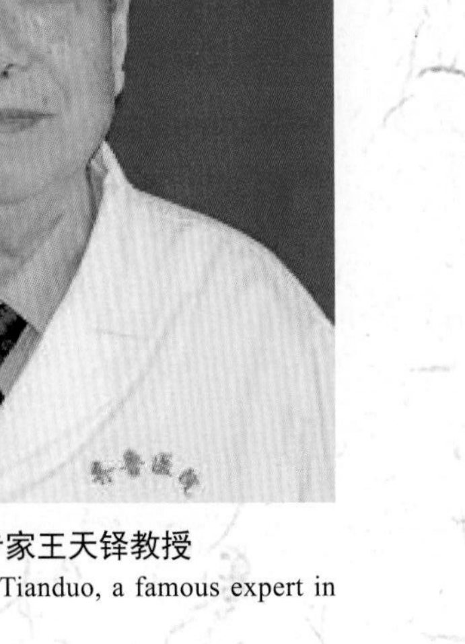

图 263 著名耳鼻喉科专家王天铎教授

Fig. 263 Professor Wang Tianduo, a famous expert in otolaryngology

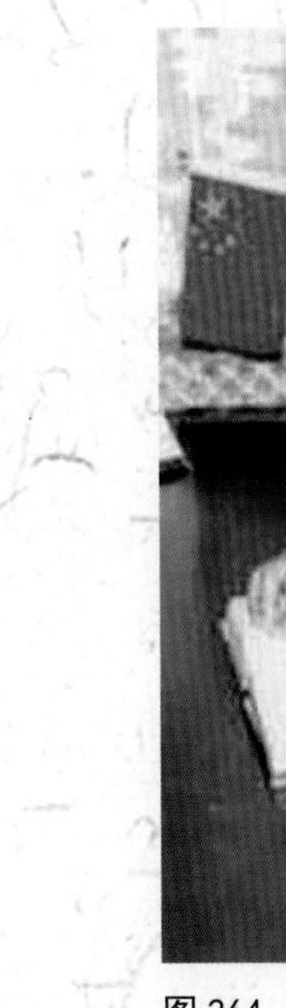

图 264 王廷础（1937 ～ 2010），耳鼻喉重点实验室首任主任，曾任山东医科大学校长

Fig. 264 Wang Tingchu (1937-2010), the first director of the Key Laboratory of Otorhinolaryngology and once served as the president of Shandong Medical University

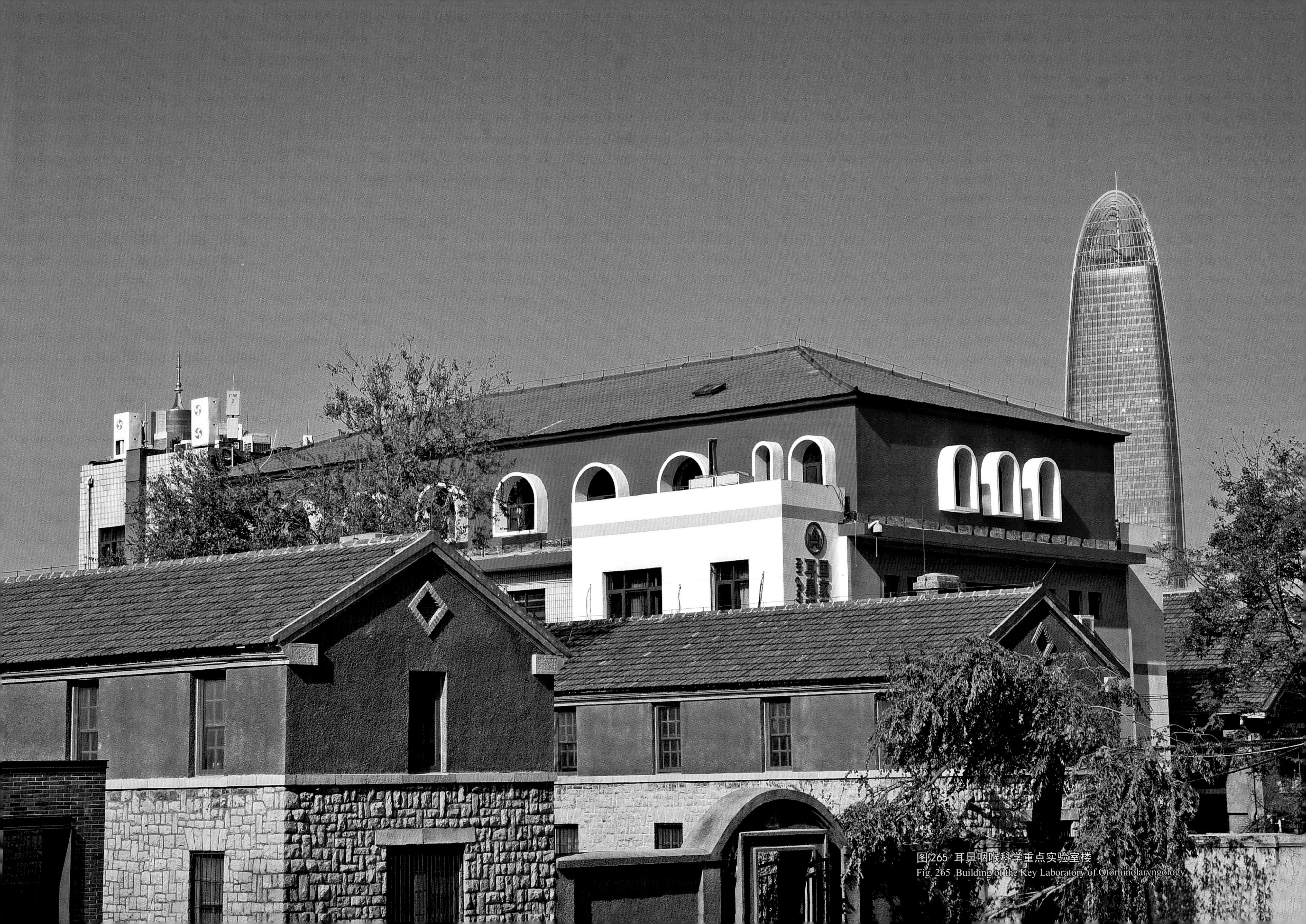

图 265 耳鼻咽喉科学重点实验室楼
Fig. 265 Building of the Key Laboratory of Otorhinolaryngology

34 实验动物楼

Laboratory Animal Building

实验动物楼建成于 2020 年 12 月，总建筑面积为 18000 平方米，分为三个功能区块，其中实验动物养殖与实验操作全部安排在地下部分，约 10000 平方米；地上部分主要为转化医学中心，将成为引领医学学科未来高端研究的重要平台。

The Laboratory Animal Building was completed in December 2020, with a total construction area of 18,000 square meters. This building is divided into three functional blocks, of which the breeding and experimental operation of laboratory animals are all arranged in the underground part, about 10,000 square meters. The above-ground part is mainly the Translational Medicine Center, which will become an important platform to lead the future high-end research of the medical discipline.

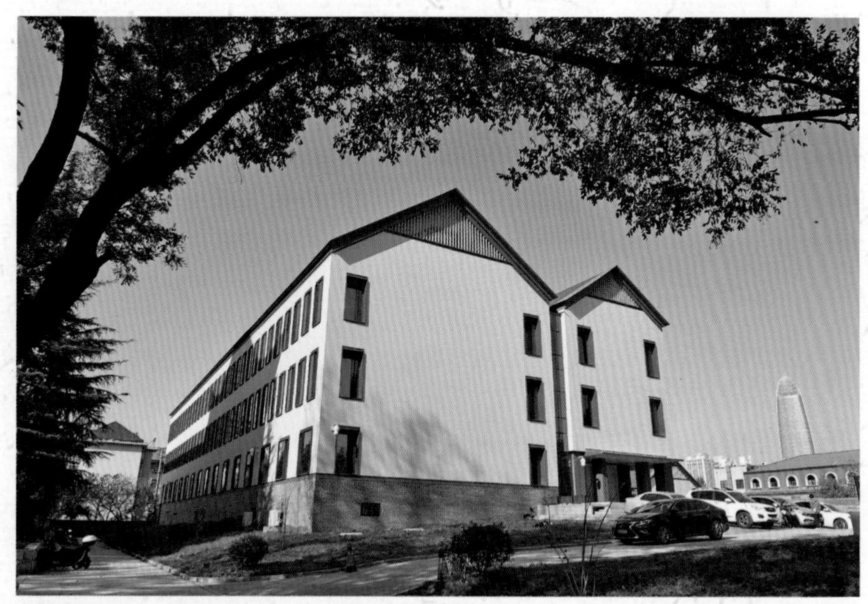

图 266 实验动物楼东面观
Fig. 266 The east view of the Laboratory Animal Building

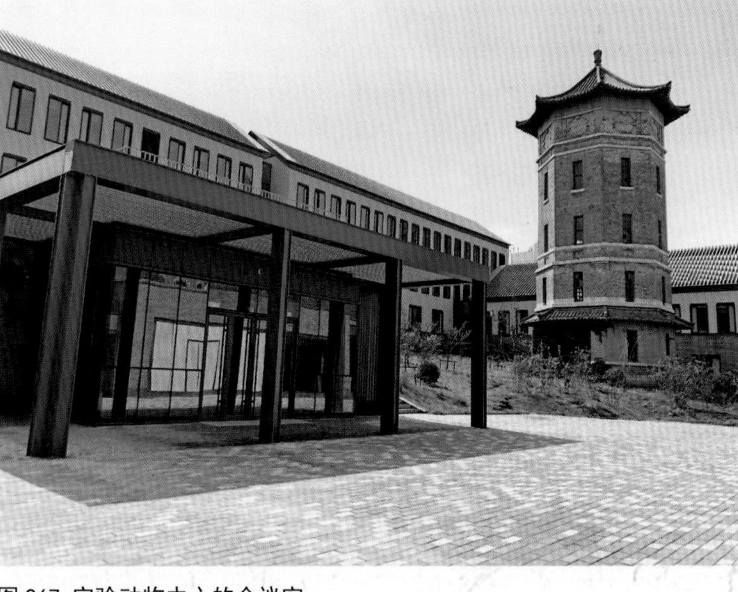

图 267 实验动物中心的会议室
Fig. 267 The meeting room of the Laboratory Animal Center

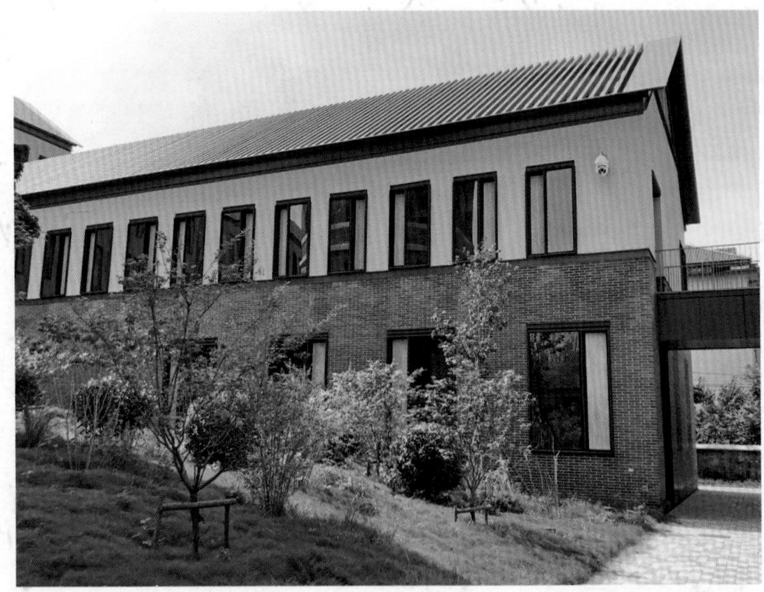

图 268 实验动物中心局部图
Fig. 268 Partial picture of the Laboratory Animal Center

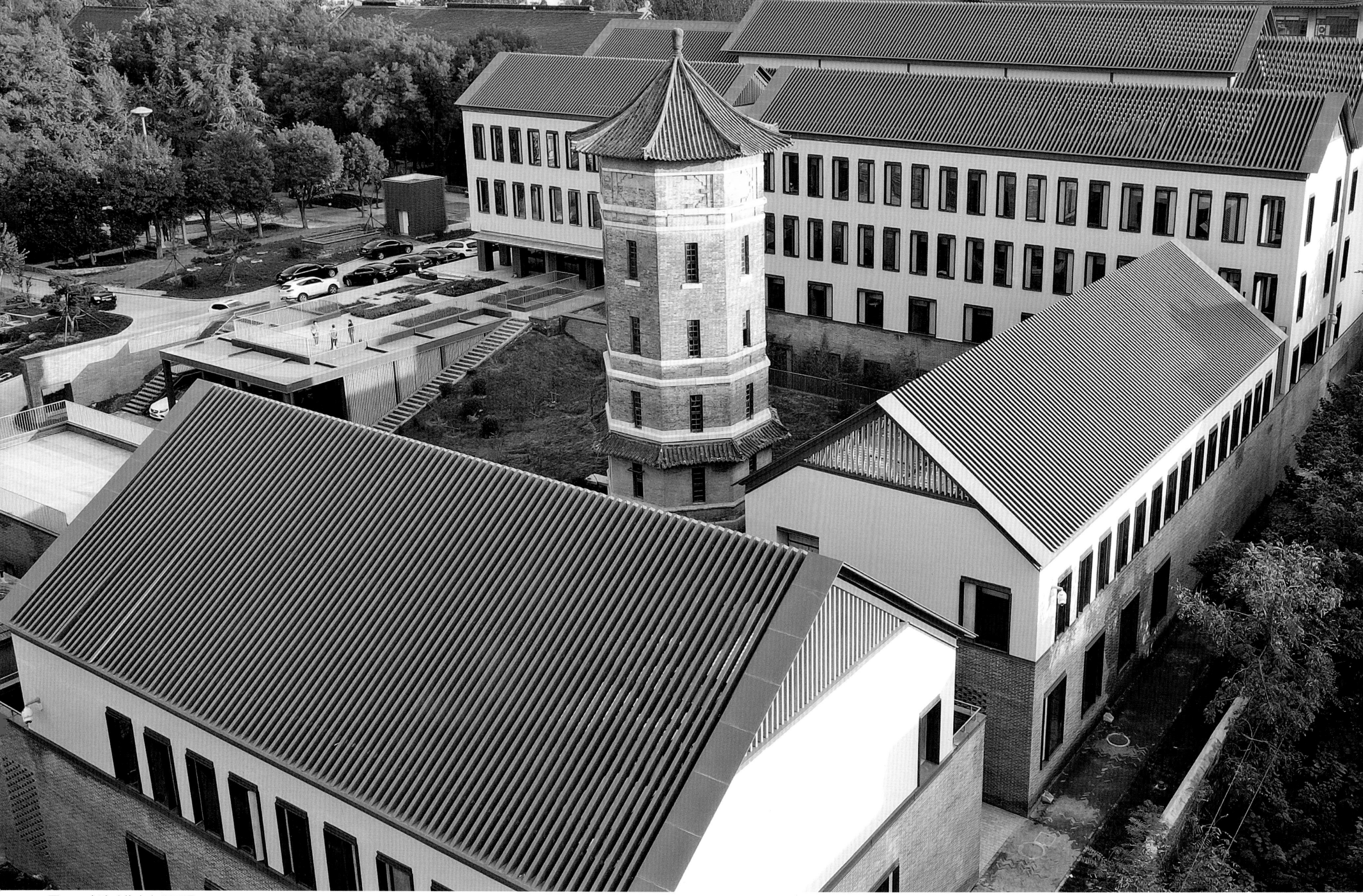

图 269 实验动物中心北面观

Fig. 269 The north view of the Laboratory Animal Center

35 药学科研楼

The Pharmaceutical Research Building

药学科研楼于2012年建成，由山东大学和鲁南制药集团联合投资，仿古风格，共五层。现由山东大学药学院使用，内有国家糖工程技术研究中心和天然产物化学生物学教育部重点实验室。国家糖工程技术研究中心于2007年4月经科技部批准组建，其目标是加强糖类资源的功能开发和资源利用，搭建糖类制备平台、糖类分析和评价平台、糖资源库平台、糖的信息交流平台，为我国糖科研成果的转化和产业化服务，推动我国糖科学技术的进步。天然产物化学生物学教育部重点实验室于2012年1月获教育部批准建立，旨在建立以天然产物的“结构、合成、功能”三要素为支撑的完整的天然产物化学生物学研究体系。实验室完成的“奥美拉唑系列产品产业化与国际化的关键技术开发”成果于2015年12月获国家科技进步奖二等奖。

The Pharmaceutical Research Building was completed in 2012, with antique style and a total of five floors. It is jointly invested by Shandong University and Lunan Pharmaceutical Group Corporation. It is now used by the School of Pharmaceutical Sciences of Shandong University, and the National Glycoengineering Research Center and the Key Laboratory of Chemical Biology of the Ministry of Education are also located here. The National Glycoengineering Research Center was established in April 2007 with the approval of the Ministry of Science and Technology of the People's Republic of China, aiming to strengthen the functional development and resource utilization of sugar resources, build a platform for sugar preparation, sugar analysis and evaluation, sugar resource library and sugar information exchange, serve the transformation and industrialization of scientific research achievements of sugar in China, and promote the science and technology progress of sugar in China. The Key Laboratory of Chemical Biology of the Ministry of Education was established in January 2012 with the approval of the Ministry of Education, aiming to establish a complete research system of chemical biology of natural products supported by the three elements of “structure, synthesis and function”. The achievement of “Key technology development for industrialization and internationalization of the series products of omeprazole” completed by the laboratory won the second prize of the National Science and Technology Progress Award in December 2015.

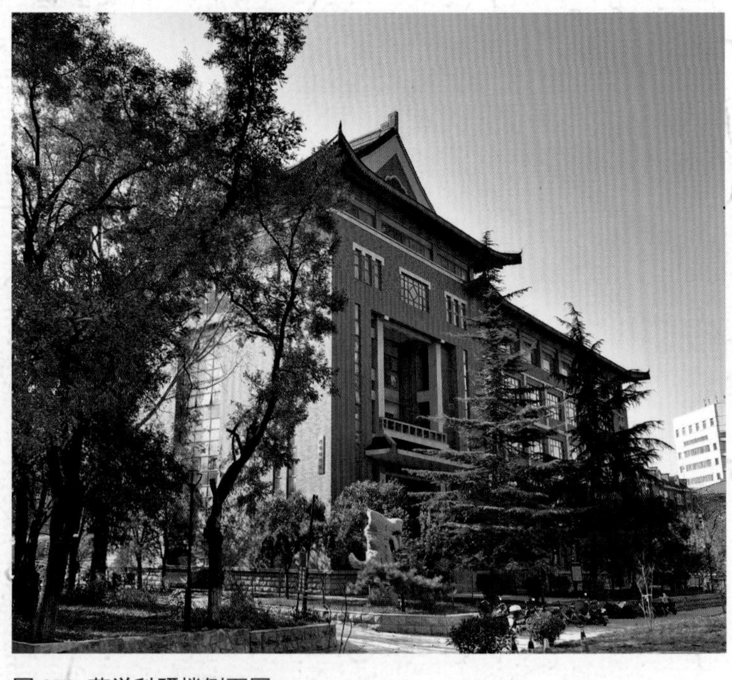

图 270 药学科研楼侧面图
Fig. 270 Side view of the Pharmaceutical Research Building

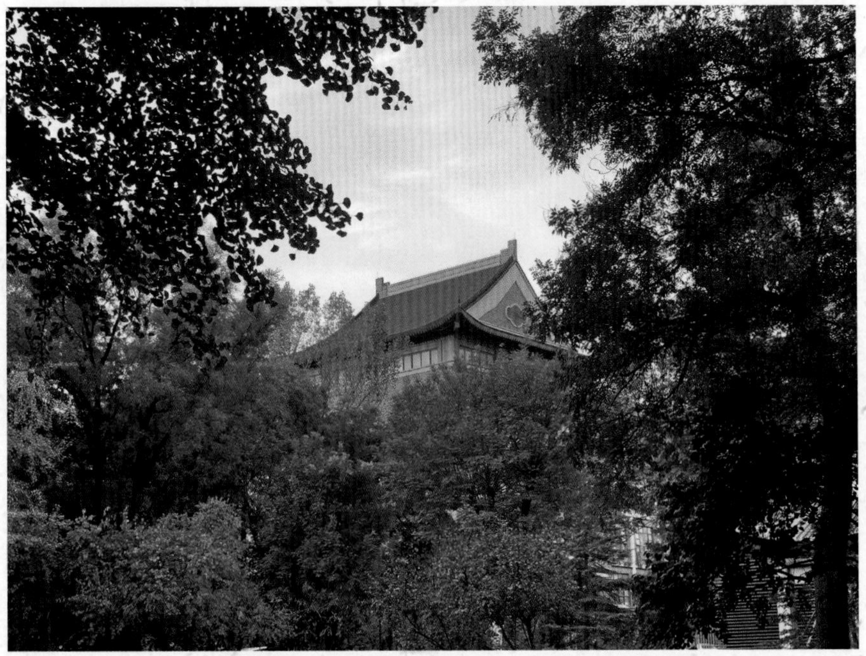

图 271 药学科研楼东北面观
Fig. 271 The northeast view of the Pharmaceutical Research Building

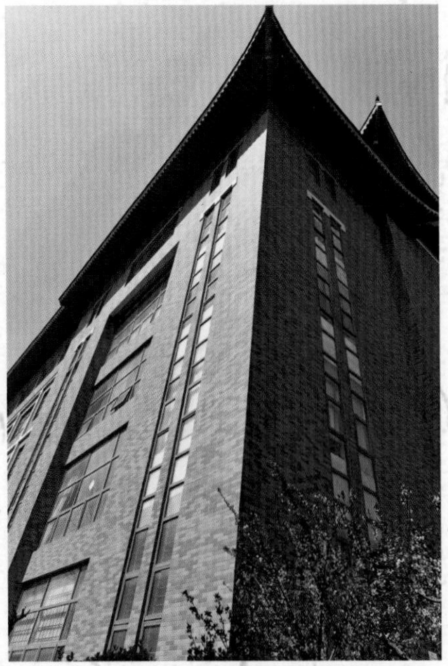

图 272 药学科研楼东南面观
Fig. 272 The southeast view of the Pharmaceutical Research Building

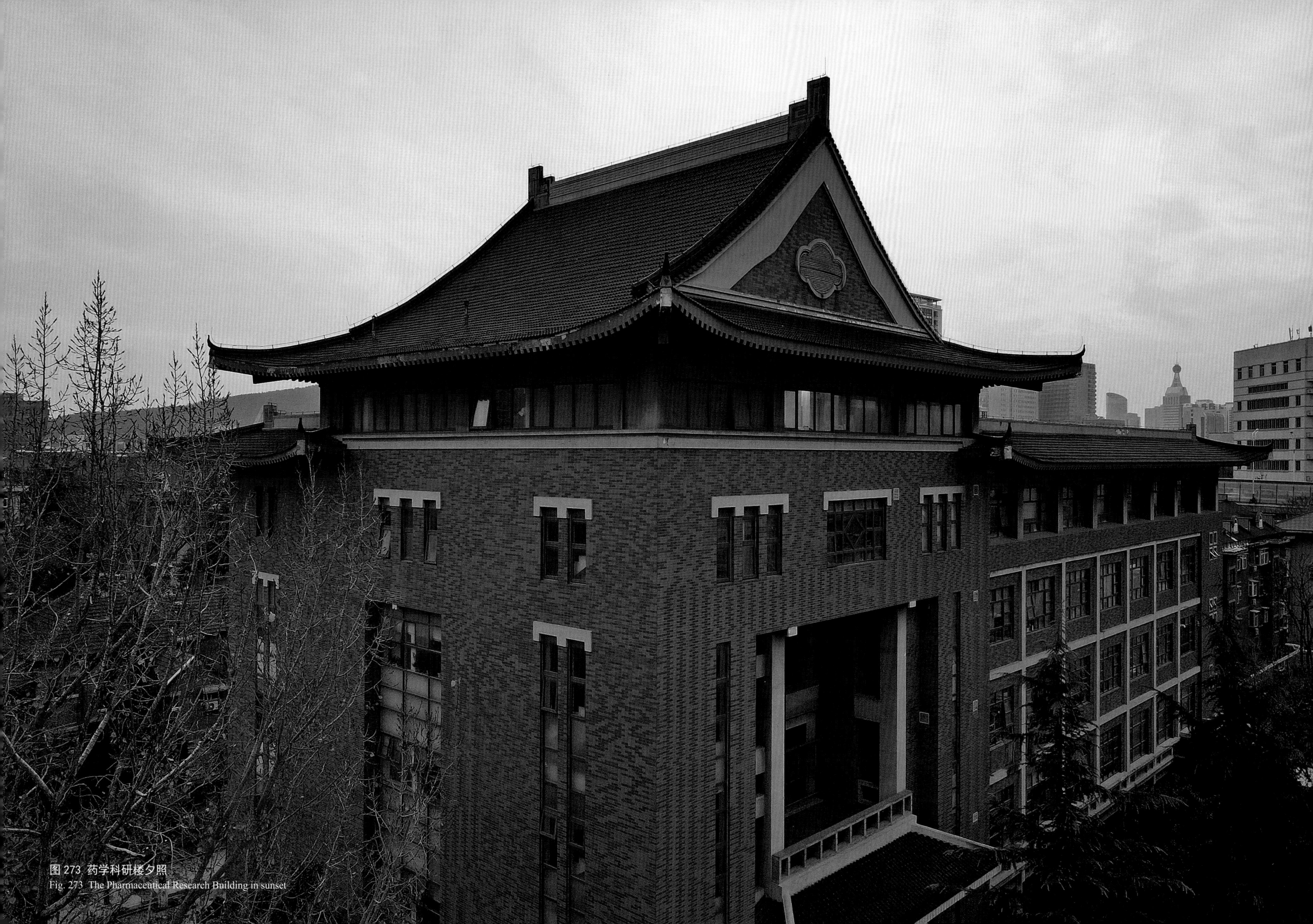

图 273 药学科研楼夕照
Fig. 273 The Pharmaceutical Research Building in sunset

36 附属卫校楼群

Complex of the Affiliated Health School

此楼群为原山东医科大学卫生学校所在地。山东医科大学卫生学校是附设在山东医科大学、隶属山东省卫生厅的一所培养护理人才的重点中等专业学校。学校校史可追溯到创建于 1914 年的山东基督教共合大学医科附设护士养成学校。1963 年，护士学校校址由附属医院迁入山东医学院校园（今山东大学趵突泉校区）的西南部，成为一个独立的院落。2000 年 6 月，山东医科大学卫生学校与山东医科大学护理系合并组建护理学院，停止中专招生。学校合并撤销后，校址归山东医科大学护理学院（后山东大学护理学院）使用。2008 年 8 月护理学院新大楼建成后，护理学院迁走，原校址被非正式地称为“老护理学院”，改建成学生宿舍楼、校医院和仓库。原办公楼位于校园院落的最东部，是一座七层的钢筋混凝土结构建筑，现为学生公寓七号楼。教学楼两座，位于校园正中，分列大门两侧，是两层砖混结构的仿古建筑，现东、西两座分别为学生公寓八号楼和九号楼。

This complex was the site of the former Health School of Shandong Medical University. The Health School of Shandong Medical University is a key secondary professional school to train nursing talents, attached to Shandong Medical University and subordinate to Shandong Provincial Health Department. The school's history can be traced back to the Nurse Training School attached to the Medical Discipline of Shantung Christian University which was founded in 1914. In 1963, the Nurse Training School was moved from the attached hospital to the southwest of the campus of Shandong Medical College (now Baotuquan Campus of Shandong University), becoming an independent courtyard. In June 2000, the Health School of Shandong Medical University and the Nursing Department of Shandong Medical University merged to form the Nursing School, and the enrollment of secondary specialized students was stopped. The site of the school belongs to the Nursing School of Shandong Medical University(later the Nursing School of Shandong University). After the completion of the new building of the Nursing School in August 2008, the Nursing School moved away and the original site was informally called the “Old Nursing School” which was transformed into the student dormitory, infirmary and warehouse. The original office building is located in the easternmost part on campus. It is a seven-storey building with reinforced concrete structure and is now the Seventh Building of Student Dormitory. There are two teaching buildings located in the middle of the campus on both sides of the gate. They are antique buildings with two-storey brick-concrete structure. Now the east and west buildings are the Eighth Building and the Ninth Building of Student Dormitory respectively.

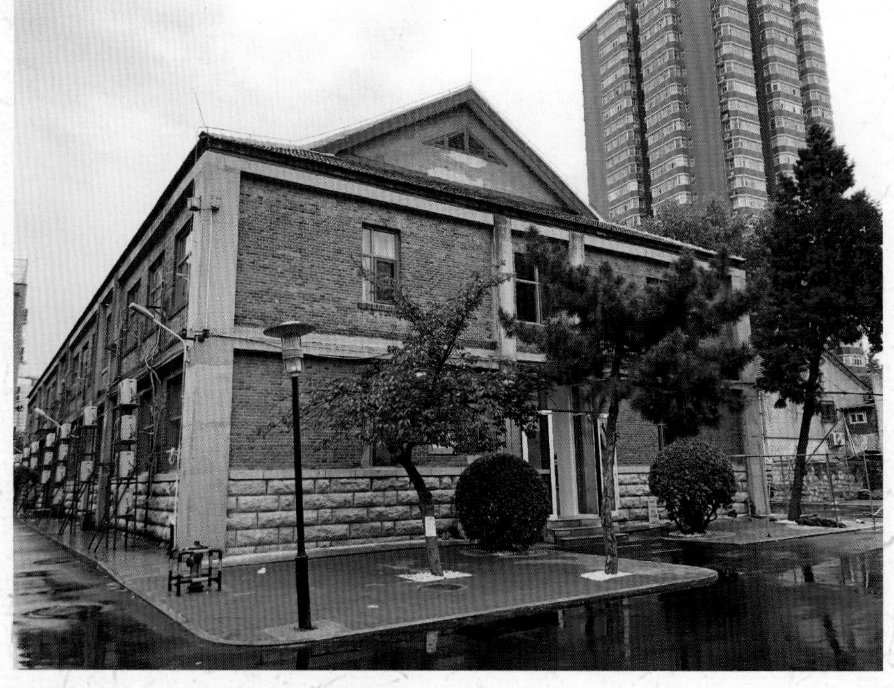

图 274 学生公寓八号楼（原东教学楼）
Fig. 274 The Eighth Building of Student Dormitory(former East Teaching Building)

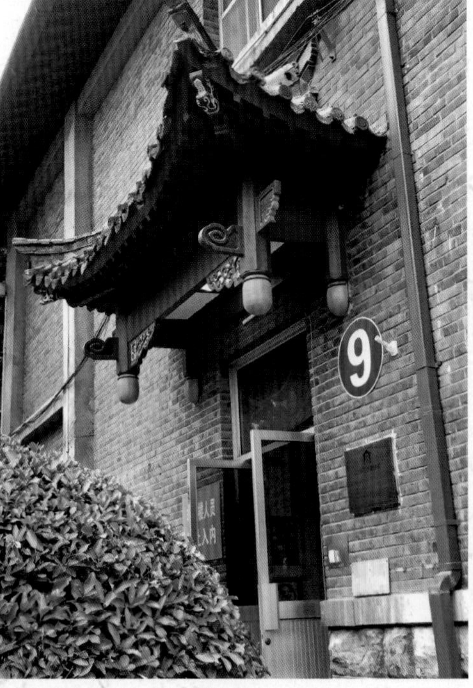
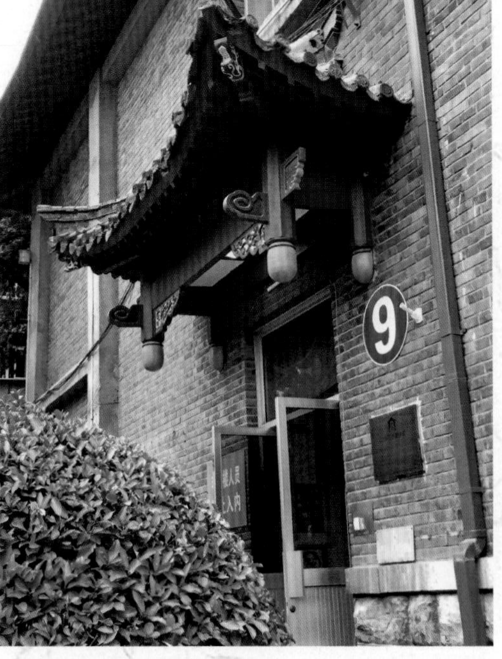

图 275 原西教学楼的门楼
Fig. 275 Gatehouse of the former West Teaching Building

图 276 校园内的南丁格尔塑像
Fig. 276 Statue of Nightingale on campus

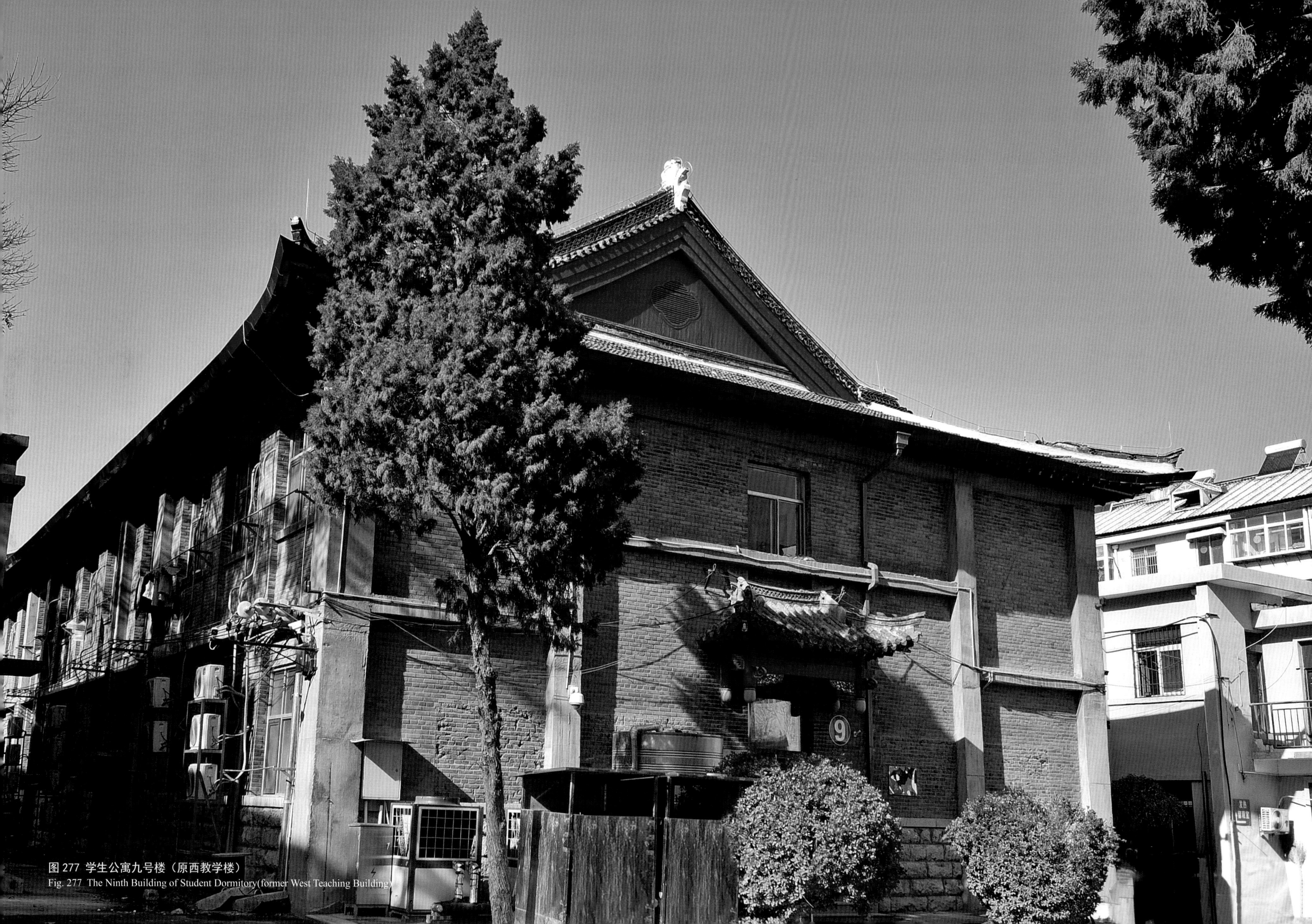

图 277 学生公寓九号楼（原西教学楼）
Fig. 277 The Ninth Building of Student Dormitory(former West Teaching Building)

37 附属小学

The Affiliated Primary School

山东大学第一附属小学为一所六年制公立小学，位于趵突泉校区东北门内，属于山东大学附属事业单位。原为山东医科大学附属小学，2003 年 6 月改为现名。学校拥有一座综合教学楼、一座辅助楼（用于学生午休等），操场为塑胶跑道和地面，建有篮球架、乒乓球台等设施。学校建立了一支学历层次高、教学水平高的教师团队，拥有多媒体讲台、语音室和图书馆等现代化教学设备，以满足对学生进行素质教育的需要。

The First Affiliated Primary School of Shandong University is a public primary school with a six-year schooling, located in the northeast gate of Baotu Spring Campus and belonging to the affiliated institutions of Shandong University. Originally as the Affiliated Primary School of Shandong Medical University, it was changed to its current name in June 2003. The school has a comprehensive teaching building, an auxiliary building (for students' lunch break and so on) and a playground with plastic track and ground, and it has also built the basketball rack, table tennis table and other facilities. The school has set up a team of teachers with high academic qualifications and teaching level, and it has also been equipped with modern teaching equipment such as multimedia platform, language laboratory and library to meet the needs of quality education for students.

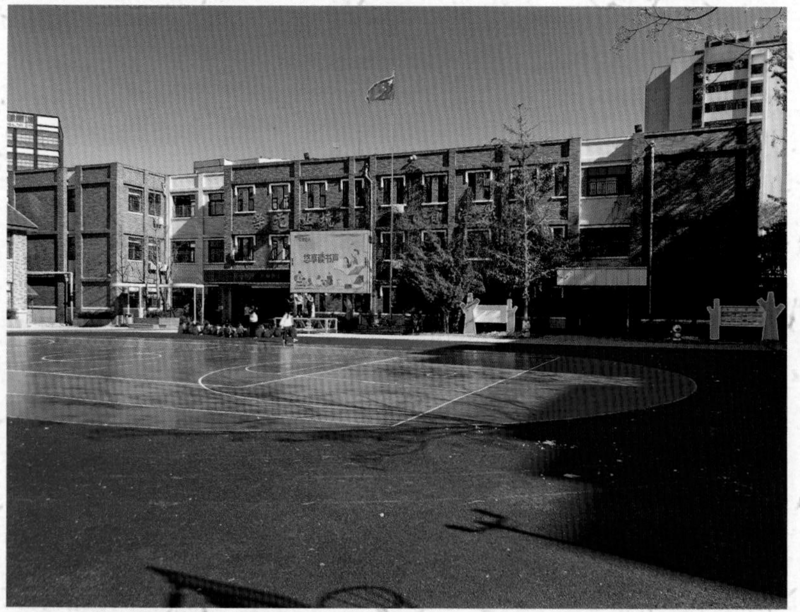

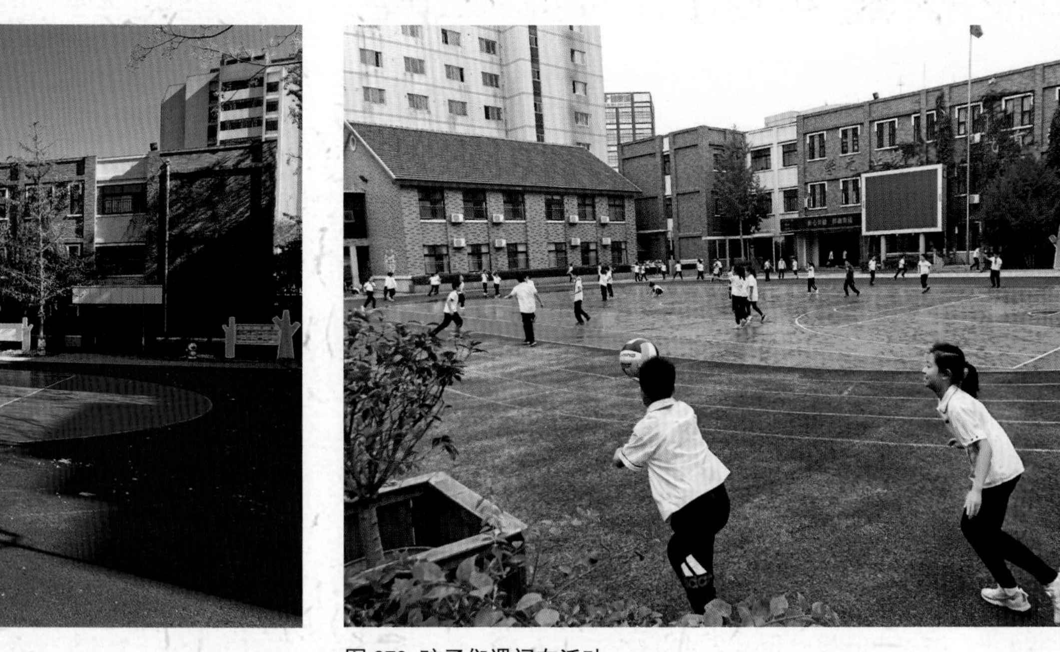

图 278 附属第一小学主楼

Fig. 278 Main building of the First Affiliated Primary School

图 279 孩子们课间在活动

Fig. 279 Children playing during recess

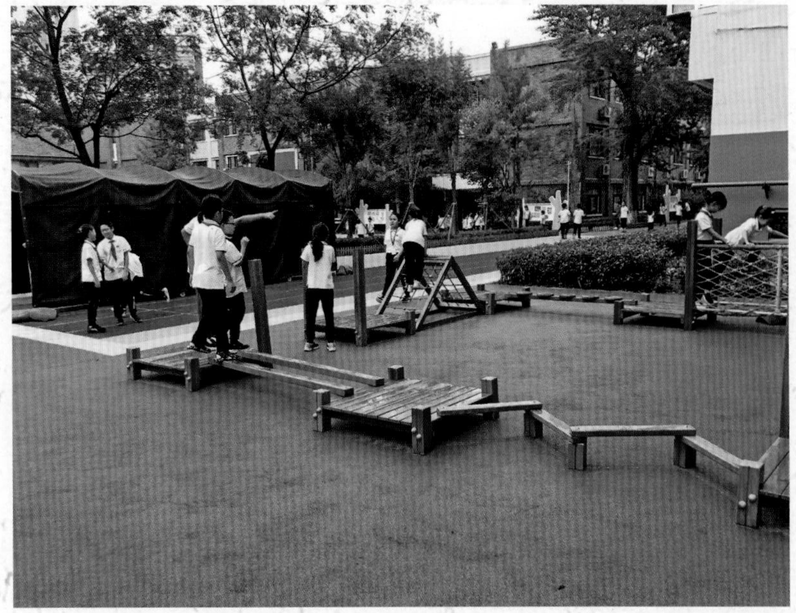

图 280 孩子们课间在做游戏

Fig. 280 Children playing games during recess

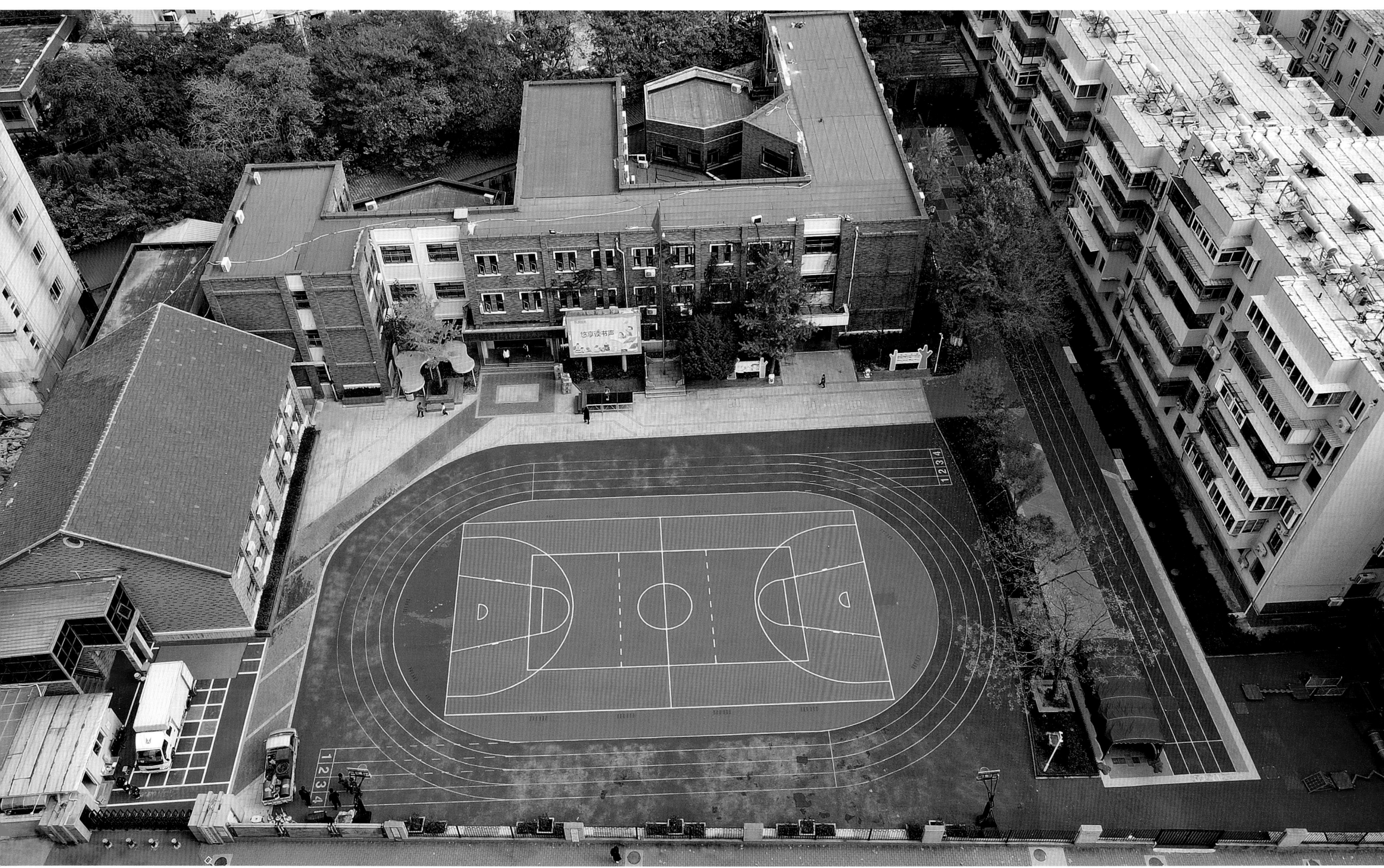

图 281 第一附属小学鸟瞰（上为东，右为南）

Fig. 281 A bird's-eye view of the First Affiliated Primary School (upper east and right south)

38 消失的齐鲁大学老建筑(1)

Lost Old Buildings of Cheeloo University (1)

康穆堂，建于 1923 年，位于中心花园中轴线的南端，是齐鲁大学标志性建筑之一。1958 年被拆除，1963 年在原址上建成第八教学楼。

康穆堂，又称康穆礼拜堂（The Kumler Memorial Chapel），以礼拜堂的捐建者美国匹兹堡的安凯尔维夫人的父母姓氏（Kumler）而命名。昔日的康穆礼拜堂是全校最讲究、最漂亮的建筑，选址在地势最高的校园南部高台之上。建筑呈东西走向，平面为拉丁十字形，主立面为西面，主入口在东面，南北两面分设次入口。外墙为一律蘑菇青石到顶，四角及窗间设有壁柱，山墙山尖处均开设玫瑰窗，其余窗户均为石砌尖券形式。内部三段分隔，室内条石铺地，中厅部分壁柱之上有石砌拱券，中厅部分为三层，顶层为钟楼；四臂部分则为二层。与校园的其他建筑相比，康穆礼拜堂风格迥异，虽具有部分中国式建筑特征，但整体以西式风格为主。仰望此楼，庄严肃穆，静中有动，给人以“飘飘乎如遗世独立，羽化而登仙”之感。

Kumler Chapel, built in 1923 and located at the southern end of the central axis of the Central Garden, is one of the landmark buildings of Cheeloo University. It was demolished in 1958 and the Eighth Teaching Building was built on the original site in 1963.

Kumler Chapel is named after the last name (Kumler) of the parents of of Mrs. Mckelvy, wife of the donor William M. Mckelvy from Pittsburgh of the United States. In the past, Kumler Chapel was the most exquisite and beautiful building in the university. It was located on the high platform in the south of the campus with the highest terrain. The building is east-west and the plane is Latin cross-shaped. The main facade is in the west, the main entrance is in the east, and the south and north sides are respectively provided with secondary entrances. The outer wall is made of blue mushroom stones to the top, and the pilasters are arranged at the four corners and between the windows. The rose windows are set at the top of the gable, and the other windows are in the form of stone pointed arch. The interior is divided into three sections, paved with dressed stones. The pilasters in the middle hall are decorated with the stone arch. The middle hall has three floors with a bell tower at the top floor, and the four sides have two floors. Compared with other buildings on campus, Kumler Chapel is in different style. Although it has some architectural characteristics of Chinese style, the overall style is mainly Western. Looking up at this building, solemn and moving in silence, you can have a feeling of “as light as if we had left the human world and become winged immortals”.

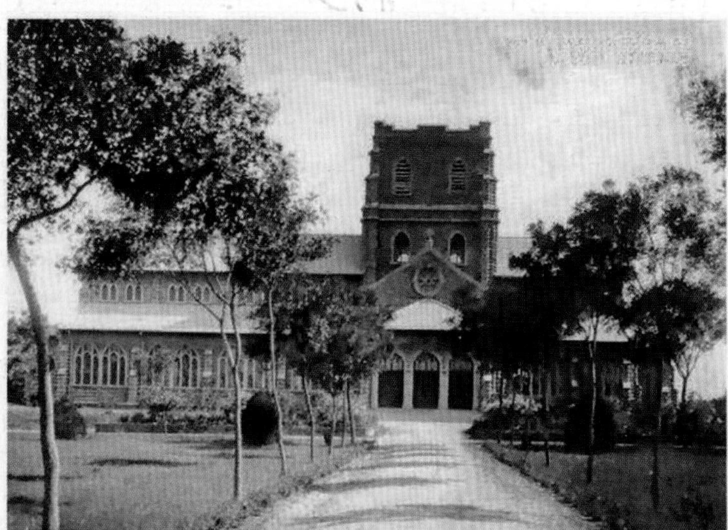

图 282 康穆堂北（正）面观
Fig. 282 The north (front) view of Kumler Chapel

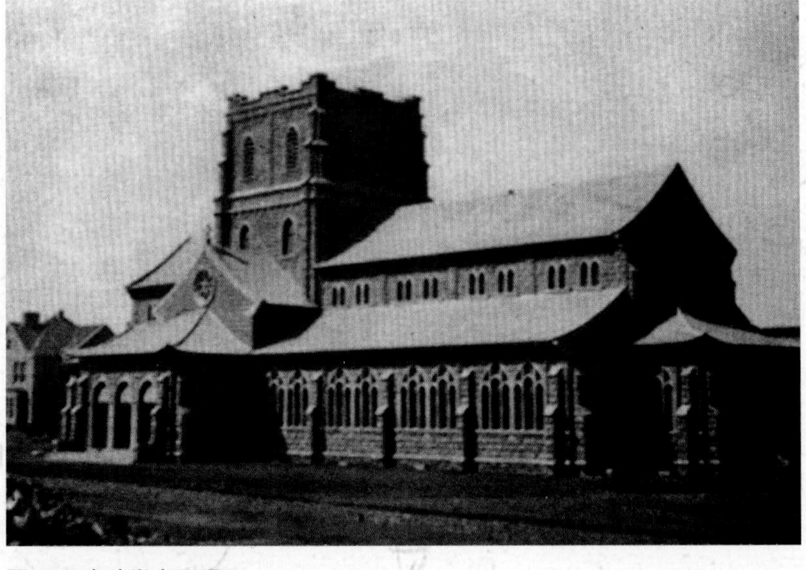

图 283 康穆堂南面观
Fig. 283 The south view of Kumler Chapel

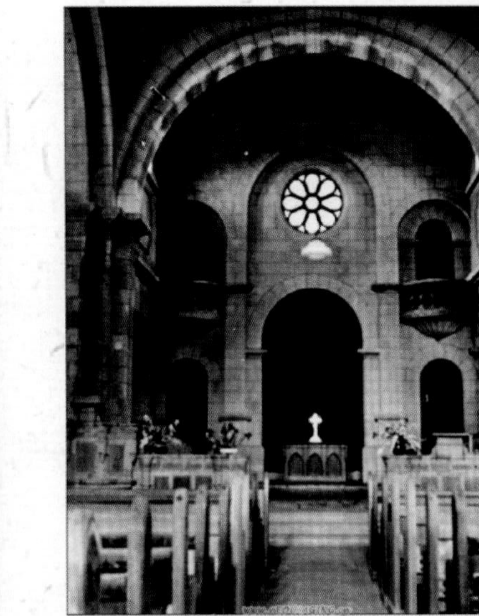

图 284 康穆堂内景
Fig. 284 The interior view of Kumler Chapel

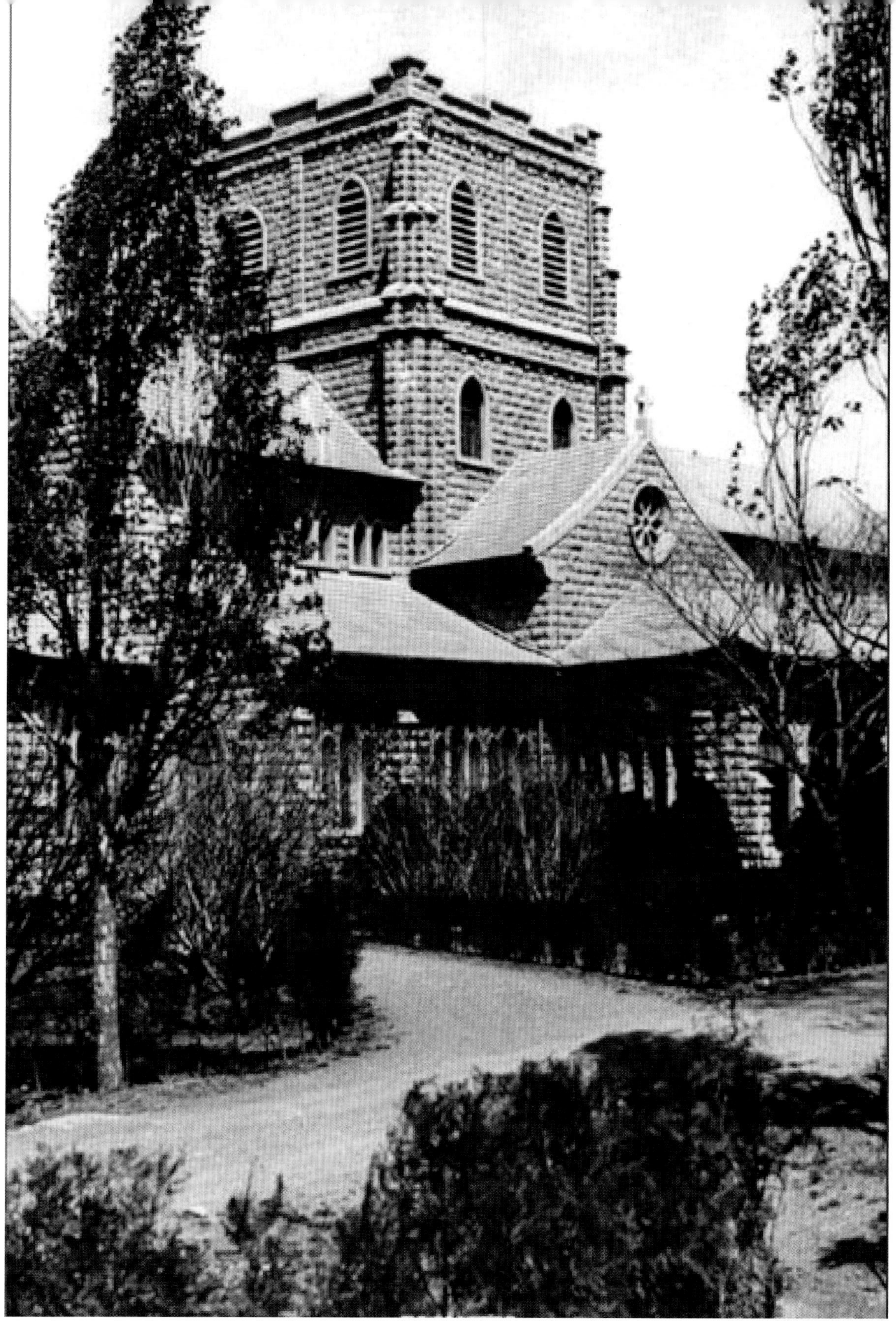

图 285 康穆堂西面观
Fig. 285 The west view of Kumler Chapel

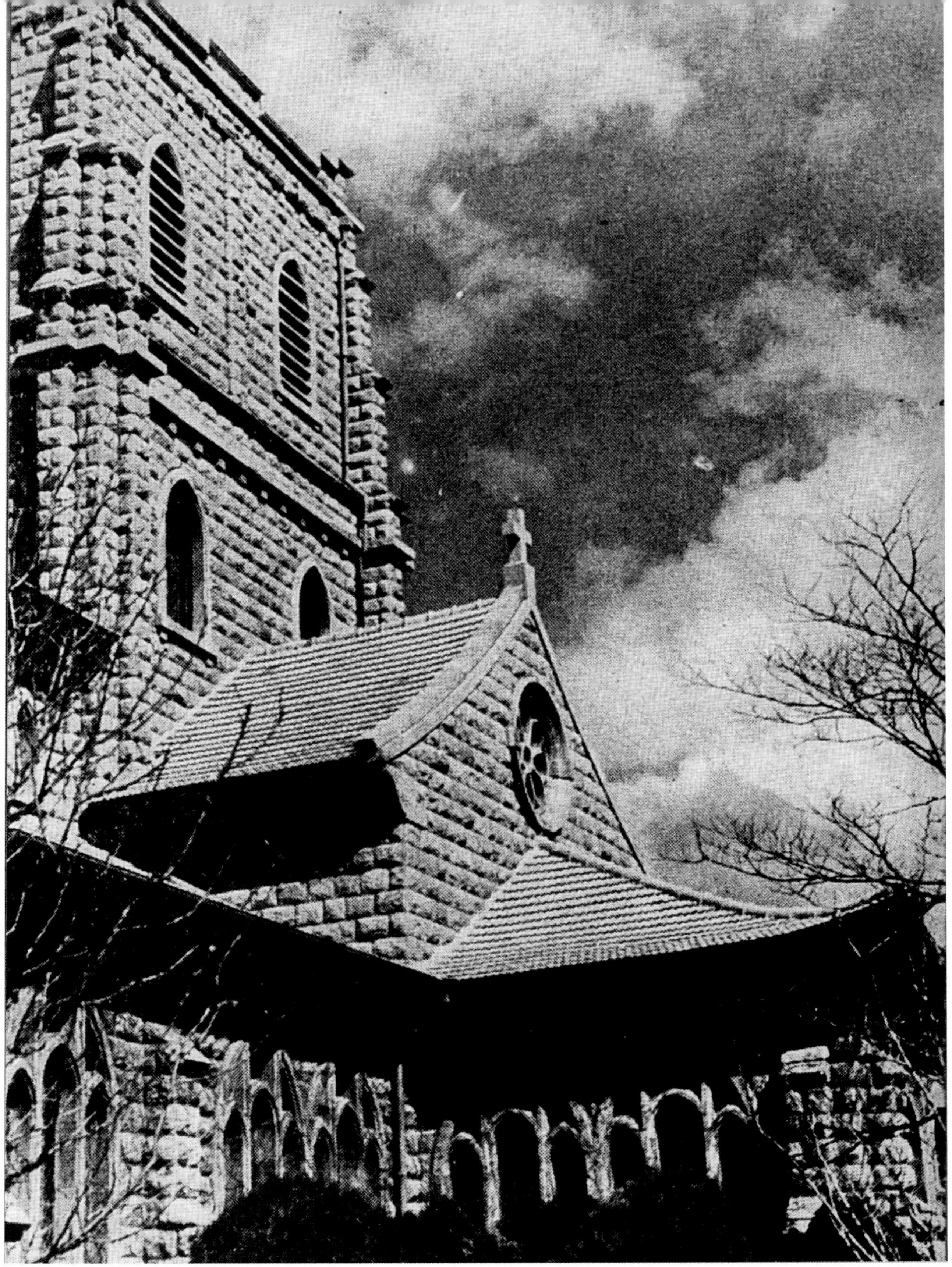

图 286 康穆堂上空风云变幻
Fig. 286 The changeable weather above Kumler Chapel

38 消失的齐鲁大学老建筑(2)

Lost Old Buildings of Cheeloo University (2)

康穆堂内建有可容纳 500 人的西式礼拜堂，除宗教活动外，也是举行重要校务活动(如毕业典礼)的场所。康穆堂有一口大钟，每当钟声响起，整个济南城的人都能听见。此钟尚在，目前存放于齐鲁医学院校史馆内。

当年齐鲁的“康穆堂”也和燕京的“未名湖”一样，闻名海内外。20 世纪 20 年代初，英国的罗素、美国的杜威、印度的泰戈尔等世界名人访华来济，都曾在此做过演讲。1924 年 4 月泰戈尔在康穆堂内作了题为“东西方文化之比较”的演讲，有“金童玉女”之称的著名诗人徐志摩和林徽因陪同来访，徐志摩同声翻译。在济南，泰戈尔遇到了高山流水式的知音，他就是被称之为“于大神仙”的于道泉（1901~1992）。当时，于道泉刚从齐鲁大学毕业，即将赴美公费留学，能用英语、梵文与泰戈尔交流，并精通佛学。后来于道泉成为著名藏学家、语言学家和教育家。于道泉一生淡泊名利，被季羡林称为没有“名利”二字的人。

Inside Kumler Chapel there is a Western-style church capable of accommodating 500 people. In addition to religious activities, it is also a place for important school activities (such as graduation ceremony). Kumler Chapel has a big bell. Whenever the bell rings, the whole city of Jinan can hear it. The bell is currently stored in the History Museum of Cheeloo College of Medicine.

As Weiming Lake in Yanjing, Kumler Chapel in Qilu was also famous at home and abroad in those days. In the early 1920s, Russell from the United Kingdom, Dewey from the United States, Tagore from India and other world celebrities visited China and came to Jinan to give speeches in Kumler Chapel. In April 1924, Tagore delivered a speech entitled “A Comparison of Eastern and Western Cultures” in Kumler Chapel. The famous poets Xu Zhimo and Lin Huiyin accompanied him on his visit and Xu Zhimo did simultaneous interpretation. In Jinan, Tagore met a bosom friend Yu Daoquan (1901-1992), known as the “Immortal Yu”. At that time, Yu Daoquan had just graduated from Cheeloo University and was about to study in the United States at public expense. He could communicate with Tagore in English and Sanskrit and was proficient in Buddhism. Later, Yu Daoquan became a famous Tibetologist, linguist and educator. Yu Daoquan was indifferent to fame and wealth all his life, and Ji Xianlin praised him as a person who did not care about fame and wealth.

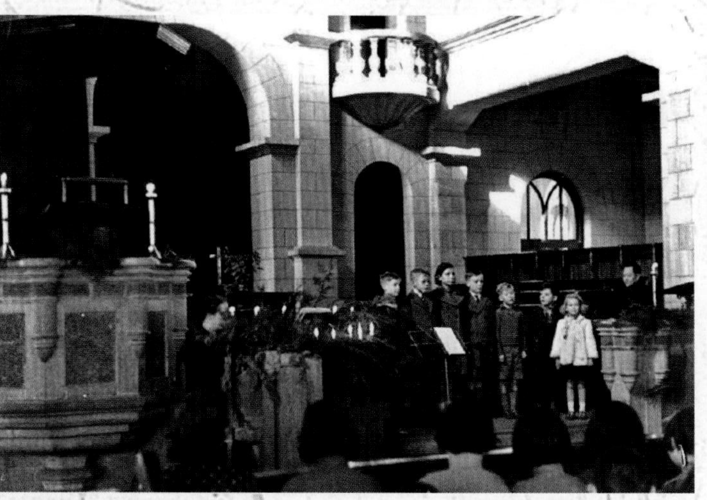

图 287 康穆堂中的唱诗班
Fig. 287 Choir in Kumler Chapel

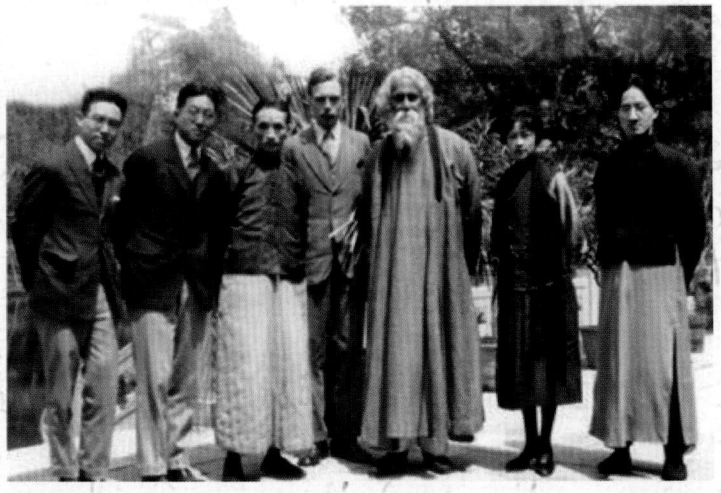

图 288 1924 年 4 月，徐志摩（右一）、林徽因（右二）、梁思成（左一）等与访问济南的泰戈尔（右三）合影。
Fig. 288 Xu Zhimo (first from right), Lin Huiyin (second from right) , Liang Sicheng (first from left) and others taking a photo with Tagore who visited Jinan in April 1924.

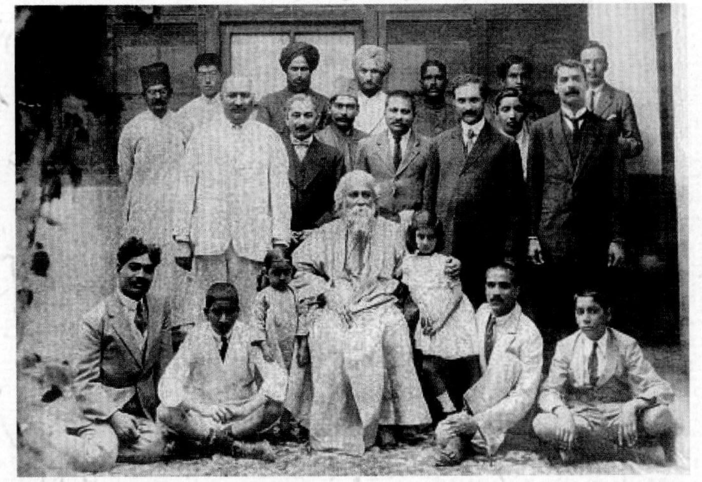

图 289 1924 年 4 月，于道泉（后排左一）与访问济南的泰戈尔（前排中）一行合影。
Fig. 289 Yu Daoquan (first from the left in the back row) taking a photo with Tagore (the middle in the front row) and his party who visited Jinan in April 1924.

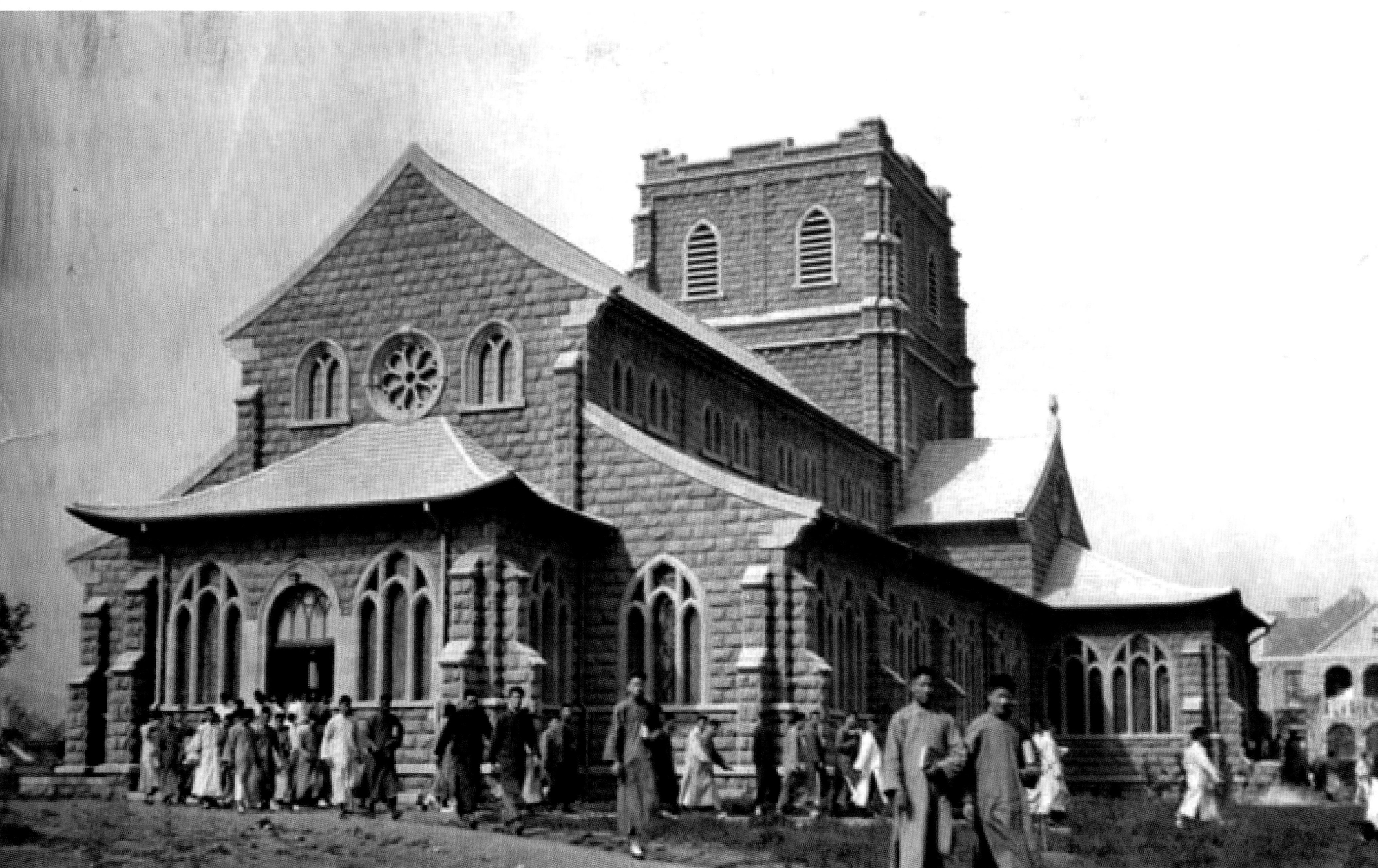

图 290 活动后师生离开康穆堂的情景

Fig. 290 Scene of teachers and students leaving Kumler Chapel after the activities

38 消失的齐鲁大学老建筑(3)

Lost Old Buildings of Cheeloo University (3)

1917 年，齐鲁大学天文台建于校园东南角，背后不远处即是白雪皑皑的千佛山。当时台内有架 25 厘米反射望远镜，为狄考文 1879 年回美国休假时所购置。这架大型精密天文望远镜 1904 年迁至潍县广文大学，1917 年搬来济南齐鲁大学，1952 年又被运到南京紫金山天文台。天文望远镜等仪器被拆走后，仅剩空壳的天文台不久即被拆除。

这座天文台隶属齐鲁大学天文算学系，该系的历史可追溯至登州文会馆时期。该会馆创办人狄考文自 1876 年就开始讲授天文算学，并设立了供学生实习用的天文台，可谓是我国第一个天文算学系。1882 年以后，文会馆第二任监督赫士（Watson M. Hayes，1857-1944）接替讲授天文算学，并著有《天文揭要》《天文初阶》等教科书。1917 年齐鲁大学设立天文算学系，第一任主任是文会馆毕业的被誉为世界六大天文学家之一的王锡恩教授。1952 年院系调整时，该天文算学系并入南京大学。齐鲁大学天文算学系名人辈出，其中 1951 年毕业生苗永瑞 1991 年当选为中国科学院学部委员（院士）。

In 1917, the Observatory of Cheeloo University was built in the southeast corner of the campus, and not far behind is the snow-capped Qianfo Hill. At that time, there was a 25-centimeter reflective telescope inside the observatory purchased by Calvin Wilson Mateer when he returned to the United States for vacation in 1879. This large precision astronomical telescope was moved to Shantung Protestant University in Weixian County in 1904, to Cheeloo University in Jinan in 1917, and then to the Purple Mountain Observatory in Nanjing in 1952. After the astronomical telescope and other instruments were removed, the observatory became an empty shell and was soon dismantled.

The observatory is part of the Department of Astronomical Arithmetic of Cheeloo University. The history of the department can be traced back to the period of Tengchow College. Calvin Wilson Mateer, the founder of Tengchow College, had been teaching astronomical arithmetic since 1876 and had set up an observatory for students to practice, which can be said to be the first Department of Astronomical Arithmetic in China. After 1882, Watson M. Hayes (1857-1944), the second supervisor of Tengchow College, took over the teaching of astronomical arithmetic and wrote textbooks such as *A Treatise on Astronomy* and *Astronomy at the First Stage*. In 1917, Cheeloo University established the Department of Astronomical Arithmetic, and the first director was Professor Wang Xi'en who graduated from Tengchow College and was known as one of the six great astronomers in the world. In 1952, the Department of Astronomical Arithmetic merged into Nanjing University during adjustment of schools and departments. The Department of Astronomical Arithmetic of Cheeloo University has many celebrities. Miao Yongrui, a 1951 graduate, was elected member (academician) of Chinese Academy of Sciences in 1991.

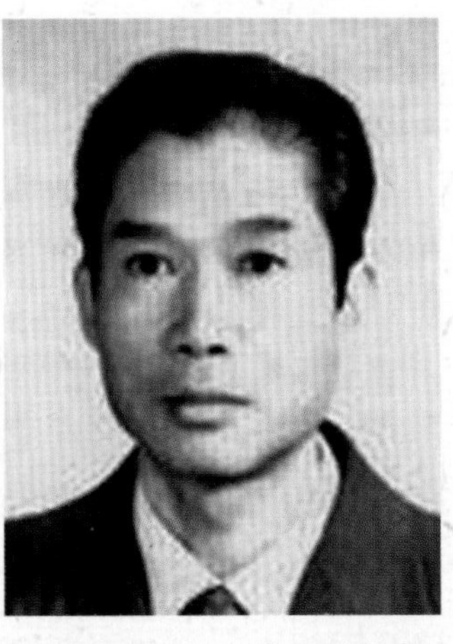

图 291 苗永瑞（1930 ～ 1999），中国科学院院士，曾任陕西天文台台长，测定了天顶星，建立了长波授时台。

Fig. 291 Miao Yongrui (1930-1999), academician of Chinese Academy of Sciences, was once the director of Shaanxi ObservatorywwHe determined the zenith star and established the long-wave time service system.

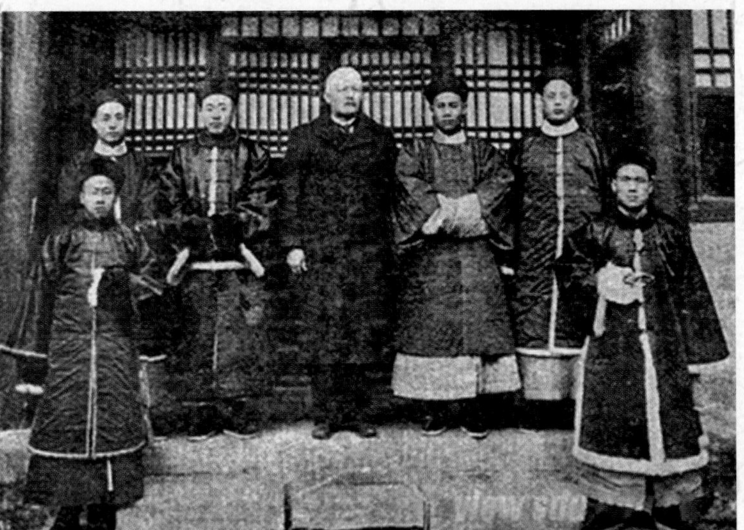

图 292 1901 年，赫士（正中）应袁世凯之邀带领王锡恩（赫士右侧）等 6 名西学教习前来济南筹办山东大学堂。

Fig. 292 In 1901, at the invitation of Yuan Shikai, Watson M. Hayes led six teachers of Western learning to Jinan to organize Shandong University and Wang Xi'en (right of Hayes) was one of them.

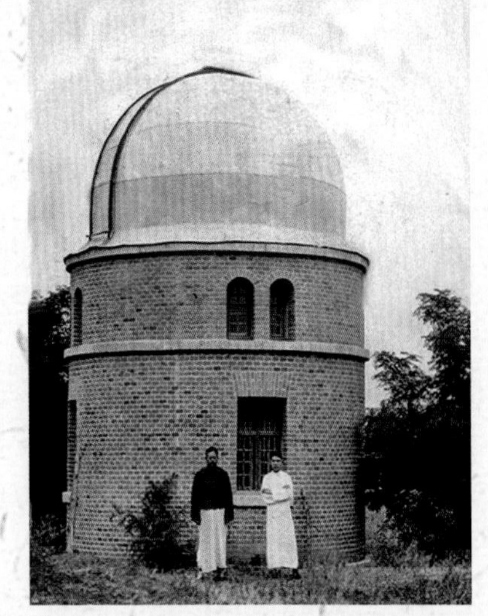

图 293 齐鲁大学新建的天文馆，馆外两位合影者中，左为天文算学系主任兼天文台台长王锡恩，右为其助手天算系副教授田冠五。

Fig. 293 Outside the newly-built planetarium of Cheeloo University, two people are taking photos. The left is Wang Xi'en, director of the Department of Astronomical Arithmetic and of the observatory; the right is his assistant Tian Guanwu, associate professor of the Department of Astronomical Arithmetic.

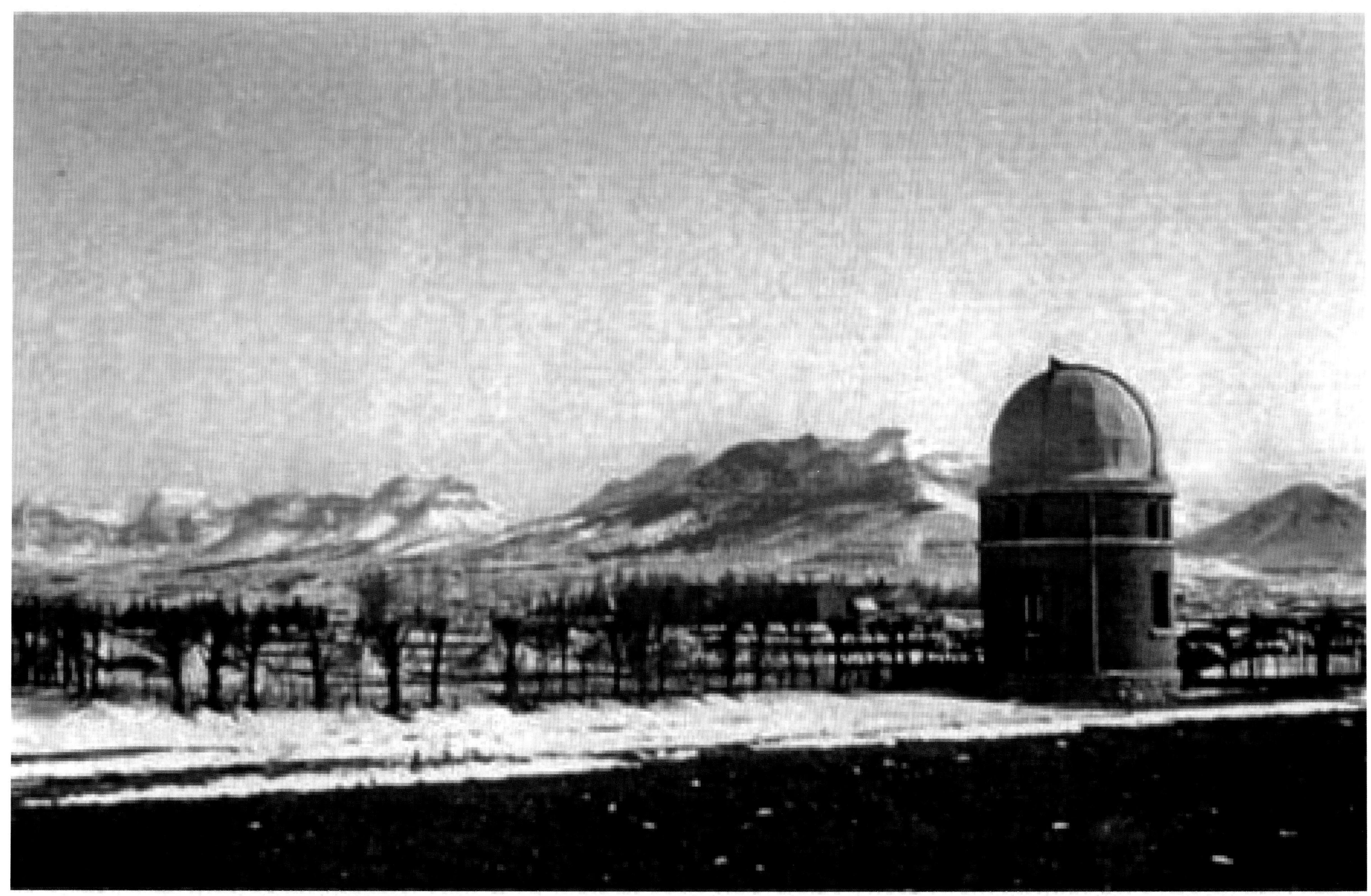

图 294 齐鲁大学天文台冬景，其南为白雪覆盖的千佛山
Fig. 294 Winter view of the Observatory of Cheeloo University, with the snow-capped Qianfo Hill in the south

38 | 消失的齐鲁大学老建筑(4)

Lost Old Buildings of Cheeloo University (4)

奥古斯丁图书馆（Augustine Library），建于1922年，为加拿大温尼伯（Winnipeg）奥古斯丁长老支会捐款修建。建筑风格与葛罗神学院楼相似，也是两层建筑。1983年因已被列为危楼而拆除，1985年在原址上建成第七教学楼。

该馆发轫时，藏书量非常有限，大多是传教士从国外带来的英文原版图书，内容除神学外，以自然科学和医学居多。20世纪30年代初，齐鲁大学顺应文化界“整理国故”思潮涌动的大势，利用美国霍尔基金给予的契机，成为参与哈佛燕京学社国学教育与研究计划的六所教会大学之一，获得15万美元专项经费，购置了大量图书。至1937年，保守估计藏书量也超过了12万册。这是奥古斯丁图书馆藏书量最丰富的时期。国学研究所还加强了对山东省及北方诸省地方志的收集及保存，由此形成了此馆藏书的地方志特色。图书馆办馆理念以人为本，设备先进。先后走出了桂质柏、皮高品等中国近代图书馆学界的重量级人物。

TAugustine Library, built in 1922, was donated by the Augustine Presbyterian Church in Winnipeg, Canada. Its architectural style is similar to that of Gotch-Robinson Theological Building and both are two-storey buildings. It was demolished in 1983 because it had been listed as a dangerous building, and the Seventh Teaching Building was completed at the original site in 1985.

In the early days of its establishment, the library had a very limited collection of books, most of which were original English books brought by missionaries from abroad. In addition to theology, the books were mostly in natural science and medicine. In the early 1930s, Cheeloo University conformed to the trend of “Sorting out the National Cultural Heritage” in the cultural circle and took advantage of the opportunity given by the Hall Fund of the United States to become one of the six missionary universities participating in the National Education and Research Program of Harvard-Yenching Institute, obtaining 150,000 US dollars of special funds and purchasing a large number of books. By 1937, at a conservative estimate, the collection exceeded 120,000 copies, and this was the most abundant period of Augustine Library. The Institute of National Studies had also strengthened the collection and preservation of the local chronicles of Shandong Province and other northern provinces, thus forming the collection characteristics of the local chronicles of this library. The concept of library management is people-oriented and the equipment is advanced. Some heavyweight figures in the field of library science in modern China such as Gui Zhibai and Pi Gaopin emerged from this library.

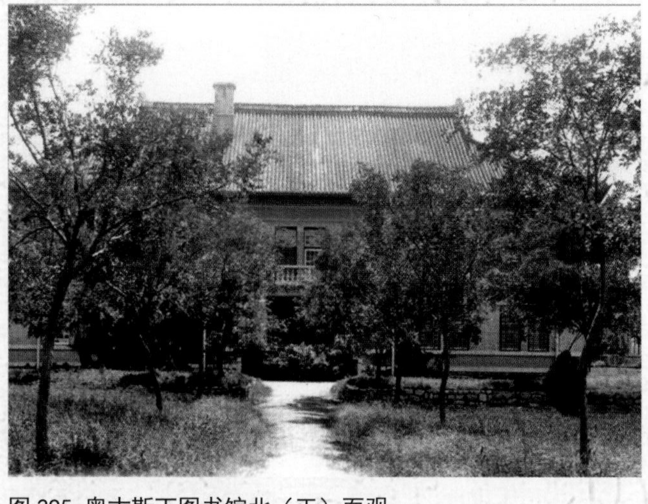

图295 奥古斯丁图书馆北（正）面观

Fig. 295 The north (front) view of Augustine Library

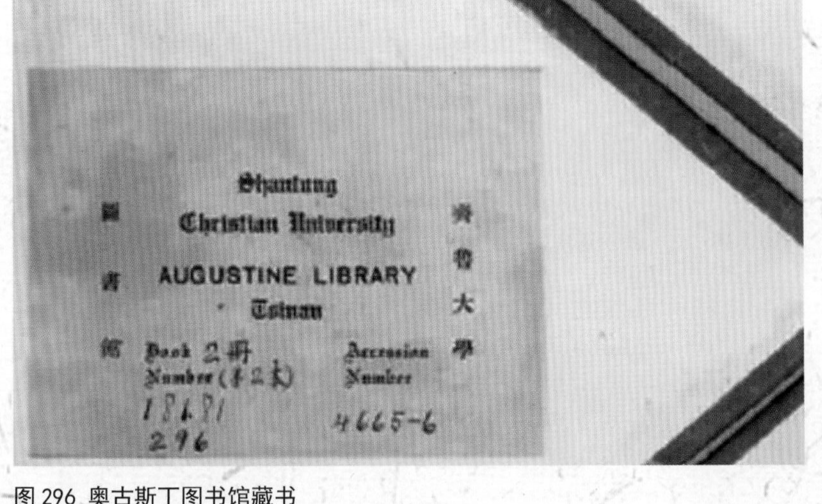

图296 奥古斯丁图书馆藏书

Fig. 296 Collection of Augustine Library

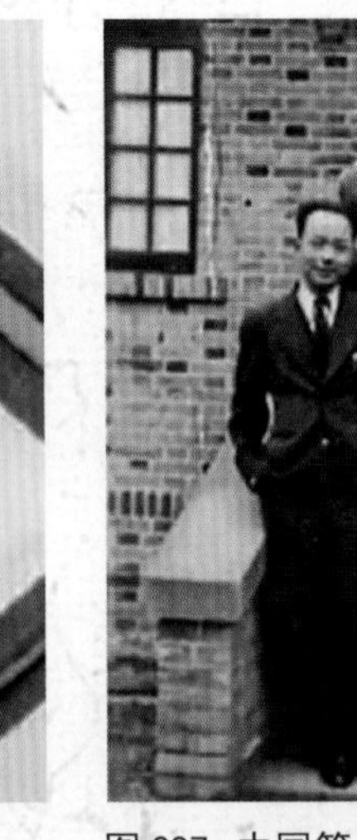

图297 中国第一位图书馆学博士桂质柏（后排左一），1922年至1925年期间担任齐鲁大学图书馆主任，后来曾任国立中央大学图书馆主任。

Fig. 297 Gui Zhibai, the first doctor of library science (first from left in the back row) in China, served as director of the Library of Cheeloo University from 1922 to 1925 and later as director of the Library of National Central University.

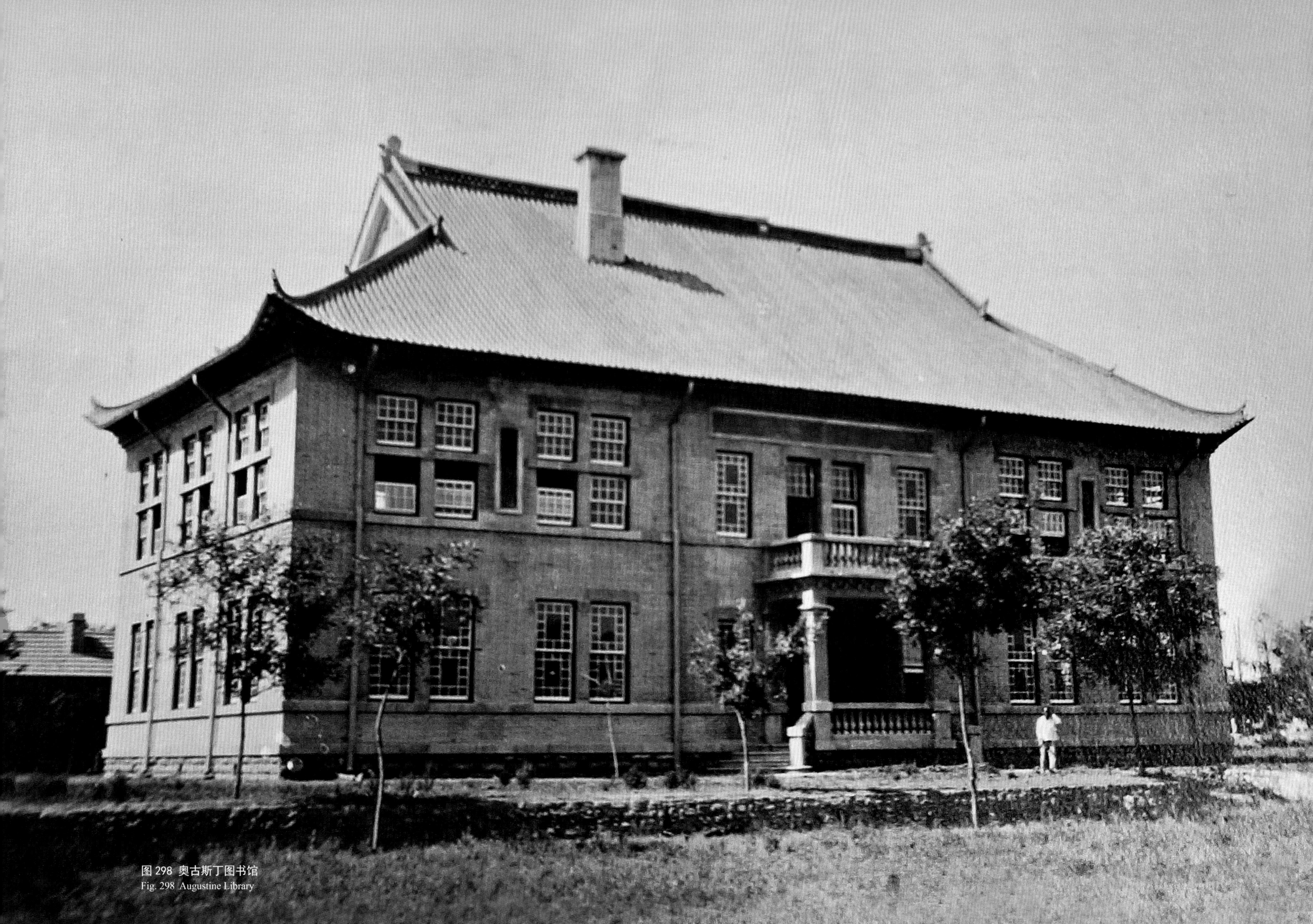

图 298 奥古斯丁图书馆
Fig. 298 Augustine Library

38 消失的齐鲁大学老建筑（5）

Lost Old Buildings of Cheeloo University (5)

齐鲁大学麻风病医院始建于 1926 年 5 月，省政府的 2500 银元被用来买地，英国麻风会的 2 万银元用于建造病房，1929 年 6 月建成，位于齐鲁大学校园东南角，占地 16 亩，建有 34 间平房，设 50 张床位。齐鲁医院院长、皮肤病学教授海贝殖兼任院长。海贝殖和他的助手尤家骏采用中西医结合疗法治疗麻风病，取得了较好效果。1934 年海贝殖回国后，尤家骏接任麻风病医院院长。1950 年人民政府接管后，院址迁往西郊，改名为济南麻风病院，后来发展为山东省皮肤病医院。

海贝殖（LeRoy F. Heimburger，1889~1960），美国密苏里州人。1929~1934 年任齐鲁医院第四任院长，是著名的皮肤性病、麻风病专家。

尤家骏（1898~1969），山东即墨人。1926 年毕业于齐鲁大学医学院，后任齐鲁大学医学院、山东医学院一级教授。出版了一系列有关麻风病的专著，是我国麻风病防治专业的开创者和奠基人。尤家骏也是山东省皮肤病医院的创始人和首任院长，该院立有尤家骏教授塑像。

The Leprosy Hospital of Cheeloo University was built in May 1926. The 2,500 silver dollars from the provincial government was used to buy the land and the 20,000 silver dollars from the Leprosy Society of the United Kingdom was used to build wards. Completed in June 1929, the hospital was located in the southeast corner on campus of Cheeloo University and covered an area of 16 mu, with 34 bungalows and 50 beds. LeRoy F. Heimburger, president of Qilu Hospital and professor of dermatology, concurrently served as the president of the Leprosy Hospital. Heimburger and his assistant You Jiajun used integrated therapy of traditional Chinese and Western medicine to treat leprosy and achieved good results. In 1934, You Jiajun took over as president of the Leprosy Hospital after Heimburger returned home. After being taken over by the People's Government in 1950, the hospital was moved to the western suburbs and renamed Jinan Leprosy Hospital. Later, it developed into Shandong Provincial Hospital of Dermatology.

LeRoy F. Heimburger (1889-1960) was a native of Missouri, the United States. He served as the fourth president of Qilu Hospital from 1929 to 1934 and he was a famous expert in dermatology and leprosy.

You Jiajun (1898-1969) was born in Jimo, Shandong Province. He graduated from the School of Medicine of Cheeloo University in 1926 and later served as a first-level professor of the School of Medicine of Cheeloo University and Shandong Medical College. He had published a series of monographs on leprosy and is the founder of the specialty in leprosy prevention and control in China. You Jiajun is also the founder and first president of Shandong Provincial Hospital of Dermatology and there is a statue of Professor You Jiajun in the hospital.

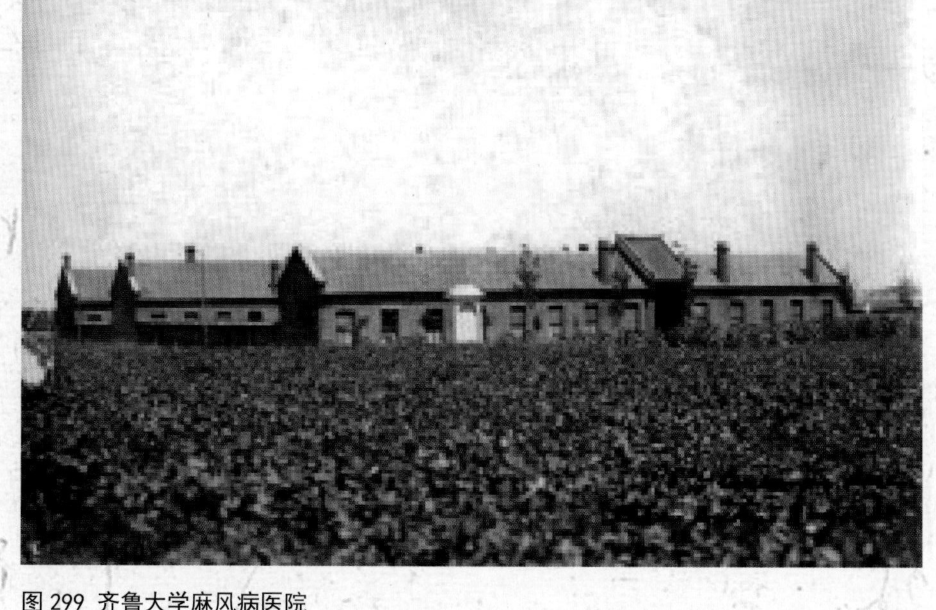

图 299 齐鲁大学麻风病医院
Fig. 299 The Leprosy Hospital of Cheeloo University

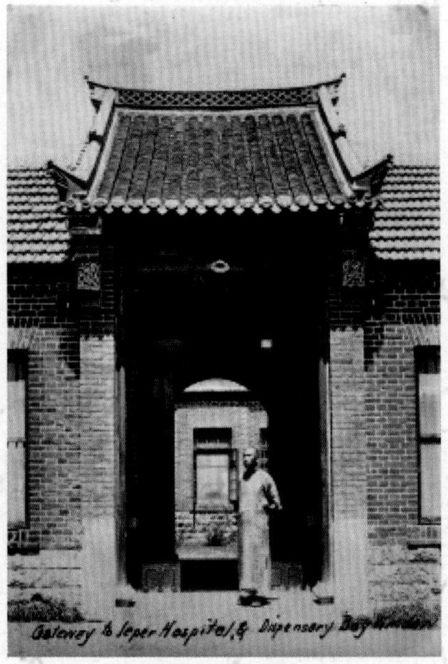

图 300 齐鲁大学麻风病医院大门
Fig. 300 Gate of the Leprosy Hospital of Cheeloo University

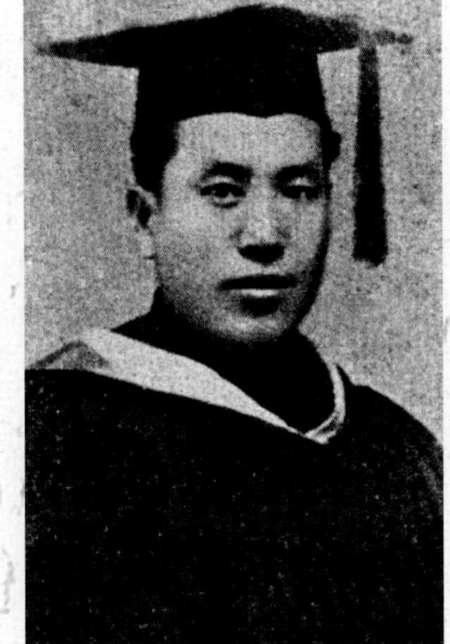

图 301 尤家骏教授
Fig. 301 Professor You Jiajun

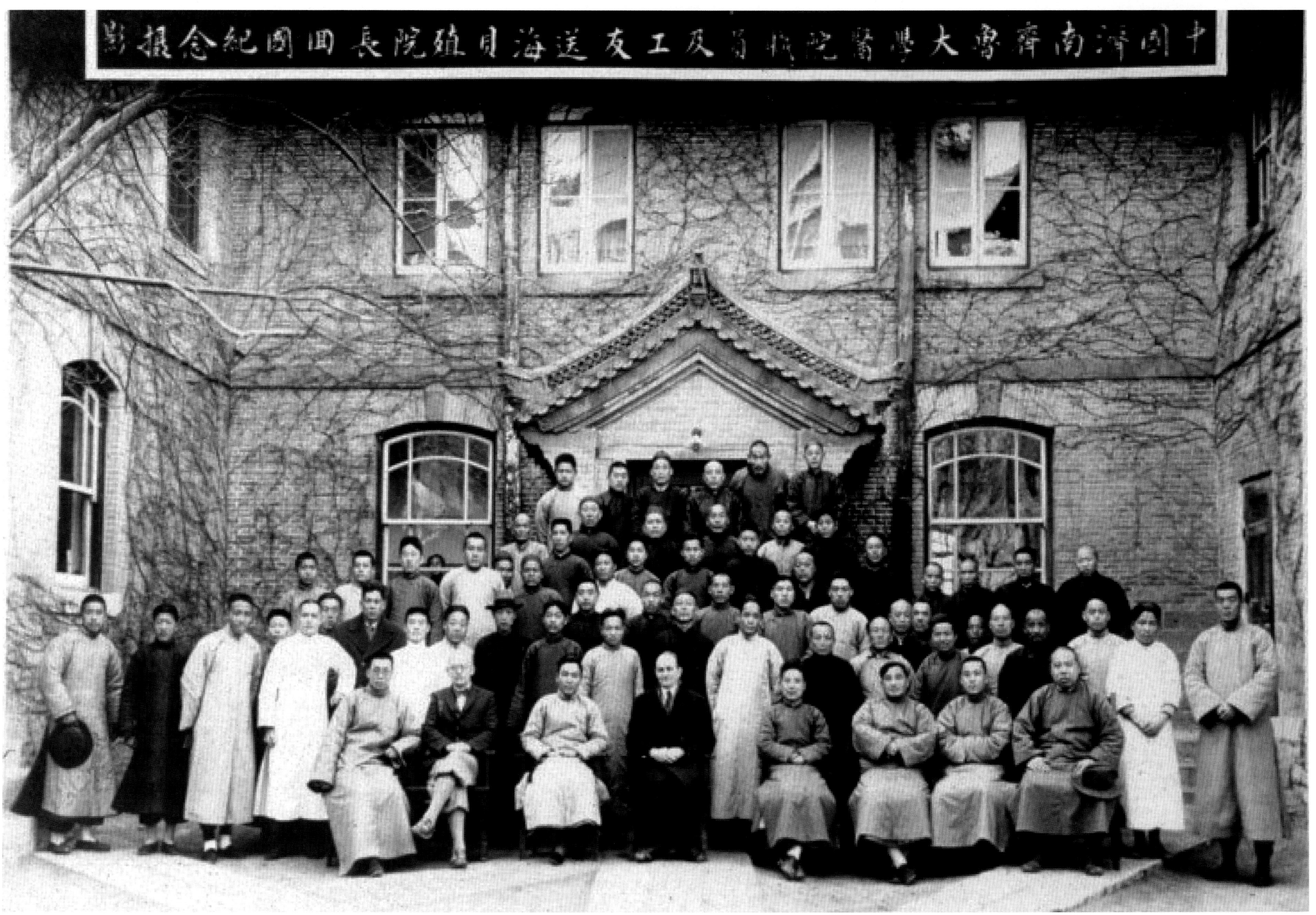

图 302 1934 年齐鲁大学医院职工及工友送海贝殖院长（前排左四着西装者）回国纪念。此后，海贝殖及其家族与齐鲁医院建立了长期友好交流关系。

Fig. 302 A photo of the hospital staff and workers of Cheeloo University seeing the Dean LeRoy F. Heimburger (the fourth from the left in Western-style clothes in the front row) off in 1934. Since then, LeRoy F. Heimburger and his family had established long-term friendly exchange relations with Qilu Hospital.

39 图书馆

Library

图书馆主楼建于 1978 年，砖混结构，四层，现为山东大学图书馆医学分馆。东西配楼建于 20 世纪 90 年代末期，砖混结构，五层（第五层为加盖钢结构），全部为教室，分别称图书楼东教室（简称图东）和图书楼西教室（简称“图西”）。当今，随着计算机技术、网络与通信技术尤其是多媒体技术的迅速发展，图书资源已实现了数字化、虚拟化、网络化和多媒体化，现代图书馆的概念已发生了巨大变化。截至 2019 年 8 月，山东大学图书馆馆藏纸质文献 587.2 万余册（含院系 48.8 万余册），各类数据库 247 个，覆盖文、理、工、医等领域；馆藏古籍 31 万余册（件），是“全国古籍重点保护单位”和“山东省古籍重点保护单位”。山东大学图书馆是首批中国高等教育文献保障系统（CALIS）成员之一、CALIS 山东省文献信息服务中心、中国高校人文社会科学文献中心（CASHL）学科中心、教育部科技查新工作站。现在在网上即可实现全校图书资源共享，非常方便。

The main building of the library was built in the 1980s, of reinforced concrete structure and with four floors. It is now the medical branch of Shandong University Library. The east and west wings were built in the 1990s, of reinforced concrete structure and with five floors (the fifth floor is of steel structure). They are all used for classrooms, being called the east classroom of the library and the west classroom of the library respectively. Nowadays, with the rapid development of computer technology, network and communication technology, and especially multimedia technology, the book resources have achieved digitization, virtualization, networking and multimedia, and the concept of modern libraries has undergone tremendous changes. By August 2019, Shandong University Library had more than 5,872,000 paper documents (including more than 488,000 copies of schools and departments) and 247 databases of various kinds, covering the fields of literature, science, industry and medicine. With a collection of more than 310,000 copies (pieces) of ancient books, Shandong University Library is rated as the “National Key Protection Unit of Ancient Books” and “Shandong Provincial Key Protection Unit of Ancient Books”. Shandong University Library is one of the first members of China Academic Library and Information System (CALIS), Shandong Provincial Library and Information Service Center of CALIS, the Discipline Center of China Academic Social Sciences and Humanities Library(CASHL), and Science and Technology Novelty Search Workstation of Ministry of Education. Now the sharing of book resources in the whole university can be realized through the Internet, which is extremely convenient.

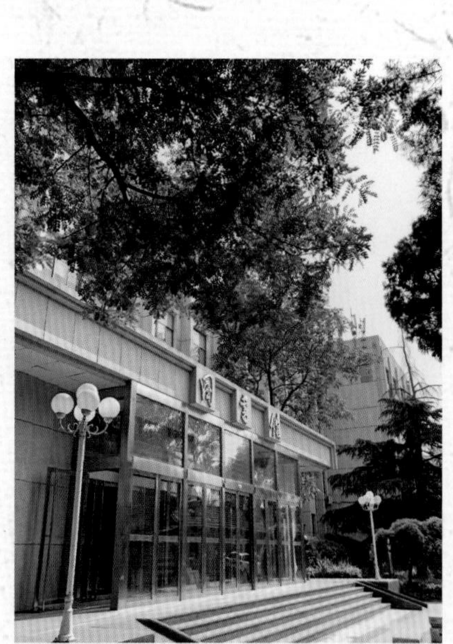

图 303 图书馆夏景
Fig. 303 The summer view of the library

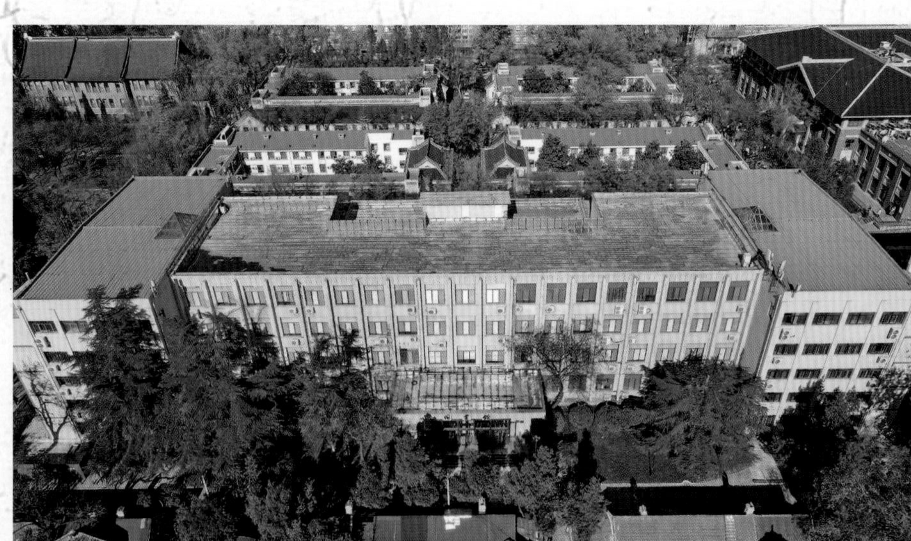

图 304 图书馆鸟瞰图
Fig. 304 A bird’s-eye view of the library

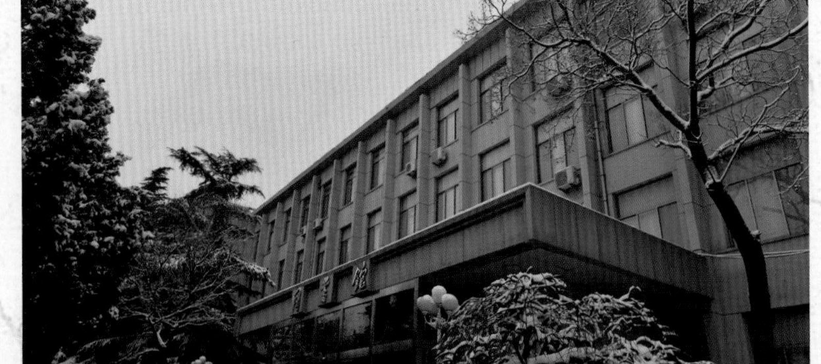

图 305 图书馆雪景
Fig. 305 Snow view of the library

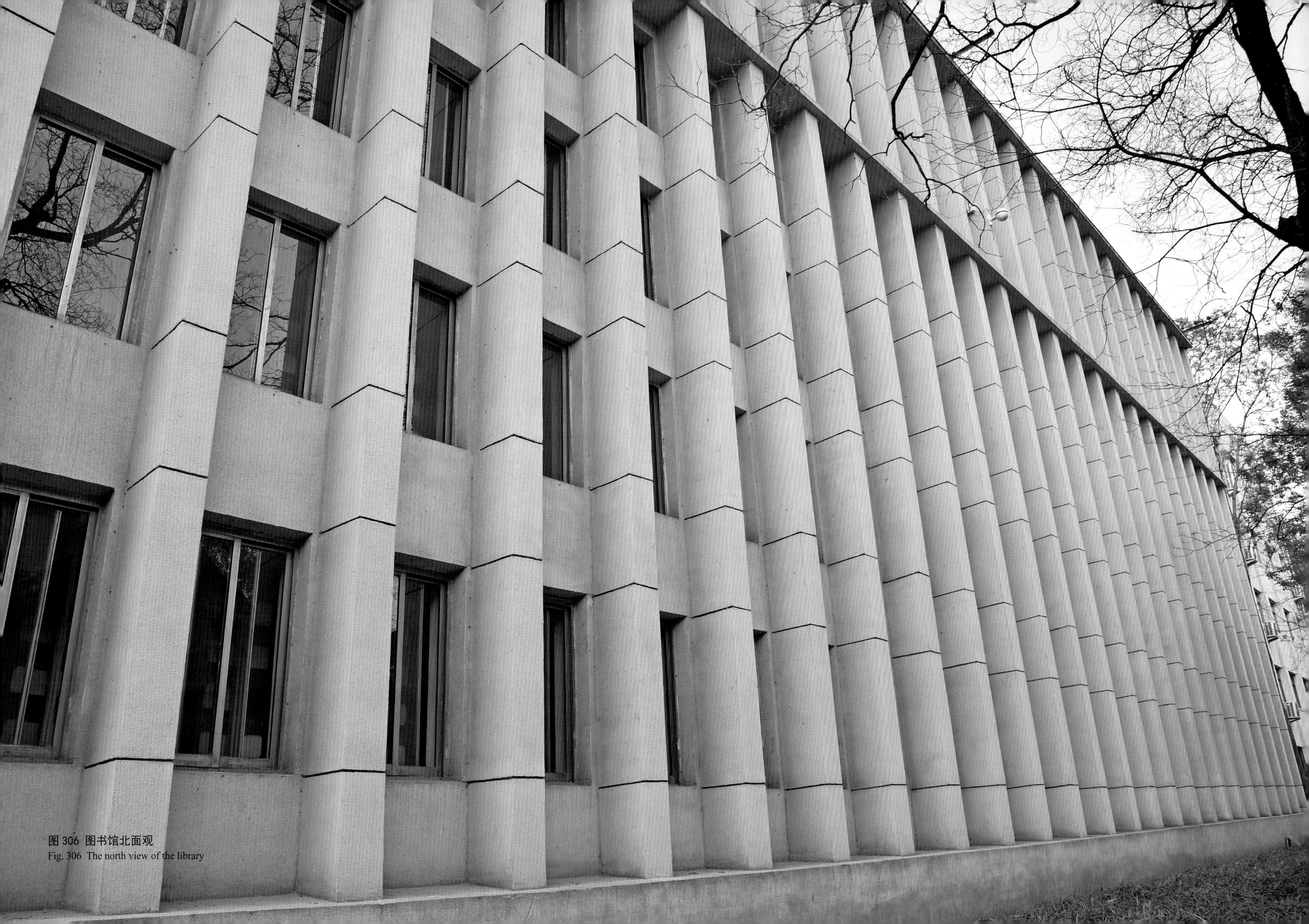

图 306 图书馆北面观
Fig. 306 The north view of the library

40 梦迪音乐厅

Mengdi Concert Hall

山东大学梦迪音乐厅，或称大学生活动中心，由医学系 1980 级校友王晨捐资建设，以其女儿王梦迪的名字命名。此建筑 2018 年 4 月开工建设，2019 年 12 月竣工，2020 年 10 月 17 日举行了启用仪式和首场音乐会。大学生活动中心总面积 12173 平方米，其中梦迪音乐厅内设观众席 560 余座，是一座集音乐演出、文化活动及学术会议于一体的综合艺术场馆，按照一流剧院、剧场及音乐厅的设施标准建造，通过装饰设计、声学控制、舞台工艺系统三方面的结合，运用先进的舞台设备创造优质的声光氛围，从各个方位、各个角度为观众呈现最佳的视听享受。

王晨，1962 年生于济南，1980 年考入山东医学院医学系，毕业后留校在齐鲁医院儿科工作。1987 年考取山东医科大学硕士研究生，1992 年下海创业，1998 年出国，主要从事医药高科技投资管理工作。近 10 年来，王晨校友先后捐赠 6000 余万元人民币用于支持母校发展，展现了对母校的赤子之心，产生了良好的示范效应。

Mengdi Concert Hall of Shandong University, also known as the Student Center, was donated by Wang Chen, a medical alumnus of 1980, and named after his daughter Wang Mengdi. The building was completed in 2020, and the opening ceremony and its first concert were held on 17 October in the same year. The Student Center covers a total area of 12,173 square meters, of which Mengdi Concert Hall has more than 560 audience seats. It is a comprehensive art venue integrating music performances, cultural activities and academic conferences. It is built according to the facility standards of first-class theaters and concert halls. Through the combination of decoration design, acoustic control and stage technology system, it uses advanced stage equipment to create a high-quality sound and light atmosphere in order to present the best audio-visual enjoyment for the audience from all directions.

Wang Chen, born in Jinan in 1962, was admitted to the Medical Department of Shandong Medical College in 1980 and stayed in Qilu Hospital to work in Pediatrics after graduation. In 1987, he was admitted to Shandong Medical University as a graduate student for a Master's degree. He started a business in 1992 and went abroad in 1998, mainly engaged in medical high-tech investment management. In the past 10 years, Wang Chen has donated more than 60 million *yuan* to support the development of his alma mater, demonstrating the attachment and devotion to his alma mater and producing a good demonstration effect.

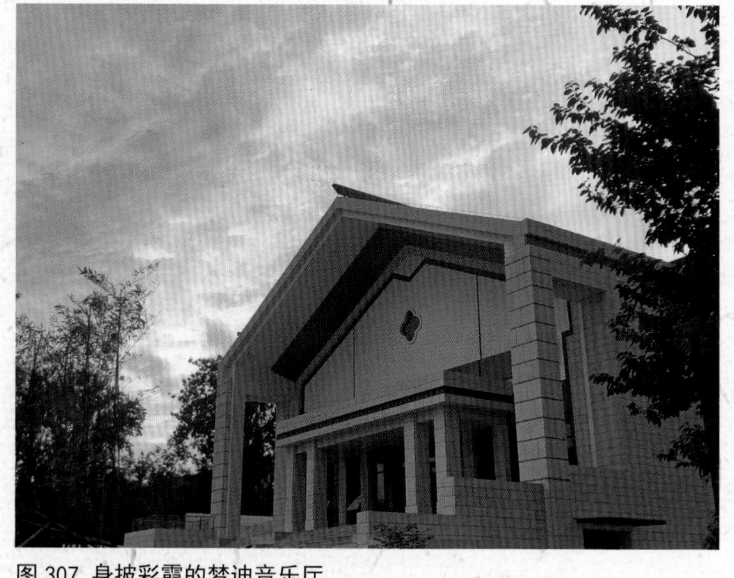

图 307 身披彩霞的梦迪音乐厅

Fig. 307 Mengdi Concert Hall in rosy clouds

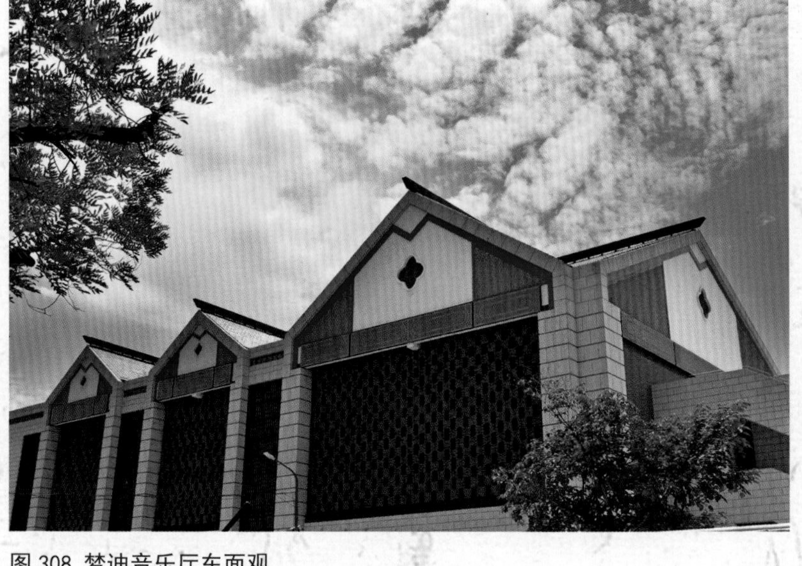

图 308 梦迪音乐厅东面观

Fig. 308 The east view of Mengdi Concert Hall

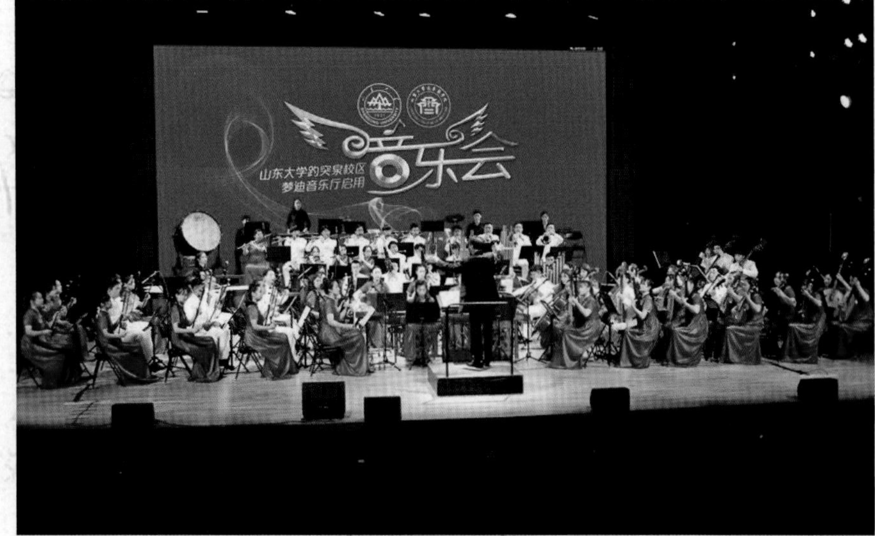

图 309 2020 年 10 月 17 日，梦迪音乐厅举行启用仪式及首场音乐会

Fig. 309 The opening ceremony and the first concert of Mengdi Concert Hall on 17 October 2020

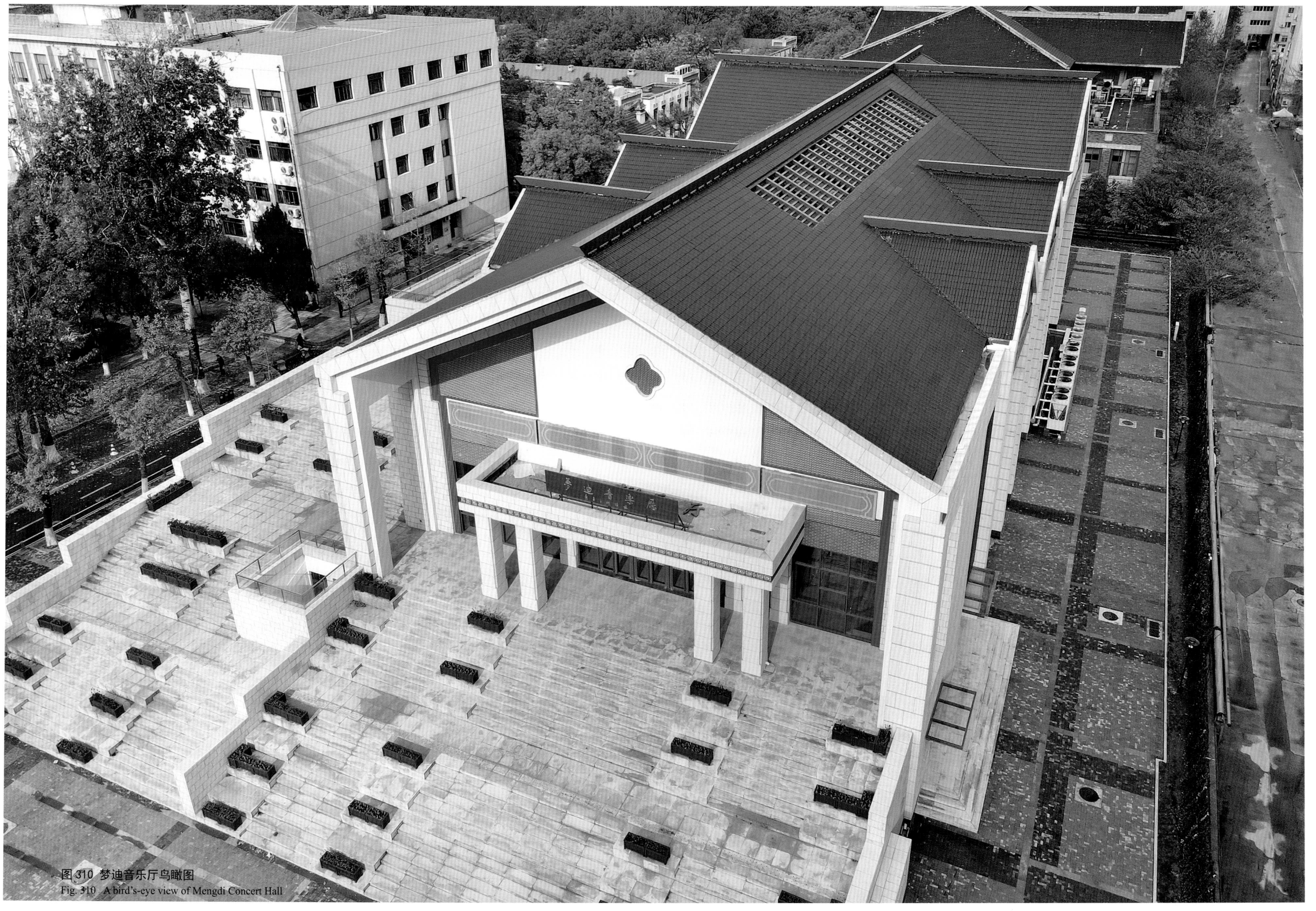

图 310 梦迪音乐厅鸟瞰图
Fig. 310 A bird's-eye view of Mengdi Concert Hall

41 体育场

Stadium

今日的体育场成形于 20 世纪 50 年代，露天结构，现分为田径场、网球场、篮球场、五人制足球场和排球场，有标准塑胶场地、草地和露天看台。

山东医学院体育教研室首任主任为我国著名体育教育家张芳梅教授（1910 ~ 1995）。他是山东德州人，早年毕业于上海东亚体育专科学校（现上海师范大学），攻读体育教育专业，当时在东亚体专篮球界被称为“东亚五虎”之一，打遍上海无敌手，多次战胜英法租界代表队。曾代表中国参加远东运动会篮球比赛。毕业后任东北大学体育教研室教授，当时的校长为张学良。新中国成立初期回到济南，在华东白求恩医学院任教，1952 年院系调整后来山东医学院体育教研室任教授、主任，是当时山东省高校为数不多的体育教授之一。

The open-air stadium today was formed in the 1950s. It is now divided into track and field ground, tennis court, basketball court, five-person football field and volleyball court, with standard plastic fields, grass and bleachers.

Professor Zhang Fangmei (1910-1995), a famous Chinese educator in physical education, was the first director of the Teaching and Research Office of Physical Education of Shandong Medical College. He was a native of Dezhou, Shandong Province. In his early years, he graduated from Shanghai East Asia Sports College (now Shanghai Normal University) and studied physical education. At that time, he was known as one of the “Five Tigers of East Asia” in the basketball session of East Asia Sports College. He played invincible in Shanghai and defeated the teams of the British and French concessions many times. He once participated in the basketball competition of the Far Eastern Championship Games on behalf of China. After graduation, he served as a professor in the Teaching and Research Office of Physical Education of Northeastern University, of which the president was Zhang Xueliang at that time. In the early days of the founding of People’s Republic of China, he returned to Jinan and taught in East China Bethune Medical College. After the adjustment of the schools and departments in 1952, he served as a professor and director of the Teaching and Research Office of Physical Education of Shandong Medical College. He was one of the few professors of physical education in colleges and universities in Shandong Province at that time.

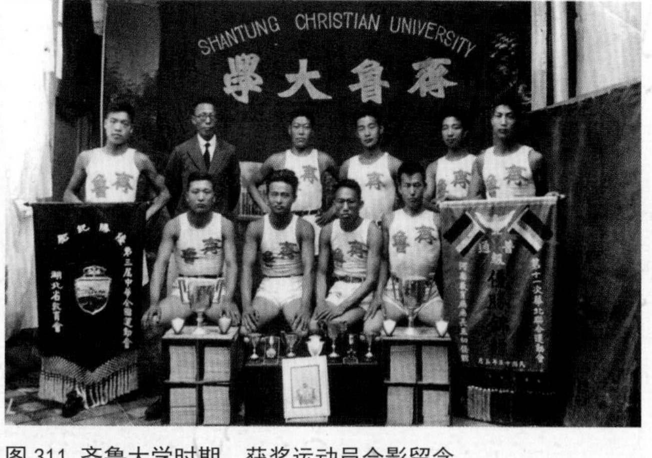

图 311 齐鲁大学时期，获奖运动员合影留念
Fig. 311 The award-winning athletes of Cheeloo University taking a photo

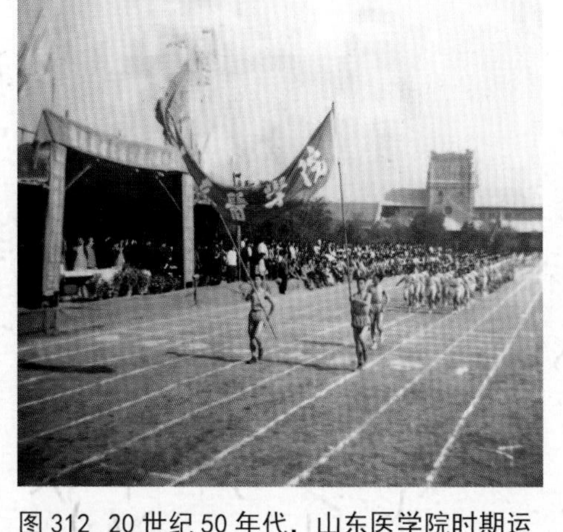

图 312 20 世纪 50 年代，山东医学院时期运动会入场式
Fig. 312 The entrance ceremony of the sports meeting in Shandong Medical College in the 1950s

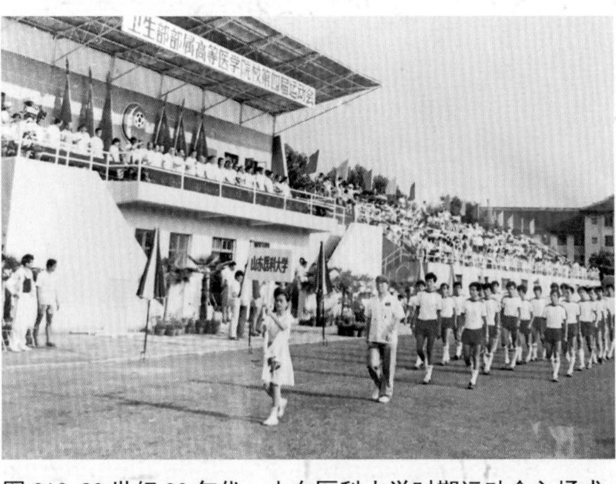

图 313 20 世纪 90 年代，山东医科大学时期运动会入场式
Fig. 313 The entrance ceremony of the sports meeting in Shandong Medical University in the 1990s

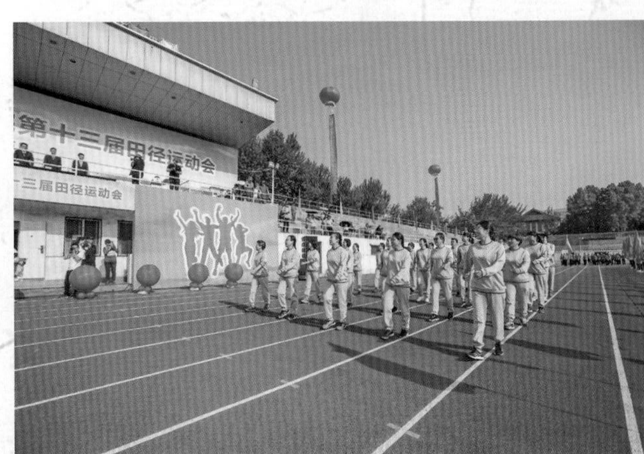

图 314 21 世纪初，山东大学时期运动会入场式
Fig. 314 The entrance ceremony of the sports meeting in Shandong University in the early 21st century

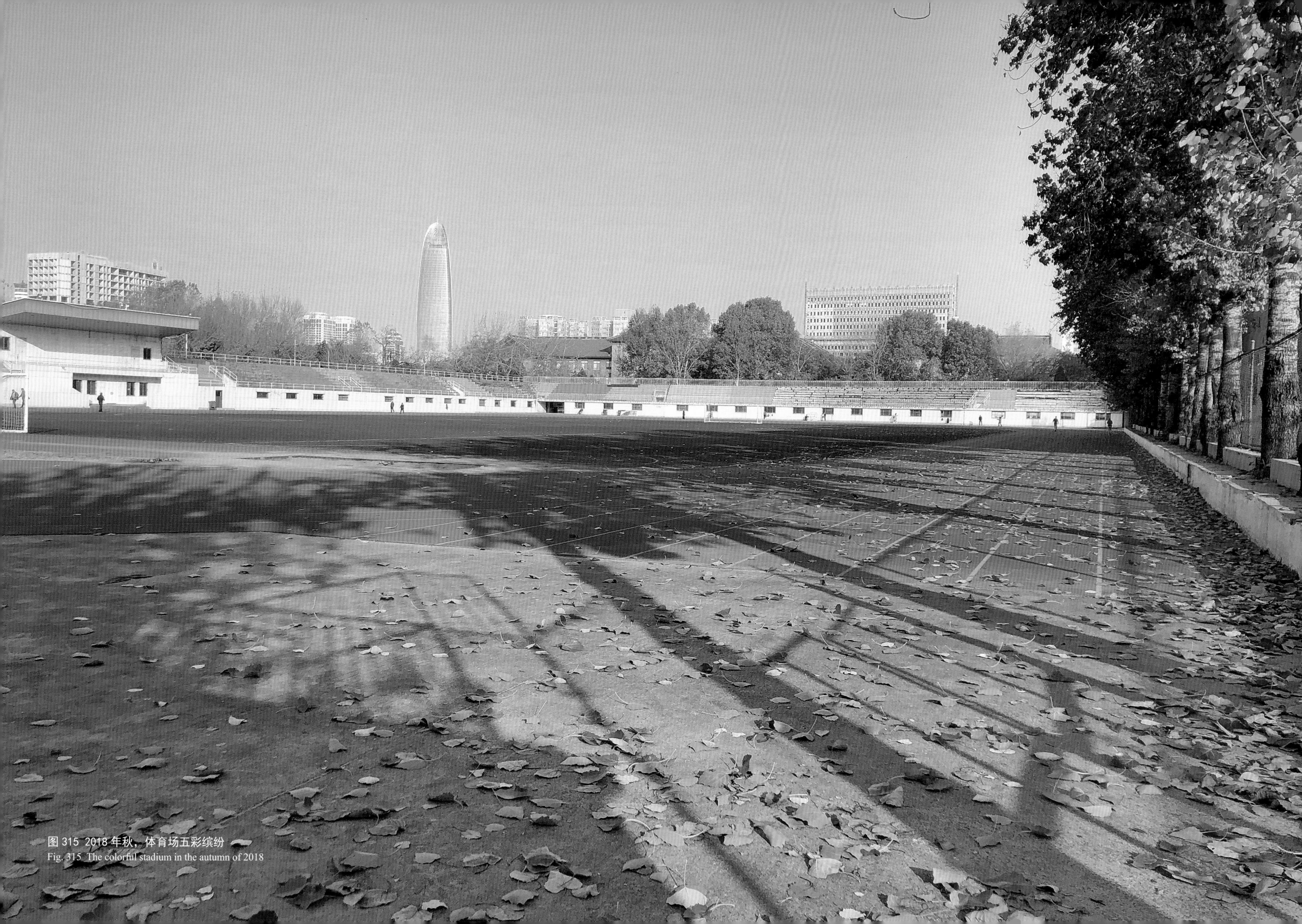

图 315 2018 年秋，体育场五彩缤纷
Fig. 315 The colorful stadium in the autumn of 2018

42 体育馆

Gymnasium

体育馆于 2001 年建成并投入使用，内部为木制地板铺装。此馆东面毗邻 3 号学生宿舍楼，西面是学校大体育场，南面有网球场，北面为校医院和老干部活动中心。体育课选羽毛球、乒乓球和健美操的同学会在这里上课。

The gymnasium was completed and put into use in 2001 and the interior is paved with wooden floors. The gymnasium is adjacent to the Third Student Dormitory Building in the east, the stadium is in the west, the tennis court is in the south, and the infirmary and the Activity Center for Veteran Cadres are in the north. Students who choose badminton, table tennis and aerobics in physical education will attend classes here.

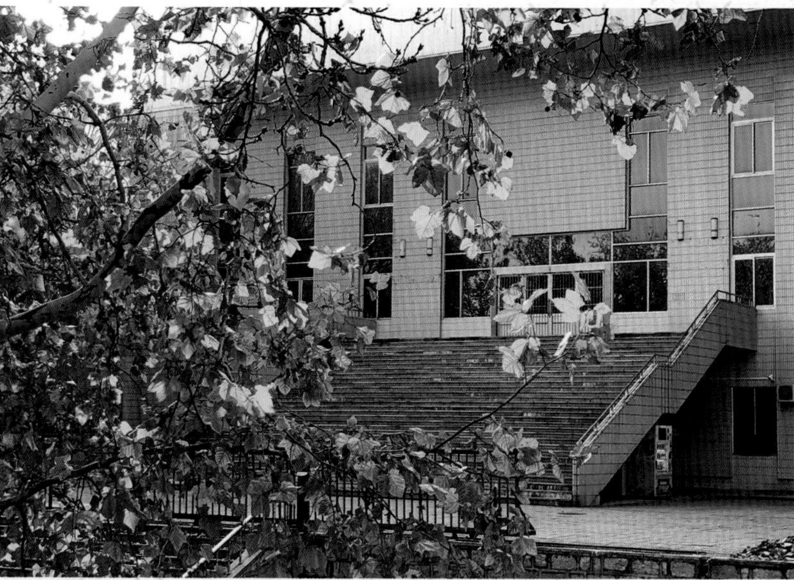

图 316 体育馆北（正）门

Fig. 316 The north (front) gate of the gymnasium

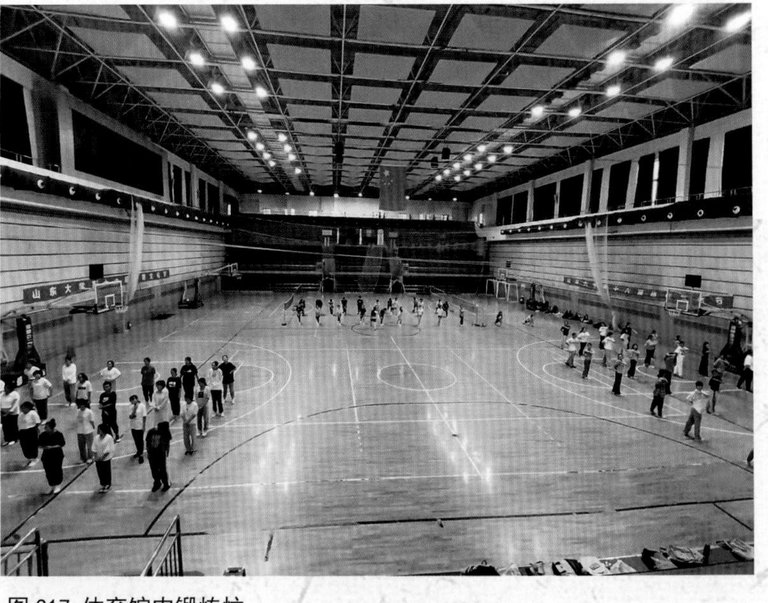

图 317 体育馆内锻炼忙

Fig. 317 People busy with exercises in the gymnasium

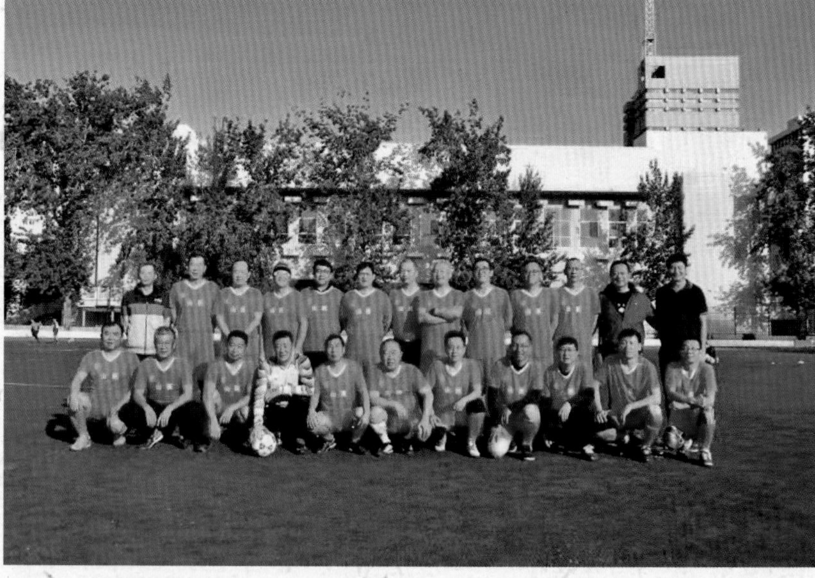

图 318 山东大学医学院足球队在体育馆外合影

Fig. 318 The football team of the School of Medicine of Shandong University taking a photo outside the gymnasium

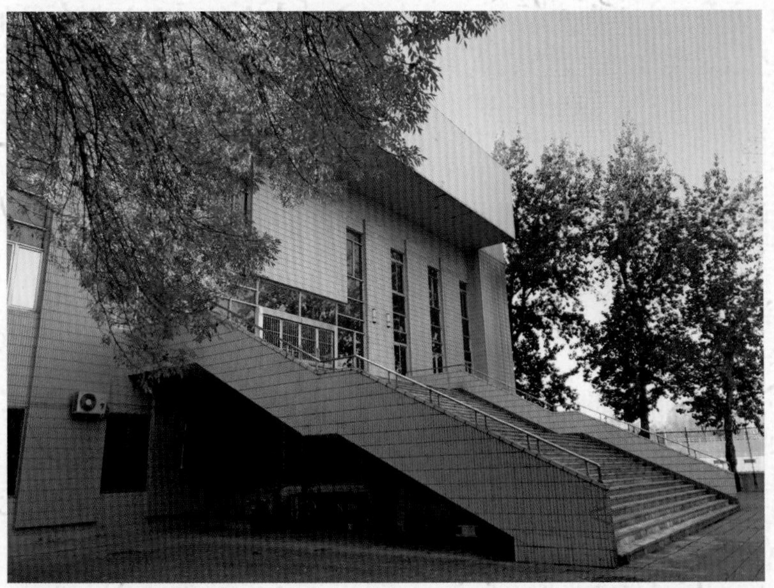

图 319 体育馆外秋色浓

Fig. 319 Deep autumn scenery outside the gymnasium

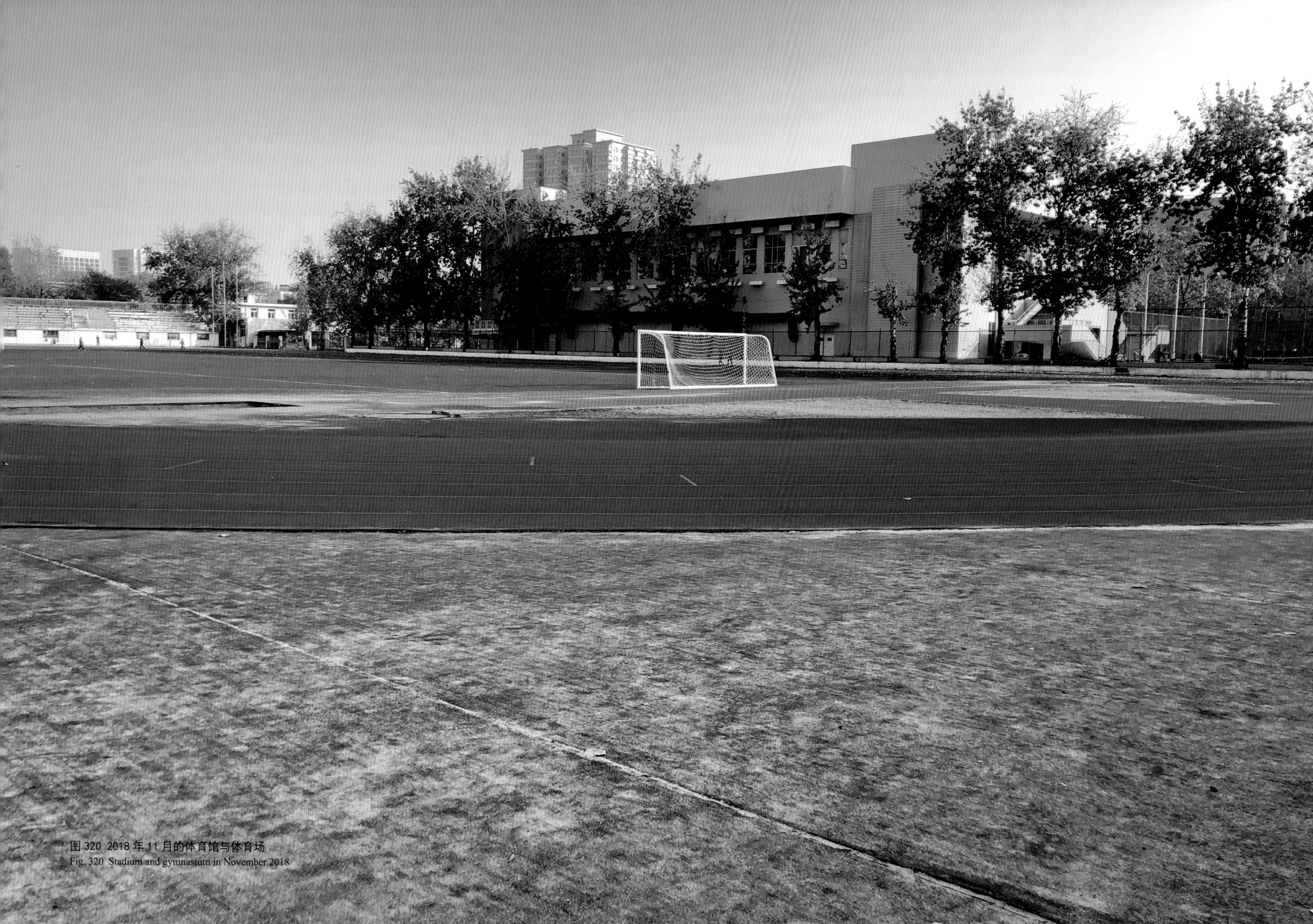

图 320 2018 年 11 月的体育馆与体育场
Fig. 320 Stadium and gymnasium in November 2018

43 食堂

Canteen

2000 年 7 月合校后，趵突泉校区的老食堂及大礼堂相继被拆除。在老食堂的位置新建了大学生活动中心（梦迪音乐厅），于原大礼堂的位置重建了食堂。现在的趵突泉校区食堂始建于 2009 年，2011 年百年院庆前夕投入使用。仿古风格，三层，南北走向。东面紧邻东村教工宿舍，设有拾阶而上的大门；西面开门于校园，正对号院中间的道路；南面是精神食堂，典雅别致的梦迪音乐厅与之并肩而立；北面设有大门与电梯，与护理和康复学院大楼隔路相望。春天是食堂周边环境最动人的时刻，成排的玉兰花迎风开放，相映于青砖红窗的墙面，显得格外醒目。

After the merging of universities in July 2000, the old canteen and auditorium of Baotuquan Campus were demolished one after another. A new Student Center (Mengdi Concert Hall) was built in the location of the old canteen, and the new canteen was built in the location of the original auditorium. The canteen of Baotuquan Campus was built in 2009 and put into use on the eve of the centennial celebration in 2011. It is of antique style, with three floors and on the south-north axis. The east is close to the faculty residence in the east village, with a gate up the steps; the west faces the road in the middle of the Courtyard; the south stands the spiritual canteen, the elegant and unique Mengdi Concert Hall; there are gate and elevator in the north, facing the Building of the School of Nursing and Rehabilitation across the road. Spring is the most moving moment in the surroundings of the canteen when rows of magnolia flowers bloom in the wind, particularly eye-catching against the wall with grey tiles and red windows .

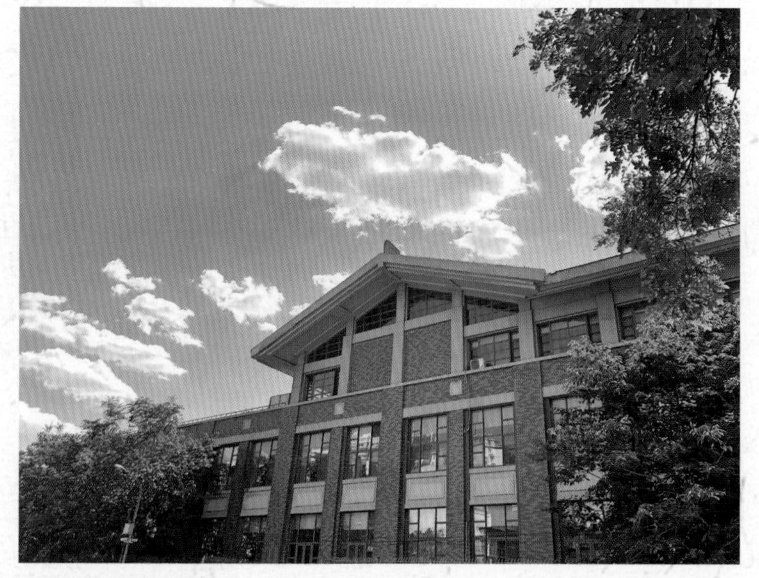

图 321 食堂东面观

Fig. 321 The east view of the canteen

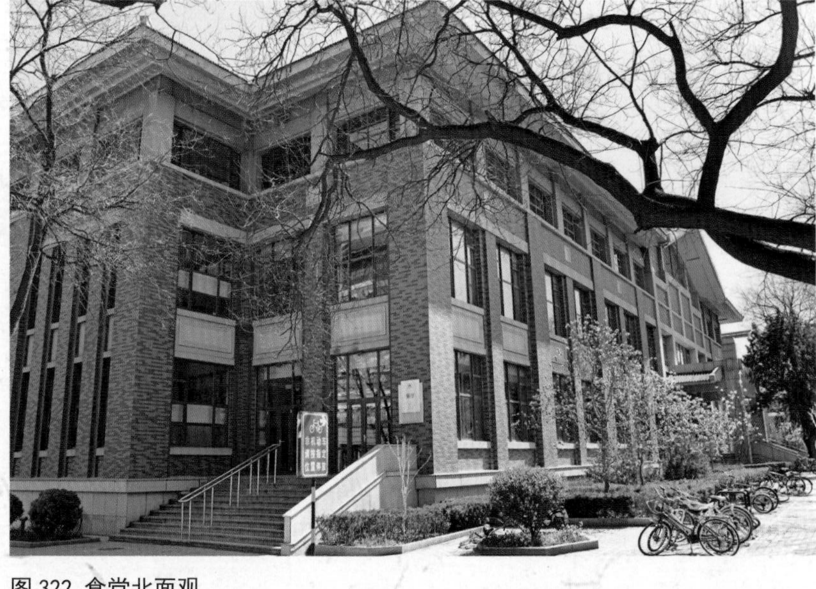

图 322 食堂北面观

Fig. 322 The north view of the canteen

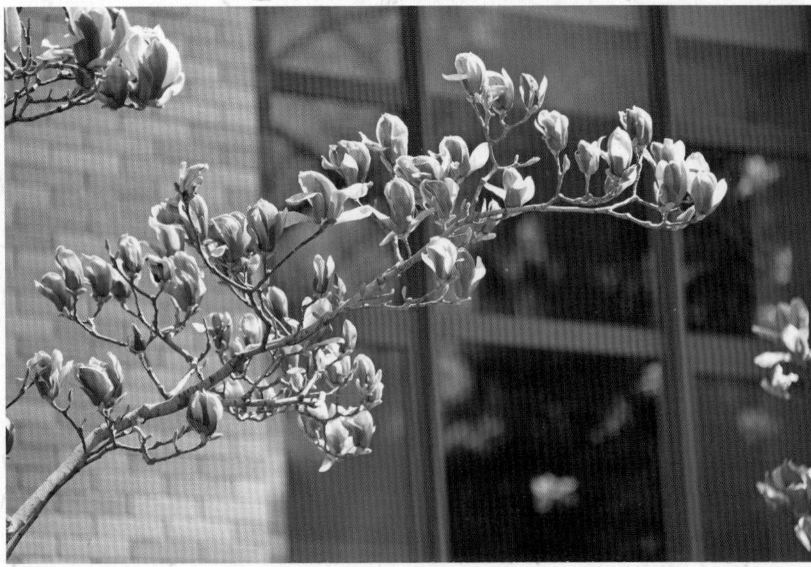

图 323 食堂窗映玉兰花

Fig. 323 Magnolia flowers against the windows of the canteen

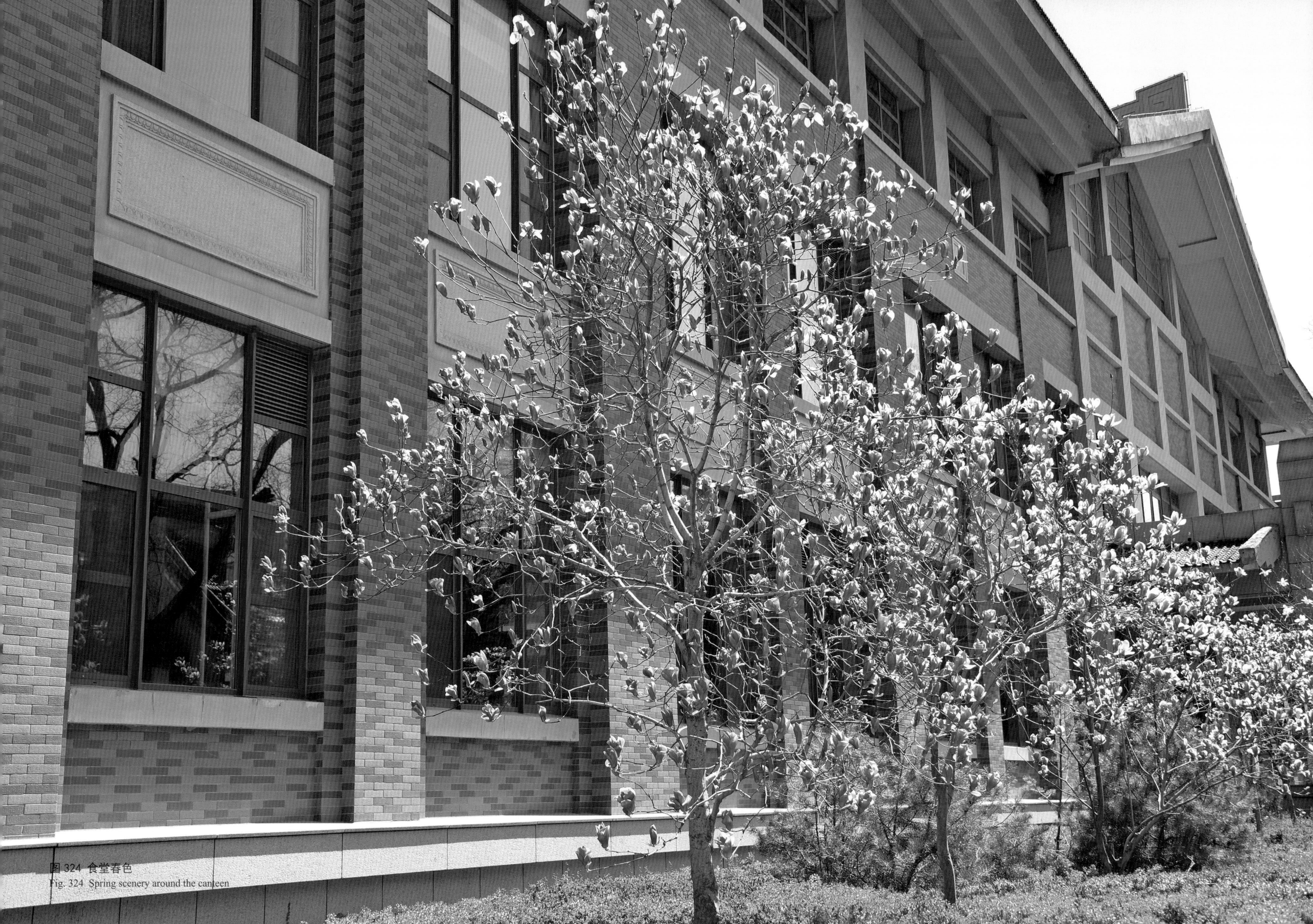

图 324 食堂春色
Fig. 324 Spring scenery around the canteen

44 水塔

Water Tower

齐鲁大学水塔建于 1917 年，砖混结构，现已无供水功能，仅供观赏。原来旁边配套的大屋顶式泵房现在早已荡然无存，只留下了这座古色古香的水塔。水塔高约 30 米，青砖砌筑。塔身呈正八角形，环绕以六条水平圈梁，稳重挺拔。塔顶覆以中国传统的八角攒尖顶，灰色筒瓦，翼角起翘，古朴中透着灵动。塔共五层，底层与二层之间环以腰檐，在一层至四层上，每一立面都留有一扇木格玻璃窗。一层墙体镶嵌有中国传统的花草图案，借以打破砖石塔身的沉重感。水塔融合了中西方建筑元素，有着重要的历史文化价值。令人感慨的是，虽然只是一座水塔，建造者却用心至极，将其整体设计构图及局部细节点缀均做得如此精良，彰显了“止于至善”的治学精神，值得后来者景仰。每当夕阳西下，如剪影般的古塔映照在橘红色的晚霞之中，给人以震撼的美感！

The Water Tower of Cheeloo University was built in 1917, of brick-concrete structure. Now it has no function of water supply and is only for viewing. The original supporting large roof-type pump house next to it has long disappeared, leaving only this antique water tower. The Water Tower is about 30 meters high and built with blue bricks. The tower body is regularly octagonal, encircled by six horizontal ring beams, stable and straight. The top of the tower is covered with traditional Chinese octagonal pyramidal roof, with grey pantiles and upturned roof-ridge, presenting a spirituality in the simplicity. The tower has five floors, with waist eaves between the bottom and second floors, and a glass window of wooden lattice on each facade from the first to fourth floors. The wall of the first floor is inlaid with traditional Chinese floral patterns to break the heavy feeling of the brick and stone tower. With the fusion of Chinese and Western architectural elements, the Water Tower has important historical and cultural values. Although it is only a water tower, the builders have made great efforts to make its overall design and local details so sophisticated, demonstrating the spirit of “aiming at absolute perfection” in learning, which deserves the admiration of the latecomers. The silhouette-like ancient tower against the afterglow at sunset gives people a shocking aesthetic feeling.

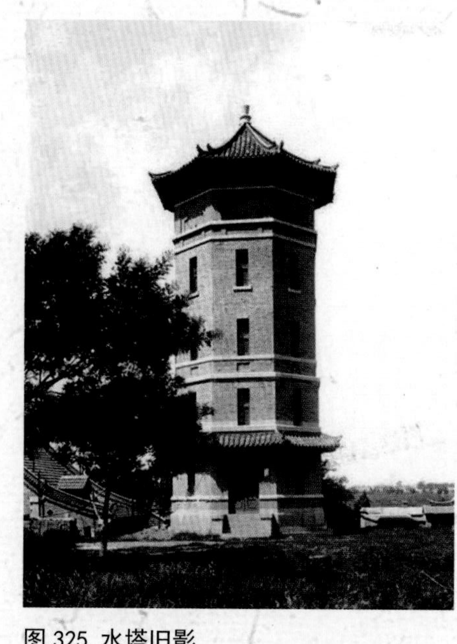

图 325 水塔旧影

Fig. 325 An old photo of the Water Tower

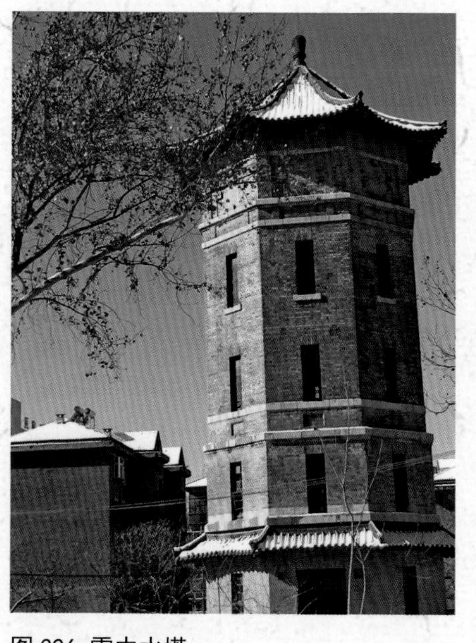

图 326 雪中水塔

Fig. 326 Water Tower in the snow

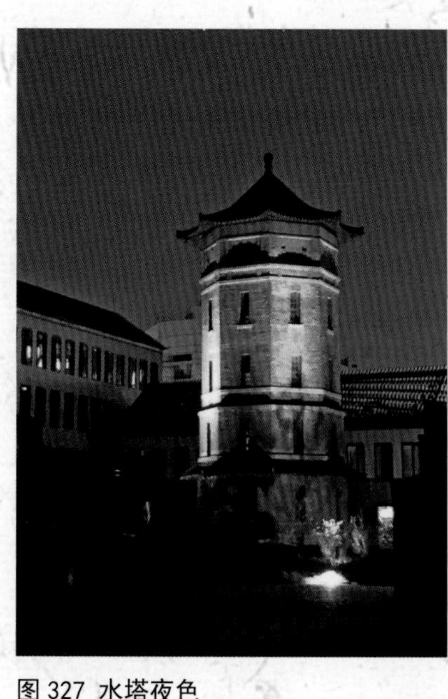

图 327 水塔夜色

Fig. 327 Water Tower at night

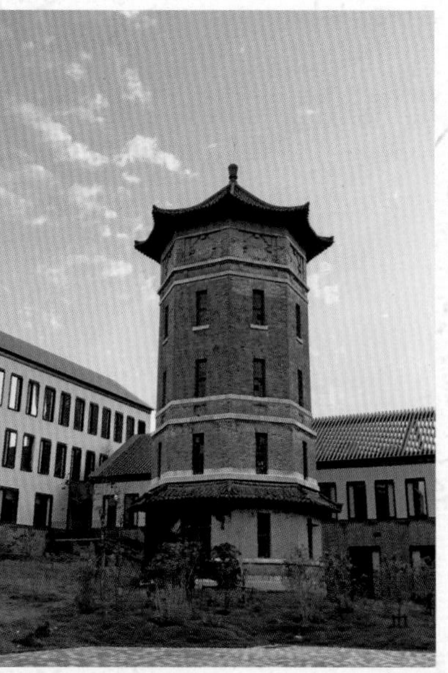

图 328 水塔夕照

Fig. 328 Water Tower at sunset

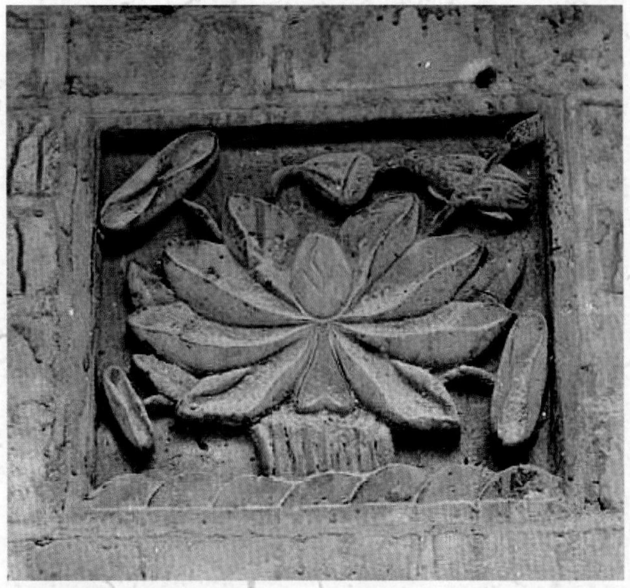

图 329 水塔一层的砖雕

Fig. 329 Tile carvings on the first floor of the Water Tower

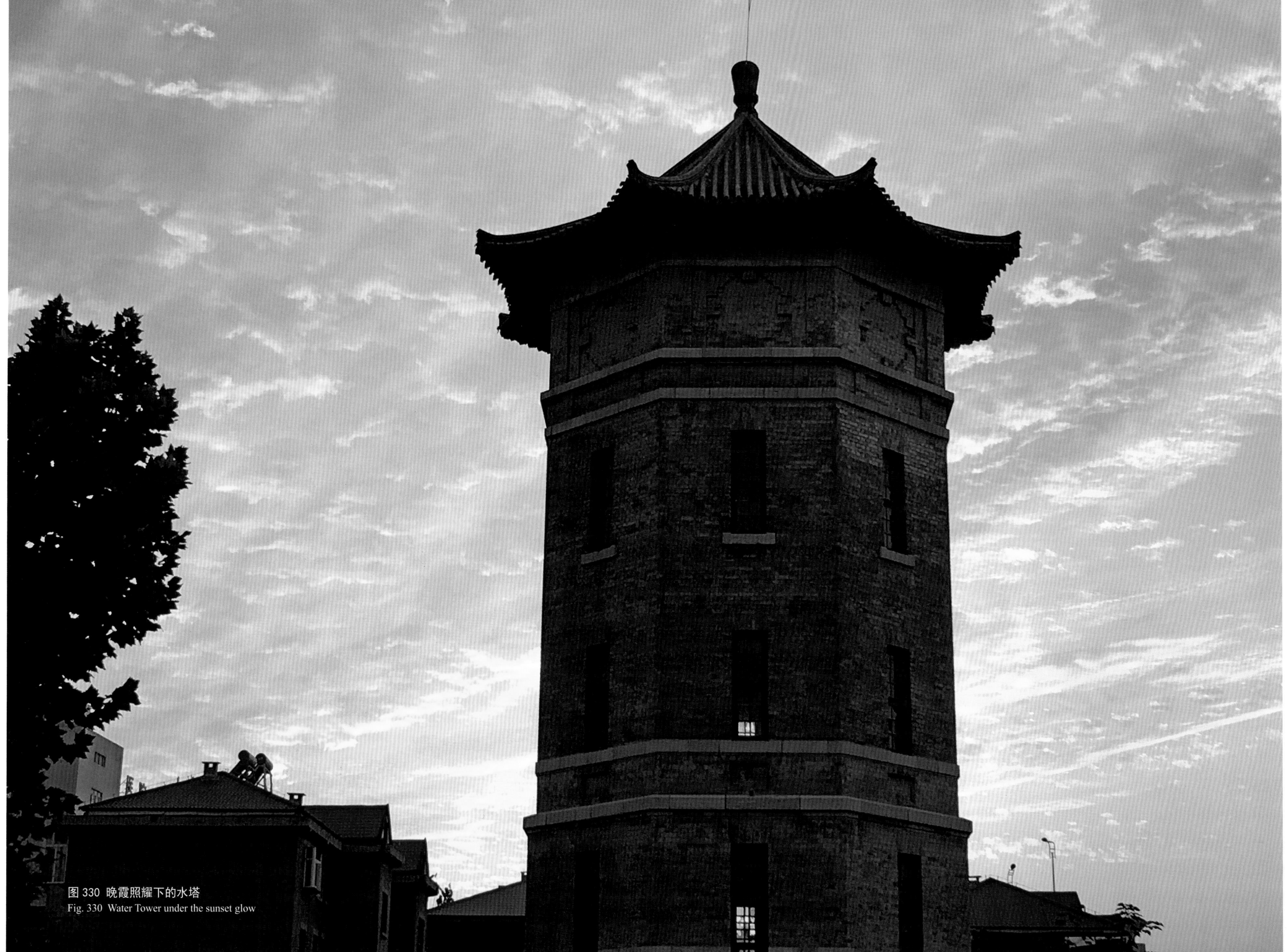

图 330 晚霞照耀下的水塔
Fig. 330 Water Tower under the sunset glow

45 圣保罗楼群（1）

St. Paul's Complex (1)

圣保罗楼群建于 1917 年，包括圣保罗楼（三座两层连体别墅）和一座小教堂，由英国圣公会所建立。圣保罗是《圣经》中的重要人物，为第一个去外邦传播福音的基督徒，对于早期基督教会的发展贡献很大，因此世界各地有很多圣保罗教堂。这里曾经是神职人员居所，也曾做过齐鲁大学招待所和女生宿舍。1952 年改名为建设楼，现为教工宿舍。

圣保罗楼与小教堂通过一处券廊相连，围成一个“L”形的开放庭院，院内栽有樱花、西府海棠等树木。小教堂设计简洁，北立面为典型的西方建筑风格。圣保罗楼上下两层共计 42 个房间，立面呈 “山”字形，节奏感强烈。屋顶与墙面呈灰色，古朴内敛。该楼的最大特点是砖雕众多，体现了经典的中华文化传统和浓郁的山东乡土气息，是齐鲁大学遗存中最华丽的建筑之一。圣保罗楼群位于校友门内西侧，是进入校园后第一个被看到的建筑，堪称齐鲁医学院的门面。

Built in 1917 by the Anglican Church, the St. Paul's Complex consists of the St. Paul's Building (three two-storey one-piece villas) and a chapel. St. Paul is an important figure in the *Bible*. He was the first Christian to spread the gospel in a foreign country and contributed greatly to the development of the early Christian church. Therefore, there are many St. Paul's churches around the world. The St. Paul's Complex used to be a residence for the clergies, and it also served as a hostel and a dormitory for girl students at Cheeloo University. In 1952, it was renamed the Construction Building and is now a faculty residence.

The St. Paul's Building and the chapel are connected by an arch corridor, forming an L-shaped open courtyard in which there are cherries, midget crabapples and other trees. The chapel is simple in design and its north facade is of a typical Western architectural style. The St. Paul's Building has a total of 42 rooms on the upper and lower floors, and the facade shows a shape of the Chinese character "shan", presenting a strong sense of rhythm. The roof and wall are grey, simple and restrained. The building is characterized by numerous tile carvings, which reflects the classical Chinese cultural tradition and rich local flavor of Shandong Province. It is one of the most gorgeous buildings in the remains of Cheeloo University. Located on the west side of the Alumni Gate, the St. Paul's Complex is the first structure you will see after entering the campus and it can be called the appearance of Cheeloo College of Medicine.

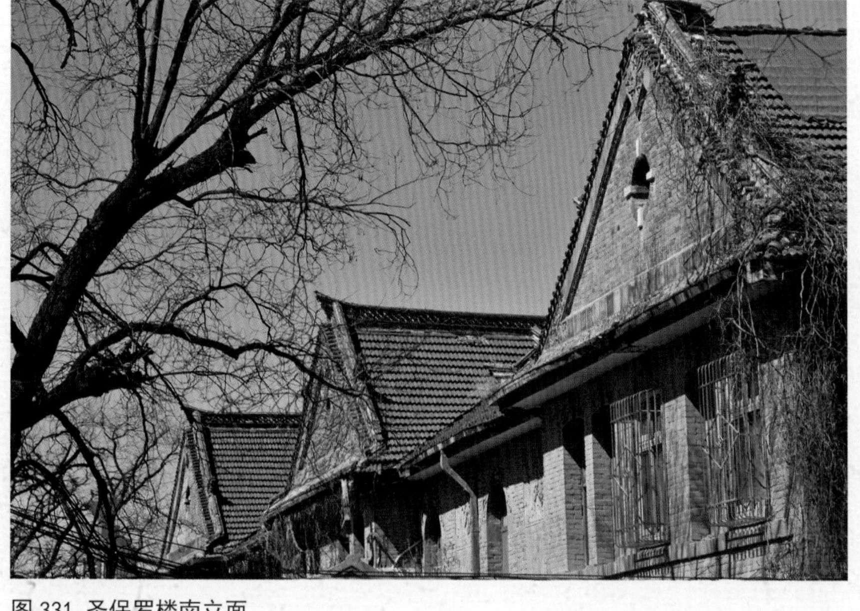

图 331 圣保罗楼南立面
Fig. 331 The south facade of the St. Paul's Building

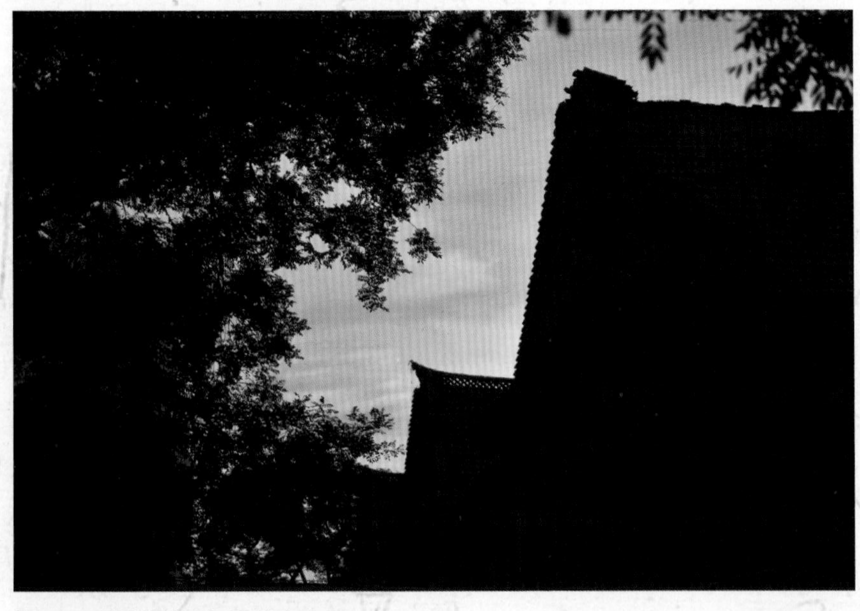

图 332 晚霞中的圣保罗楼南立面
Fig. 332 The south facade of the St. Paul's Building against the afterglow

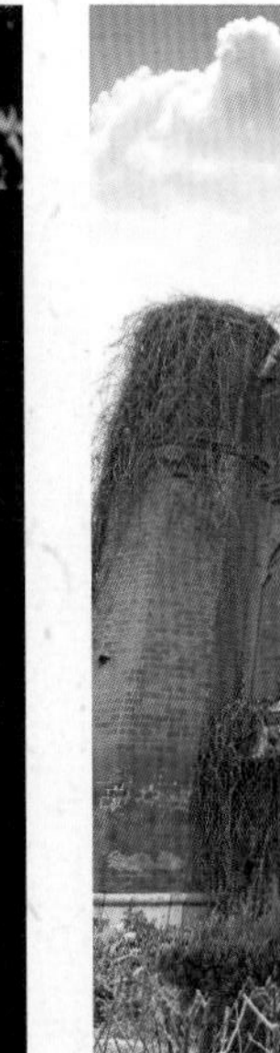

图 333 圣保罗楼北立面
Fig. 333 The north facade of the St. Paul's Building

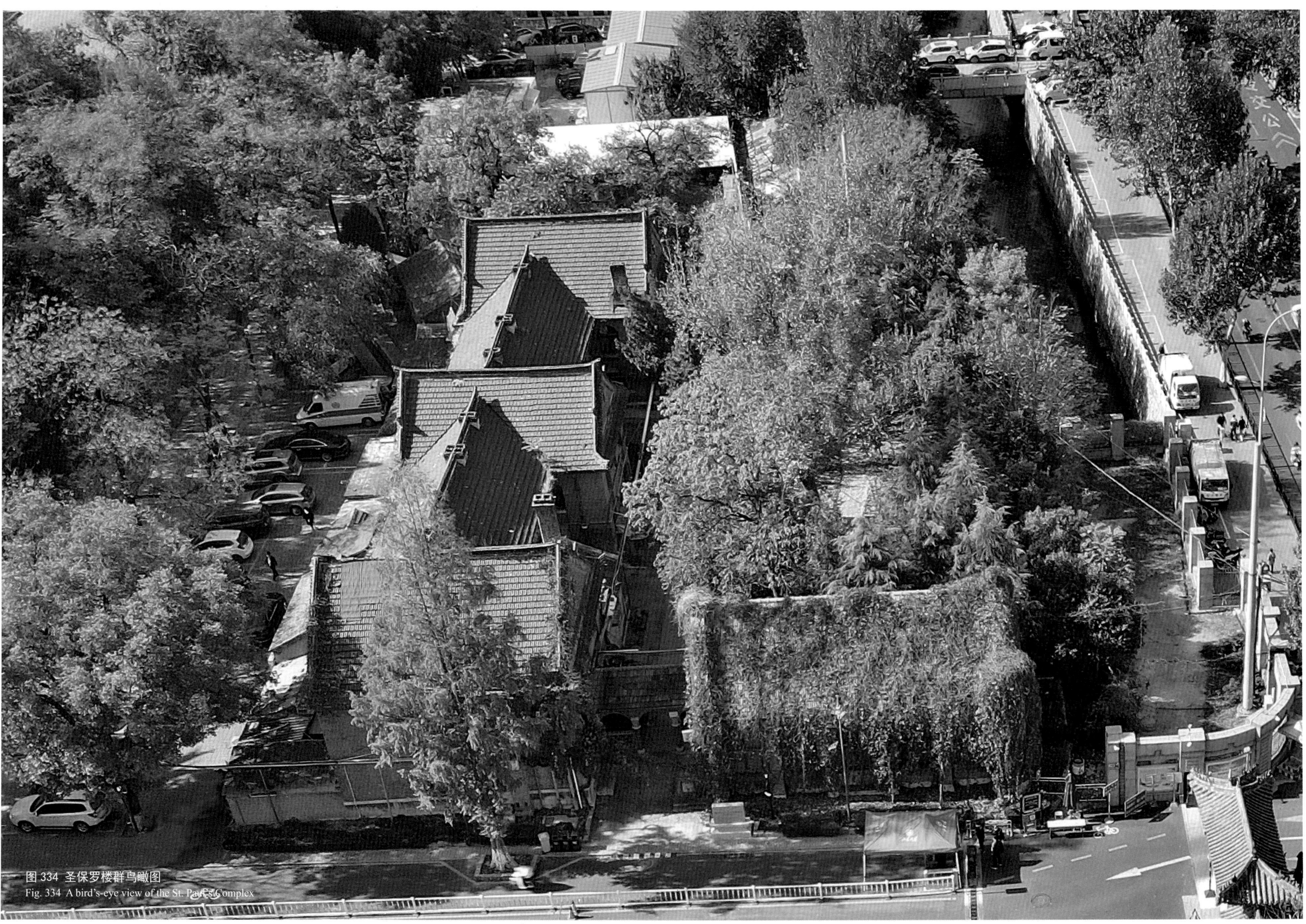

图 334 圣保罗楼群鸟瞰图
Fig. 334 A bird's-eye view of the St. Paul's Complex

45 圣保罗楼群（2）

St. Paul's Complex (2)

圣保罗小教堂有以下三点不得不提。第一，北立面模仿了罗曼式教堂的正立面，西式韵味明显。但在手法上十分简略，用红砖侧排并弯曲砌筑成拱形，模仿教堂的“拱券”，用砖直线侧砌模仿西式建筑常用的“柱子”，甚至在“拱券”与“柱子”之间用砖的叠涩模拟了“柱头”。第二，南立面屋脊留存有一个六边形的叠涩，状似蜂巢。其实该处原本筑有一个小塔楼，而现在的叠涩应该是其基座。第三，小教堂楼体密密麻麻布满了“爬山虎”，而使其颜色四季分明。无怪乎曾两度在齐鲁大学任教的老舍先生在他那篇著名的散文《非正式的公园》中写道：“当夏天，进了校门便看见一座绿楼，楼前一大片绿草地，楼的四围全是绿树，绿树的尖上浮着一两个山峰……绿楼？真的，‘爬山虎’的深绿肥大的叶一层一层地把楼盖满，只露着几个白边的窗户；每阵小风，使那层层的绿叶掀动，横着竖着都动得有规律，一片竖立的绿浪。”

The following three points have to be mentioned about the St. Paul's Chapel. First, the north facade imitates the front facade of the Roman church, with obvious Western flavor but simple in the technique. Red bricks are laid on edge and bent to build an arch like that of the church. Bricks are laid on edge in linear way to build the columns of the western architecture. Even the brackets of bricks are built to imitate the capitals between the arch and the columns. Second, there is a hexagonal bracket on the south facade of the ridge like a honeycomb. In fact, there was originally a small tower built there and the bracket should be its base. Third, the building of the chapel is densely covered with creepers, showing the four distinct seasons. No wonder Mr. Lao She who taught at Cheeloo University twice wrote in his famous essay "An Informal Park": "When you enter the university in summer, you will see a green building, with a large green grass ahead. The building is surrounded by green trees, on the tip of which floating a peak or two... Green building? Really. The dark green fat leaves of the creepers cover the building layer by layer, leaving only a few white-edged windows exposed. The gust of breeze lifts the layers of green leaves, moving regularly horizontally and vertically and presenting a vertical green wave."

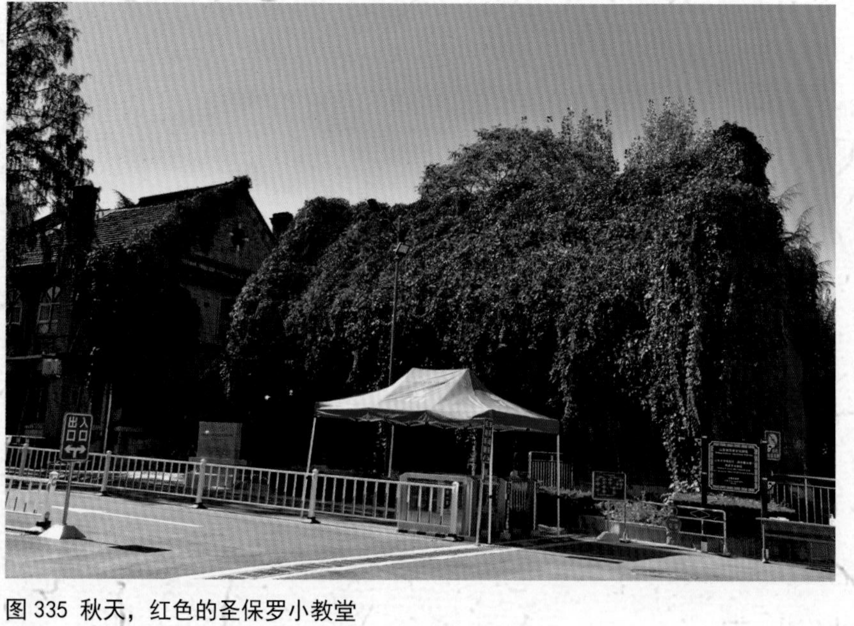

图 335 秋天，红色的圣保罗小教堂
Fig. 335 Red St. Paul's Chapel in autumn

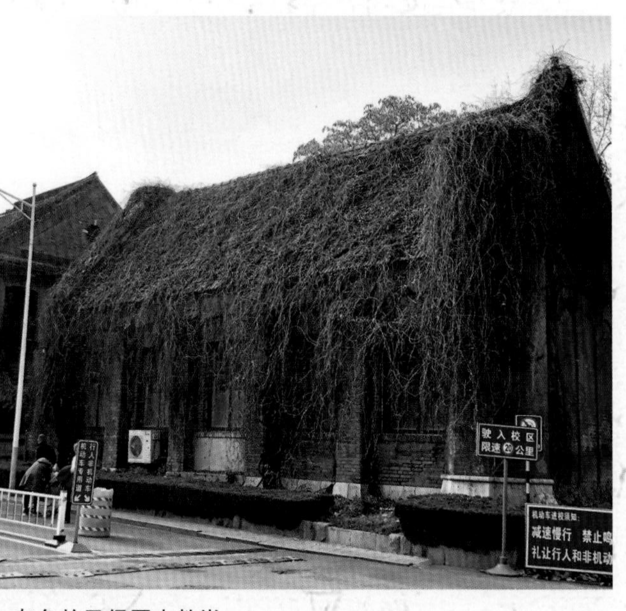

图 336 冬天，灰色的圣保罗小教堂
Fig. 336 Grey St. Paul's Chapel in winter

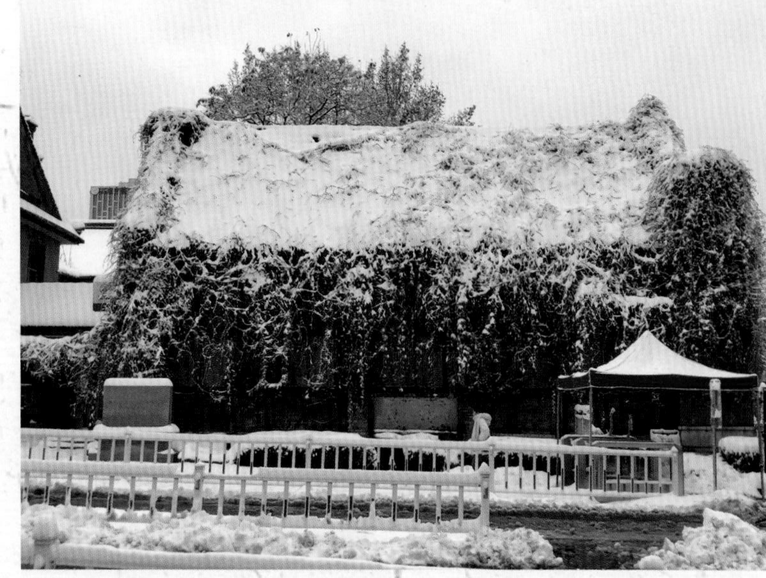

图 337 春雪覆盖的白色圣保罗小教堂
Fig. 337 White St. Paul's Chapel covered with spring snow

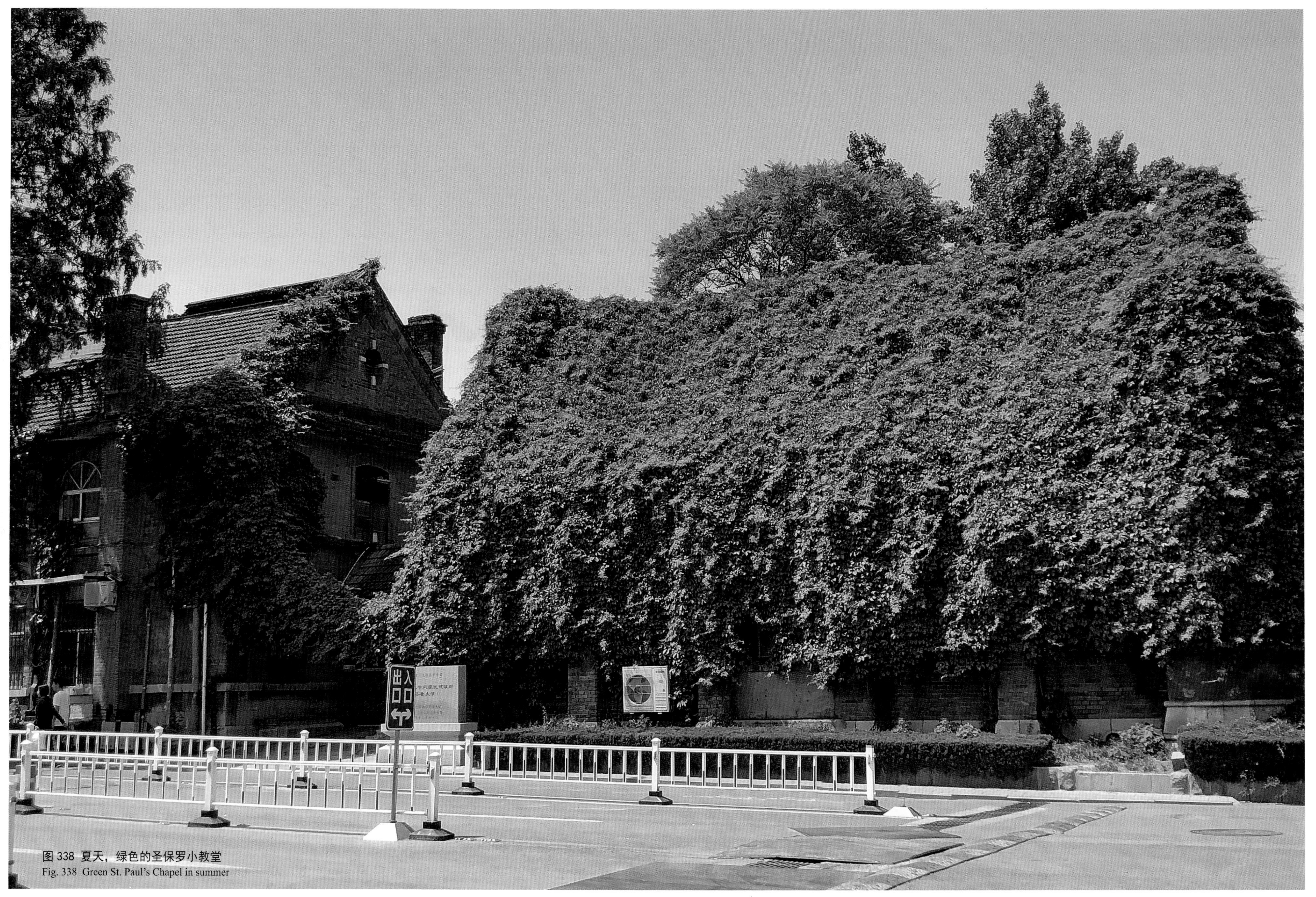

图 338 夏天，绿色的圣保罗小教堂
Fig. 338 Green St. Paul's Chapel in summer

45 圣保罗楼群（3）

St. Paul's Complex (3)

圣保罗楼的南立面构图方式极具中西合璧特色，中央与两端均有垂直交叉的部分，东西方向上分为五段，为典型西式做法。与西式古典主义相似，圣保罗楼南立面上下构图也是“三段式”组合，即屋顶、屋身、台基，但在比例上圣保罗楼的屋顶与屋身的比例增加，适当地向传统中式建筑的构图尺度倾斜。

圣保罗楼的最大特点是外墙装饰极为精致，在窗楣、窗槛、门楣、山花等位置分布有大小与形态各异的 70 多个砖雕。与考文楼与柏根楼的砖雕较为简洁、几何化不同，圣保罗楼的砖雕尺寸要略大一些，其雕刻手法借鉴了中式传统民居的浮雕方式，内容均为构图完整的、传统民居中常见的梅花、葡萄、牡丹、荷花、灵芝、雄鸡、喜鹊、蝙蝠、狮子等花草鸟兽图案。还使用谐音以及花鸟的象征意义来表达吉祥富贵的寓意，如：在建筑北立面山花一侧有喜鹊站立在梅树上的雕刻，寓意喜（喜鹊）上眉（梅树）梢。

The design of the south facade of the St. Paul's Building is of Chinese and Western features. There are vertical intersections between the center and both ends. It is divided into five sections from east to west, which is a typical Western style. Similar to the Western classicism, the design of the south facade of the St. Paul's Building is also a "three-section" combination, namely the roof, the body and the foundation. However, the roof and body of the St. Paul's Building increase in proportion, appropriately inclined to the design of traditional Chinese architecture.

The most important feature of the St. Paul's Building is that the decoration of the exterior wall is extremely exquisite. There are more than 70 tile carvings of different sizes and shapes distributed in the window lintel, window sill, door lintel, pediments and other positions. Different from the simple geometric tile carvings of Calvin Mateer Hall and Bergen Hall, the tile carvings of the St. Paul's Building are slightly larger in size. As to the carving techniques, the reliefs of traditional Chinese dwellings are used for reference. The patterns are the species of flora and fauna such as the plum blossom, grape, peony, lotus, Ganodorma lucidum, rooster, magpie, bat, lion and so on that are common in traditional dwellings with complete composition. The homophonic sounds and symbolic meanings of flowers and birds are also used to express the meaning of good luck and wealth. The following is an example: On the side of the pediment on the forth facade of the building, there is a carving of the magpie standing on the plum tree, implying that "happiness (magpie) appears on the eyebrows (plum tree)".

图 339 屋山左下角上的砖雕
Fig. 339 Tile carvings on the lower left corner of the gable

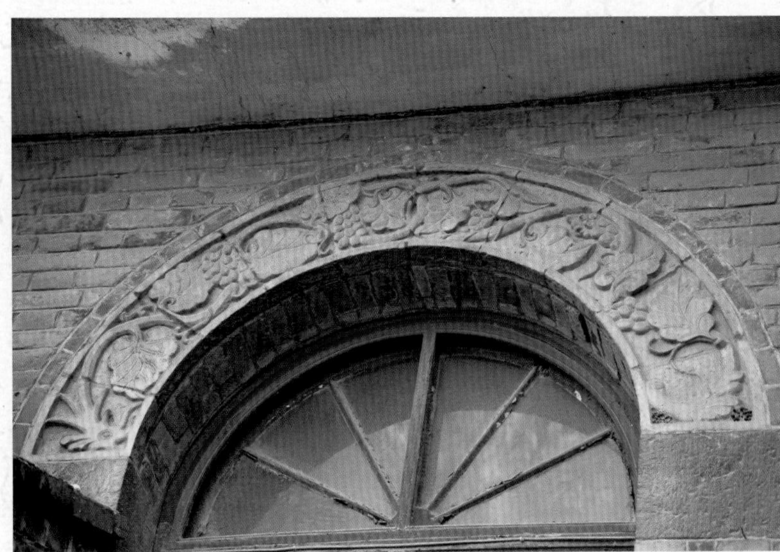

图 340 窗楣上的砖雕
Fig. 340 Tile carvings on the lintel

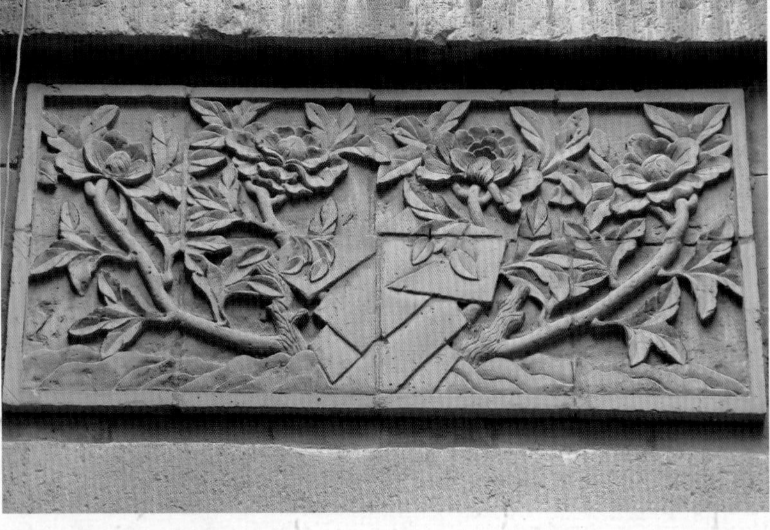

图 341 窗下方的砖雕
Fig. 341 Tile carvings under the window

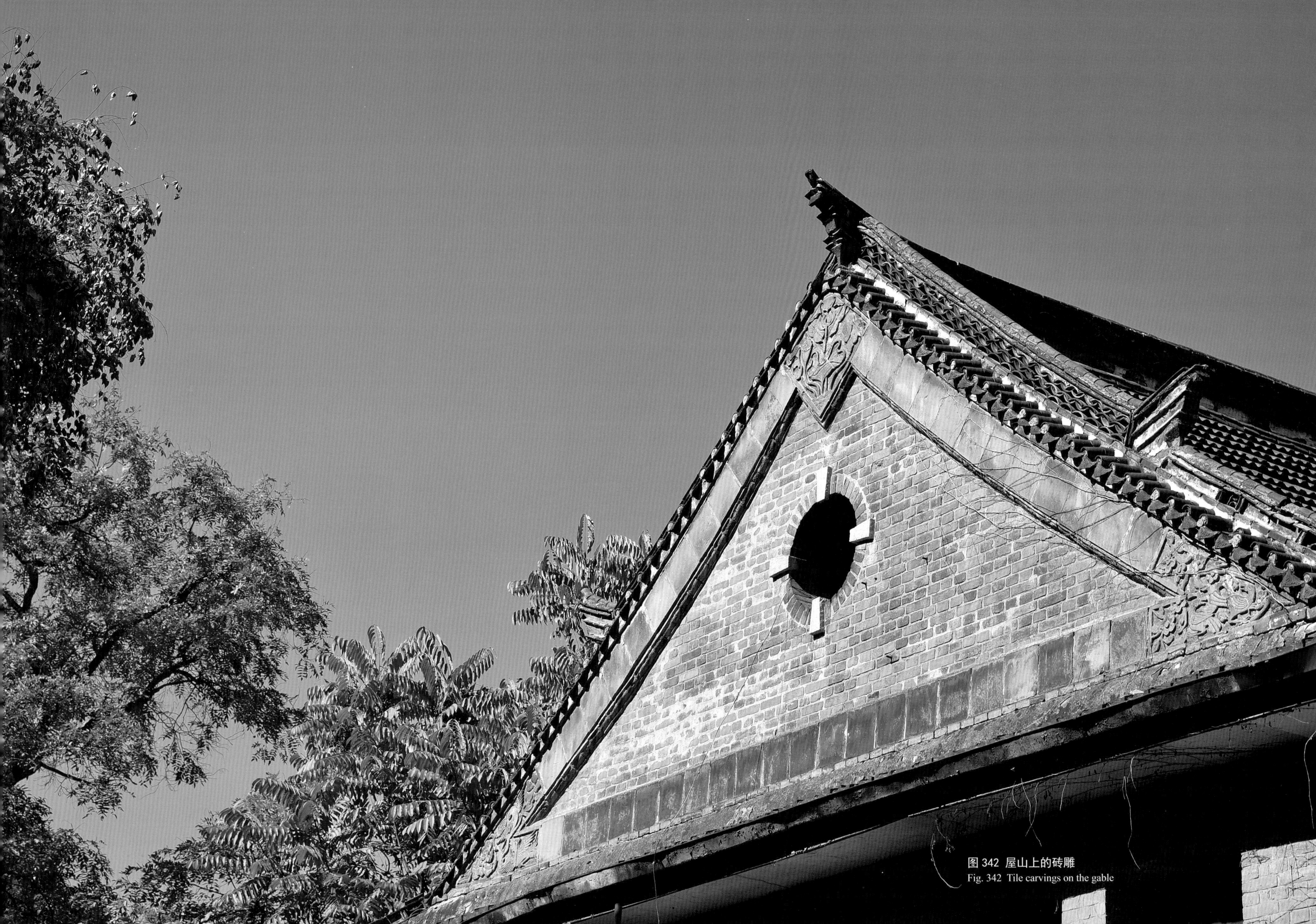

图 342 屋山上的砖雕
Fig. 342 Tile carvings on the gable

45 圣保罗楼群（4）

St. Paul's Complex (4)

圣保罗楼与小教堂通过一处券廊相连。券廊三开间，半圆拱形，有八根用青砖构成的圆形廊柱支撑，柱脚座落在白色圆柱石上。圆柱石四周刻有精致的浮雕图案，为暗八仙纹与鸟纹，极具中国传统文化特色。其中，暗八仙纹是由传统八仙纹延伸而来的宗教纹样，这种纹样以道教神话中的八仙过海为题材，以八仙所持的法器来暗喻仙人，借八仙帮助世人的故事来表达人们对美好生活的向往与追求。在券廊白色圆柱石上可以清晰地辨认出暗八仙纹中的宝剑、葫芦、阴阳板、团扇、花篮、渔鼓、横笛与荷花，还有代表吉祥如意的仙鹤、葡萄等纹样。与此同时，为了丰富暗八仙纹的表现性，石雕图案中还增添了飘带、云纹、海波纹、花卉等纹样，让八仙纹样构图更加饱满。

The St. Paul's Building is connected to the chapel by an arch corridor. The arch corridor has three bays with semi-circular arch, supported by eight round columns made of blue bricks, with the column feet located on white cylindrical stones. The cylindrical stones are engraved with exquisite reliefs around it such as the patterns of the emblems of the Eight Immortals and birds with the characteristics of traditional Chinese culture. Among them, the patterns of the emblems of the Eight Immortals are religious patterns extended from the traditional patterns of the Eight Immortals. The Taoist mythology of "The Eight Immortals Crossing the Sea" is taken as the theme of such patterns and the emblems held by the Eight Immortals are used to represent the immortals to express people's yearning for and pursuit of a better life through the stories of the Eight Immortals helping people. The patterns of the emblems of the Eight Immortals, that is, the sword, gourd, jade plate, palm-leaf fan, basket of flowers, percussion instrument, flute and lotus, can be clearly identified on the white cylindrical stones of the arch corridor; and there are also patterns of the cranes and grapes representing good luck and happiness. In the meanwhile, in order to enrich the expression of the patterns of the emblems of the Eight Immortals, patterns of ribbon, clouding, ripple, flowers, plants and so on have been added to the stone carvings.

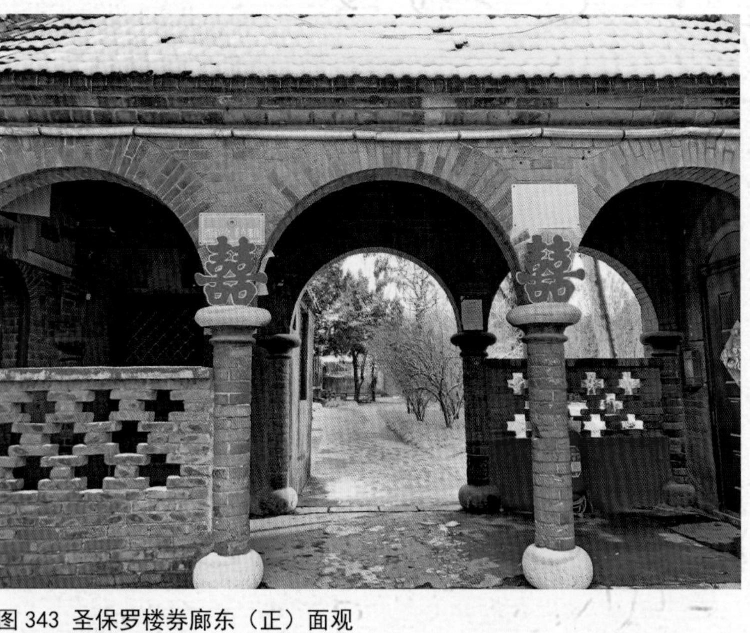

图 343 圣保罗楼券廊东（正）面观

Fig. 343 The east (front) view of the arch corridor of the St. Paul's Building

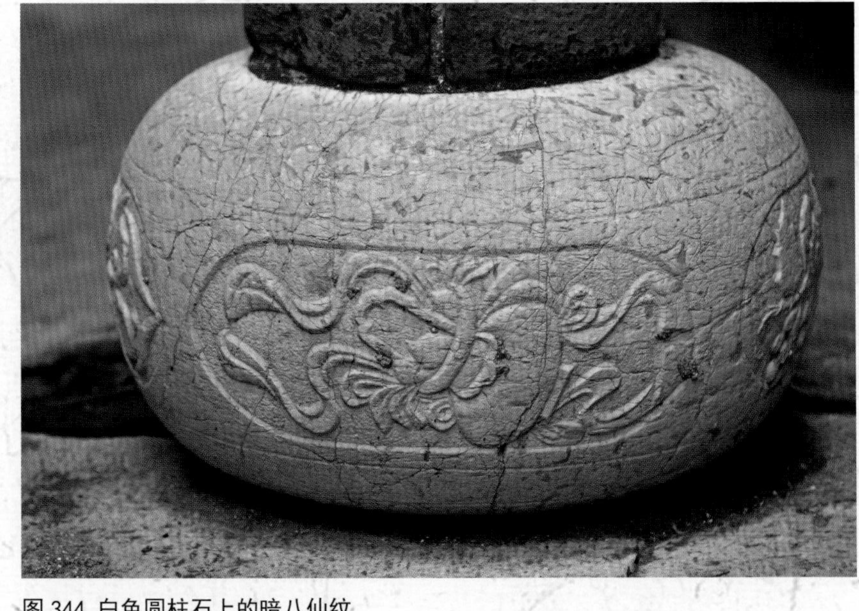

图 344 白色圆柱石上的暗八仙纹

Fig. 344 Patterns of the emblems of the Eight Immortals on the white cylindrical stone

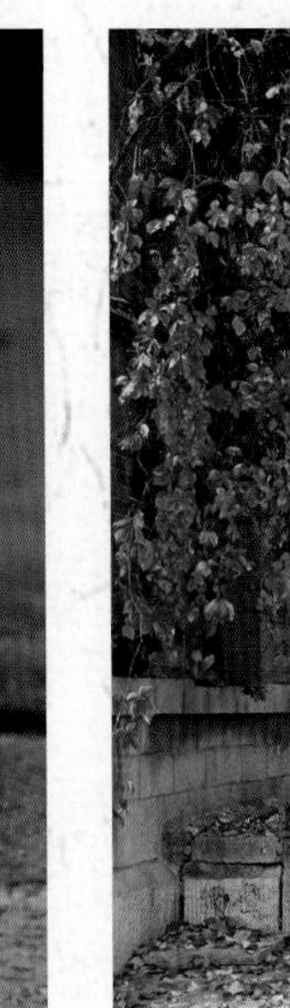

图 345 圣保罗楼券廊的中间门洞

Fig. 345 The middle doorway of the arch corridor of the St. Paul's Building

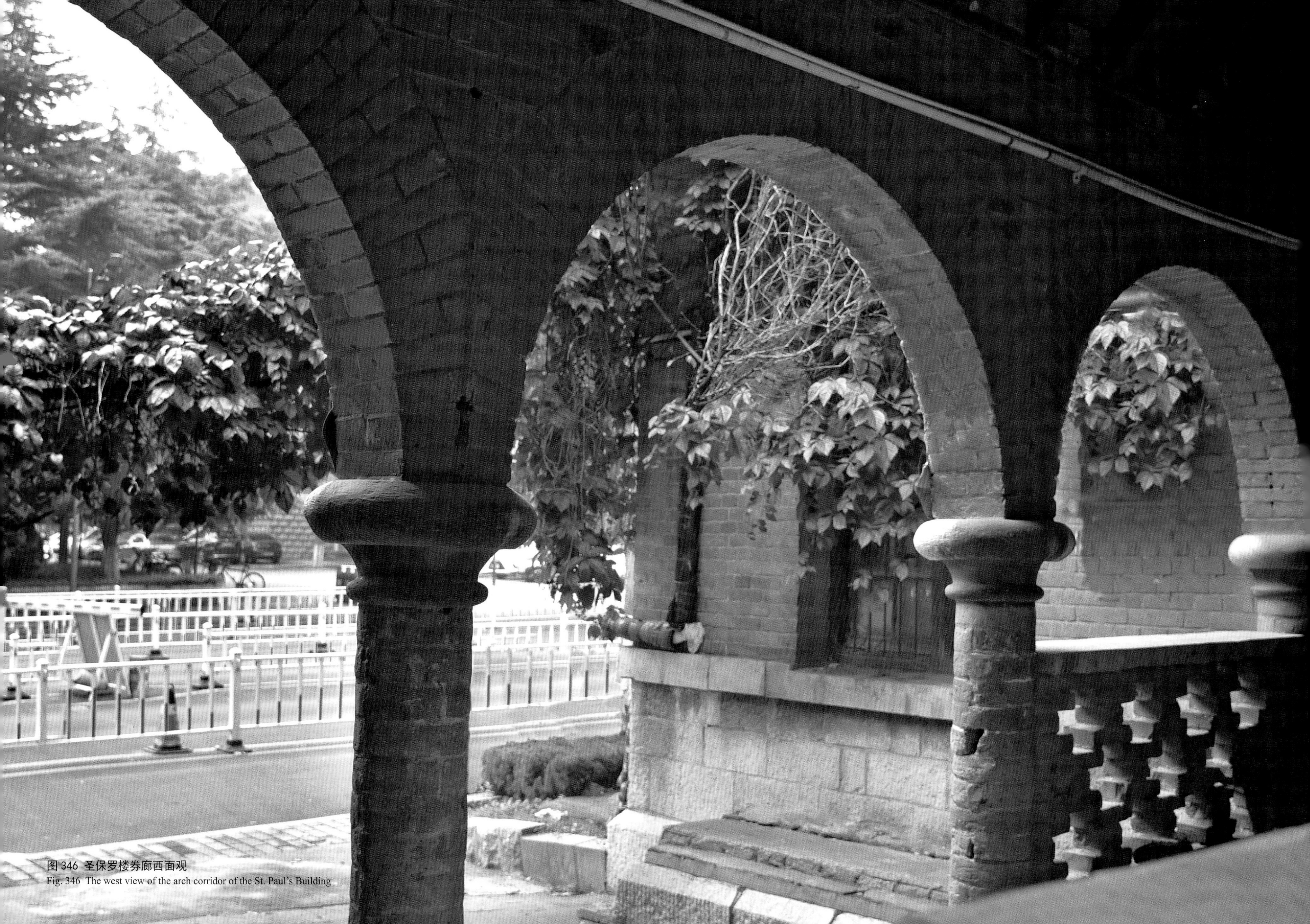

图 346 圣保罗楼券廊西面观
Fig. 346 The west view of the arch corridor of the St. Paul's Building

46 四百号院（1）

No. 400 Courtyard (1)

四百号院，简称号院，1916年建成，是齐鲁大学建校初期的重要建筑，为男生宿舍，由两列八栋二层的砖木宿舍楼组成，围成六个院落。东西各设一个宿舍院的总入口，入口处有一个中国传统木结构建筑屋顶和西洋式圆券洞门组合而成的门楼。号院每幢楼有学生宿舍 30 间，学生一人一室，每室 7~8 平方米，室内有壁柜、书橱、桌、椅、床铺等设施，冬天还有暖气，居住条件十分优越。号院建筑中西合璧，古朴浑厚，典雅大气。建筑的门窗组合，用毛石砌筑的墙角隅石处理，山墙尖上有圆、方、椭圆等各式通风孔，都是西洋古典建筑的手法。

No. 400 Courtyard, or Courtyard for short, was completed in 1916 and it is an important building in the early days of Cheeloo University. Being used for boys' dormitory, it consists of two rows of eight two-storey brick and wood dormitory buildings, enclosing six yards. The east and west are respectively provided with a main entrance of the dormitory buildings, and there is an arch with a traditional Chinese roof of wood structure and a Western-style circular gate in the entrance. Each building of the courtyard has 30 dormitories, with one room for one student. The area of the room is 7-8 square meters and each room is equipped with wall cabinets, bookcases, tables, chairs, beds and other facilities. In winter, there is heating, and the living conditions are very superior. The courtyard is of both Chinese and Western architectural style, simple but elegant. The combination of doors and windows, the cornerstones built with the rubble, and the round, square and oval ventilation holes on the gable tip all present Western classical architectural techniques.

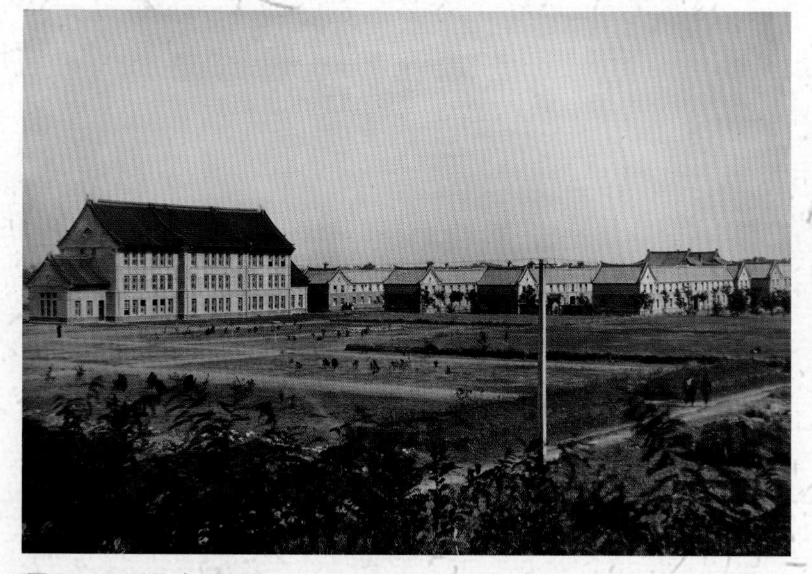

图 347 四百号院西面观
Fig. 347 The west view of No. 400 Courtyard

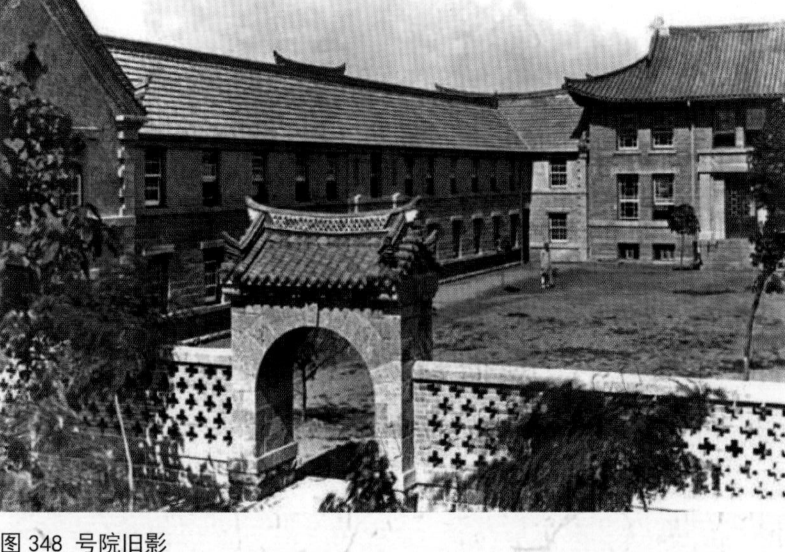

图 348 号院旧影
Fig. 348 An old photo of the Courtyard

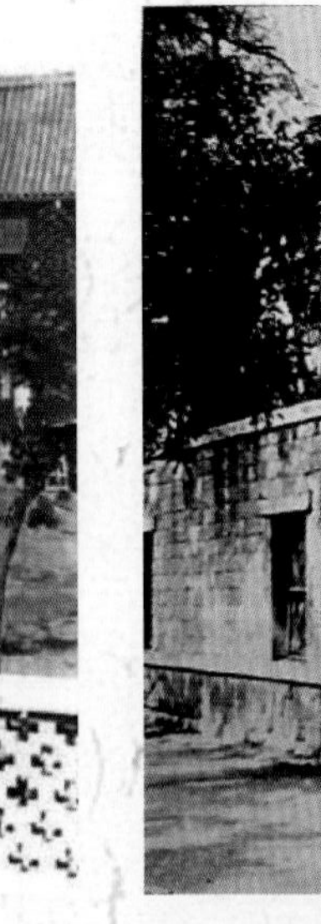

图 349 号院的老门楼
Fig. 349 Old arch of the Courtyard

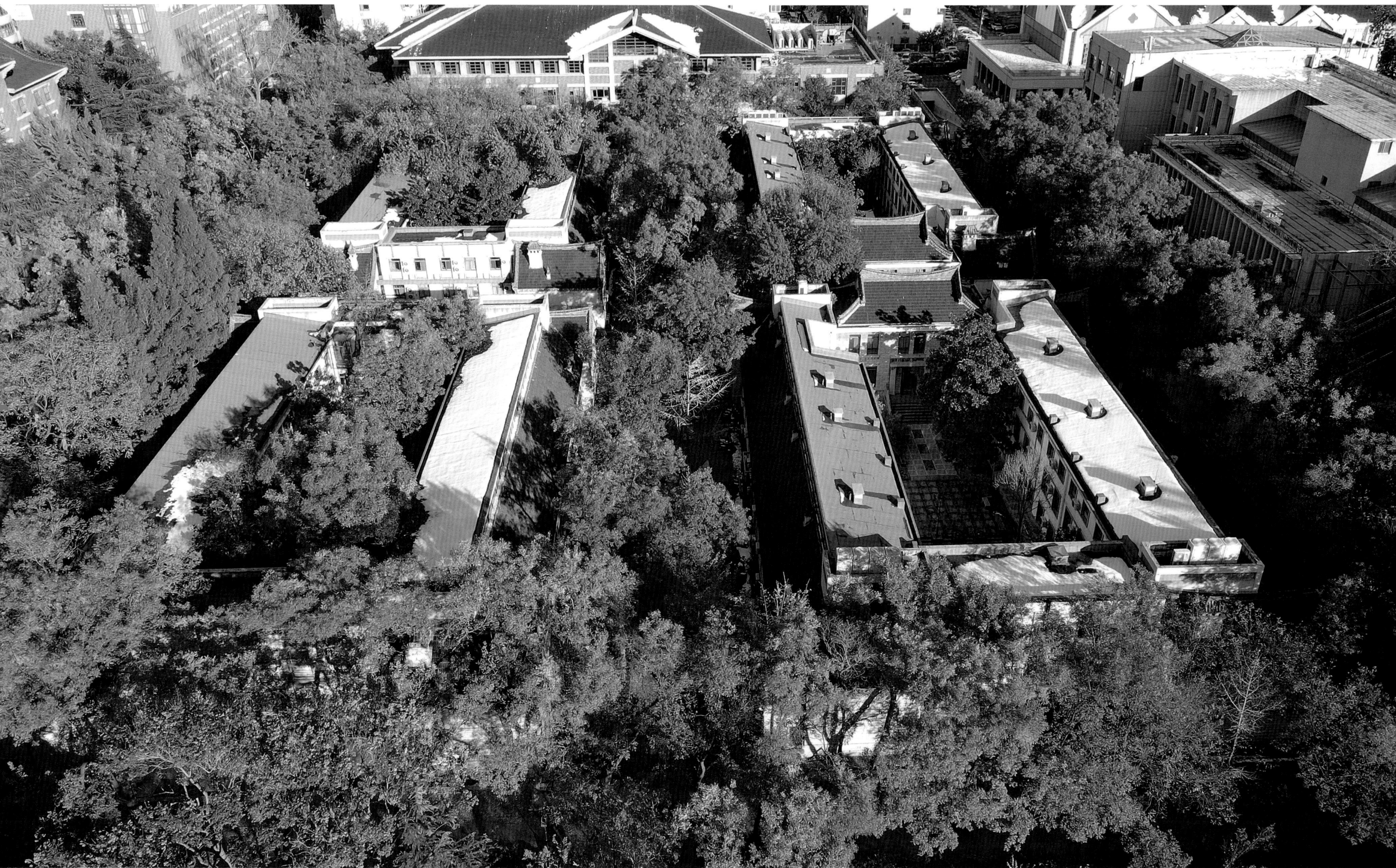

图 350 号院鸟瞰图
Fig. 350 A bird's-eye view of the Courtyard

46 四百号院（2）

No. 400 Courtyard (2)

2003 年对号院进行了全面翻修和内部现代化改造，将六个院落改为四个院落，以十字路隔开，去掉门楼，房间数由原 304 间增为 656 间；所有学生公寓内增设公共厨房、卫生间、活动室（棋牌、书画等）、储藏间等；设施方面增加了采暖空调、有线电视网络、综合布线等。现为山东大学留学生公寓和博士生公寓。

In 2003, the courtyard was completely renovated and modernized internally, with six yards replaced by four yards separated by cross roads. The arch was removed and the number of rooms increased from 304 to 656. Public kitchens, toilets, activity rooms (board games, painting and calligraphy and so on) and storerooms are added in the dormitories. The air conditioning of heating, cable television network, comprehensive wiring and other facilities are also added. The Courtyard now serves as the apartment for overseas students and doctoral students of Shandong University.

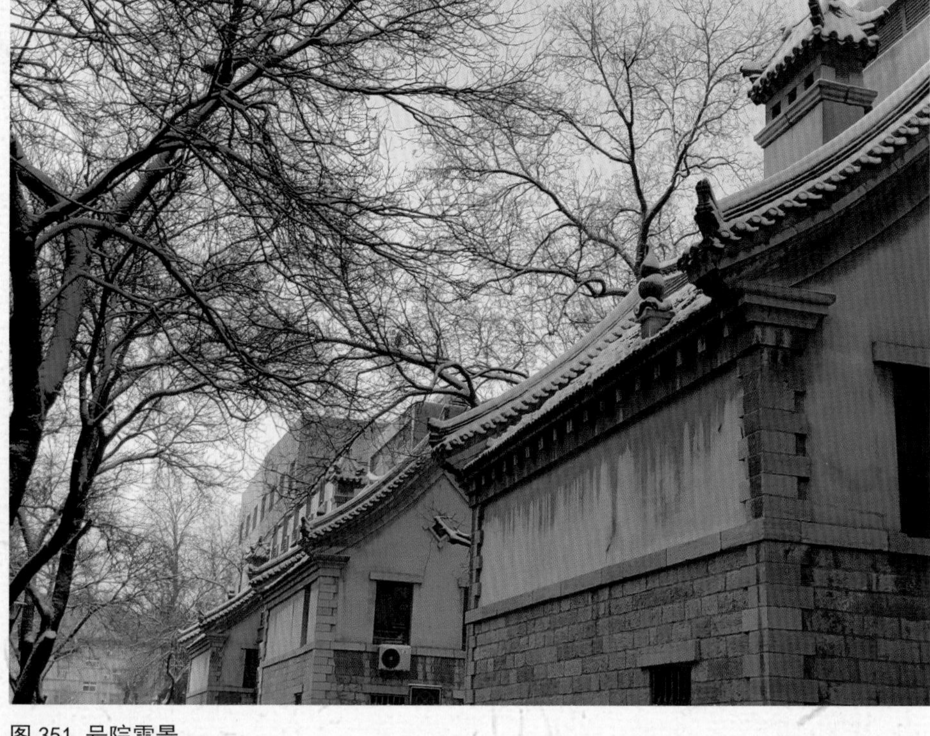

图 351 号院雪景
Fig. 351 Snow view of the Courtyard

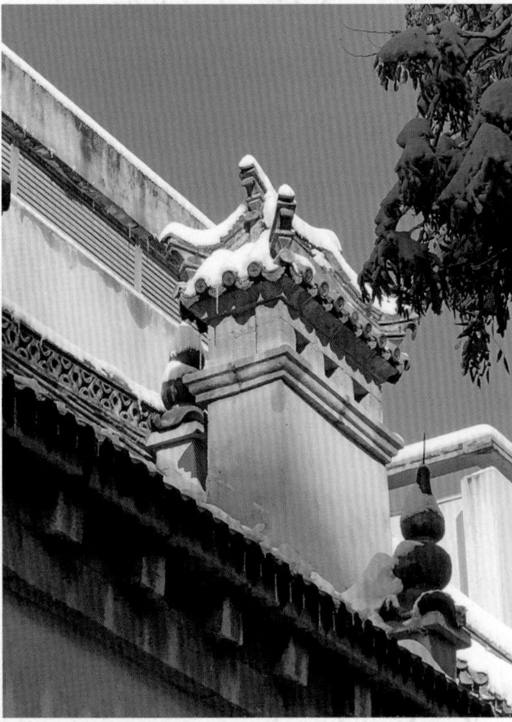

图 352 号院的天窗
Fig. 352 Skylight of the Courtyard

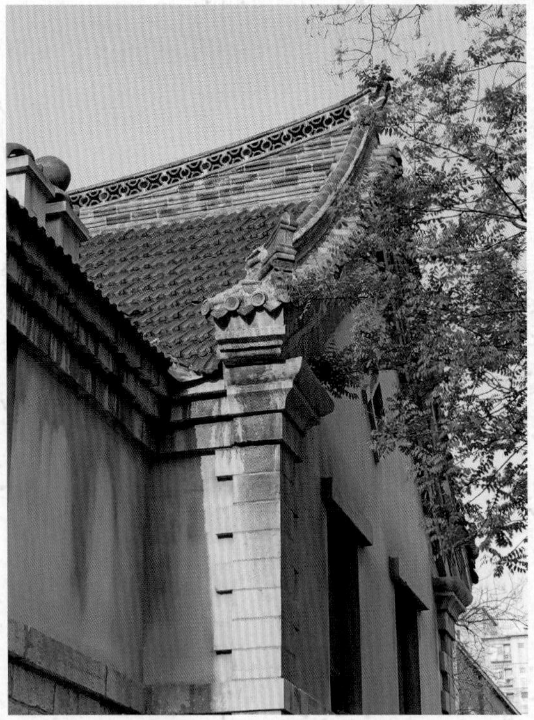

图 353 号院夕晖
Fig. 353 The Courtyard at sunset

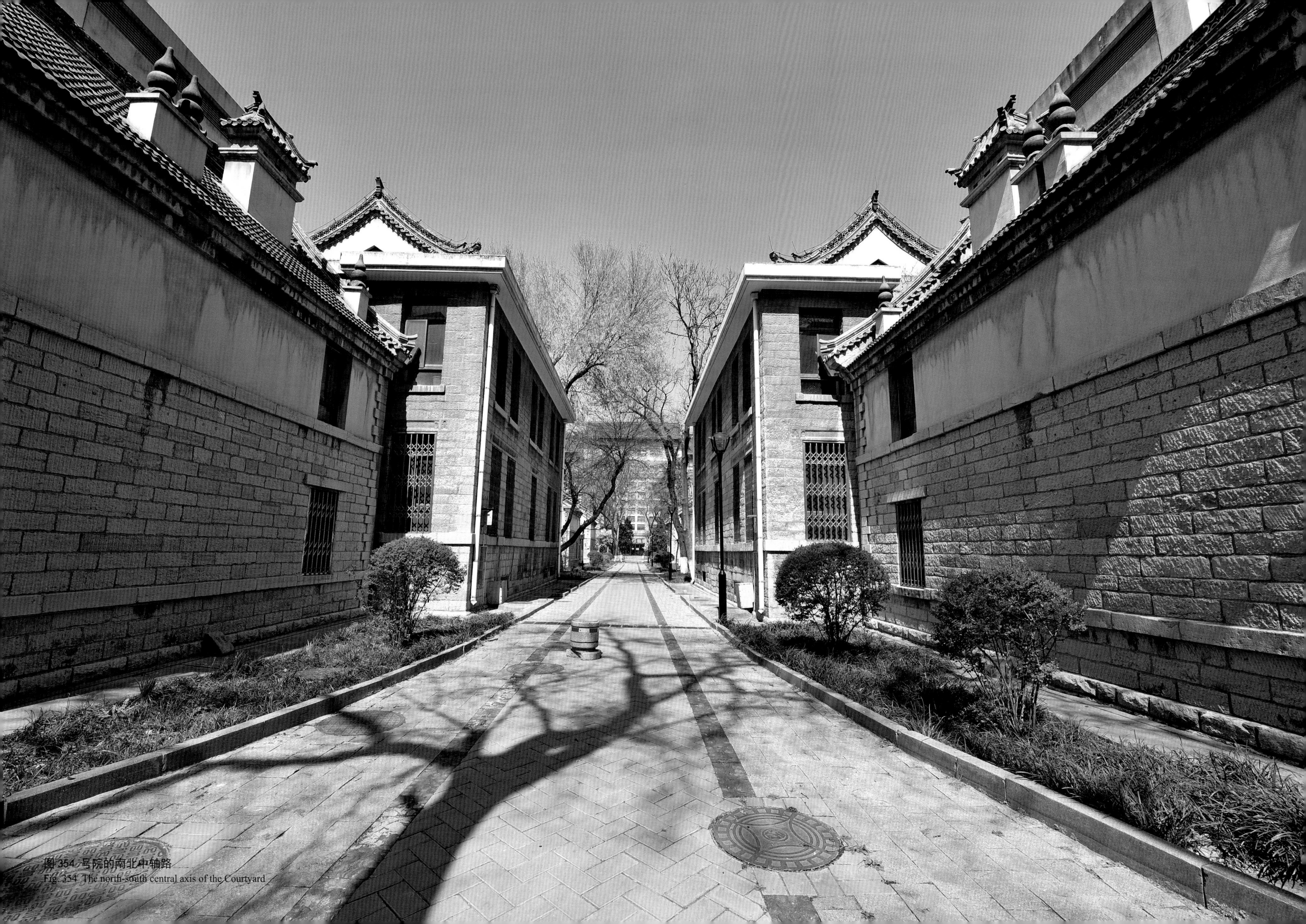

图 354 号院的南北中轴路
Fig. 354 The north-south central axis of the Courtyard

47 | 景蓝斋（1）

Jinglan Building (1)

景蓝斋建成于 1924 年，为纪念齐鲁大学女生部首任主任蓝娜德博士而命名，取景（敬）仰蓝主任之意。景蓝斋是纯粹的欧式建筑，楼体两侧高，中间偏低，屋顶阁楼上几个日耳曼式曲线形老虎窗尤其引人注目。整座楼为砖木结构，蘑菇石墙基，灰砖清水墙，石窗台，石门楣，木楼板，红瓦顶。东立面南北两端的折线形屋面、门罩及正中曲线形檐口，简洁而富有装饰感的烟囱等，均显出欧式建筑手法和特色。景蓝斋基本上是一个四合院，齐鲁大学时期为女生宿舍，每两人一间，20 多平方米，室内设施齐全，居住条件比男宿舍优越。1952 年后为山东省耳鼻咽喉科学研究所使用，现改为临床医学模拟中心。

蓝娜德（Eliza Leonard，生卒年月不详）博士，女，美北长老会传教医生，初来华时在华北协和女子大学医科任职。该女子大学创始人为麦美德博士，后任齐鲁大学女生部第二任主任。1924 年初，蓝娜德博士被齐鲁大学任命为女生部首任主任。

Jinglan Building was completed in 1924 and it was named in memory of Dr. Leonard, the first director of the Girls' Department of Cheeloo University. Jinglan Building is a pure European architecture, high on both sides and low in the middle, and a few Germanic curved roof windows on the attic are especially eye-catching. The whole building is of brick-wood structure, with wall base of mushroom stones, fair-faced wall with grey bricks, stone windowsill, stone lintel, wood floor and roof of red tiles. The broken-line roof at the north and south ends of the east facade, the arch, the curved cornice in the middle and the simple but decorative chimney all show the European architectural techniques and characteristics. Jinglan Building is basically a quadrangle courtyard, and it was once used for girl students' dormitory at Cheeloo University. The area of one room is more than twenty square meters, with well-equipped indoor facilities for two students, and the living conditions are superior to boys' dormitory. After 1952, Jinglan Building was used by Shandong Provincial Institute of Otolaryngology, and now it is changed into Medical Simulation Center.

Dr. Eliza Leonard (date of birth and death unknown), female, missionary physician of American Presbyterian Missions, North, worked in the Medical Department of North China Union College for Women when she first came to China. This college was founded by Dr. S. Luella Miner and later she served as the second director of the Girls' Department of Cheeloo University. In early 1924, Dr. Leonard was appointed as the first director of the Girls' Department by Cheeloo University.

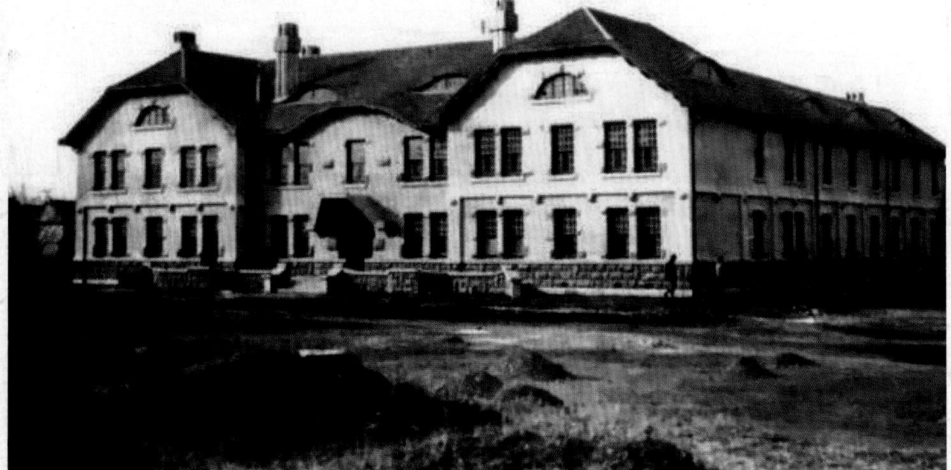

图 355 景蓝斋旧影（东立面）
Fig. 355 An old photo of Jinglan Building (the east facade)

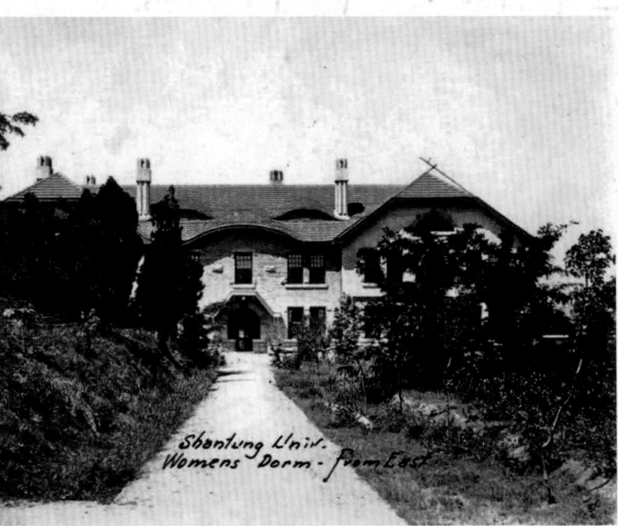

图 356 景蓝斋东（正）门前旧时风景
Fig. 356 Old scenery in front of the east (front) gate of Jinglan Building

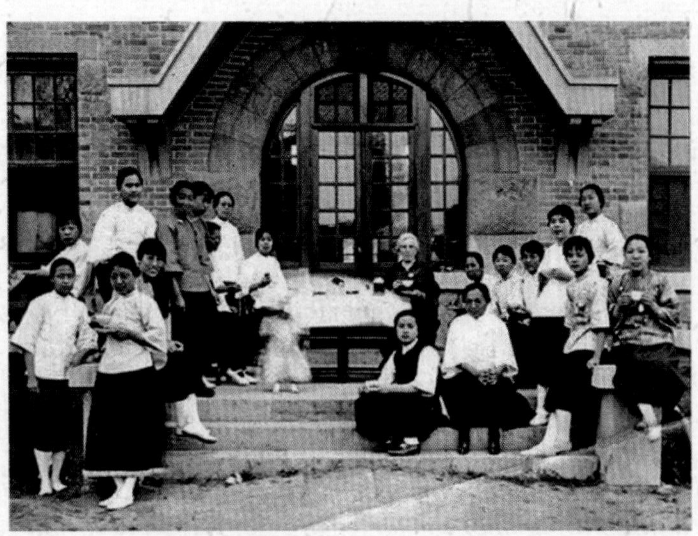

图 357 1927 年，景蓝斋前麦美德博士主持的师生茶话会
Fig. 357 A tea party for teachers and students presided over by Dr. S. Luella Miner in front of Jinglan Building in 1927

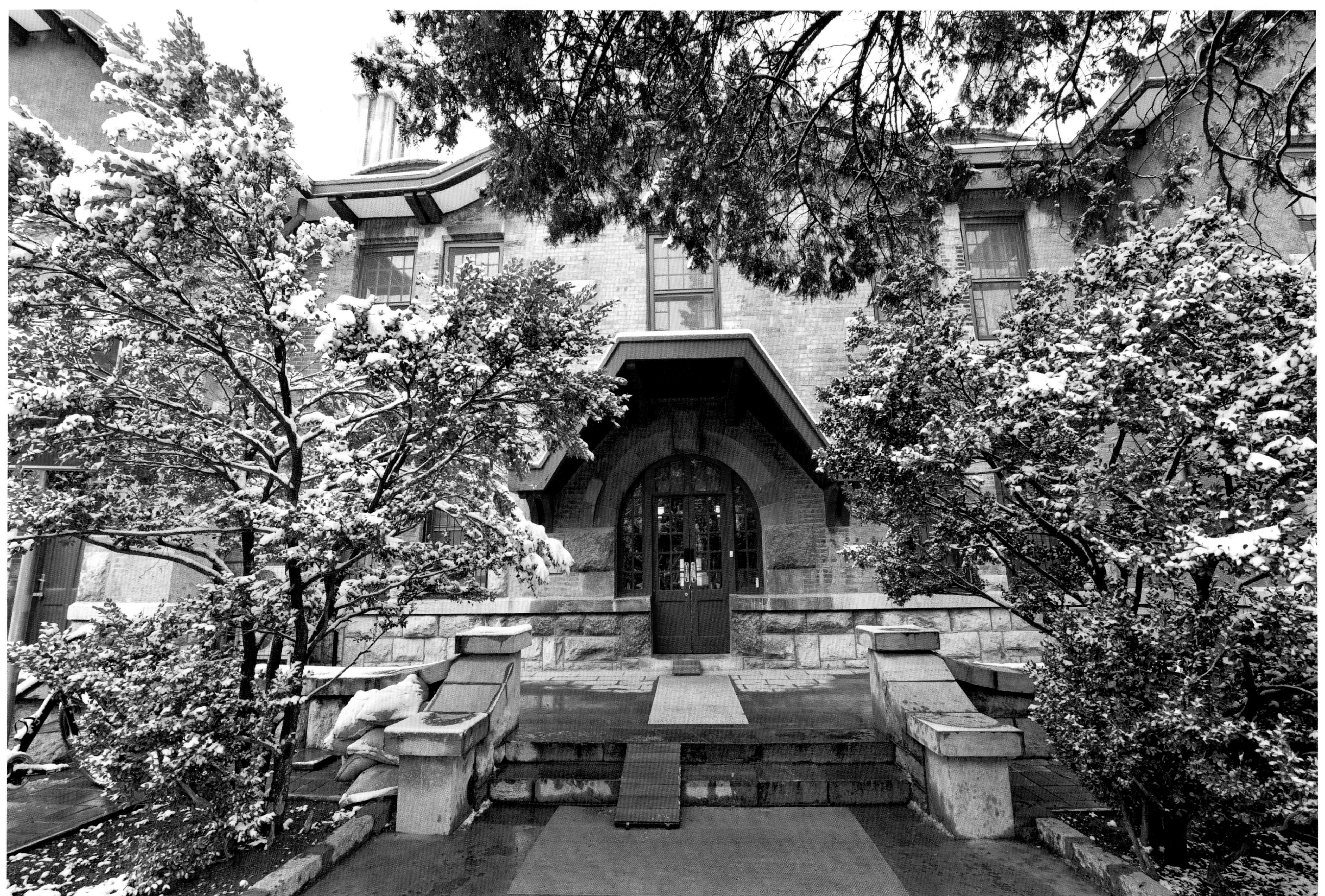

图 358 景蓝斋雪景
Fig. 358 Snow view of Jinglan Building

47 景蓝斋（2）

Jinglan Building (2)

1952 年以来，景蓝斋一直是山东省耳鼻咽喉科学研究所驻地，杨仁中教授首创的我国第一个人工喉就是在这里研制成功并用于临床的。

杨仁中，1933 年生，山东济宁人，我国著名语音康复专家。1957 年毕业于山东医学院。1958 年首创中国第一个人工喉，创建第一个语音康复基地——中国人工喉科研组。他发明的人工喉等系列语音康复设施，使失去发音能力的 3000 余例国内外“半路哑人”重新开口讲话，先后接待了 100 多个国家、地区的访问学者，至今仍被赞誉为“历史久、方法多、效果好、形成系列、技术先进”。他提出的“食管发音讲话训练法”和发明的“中国人工喉 8-5 型”均于 1978 年获得全国科学大会奖，曾七次受到毛泽东、周恩来等党和国家领导人接见，三次登上天安门参加国庆大典。曾任山东省卫生厅副厅长、山东医学院附属医院副院长、山东省耳鼻咽喉科学研究所所长等职。历任第四、五届全国人大代表，享受国务院特殊津贴和全国劳模津贴。

Since 1952, Jinglan Building has been the residence of Shandong Provincial Institute of Otolaryngology and this is the very place where the first Chinese artificial larynx initiated by Professor Yang Renzhong was successfully developed for clinical use.

Yang Renzhong, born in 1933 in Jining, Shandong Province, is a famous expert in speech rehabilitation in China. In 1957, he graduated from Shandong Medical College. In 1958, he initiated the first Chinese artificial larynx and established the first speech rehabilitation base—The Research Group of the Chinese Artificial Larynx. He invented a series of speech rehabilitation facilities such as the artificial larynx to enable more than 3,000 “halfway dumb people” at home and abroad who had lost their pronunciation ability to speak again. He had successively received visiting scholars from more than 100 countries and regions. He is now still praised for his contribution of “a long history, many methods, good results, series formation and advanced technology”. He put forward the “training method of esophageal speech” and invented the “type 8-5 of Chinese artificial larynx”. Both won the award of the National Science Conference in 1978. He was received by Mao Zedong, Zhou Enlai and other Party and State leaders seven times, and boarded the rostrum of Tian’anmen three times to celebrate the National Day. He once served as deputy director-general of the Health Department of Shandong Province, vice president of the Affiliated Hospital of Shandong Medical College and director of Shandong Provincial Institute of Otolaryngology. He is the representative of the fourth and fifth National People’s Congress and enjoys the special government allowances of the State Council and an allowance for the National Model Worker.

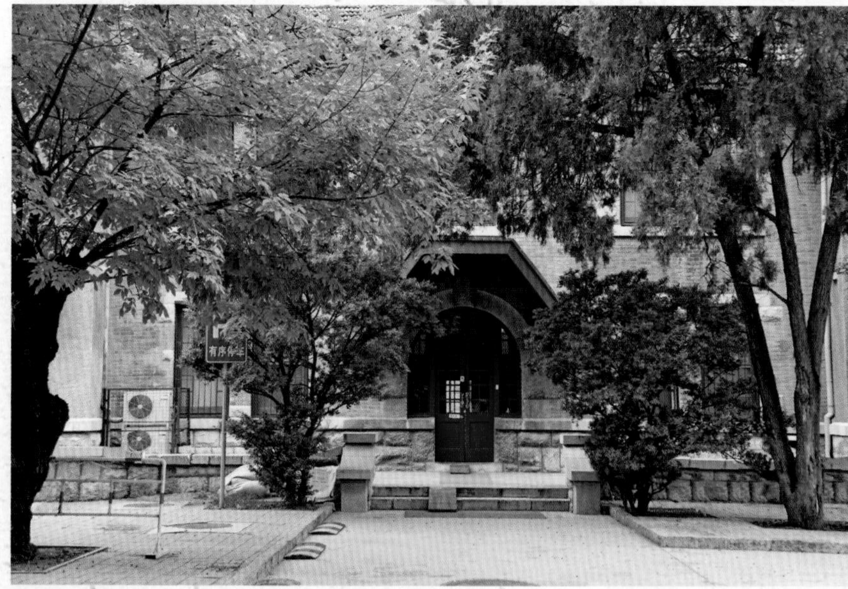

图 359 景蓝斋大门近影
Fig. 359 A recent photo of the gate of Jinglan Building

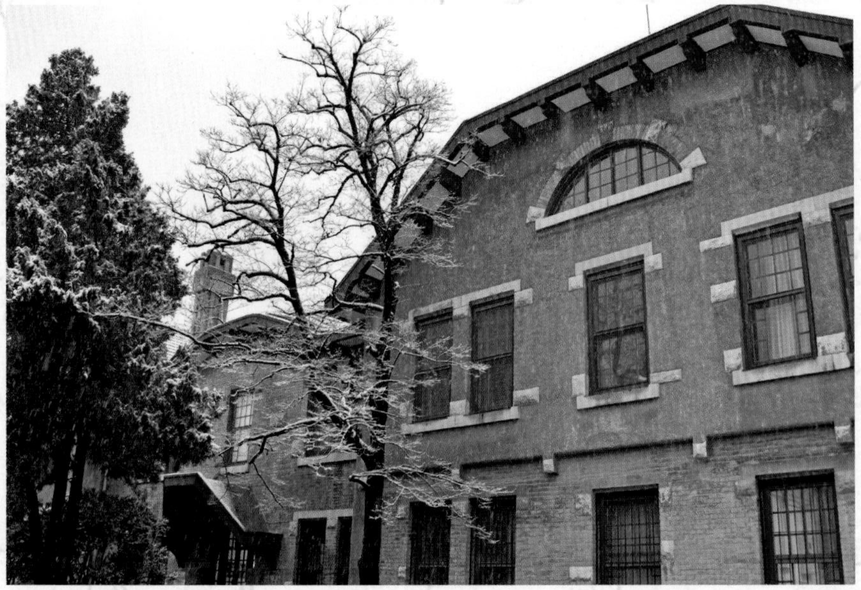

图 360 身披瑞雪的景蓝斋
Fig. 360 Jinglan Building covered with snow

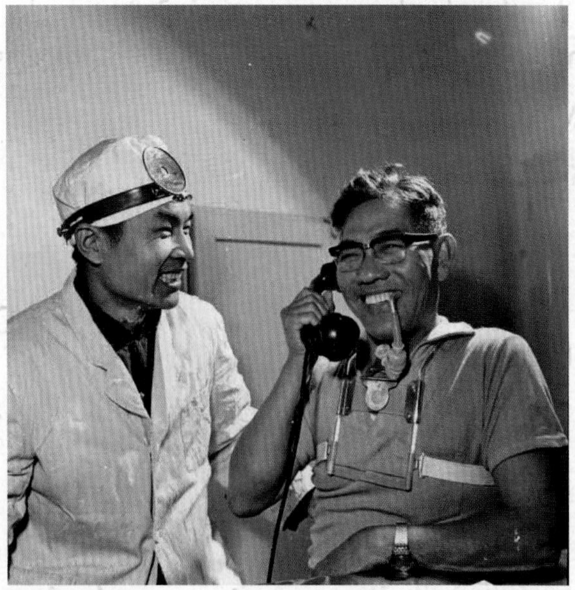

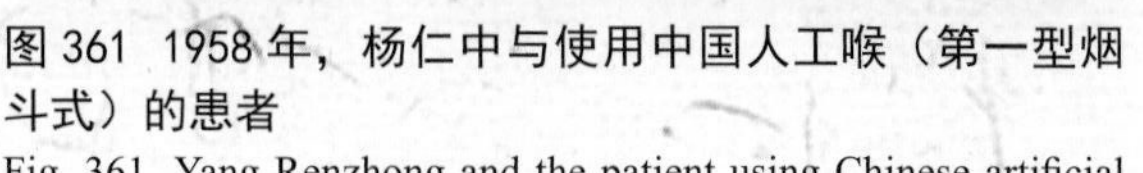

图 361 1958 年，杨仁中与使用中国人工喉（第一型烟斗式）的患者
Fig. 361 Yang Renzhong and the patient using Chinese artificial larynx (a pipe type) in 1958

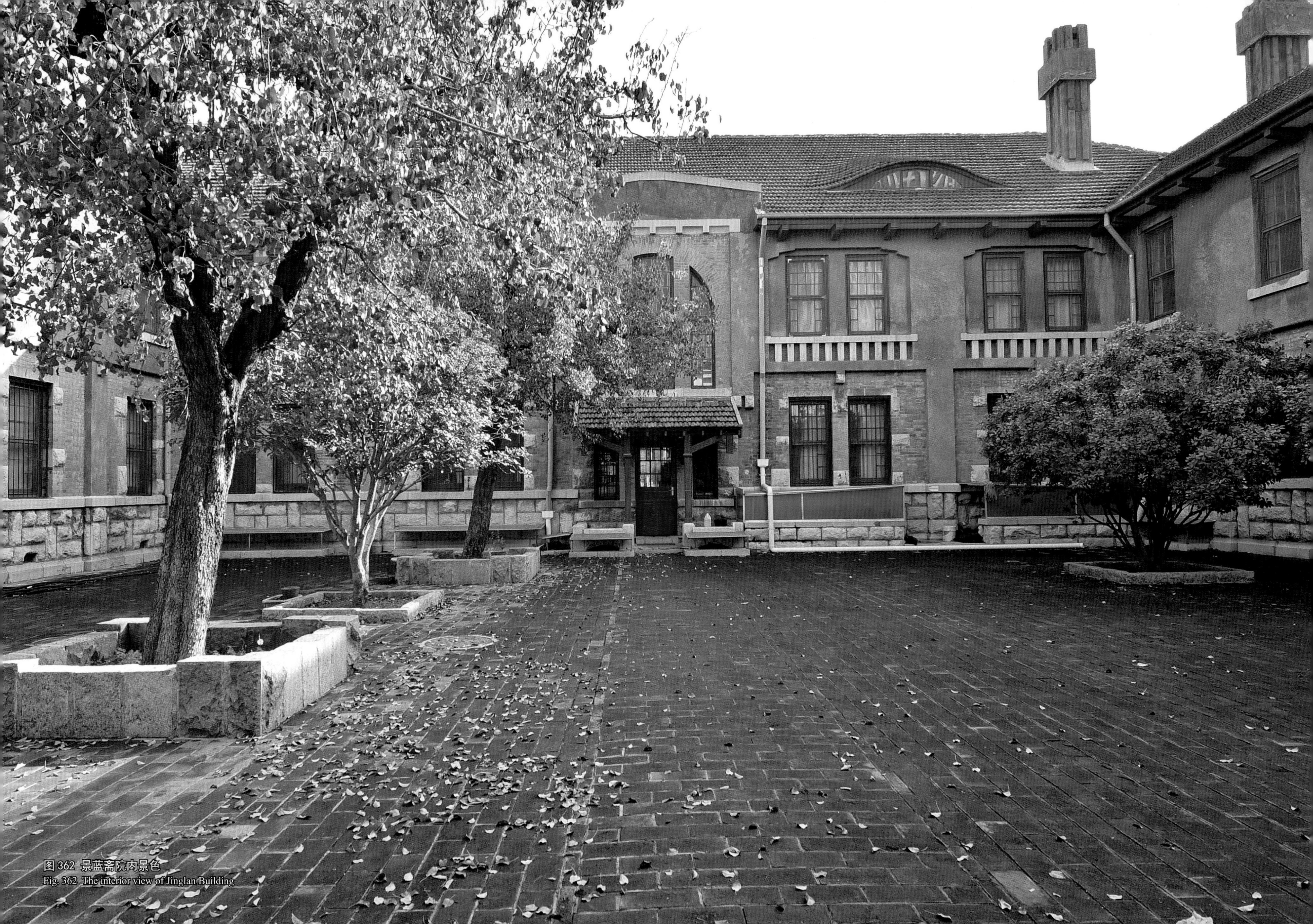

图 362 景蓝斋院内景色
Fig. 362 The interior view of Jinglan Building

48 美德楼

Miner Building

1931 年，齐鲁大学在南京国民政府教育部成功立案，自此学校各科大发展，女生也迅速增多，原女生宿舍景蓝斋已无法容纳。1933 年，在女生部第三任主任刘兰华（1889 ~ 1969）的筹措下建起第二座女生宿舍，取名“美德楼”，意为纪念女生部第二任主任麦美德博士，建筑资金为女生部历年结余的 2000 余美元日常经费。美德楼与景蓝斋的建筑风格相似，都是纯粹的欧式建筑。但与景蓝斋的雍容大度相比，美德楼显得十分简约，自有一番精致玲珑的韵味。

麦美德（S. Luella Miner，1861~1935）博士是推动中国教会大学发展的重要人物，同时也是近代女性高等教育史中的元勋。1905 年在北京创办华北协和女子大学，1920 年出任燕京大学女子部主任，1925 年被聘为齐鲁大学女生部第二任主任兼神学院教授，并一直留任齐鲁大学至 1935 年去世。以麦美德博士命名的建筑还有燕京大学校园内的麦风阁（Miner Hall）和齐鲁大学在华西坝的女生宿舍楼美德斋。

In 1931, Cheeloo University was successfully registered in the Ministry of Education of Nanjing National Government. Since then, various disciplines had greatly developed. The number of girl students had also increased rapidly and the original girls' dormitory Jinglan Building can not accommodate it. In 1933, under the fundraising of Liu Lanhua (1889-1969), the third director of the Girls' Department, the second girls' dormitory building was built, and it was named “Miner Building” to commemorate Dr. S. Luella Miner, the second director of the Girls' Department. The construction fund, more than 2,000 US dollars, is the daily fund saved by the Girls' Department over the years. The architectural styles of Miner Building and Jinglan Building are similar and both of them are pure European-style architecture. But compared with the grace of Jinglan Building, Miner Building appears very simple, with its own exquisite charm.

Dr. S. Luella Miner (1861-1935) is an important figure in promoting the development of missionary universities in China and in the history of women's higher education in modern China. In 1905, she founded North China Union College for Women in Beijing. In 1920, she became the director of the Girls' Department of Yenching University. In 1925, she was appointed as the second director of the Girls' Department of Cheeloo University and professor of the School of Theology. She remained in Cheeloo University until death in 1935. The buildings named after Dr. S. Luella Miner also include Miner Hall on campus of Yenching University and Miner House, the girls' dormitory building of Cheeloo University in Huaxiba, Chengdu.

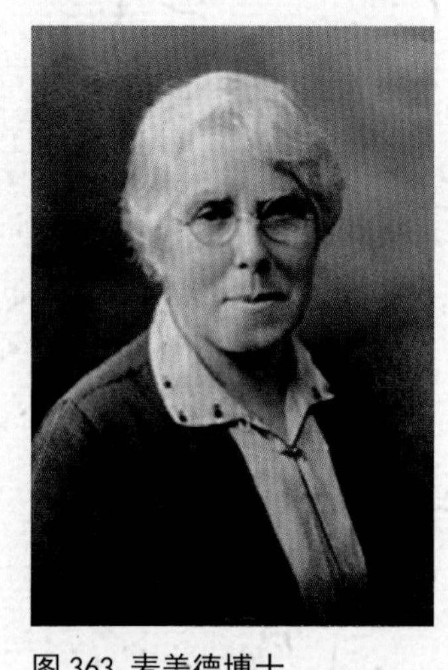

图 363 麦美德博士
Fig. 363 Dr. S. Luella Miner

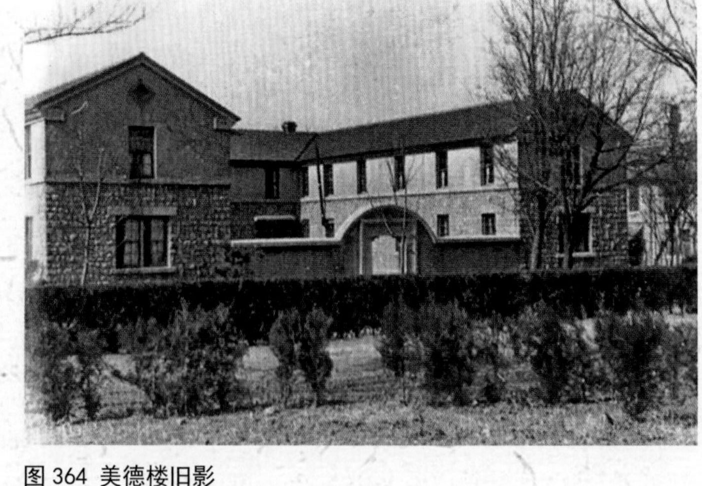

图 364 美德楼旧影
Fig. 364 An old photo of Miner Building

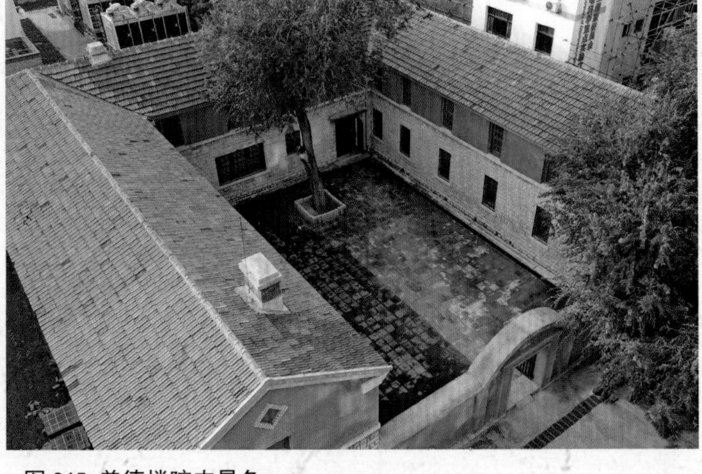

图 365 美德楼院内景色
Fig. 365 The interior view of Miner Building

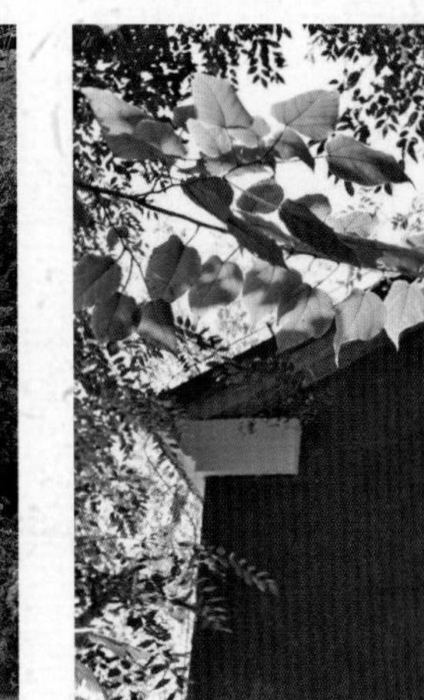

图 366 美德楼东面屋山
Fig. 366 The east gable of Miner Building

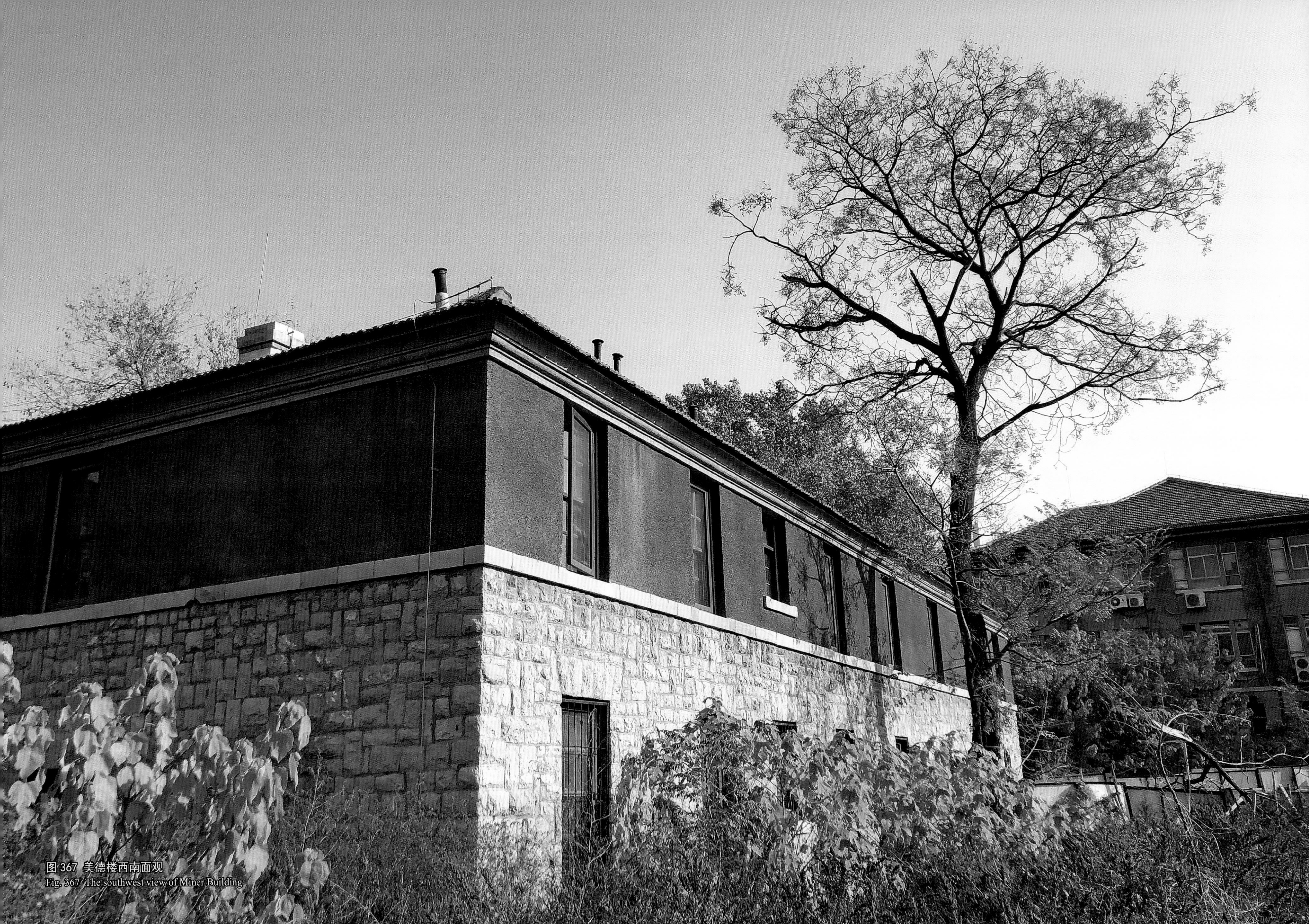

图 367 美德楼西南面观
Fig. 367 The southwest view of Miner Building

49 教授别墅（1）

Professors' Villas (1)

1917 年 9 月，齐鲁大学正式开学。为招贤纳士，从而提高教学质量和社会声誉，学校修建了 30 余幢欧式别墅，供教授们居住。目前尚存 17 幢完好的齐鲁大学教授别墅，集中分布于两处。一处在长柏路与青杨路之间，共 11 幢，分列教学八楼东西两侧；另一处在青杨路以南，6 幢，混杂在现代住宅之中。

在长柏路与青杨路之间，原有 13 幢别墅楼，自西向东编为 1 至 13 号，后来为建食堂拆除了 13 号，7 号则因建教学八楼而被拆除，因此现仅存有 11 幢。现在的门牌号自东向西排列，为 1 至 12 号，其中 7 号和 8 号是一栋楼分东西挂了两个门牌号，东 7 西 8。这 11 幢西式别墅，从东到西一字排开，仿佛一处规模宏大的别墅建筑展览，是济南市最集中的西式别墅建筑群。每栋别墅多是独门独院，绿树环绕。

In September 1917, Cheeloo University officially opened. In order to improve the teaching quality and social reputation, the university had built more than thirty European villas for professors to recruit the celebrated scholars. At present, there are still seventeen intact professors' villas of Cheeloo University which are distributed in two places. There are eleven buildings in the place between Changbai Road and Qingyang Road, on the east and west sides of the Eighth Teaching Building. The other six buildings are in the south of Qingyang Road, mixed with the modern housing.

Originally there were thirteen villas in the place between Changbai Road and Qingyang Road, numbered from 1 to 13 from west to east. Later, villas No. 13 and No. 7 were demolished for the construction of a canteen and the Eighth Teaching Building respectively. Therefore, there are only eleven villas left. The villas are numbered from 1 to 12 from east to west, of which No. 7 and No. 8 are two house numbers hung in the same building, East 7 and West 8. The eleven Western-style villas lined up from east to west like a large-scale villa exhibition, which is the most concentrated Western-style villa complex in Jinan City. Each villa has its own entrance and courtyard, surrounded by green trees.

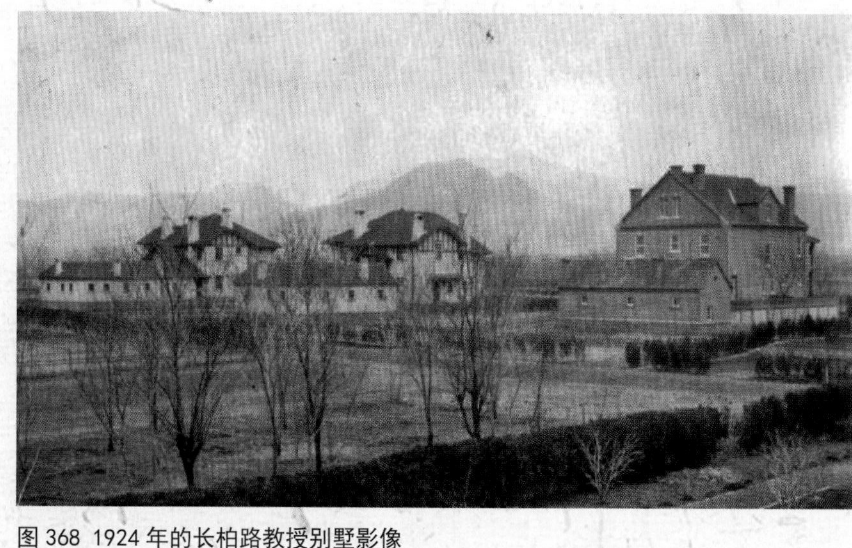

图 368 1924 年的长柏路教授别墅影像

Fig. 368 An image of the professors' villas on Changbai Road in 1924

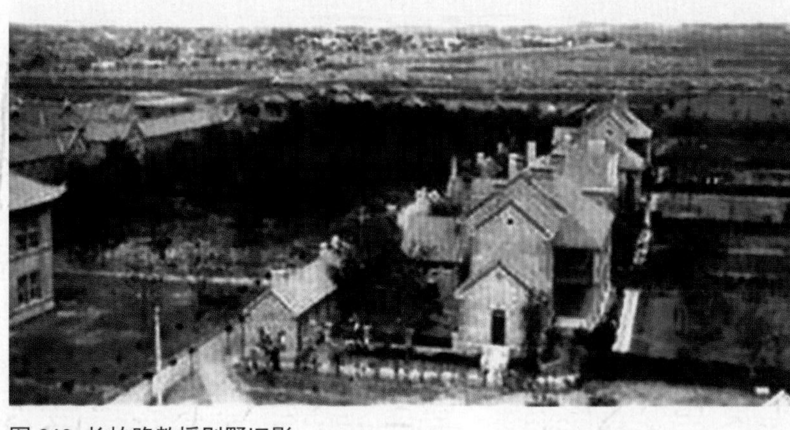

图 369 长柏路教授别墅旧影

Fig. 369 An old photo of the professors' villas on Changbai Road

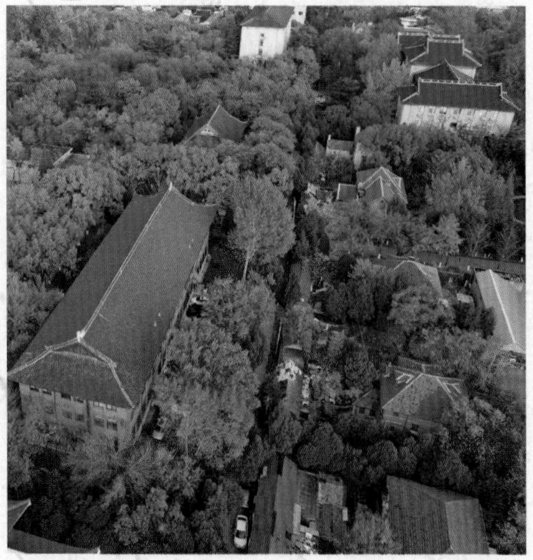

图 370 长柏路南、教学八楼西的教授别墅，由东至西编为 6 ～ 12 号

Fig. 370 Professors' villas numbered from 6 to 12 from east to west in the south of Changbai Road and west of the Eighth Teaching Building

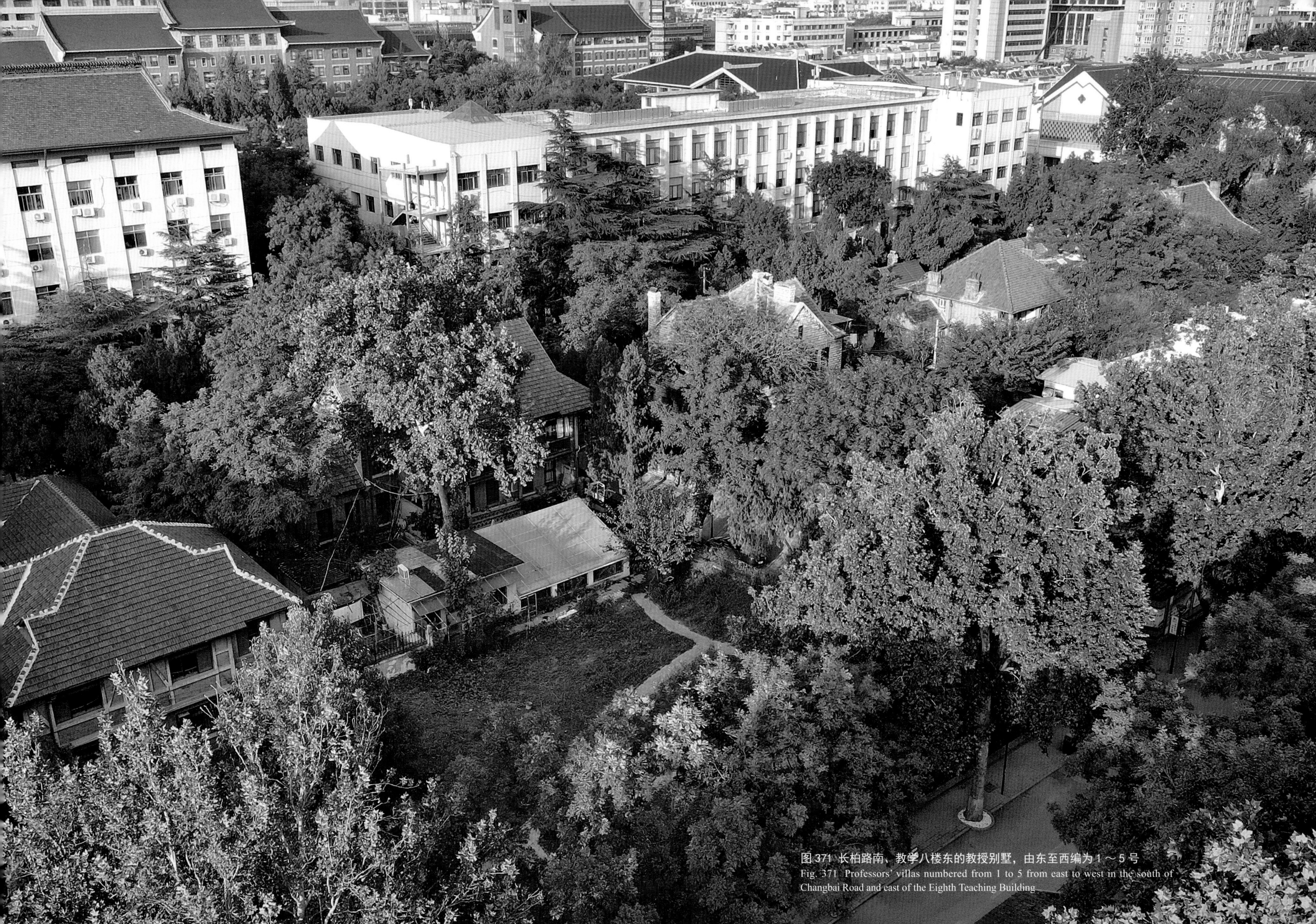

图 371 长柏路南、教学八楼东的教授别墅，由东至西编为 1 ～ 5 号

Fig. 371 Professors' villas numbered from 1 to 5 from east to west in the south of Changbai Road and east of the Eighth Teaching Building

49 教授别墅（2）

Professors' Villas (2)

这些教授别墅，其建筑风格各有特色，大致可区分为围廊式或前廊式、欧洲本土式、老摩登式和庭院平房式四种类型；其结构有砖木混合的、纯石头结构的、全砖砌成的等。真可谓形态各异，姿态万千。

现长柏路第 1 号、2 号、4 号、7 号、8 号、12 号别墅是围廊式或前廊式别墅的典型代表。这种住宅的特点是有附加的外廊，外廊有三面、二面和一面多种形式。这种平面形式，尤其是全围廊的平面形式是西方近代建筑传入中国最早期的形式，是研究西方建筑文化与中国文化交流最具代表性的实例。

These professors' villas have their own distinctive architectural styles, which can be roughly divided into four types: the style of corridor or front corridor, European style, old modern style and the style of bungalow with courtyard. Their building structures are multifarious, including mixed brick and wood, pure stones, all bricks and so on.

At present, villas No. 1, No. 2, No. 4, No. 7, No. 8 and No. 12 on Changbai Road are typical representatives of corridor-type or front corridor-type villas. This kind of residence is characterized by an additional outer corridor which has various forms of three planes, two planes and one plane. This kind of plane form, especially of the full corridor, is the earliest form of modern Western architecture introduced into China, and is the most representative example of the study of the exchange between Western architectural culture and Chinese culture.

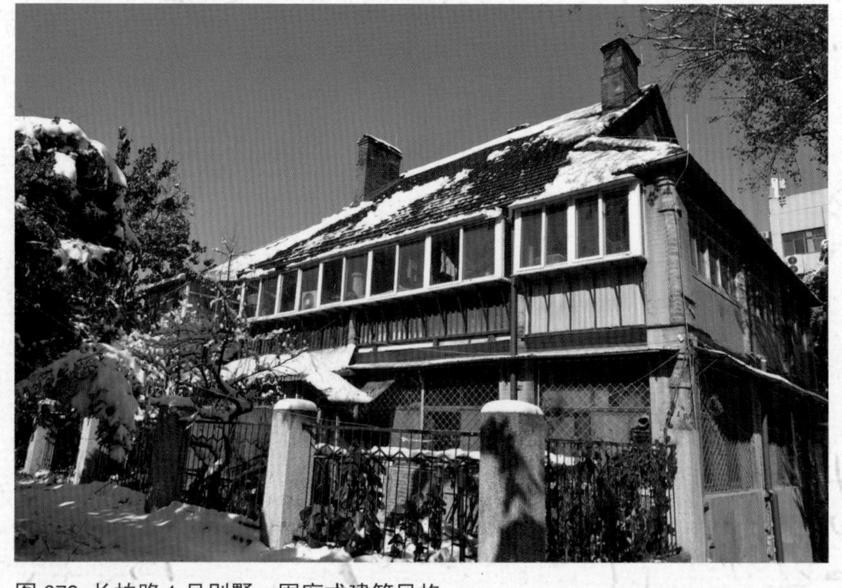

图 372 长柏路 1 号别墅，围廊式建筑风格
Fig. 372 Villa No. 1 on Changbai Road, with the corridor

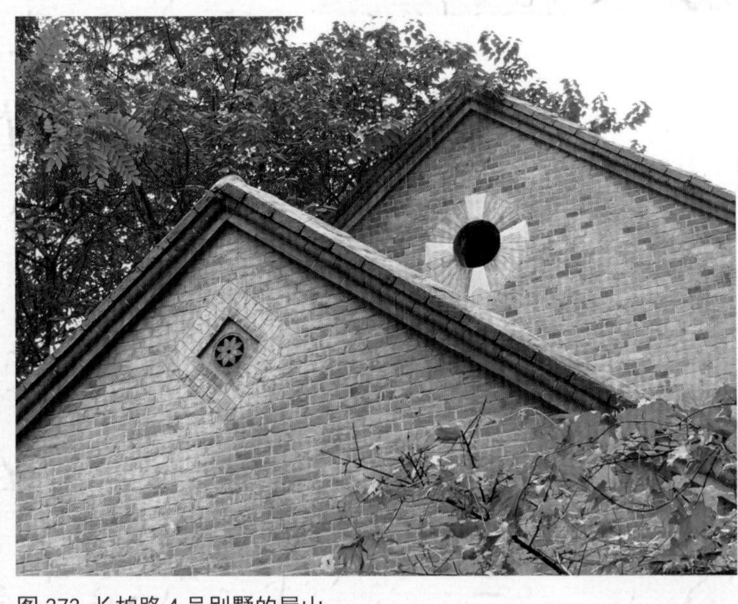

图 373 长柏路 4 号别墅的屋山
Fig. 373 Gable of Villa No. 4 on Changbai Road

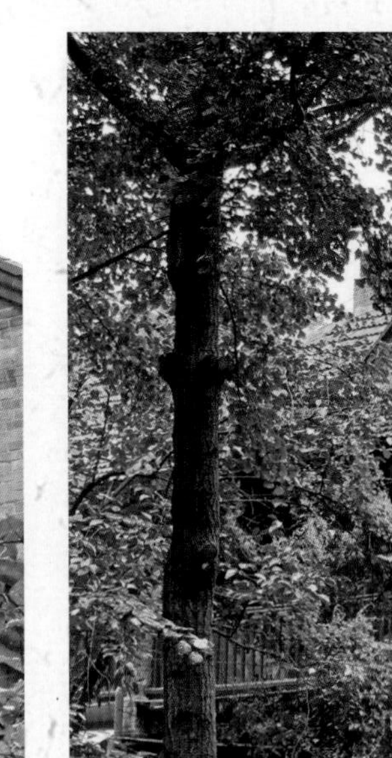

图 374 长柏路 7、8 号别墅南面观
Fig. 374 The south view of Villa numbered 7 and 8 on Changbai Road

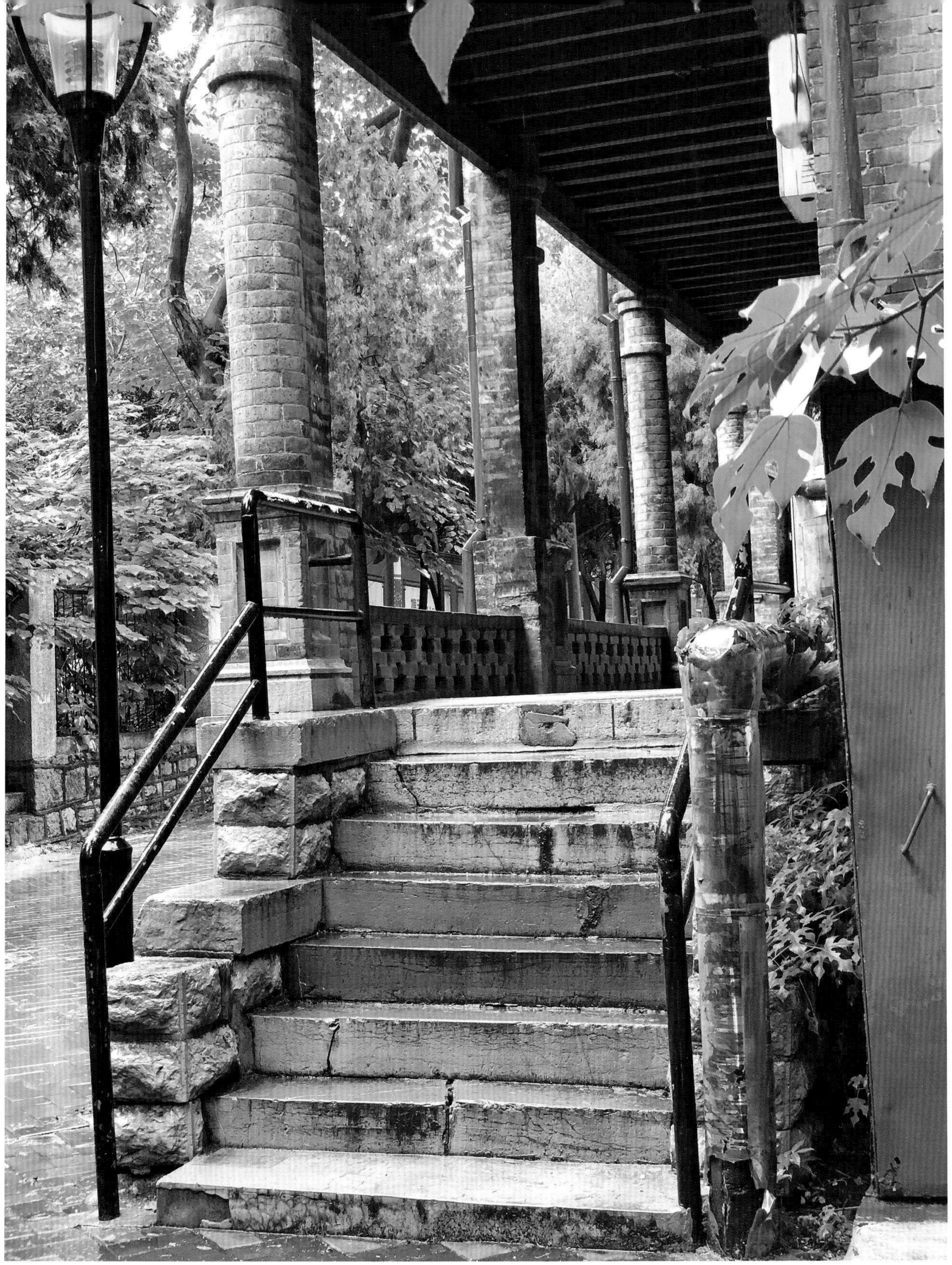

图 375 长柏路 4 号别墅东面围廊
Fig. 375 The east corridor of Villa No. 4 on Changbai Road

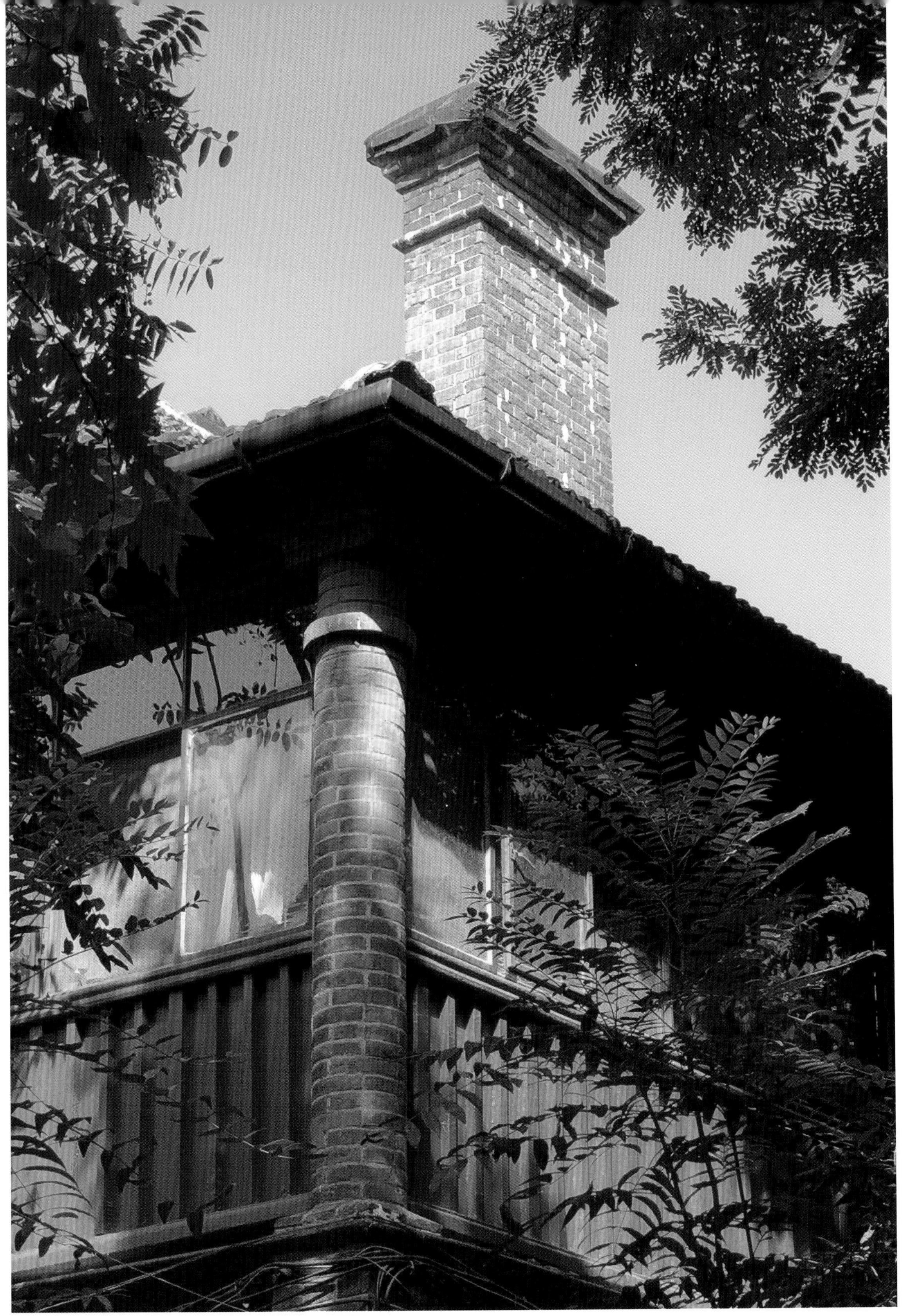

图 376 长柏路 12 号别墅南面观
Fig. 376 The south view of Villa No. 12 on Changbai Road

49 教授别墅（3）

Professors' Villas (3)

现长柏路第 3 号、5 号、6 号和 9 号别墅基本上为欧洲本土式别墅。这种住宅从平面到造型完全按照原户主的母国样式建造，故地域性和民族性比较突出。有北欧类半木结构式、德国城堡式等。

当时居住以上两种类型别墅的都是齐鲁大学地位最高的人。如海贝殖居住的 3 号别墅（原 10 号别墅）、巴慕德居住的 6 号别墅（原 6 号别墅）均为城堡式别墅，不仅材质坚固、体量大，设计也更有特色。吴克明校长和杨德斋校长住过的 9 号别墅（原 4 号别墅）则是北欧类半木结构式建筑。

At present, villas No. 3, No. 5, No. 6 and No. 9 on Changbai Road basically belong to European-style villas. From the plane to the shape, this kind of residence is completely built in accordance with the architectural style of the original householder's home country, so the regional and national characteristics are more prominent. Such villas are in Nordic half-timbered style and style of German castles.

At that time, people living in both types of villas were the highest-ranking people at Cheeloo University. For example, Villa No. 3 (former Villa No. 10) inhabited by LeRoy Francis Heimburger and Villa No. 6 (former Villa No. 6) inhabited by Harold Balme are castle-style villas which are not only solid in material and large in size, but also more distinctive in design. Villa No. 9 (former Villa No. 4) once inhabited by President Wu Keming and President Yang Dezhai is a Nordic half-timbered building.

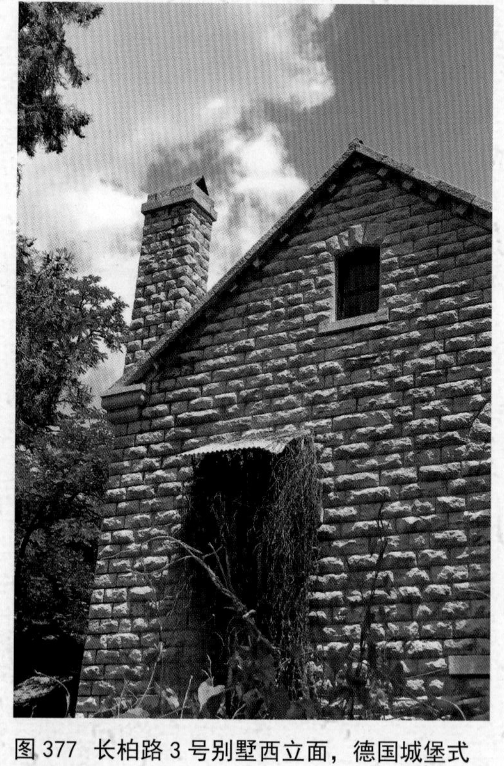

图 377 长柏路 3 号别墅西立面，德国城堡式建筑风格

Fig. 377 The west facade of Villa No. 3 on Changbai Road, in the architectural style of German castles

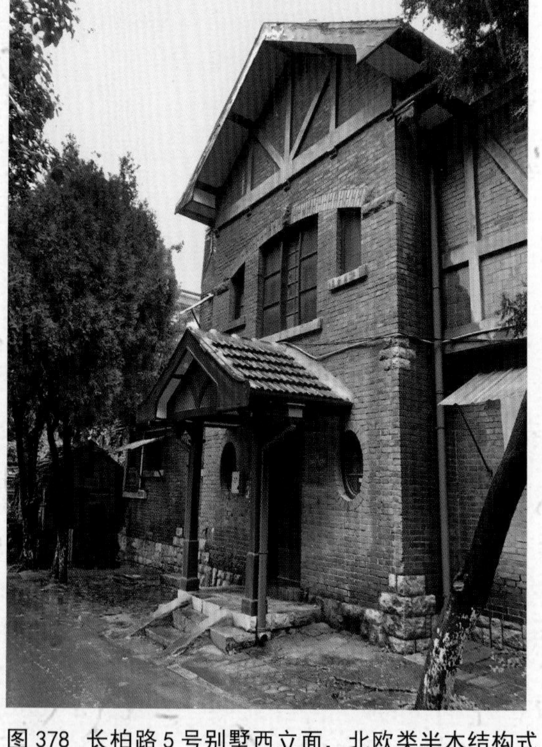

图 378 长柏路 5 号别墅西立面，北欧类半木结构式风格

Fig. 378 The west facade of Villa No. 5 on Changbai Road, in Nordic half-timbered style

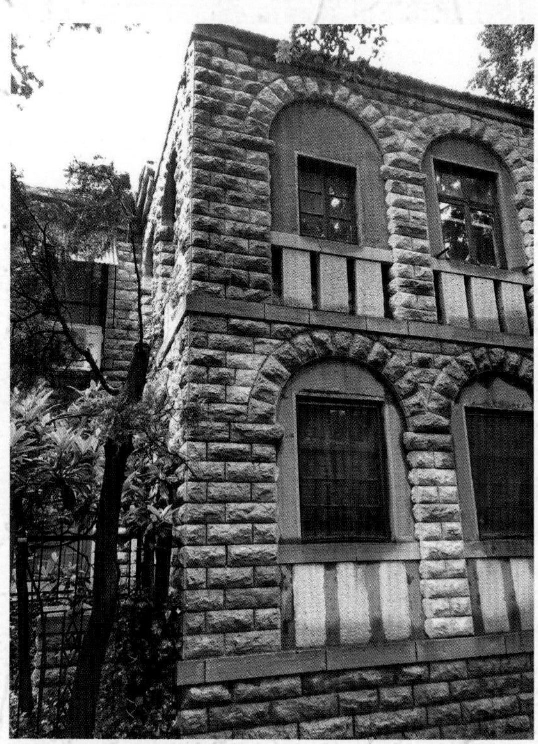

图 379 长柏路 6 号别墅东立面

Fig. 379 The east facade of Villa No. 6 on Changbai Road

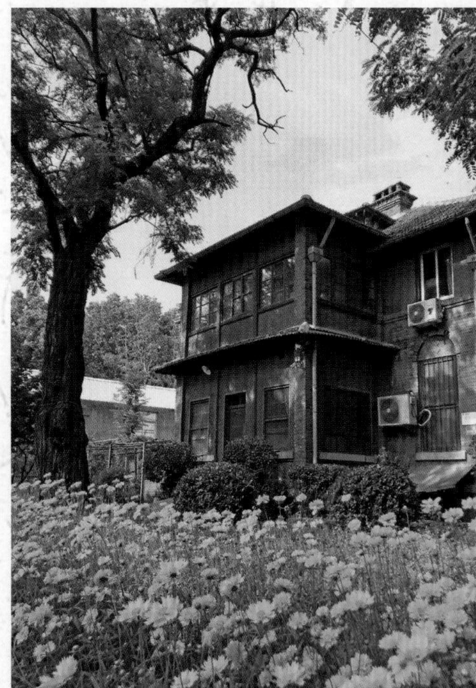

图 380 长柏路 9 号别墅东面观

Fig. 380 The east view of Villa No. 9 on Changbai Road

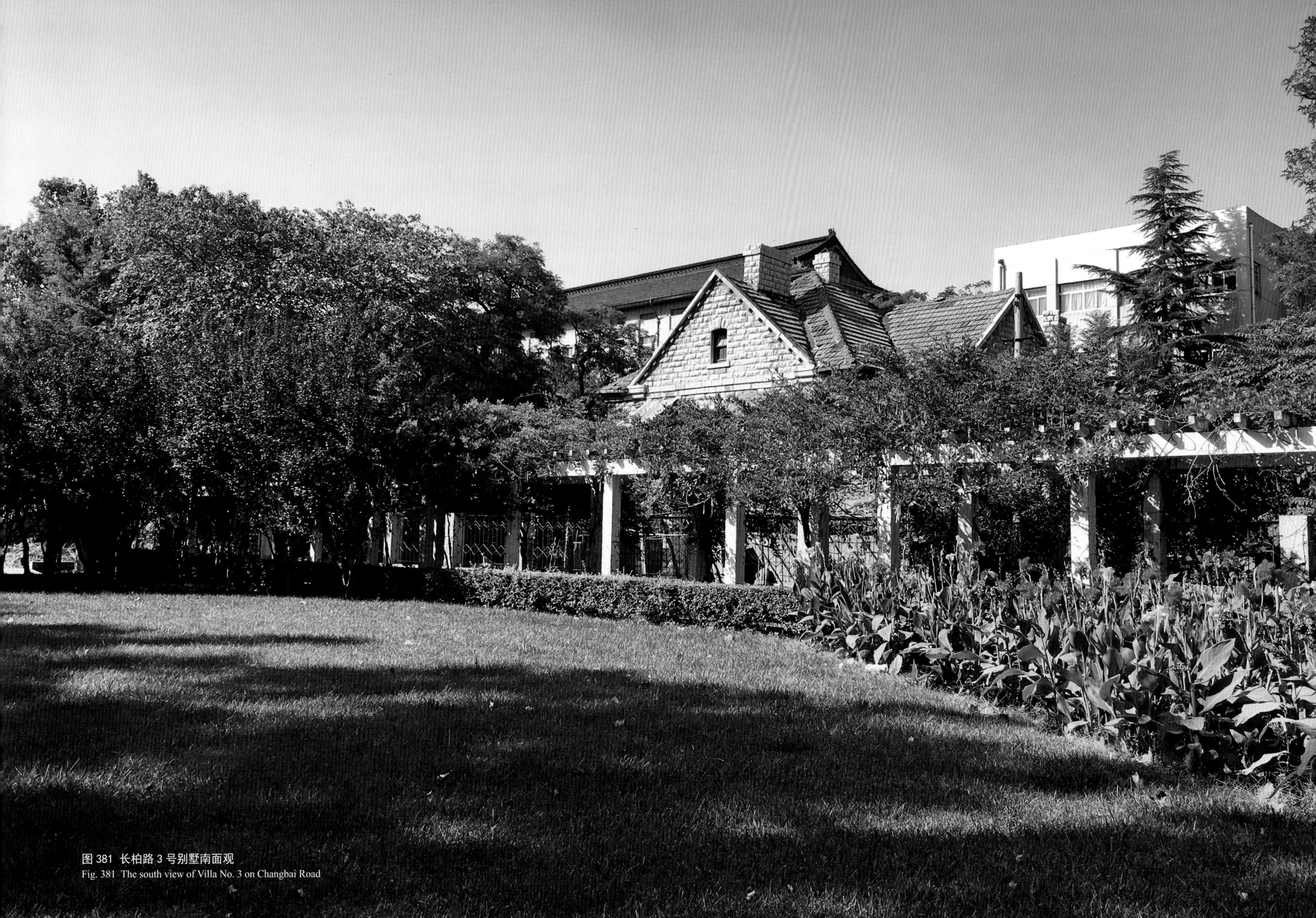

图 381 长柏路 3 号别墅南面观
Fig. 381 The south view of Villa No. 3 on Changbai Road

49 教授别墅（4）

Professors' Villas (4)

现长柏路第 10 号、11 号别墅是老摩登式别墅，造型较简洁，装饰比较少，强调功能的合理性和技术的先进性，属于欧洲古典建筑向近现代建筑转换的类型。

1937 年，老舍先生二进齐鲁大学，居住在第 11 号别墅（原 2 号别墅）。据老舍夫人胡絜青叙述："这座灰色砖楼的结构颇为别致：由当中并列的两个楼门和平行上升的两个楼梯，把小楼一分为二，东西各半。我们住的是东半楼。楼下的两大开间作为客厅和书房，楼上三间作为卧室，厨房在楼下。这一带有好几座式样不同的小楼，住的多是外籍教授，环境很美。楼前楼后有不少苍翠的松柏。站在我们的卧室里，又可以在晴空下远眺千佛山和马鞍山的秀色了。……"现在，这里颇为冷清，只有屋顶上的鸽子还在那里张望，仿佛在等待着这座房子故主的归来。

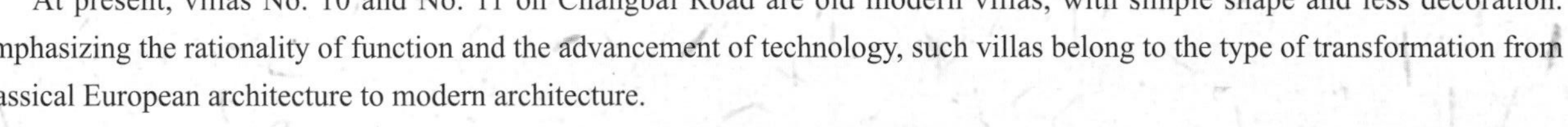

At present, villas No. 10 and No. 11 on Changbai Road are old modern villas, with simple shape and less decoration. Emphasizing the rationality of function and the advancement of technology, such villas belong to the type of transformation from classical European architecture to modern architecture.

In 1937, Mr. Lao She joined Cheeloo University for the second time and lived in Villa No. 11 (former Villa No. 2). According to Lao She's wife Hu Jieqing: "This grey brick building is quite unique in structure: this building is divided into east and west parts by two parallel doors and two stairs rising in parallel in the middle. We live in the east. The two large rooms downstairs serve as the living room and the study, the three upstairs serve as bedrooms, and the kitchen is downstairs. There are several buildings of different styles in this area, mostly inhabited by foreign professors. The environment is very beautiful. There are many verdant pines and cypresses in front of and behind the buildings. Standing in our bedroom, we can overlook the beauty of Qianfo Hill and Ma'an Hill in the clear sky." Now this building looks rather deserted and only the pigeons on the roof are still looking around, as if waiting for the return of the original householder.

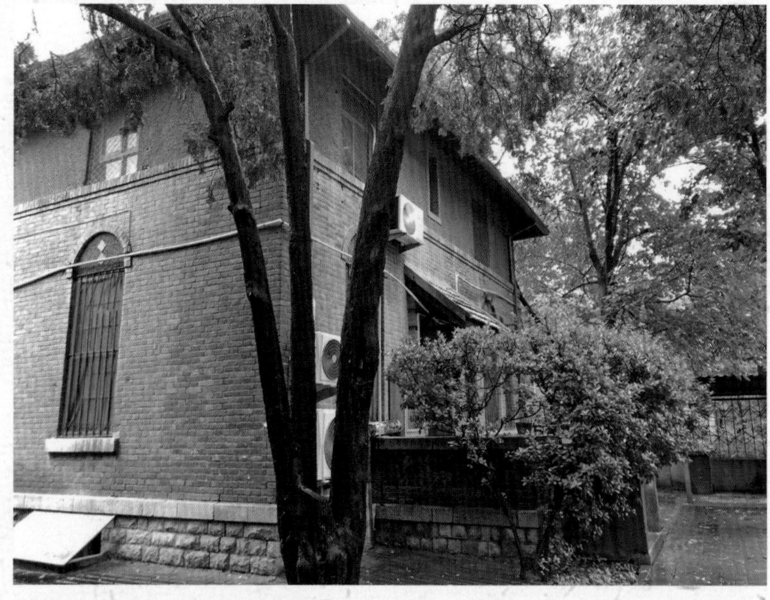

图 382 长柏路 10 号别墅西面观
Fig. 382 The west view of Villa No. 10 on Changbai Road

图 383 长柏路 11 号别墅屋顶的鸽子
Fig. 383 Pigeons on the roof of Villa No. 11 on Changbai Road

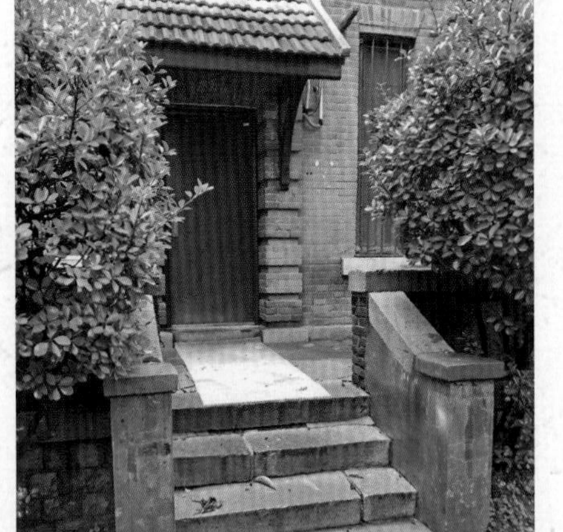

图 384 长柏路 10 号别墅南门
Fig. 384 The south gate of Villa No. 10 on Changbai Road

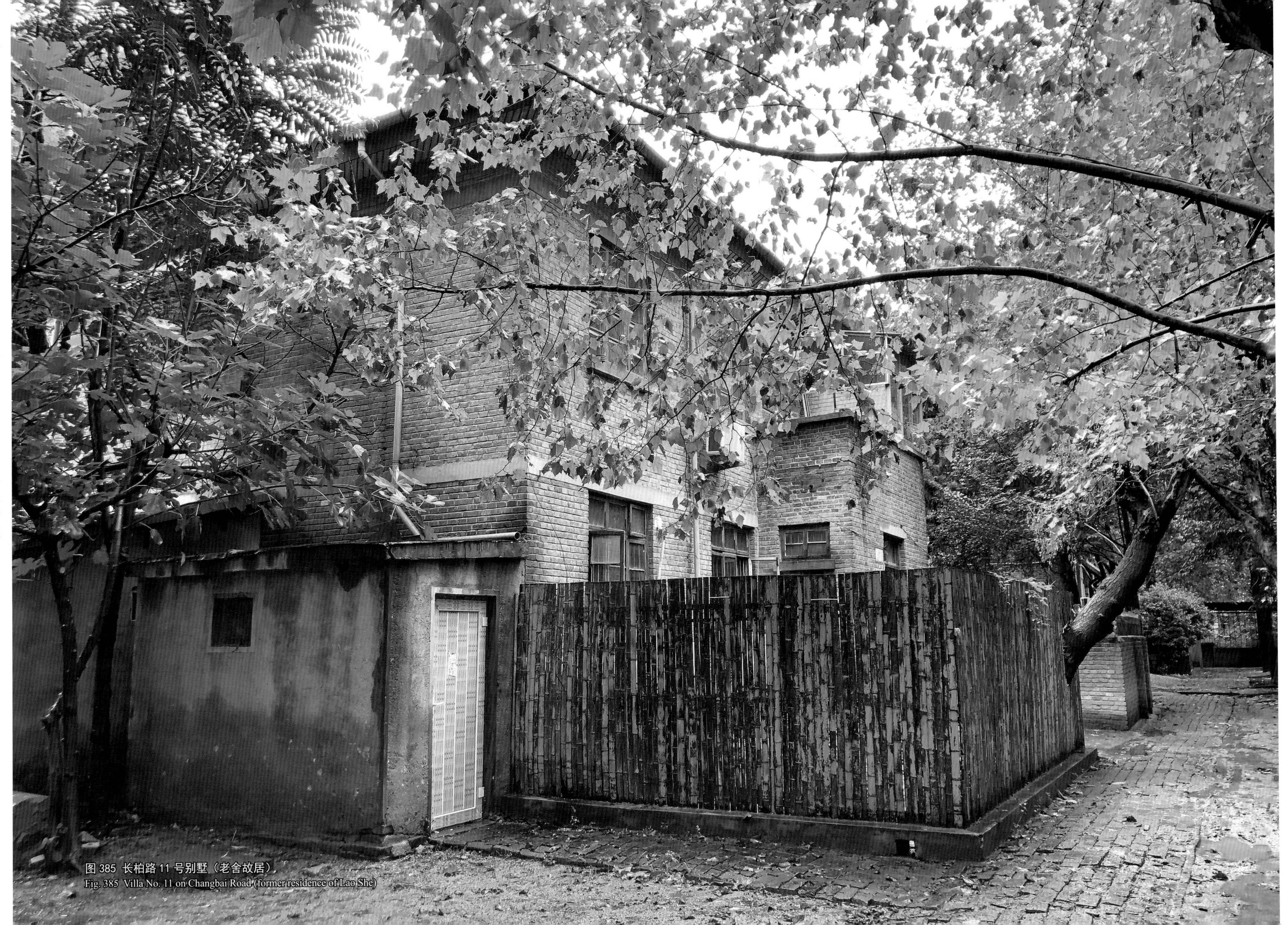

图 385 长柏路 11 号别墅（老舍故居）
Fig. 385 Villa No. 11 on Changbai Road (former residence of Lao She)

49 教授别墅（5）

Professors' Villas (5)

第四种类型的别墅为庭院平房式，用院落组织建筑空间，强调居住环境的质量，占地面积相对比较大，现门牌为青杨路 2 号的别墅应为这一种类型。

在西村，青杨路以南，在 1 号楼与 2 号楼之间和 3 号楼与 4 号楼之间，各有两座风格别致的教授别墅，有的尚有人居住，有的已破损不堪。现 18 号楼（原外籍教师宿舍）北侧，还有一座身披绿色植被的别墅。它们在现代楼群之中，仍然屹立在风雨之中，以坚强的毅力强忍寂寞，在翘首等待着千古知音的到来。

The fourth type of villa is the bungalow with courtyard, which builds the space with the organization of the courtyard, emphasizes the quality of the living environment, and occupies a relatively large area. Now the villas at No. 2 Qingyang Road belong to this type.

In the West Village south of Qingyang Road, there are two professors' villas of unique style between Buildings No. 1 and No. 2 and Buildings No. 3 and No. 4 respectively, either being inhabited or having been damaged. Now on the north side of Building No. 18 (former foreign teachers' dormitory), there is also a villa covered with green vegetation. Mixed in the modern buildings, they are still standing in the wind and rain to endure loneliness with strong perseverance, eagerly awaiting the arrival of the understanding people.

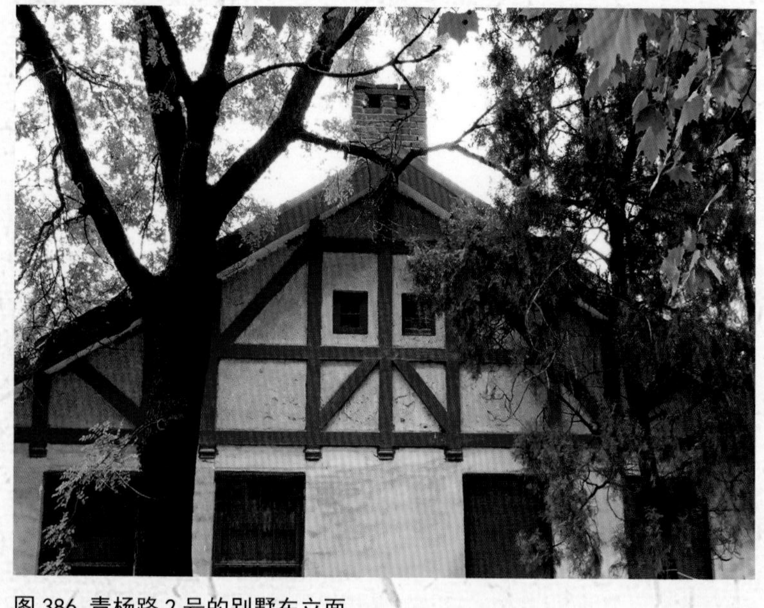

图 386 青杨路 2 号的别墅东立面

Fig. 386 The east facade of the villa at No. 2 Qingyang Road

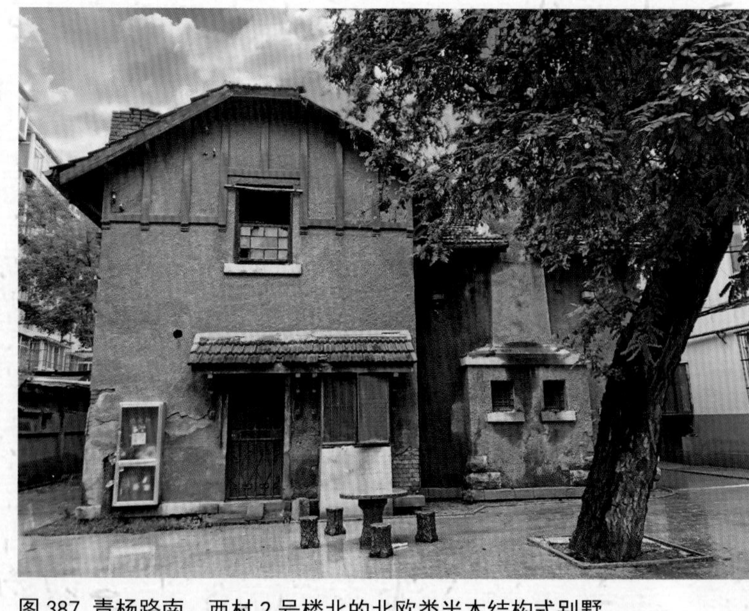

图 387 青杨路南、西村 2 号楼北的北欧类半木结构式别墅

Fig. 387 Nordic half-timbered villa in the north of Building No.2 in the West Village south of Qingyang Road

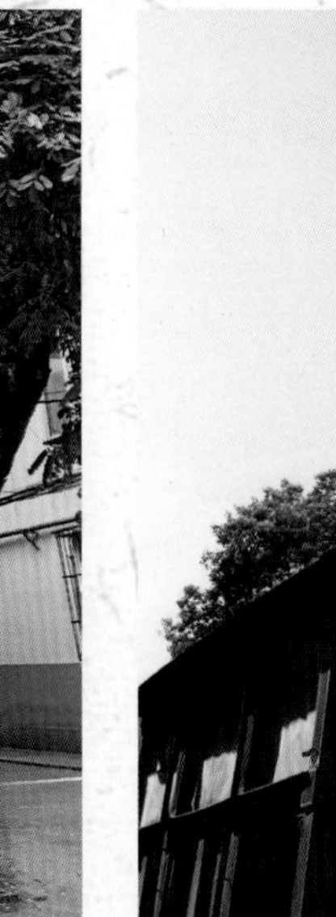

图 388 青杨路南、西村 3 号楼北的东侧别墅

Fig. 388 The east side of the villa in the north of Building No. 3 in the West Village south of Qingyang Road

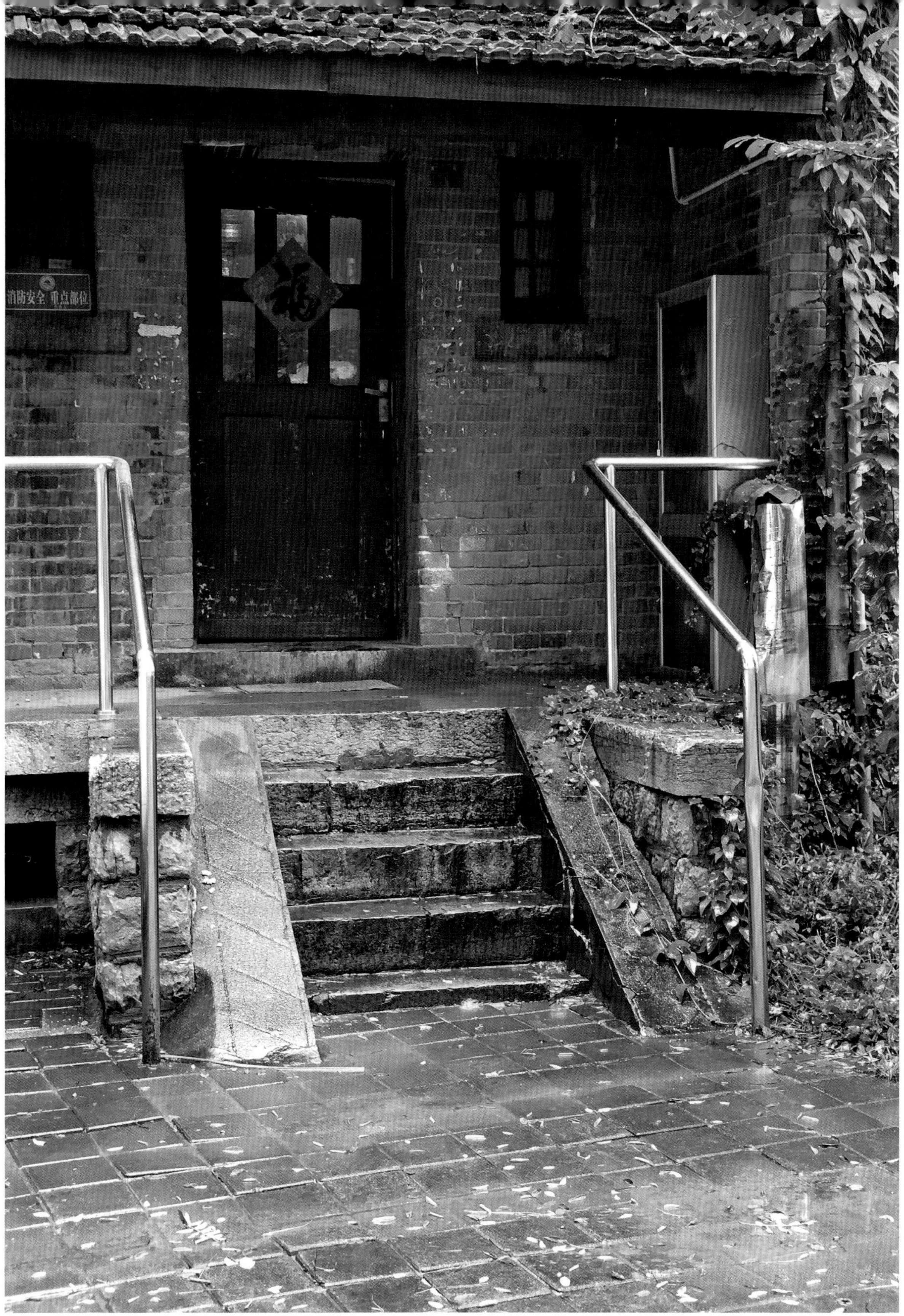

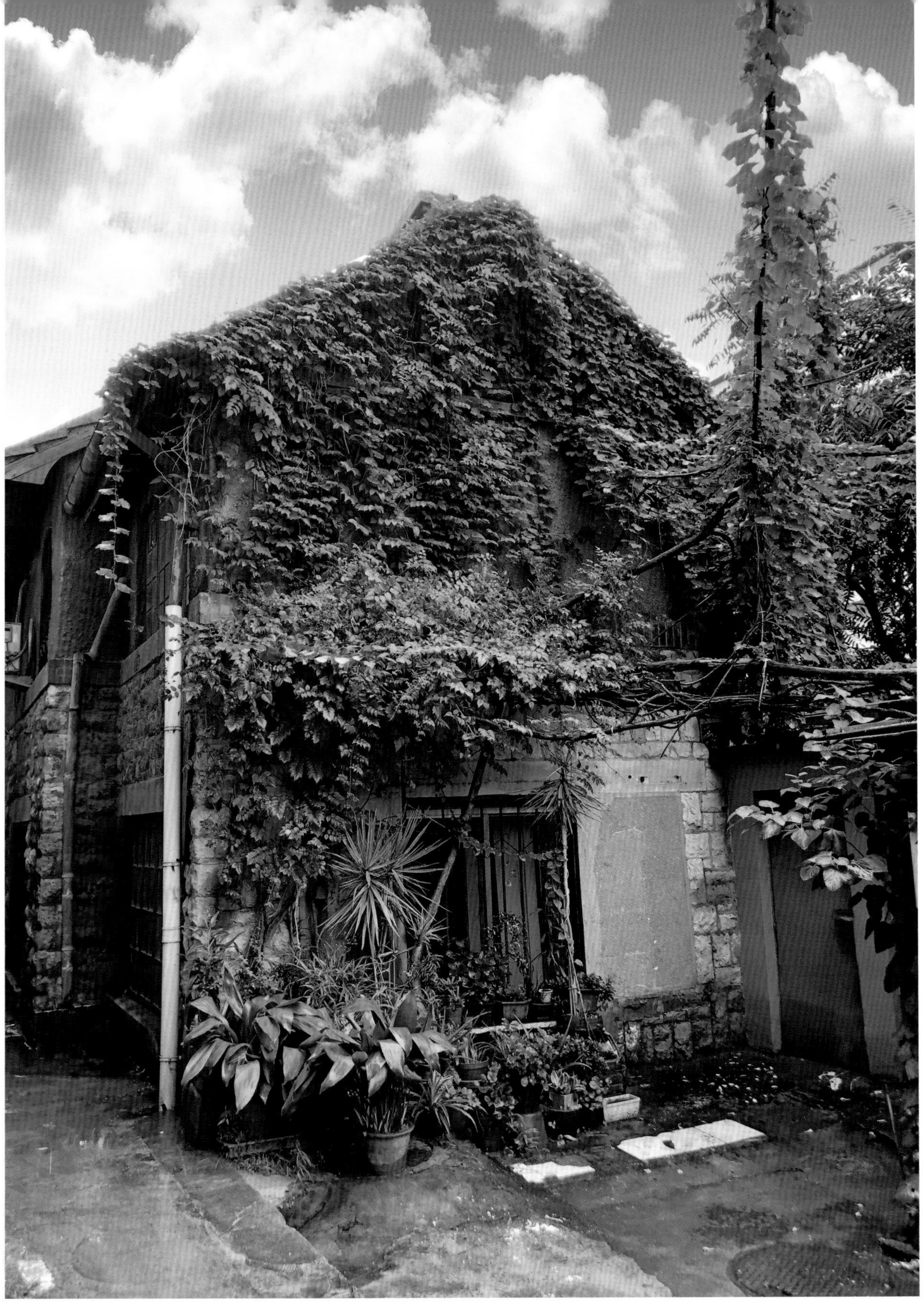

图 389 青杨路南、西村 3 号楼北的西侧别墅
Fig. 389 The west side of the villa in the north of Building No.3 in the West Village south of Qingyang Road

图 390 青杨路南、西村 18 号楼（原外籍教师宿舍）北侧别墅
Fig. 390 The villa in the north of Building No.18 in the West Village (former foreign teachers' dormitory) south of Qingyang Road

50 | 教工与学生宿舍

Faculty and Student Dormitory Buildings

现在的教工宿舍主要分布在校园周边的东村、西村和南村，学生宿舍主要位于体育场东侧、附属卫校和号院。随着社会的变迁，教工住房制度已发生了巨大变化，与齐鲁大学时期已完全不同了。

Now the faculty dormitories are mainly distributed in the East Village, the West Village and the South Village around the campus, and the student dormitories are mainly located on the east side of the stadium and in the affiliated Health School and the Courtyard. With the changes of society, the housing system for the faculty has undergone great changes, which is completely different from that of Cheeloo University.

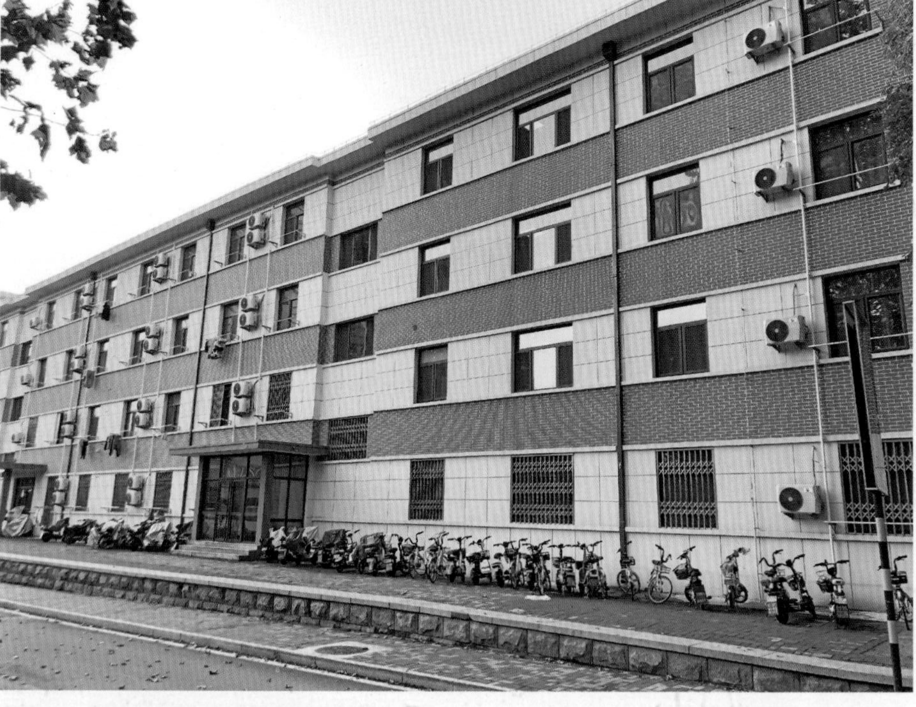

图 391 1 号学生宿舍楼南面观
Fig. 391 The south view of the No.1 Student Dormitory Building

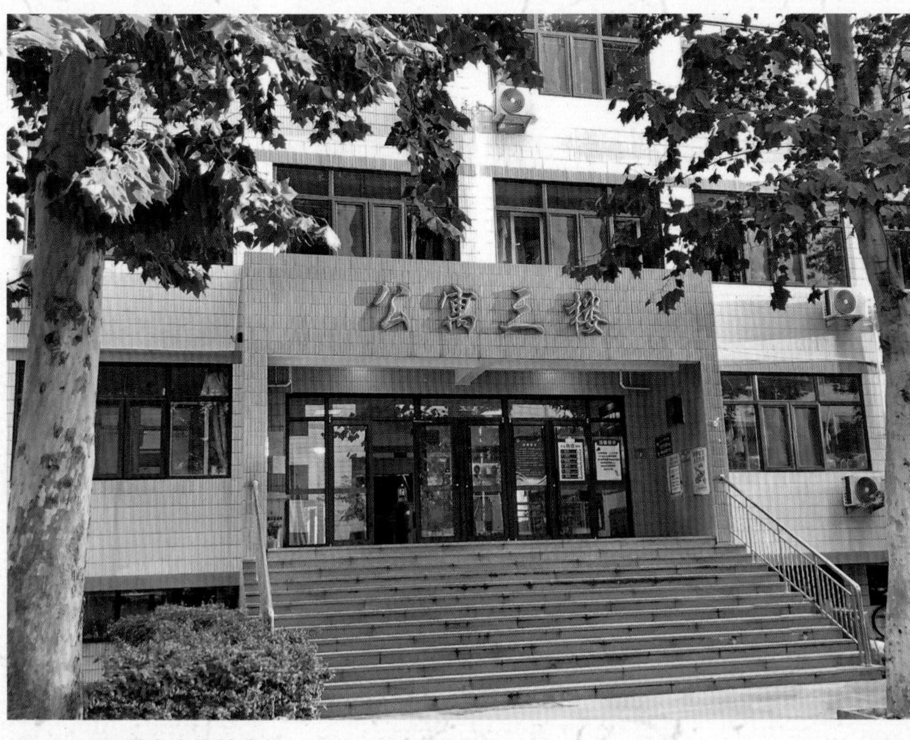

图 392 3 号学生宿舍楼南门
Fig. 392 The south gate of the No.3 Student Dormitory Building

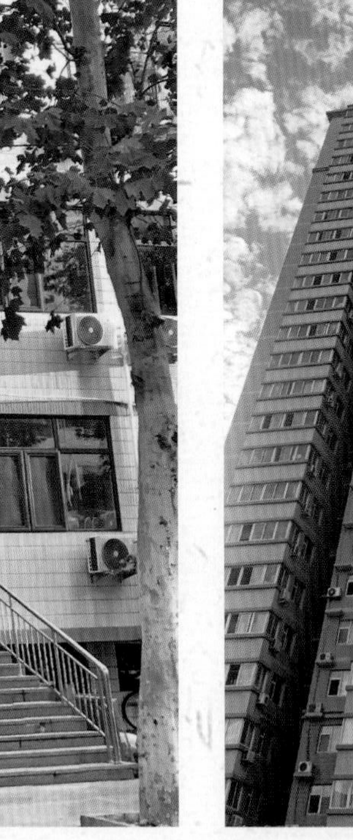

图 393 教工东村 8 号宿舍楼
Fig. 393 No. 8 Faculty Dormitory Building in the East Village

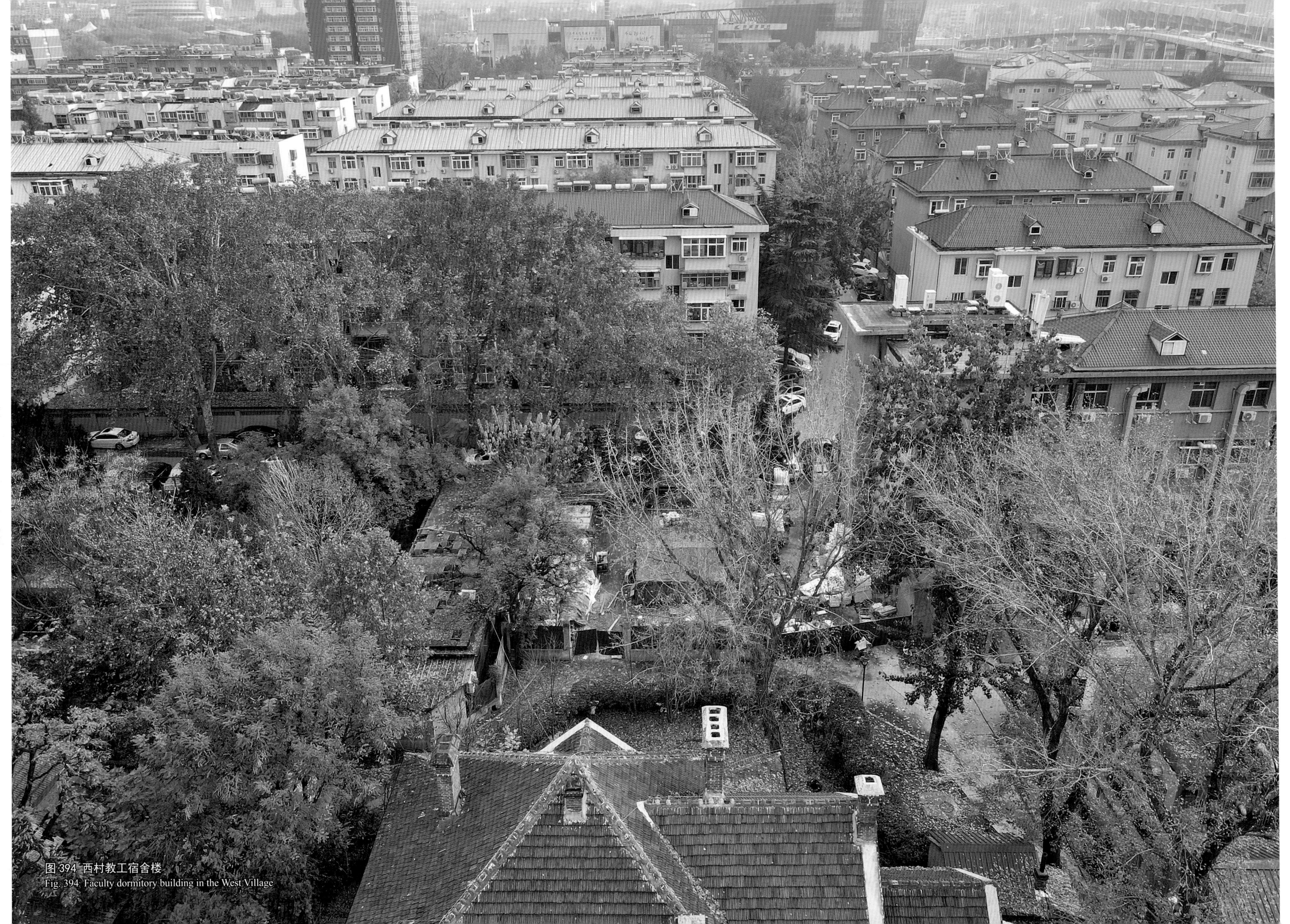

图 394 西村教工宿舍楼
Fig. 394 Faculty dormitory building in the West Village

51 春花烂漫（1）
Spring Flowers in Full Bloom (1)

梅花是中国十大名花之首，与松、竹并称为“岁寒三友”，以其高洁、耐寒、坚强、谦虚的品格，给人以立志奋发的激励。古往今来，仁人志士咏梅、画梅、摄梅，以表达对梅花的热爱。趵突泉校区的梅花主要位于校友门东侧的梅园内。最早开放的当然是蜡梅，花期足足有五个月，涵盖冬春两季。春节一过，红梅、朱砂梅、宫粉梅、绿萼梅、单瓣早白梅、六瓣白梅和单瓣跳枝梅等竞相开放，梅园一下子热闹起来。赏梅的人络绎不绝，连蜜蜂也不怕冷了，犹恐错过了采蜜的大好时光。大致三月中旬，杏梅、美人梅和榆叶梅怒放，远远望去满树的白云和红霞，交映生辉，美不胜收。这时，梅花交响曲迎来了高潮，梅园也到了一年的鼎盛时期。有《一剪梅》词一首为证：“前夜春来几树彤，梅放盈盈，蜂叫嗡嗡。今晨再探满园空，残萼仍红，幼子还绒。花似流云人似风，云逝轻轻，风过匆匆。落英潇洒去无踪，香尚朦胧，情更醇浓。”

Plum blossom ranks the first among ten famous flowers in China and is known as “three durable plants of winter” with pine and bamboo. With noble and unsullied, cold-resistant, strong and modest character, the plum blossom gives people the incentive to be determined to work hard. Throughout the ages, people with lofty ideals have eulogized, painted and photographed plum blossoms to express their love for them. The plum blossoms on Baotuquan Campus are mainly located in the Plum Garden on the east side of the Alumni Gate. The earliest to bloom is the wintersweet which flowers for five months, covering winter and spring. After the Spring Festival, varieties of the plum blossom compete to put forth their blossoms and the Plum Garden suddenly becomes lively. There is an endless stream of plum-enjoying people, and even bees are not afraid of the cold in order not to miss the good time of collecting honey. Around the middle of March, the plum blossoms of bungo Makino, Prunus blireana and Prunus triloba are in full bloom, with the branches full of white and rosy clouds being a feast for the eyes looking from afar. At this time, the symphony of plum blossoms comes to a climax and the Plum Garden also reaches the peak of the year. There is a poem “A Spray of Plum Blossoms” as evidence: “After one night of spring breeze, the plum blossoms were in bloom. The plum blossoms bloomed gracefully, and the bees buzzed in the clover. I went to the garden this morning and found all the plum blossoms had fallen, leaving the red remnants and budding blossoms. The flowers like drifting clouds that floated away gently, and people like the wind that passes in a hurry. The fallen petals were gone without a trace, leaving a faint aroma and strong feelings.”

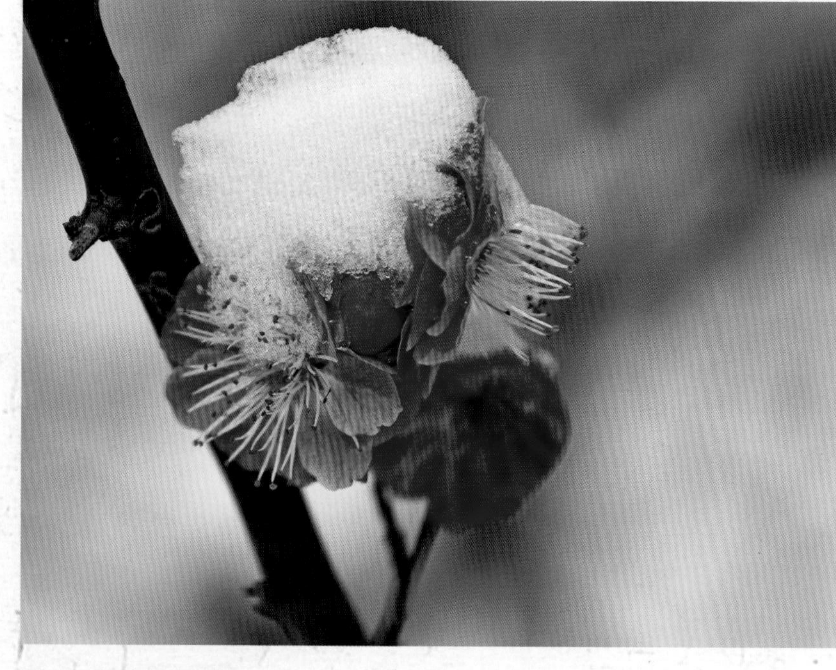
图 395 红梅笑迎春雪
Fig. 395 Red plum blossoms against the spring snow

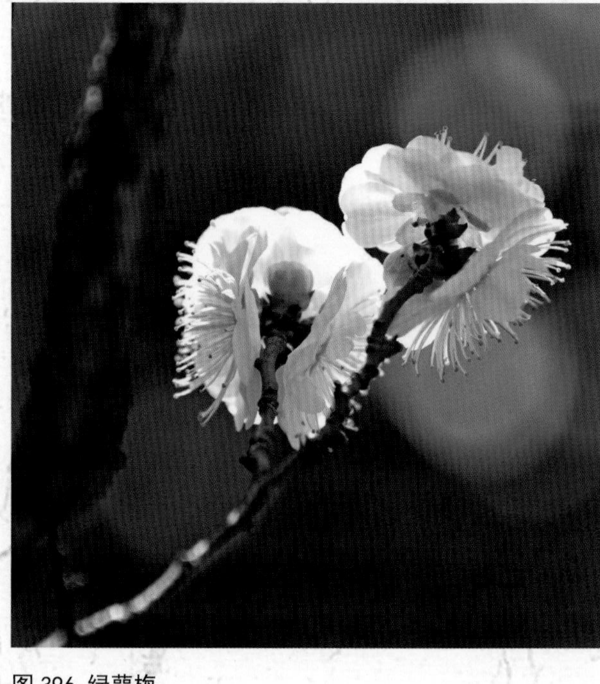
图 396 绿萼梅
Fig. 396 Armeniaca mume f. viridicalyx

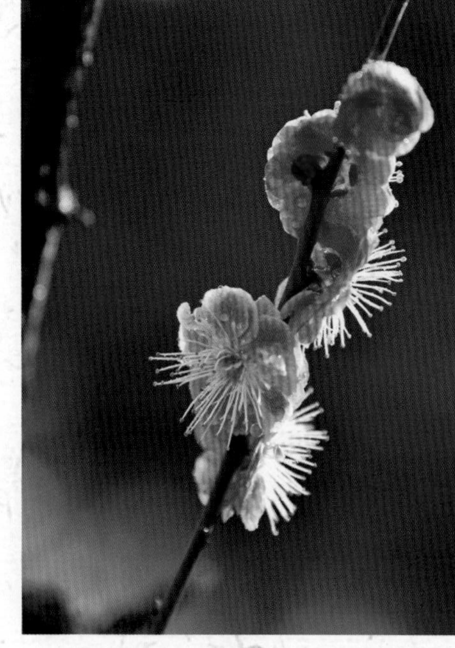
图 397 红梅不与群花同
Fig. 397 Red plum blossoms different from other flowers

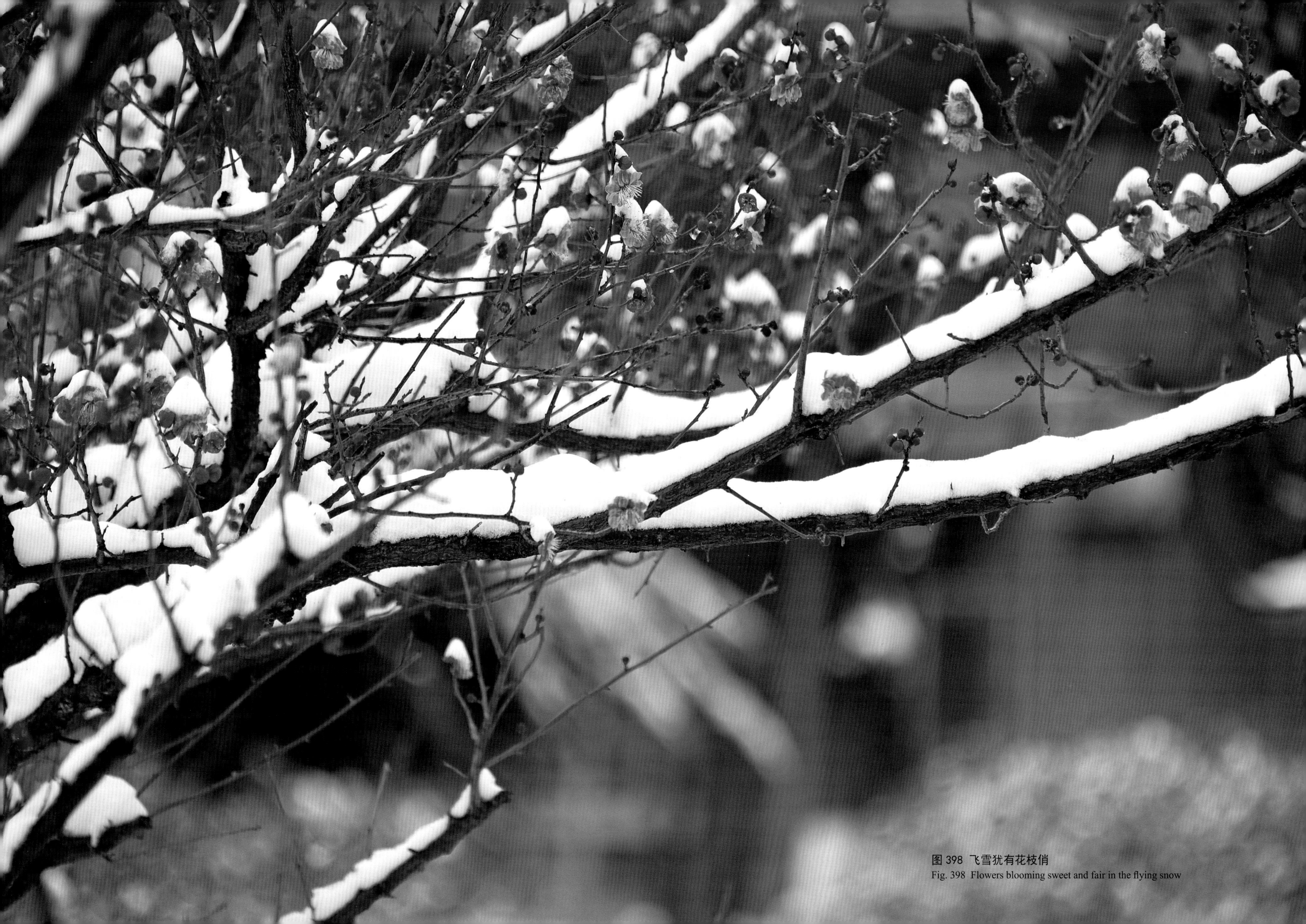

图 398 飞雪犹有花枝俏
Fig. 398 Flowers blooming sweet and fair in the flying snow

51 春花烂漫（2）

Spring Flowers in Full Bloom (2)

每到清明节前后，正是丁香花开的时候。远远望去，满树的丁香花像昨夜忽然飘落的白雪，在路旁和楼宇间摇弋。丁香花没有红梅花的夺目妖艳，更不具海棠花的婆娑多姿。它更像月光下的素衣仙子，静雅而恬淡。但它的香气却十分浓郁，犹如醇厚的陈年老酒，酯润咽喉，令人陶醉。丁香花花瓣很小，但万千朵白玉般的花儿一起开放，则显得十分热烈，整个校园仿佛都沸腾了。过往的行人也十分兴奋，激情被丁香花所点燃，喷薄四射。有诗为证：“翩翩素艳来，恍若舞瑶台。郁馥春风醉，清姿月影徊。云升花径亮，雪照玉楼白。此物通人意，应知为谁开。”

Lilac flowers bloom around the Tomb-Sweeping Day. From a distance, the lilac flowers look like the snow that suddenly fell last night, swaying by the roadside and between buildings. Different from red plum blossoms that are dazzlingly chanting and begonia flowers that are gracefully slender, lilac flowers like a plain fairy in the moonlight, quiet and graceful. But their aroma is very rich like the mellow wine of many years' standing that makes you intoxicating when you drink it. Although the petals are very small, it is a great scene when tens of thousands of white jade-like flowers bloom together and the whole campus seems to seethe with excitement. Passers-by are also very excited and burst with passion ignited by lilac flowers. There is a poem as evidence: “The white lilac flowers bloom in profusion, just like dancing in the terrace made of jade. The strong fragrance intoxicates the spring breeze, and the slender figure sways under the moon. The lilac flowers become bright as the clouds rise, and they shine on the building as white as jade. The lilac flowers thoroughly understand people's mind and they should know whom they bloom for.”

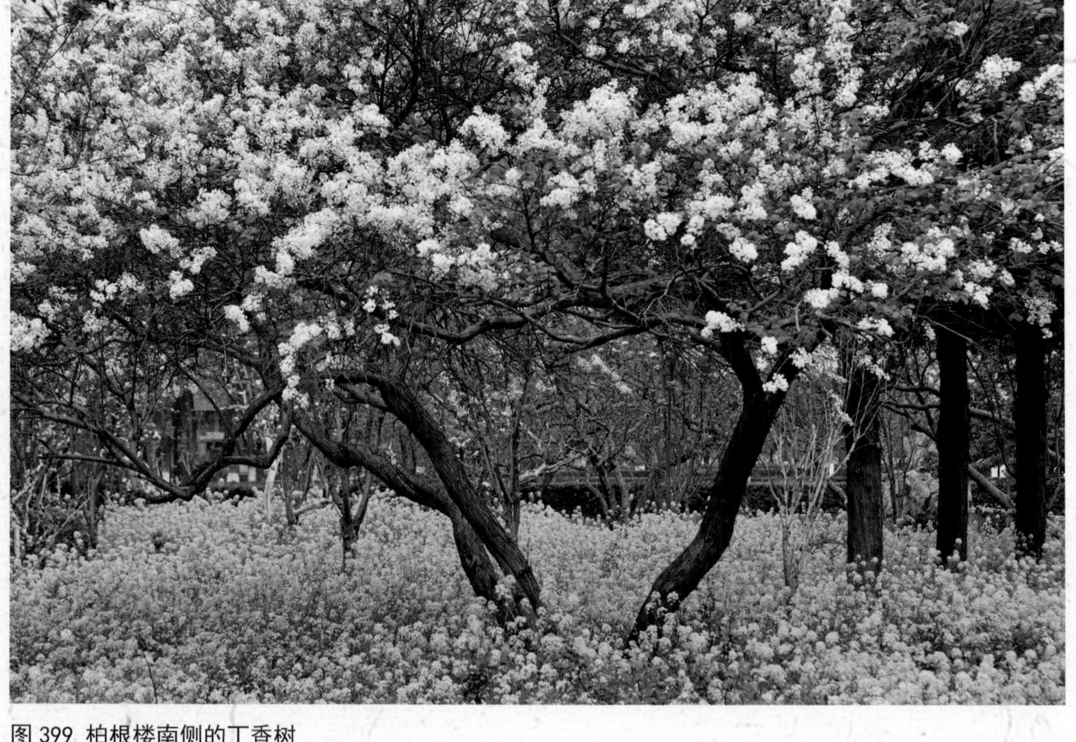

图 399 柏根楼南侧的丁香树
Fig. 399 Lilacs on the south side of Bergen Hall

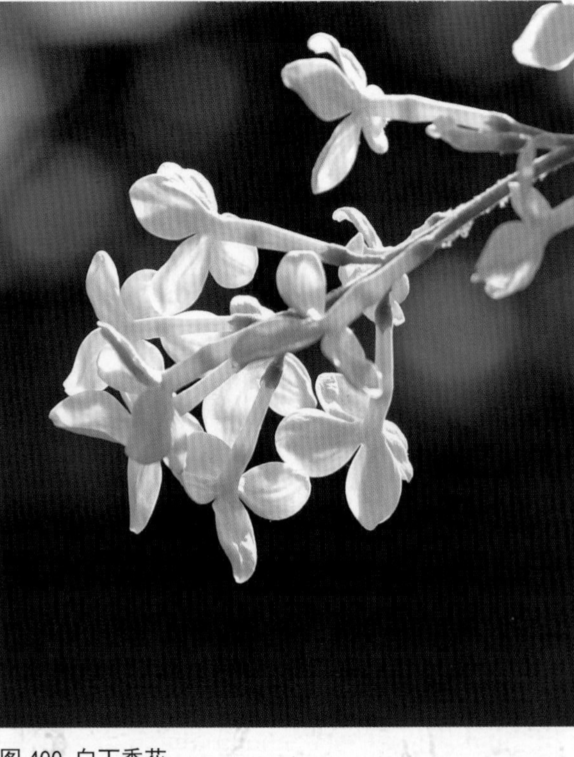

图 400 白丁香花
Fig. 400 White lilac flowers

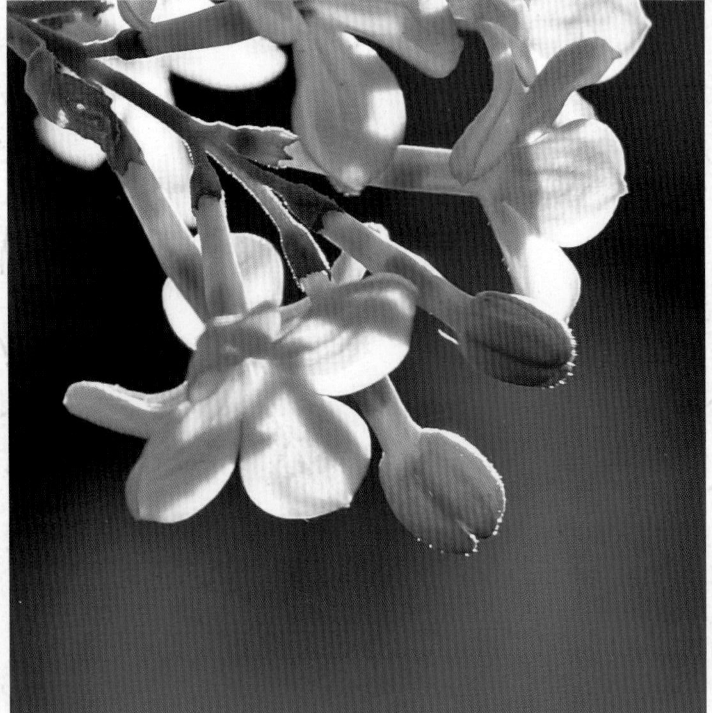

图 401 紫丁香花
Fig. 401 Purple lilac flowers

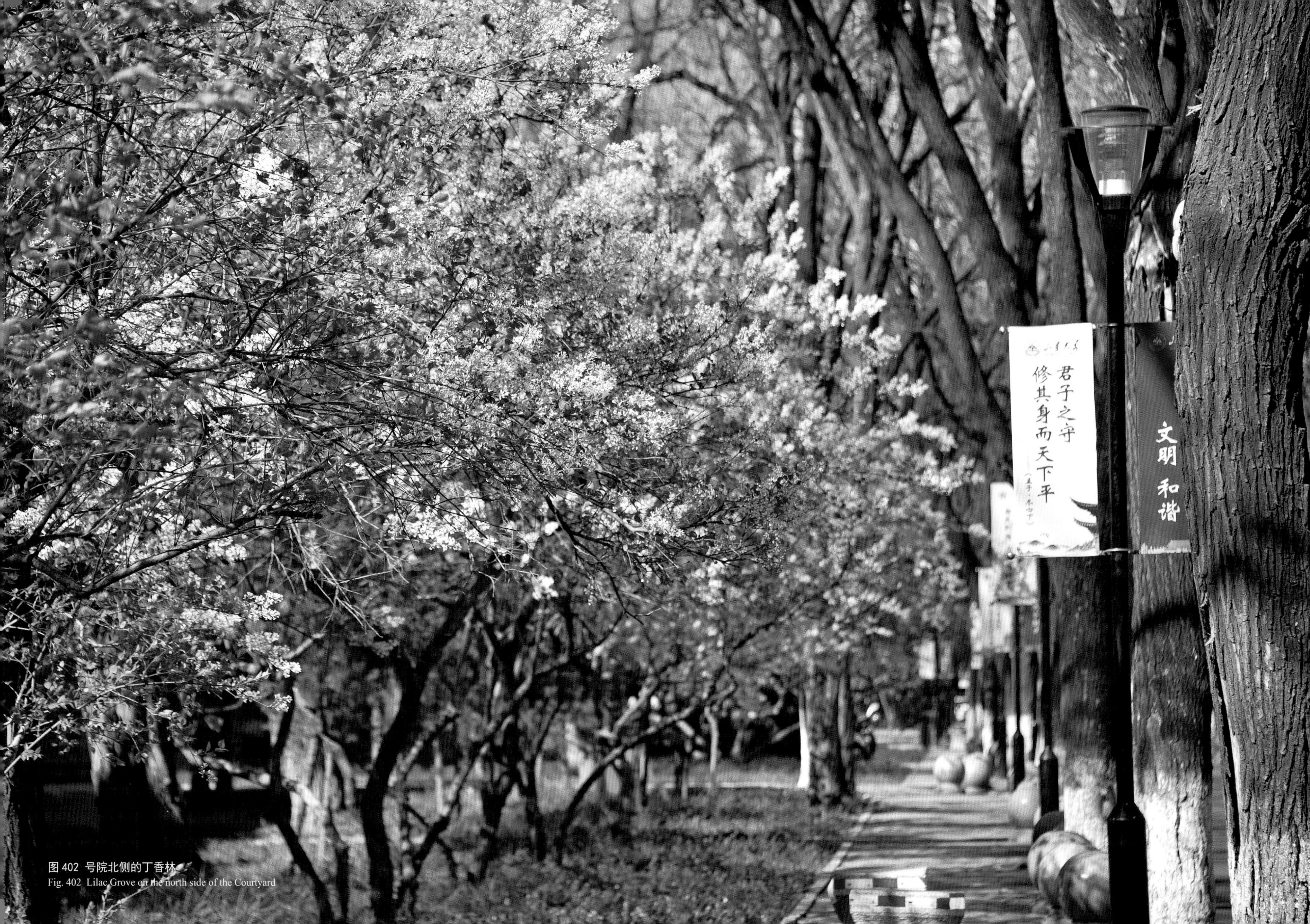

图 402 号院北侧的丁香林
Fig. 402 Lilac Grove on the north side of the Courtyard

51 春花烂漫（3）

Spring Flowers in Full Bloom (3)

春天一到，趵突泉校区就变成了花的世界。仰望树上，最为雅致靓丽的非海棠莫属。一朵朵，一簇簇，满树繁花盛开，微风拂来，若彩云飘动，甚是喜人。无怪乎苏东坡亦为之倾倒，写下了“只恐夜深花睡去，故烧高烛照红妆”的千古名句。被称为“海棠四品”的贴梗海棠、木瓜海棠、西府海棠和垂丝海棠校园内全有，另外在梅园内还能看到美洲海棠的身影。贴梗海棠主要栽培于花园两翼，每当春天，成千上万朵红花齐放，天都被照红了半边。木瓜海棠开在柏根楼南侧和药圃内，给人以悠然自得的感觉，微雨中娇艳欲滴，楚楚动人。西府海棠和垂丝海棠依旧含笑于柏根楼、教学一楼、圣保罗楼和梅园等处，尤其是西府海棠，花未开时，花蕾红艳上扬，似点点胭脂升起，开后则渐变粉红，犹如晓天明霞，高贵而典雅。正如陆游所描写的那样，“虽艳无俗姿，太皇真富贵”。所以，海棠素有“花中神仙”和“花贵妃”之称。

When spring arrives, Baotuquan Campus becomes a world of flowers. Looking up at the trees, you will find the begonia flowers are the most elegant and beautiful. When the breeze blows, clusters of begonia flowers in full bloom look like the floating iridescent clouds, which is very gratifying. No wonder Su Dongpo also fell for it and wrote the immortal words: “Fearing the flowers would go to sleep towards deep night, I burnt thick candles aloft to shine the beauties bright.” The four famous species of begonia flowers, Chaenomeles speciosa, Chaenomeles cathayensis, Malus micromalus and Malus halliana all can be found on the campus, and you can also find the American begonia in the Plum Garden. Chaenomeles speciosa is mainly cultivated on both wings of the garden. In spring, tens of thousands of red flowers bloom together, making half the sky red. Chaenomeles cathayensis blooms leisurely on the south side of Bergen Hall and in the Medicinal Garden, delicate and attractive in the drizzle. Malus micromalus and Malus halliana bloom around Bergen Hall, the First Teaching Building and St. Paul Building and in the Plum Garden. When Malus micromalus has not bloomed, the brilliant red buds rise like a little rouge. After blooming, the flowers gradually become pink like a bright glow in the morning, noble and elegant. Lu You once described begonia flowers as “gorgeous but not gaudy, rich and honored”. Therefore, begonia flowers are honored as “Fairy of Flowers” and “High-Ranking Imperial Concubine of Flowers”.

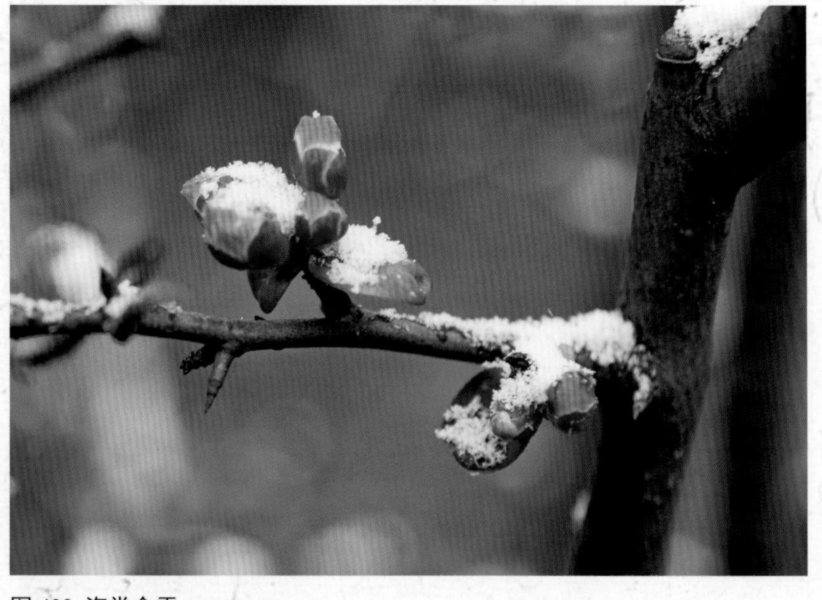

图 403 海棠含雪

Fig. 403 Snow-covered begonia flowers

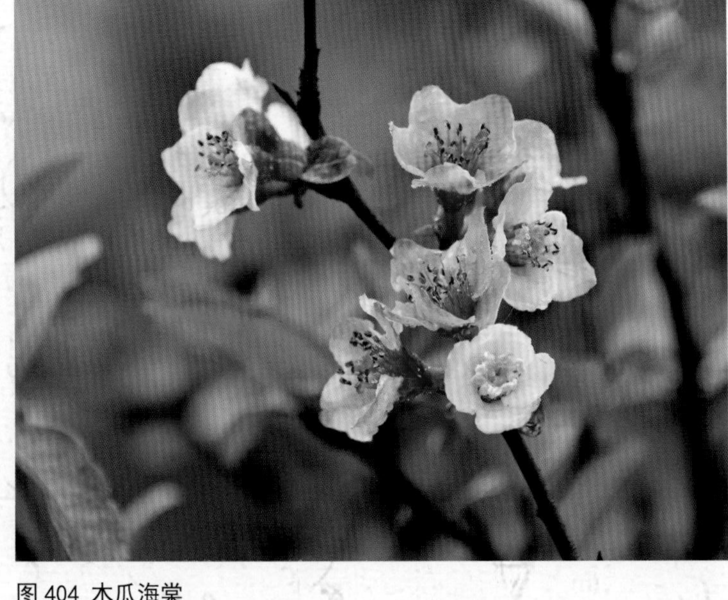

图 404 木瓜海棠

Fig. 404 Chaenomeles cathayensis

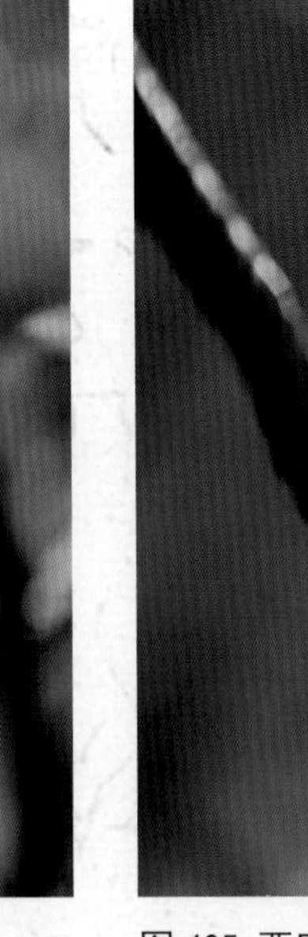

图 405 西府海棠含苞欲放

Fig. 405 Malus micromalus in bud

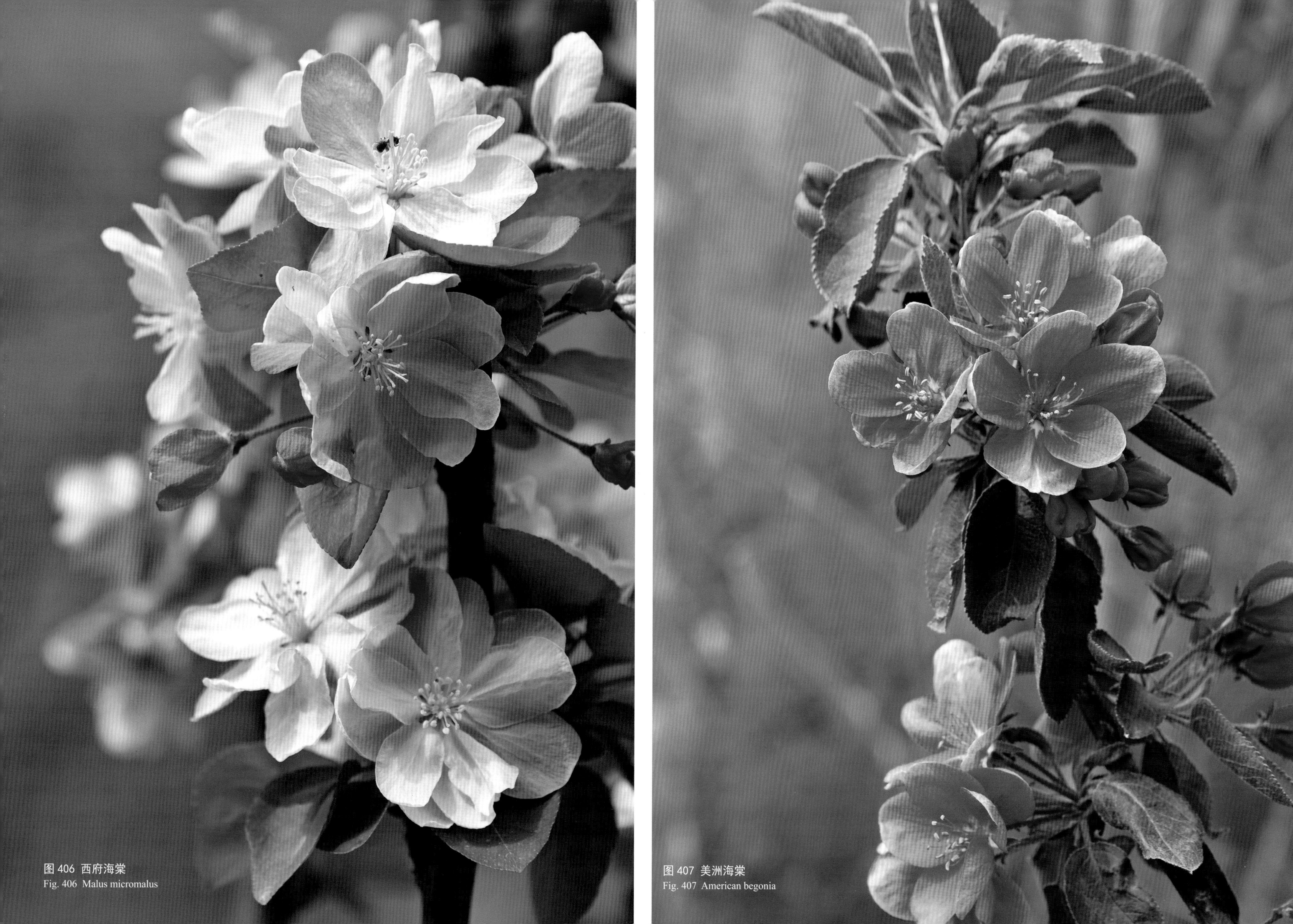

图 406 西府海棠
Fig. 406 Malus micromalus

图 407 美洲海棠
Fig. 407 American begonia

51 春花烂漫（4）

Spring Flowers in Full Bloom (4)

一看到樱花，总是想到鲁迅先生在《藤野先生》一文中所写的那句话：“上野的樱花烂漫的时节，望去确也像绯红的轻云”。据文献记载，樱花起源于中国，原产于喜马拉雅山脉。秦汉时期，宫廷皇族就已种植樱花，距今已有 2000 多年的栽培历史。唐朝时期樱花传入日本，并在日本发扬光大，成为其国花。

三月是樱花开放的季节，热烈而奔放，像一片薄薄的彩云在考文楼南面流动。在粉红色的花海中，白色往往被人忽视。那株硕大的白色樱花树在考文楼灰砖红窗的背景下，显得冰清玉洁，熠熠生辉。走近樱花，一股淡淡的清香入鼻，如锦似缎的花瓣开放得十分整齐，有一种昂扬向上的力量和生机勃勃的气势，催人奋进。樱花似乎凋零得很快，一阵清风袭来，万千片花瓣飘落，形成了一道“山樱花落红飘雨”的壮丽景观。

Seeing the cherry blossoms, I always think of Mr. Lu Xun's words in the article “Mr. Fujino”: “During the season when cherry blossoms were in full bloom around the Ueno Region, the sight seemed like patches of light crimson clouds.” According to literature, cherry blossoms originated in China and are native to the Himalayas. During the Qin and Han Dynasties, the royal family had planted cherry blossoms, which has a cultivation history of more than 2,000 years. Cherry blossoms were introduced to Japan during the Tang Dynasty and flourished there to become its national flower.

March is the season for cherry blossoms to bloom. Blooming in profusion, the cheery blossoms flow in the south of Calvin Mateer Hall like a piece of thin iridescent cloud. In the sea of pink flowers, the white ones are often ignored. That large white flowering cherry radiates purity against the grey bricks and red windows of Calvin Mateer Hall. Approaching the cherry blossoms, you will smell a delicate fragrance. The high-spirited strength and vigorous momentum of the neatly open brocade-like petals inspire people to forge ahead. Cherry blossoms seem to wither very quickly, and hit by a cool breeze, tens of thousands of petals fall, forming a magnificent scenery of “the red cherry blossoms falling like rain”.

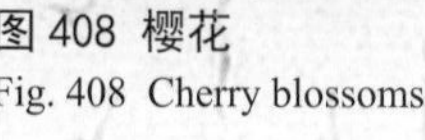

图 408 樱花
Fig. 408 Cherry blossoms

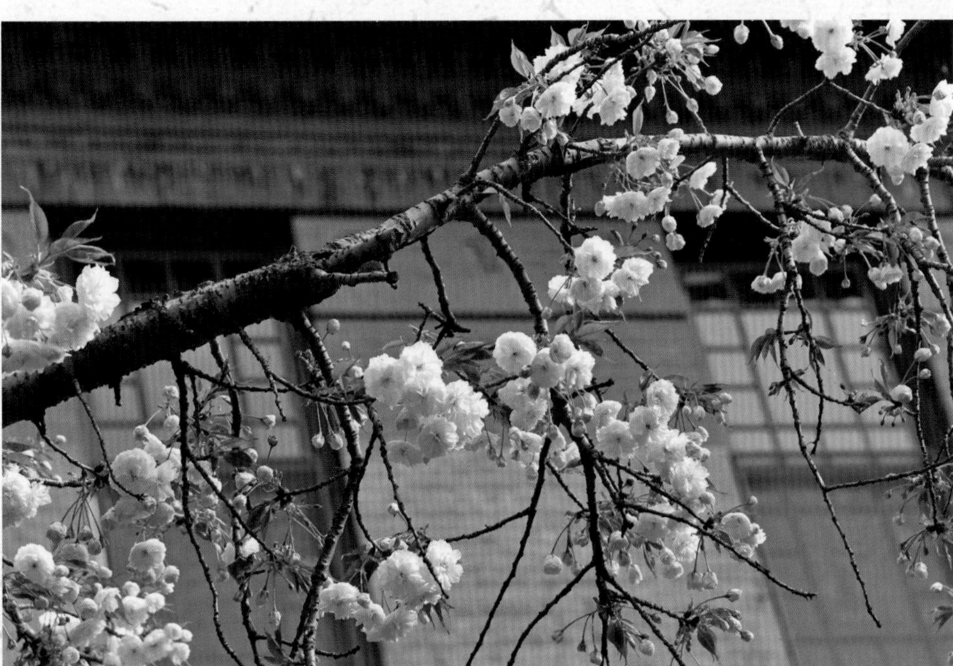

图 409 考文楼南侧的白色樱花
Fig. 409 White cherry blossoms on the south side of Calvin Mateer Hall

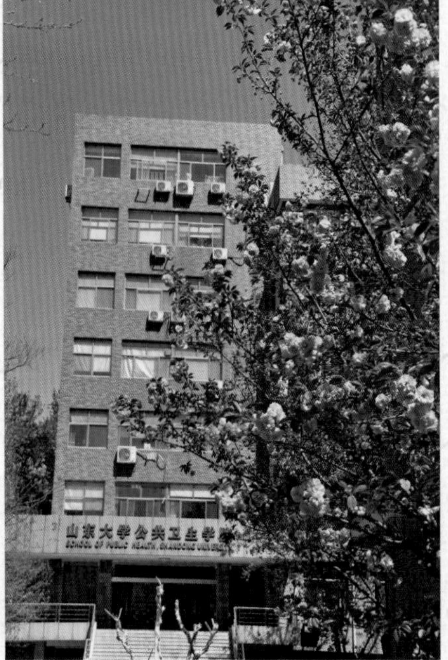

图 410 教学九楼南面的樱花
Fig. 410 Cherry blossoms in the south of the Ninth Teaching Building

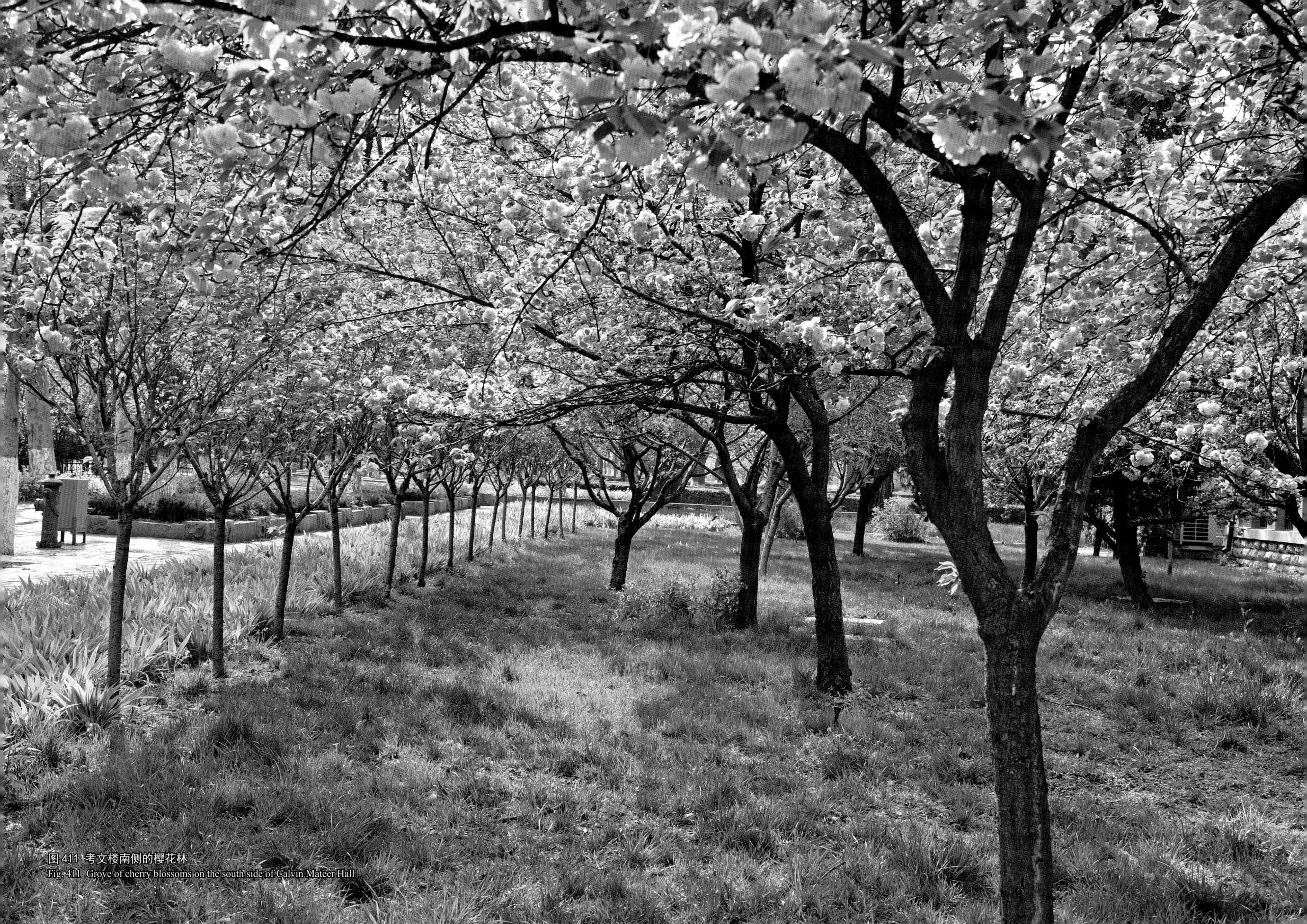

图 411 考文楼南侧的樱花林

Fig. 411 Grove of cherry blossoms on the south side of Calvin Mateer Hall

51 春花烂漫（5）

Spring Flowers in Full Bloom (5)

“四瓣蓝花碧叶出，氤氲梦幻艳泉都。一株虽可成风景，连片方能惊世殊。”这种开着四个紫蓝色花瓣的植物学名叫诸葛菜，俗称二月兰。仅仅一株二月兰虽然好看，但引不起多少人的注意。若是连片而生则令人大为震憾，这些紫蓝色的花瓣顿时汇合成了紫色海洋，在微风中翻着细浪，如梦如幻。我记得有一年，在中心花园的路边、柏根楼南侧、电镜楼南侧、教学二楼北侧、教学八楼北侧与西侧、图书馆南侧以及学生宿舍路旁，到处铺满了二月兰，一片片紫色的烟雾从地面上升腾，直冲云霄。二月兰花色多变，一开始为紫蓝色，继而变成了浅红色，最后褪色而成白色，颇为神奇。二月兰花期很长，接近两个月，真是一种美化地面的好植物。

“Blue flowers of four petals bloom among the leaves, and the dense blossoms amaze the Spring City. Although a plant can become a scenery, large areas of orchids can surprise the world.” The botanical name of the plant with four indigo petals is Orychophragmus violaceus. Although one plant of Orychophragmus violaceus is beautiful, it can not attract much attention. Large areas of Orychophragmus violaceus are really shocking. These indigo petals merge into a purple ocean and billow in the breeze. What a dreamlike scene! One year, the Orychophragmus violaceus bloomed at the roadside of the Central Garden and the student dormitories, on the south side of Bergen Hall, Building of Electron Microscopy and the library, on the north side of the Second Teaching Building, and on the north and west sides of the Eighth Teaching Building. Patches of purple mist rose from the ground to the sky. The color of Orychophragmus violaceus is changeable: at first it is indigo, then changes to light red, and finally fades into white, which is quite magical. The flowering phase of Orychophragmus violaceus is very long, nearly two months, and it is really a good plant to beautify the ground.

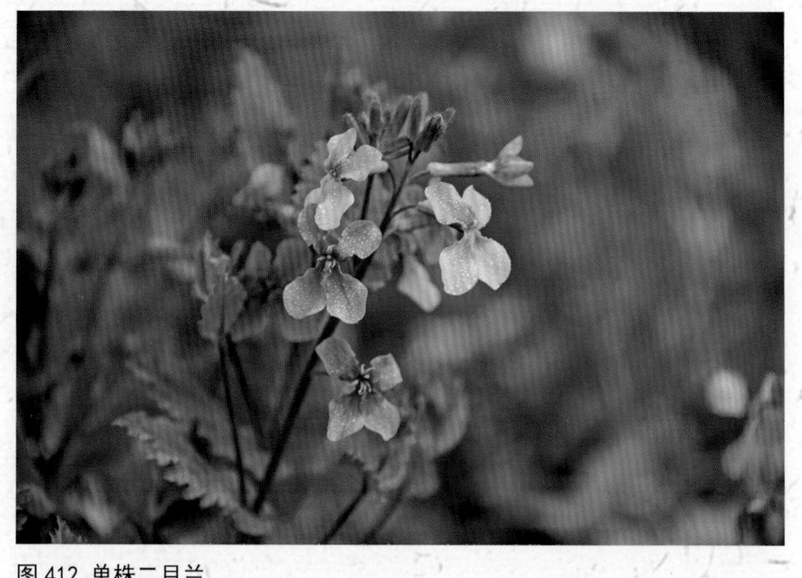

图 412 单株二月兰

Fig. 412 Single-plant Orychophragmus violaceus

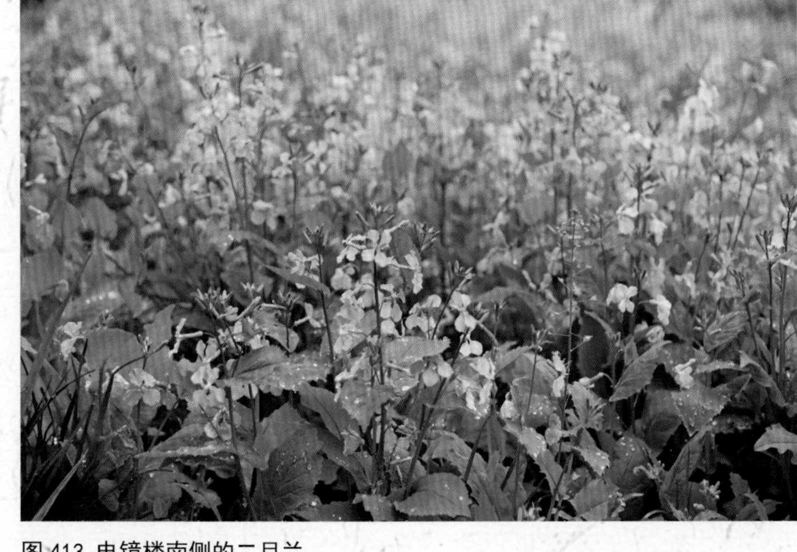

图 413 电镜楼南侧的二月兰

Fig. 413 Orychophragmus violaceus on the south side of the Building of Electron Microscopy

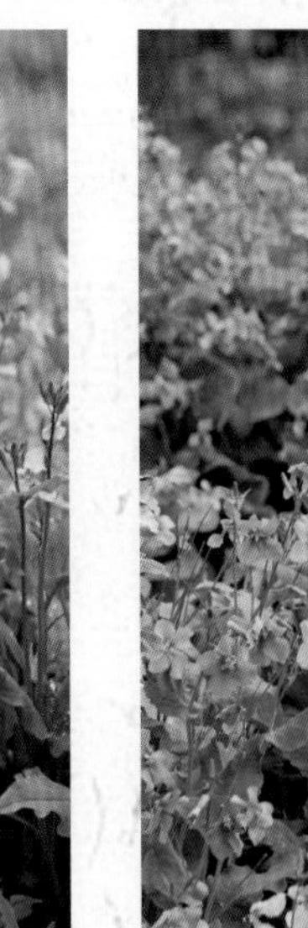

图 414 如紫色海洋般的二月兰

Fig. 414 Orychophragmus violaceus like a purple ocean

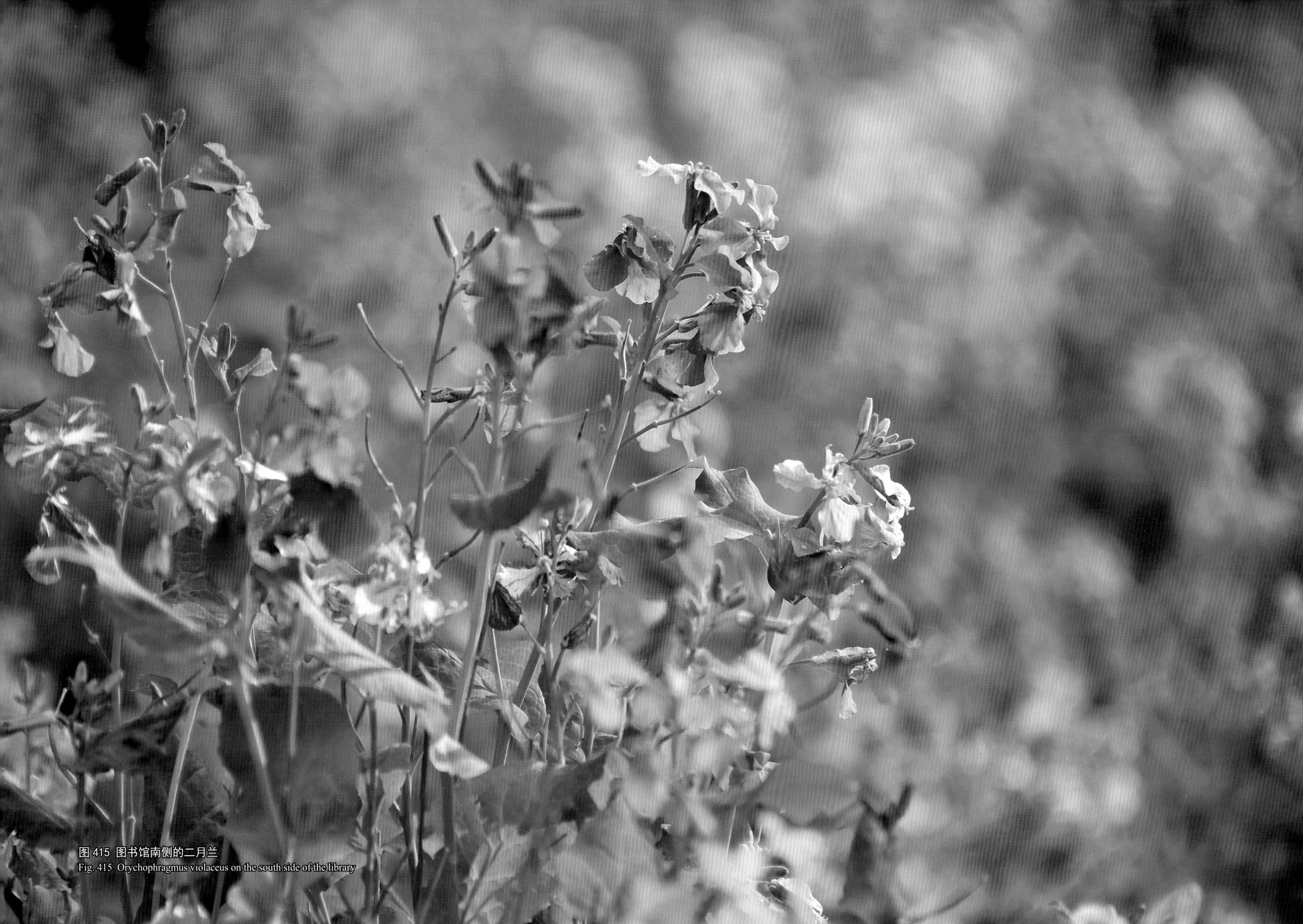

图 415 图书馆南侧的二月兰
Fig. 415 Orychophragmus violaceus on the south side of the library

51 春花烂漫（6）

Spring Flowers in Full Bloom (6)

牡丹，为多年生落叶灌木，有百花之王、国色天香等美誉，民间素认牡丹为中国国花。唐代著名诗人刘禹锡以“唯有牡丹真国色，花开时节动京城”的千古名句来盛赞牡丹。牡丹花朵硕大、形态优美、色泽鲜艳、香气浓郁，为历代人们所称颂，具有很高的观赏和药用价值。趵突泉校区，在护理学院大楼前、药圃内、教授别墅旁等处栽培有牡丹，花色有红色、紫色、白色、粉色和黄色不等。红色牡丹热情奔放，朝气蓬勃；紫色牡丹姹紫嫣红，娇艳动人；白色牡丹姣洁如玉，浩然大气；粉色牡丹雍容华贵，仪态万方；黄色牡丹高贵典雅，魅力四射。牡丹文化的起源，若从《诗经》牡丹进入诗歌算起，距今约 3000 年历史。秦汉时代以药用植物将牡丹记入《神农本草经》，牡丹从此进入药物学领域。南北朝时，北齐杨子华画牡丹，牡丹进入了艺术领域。

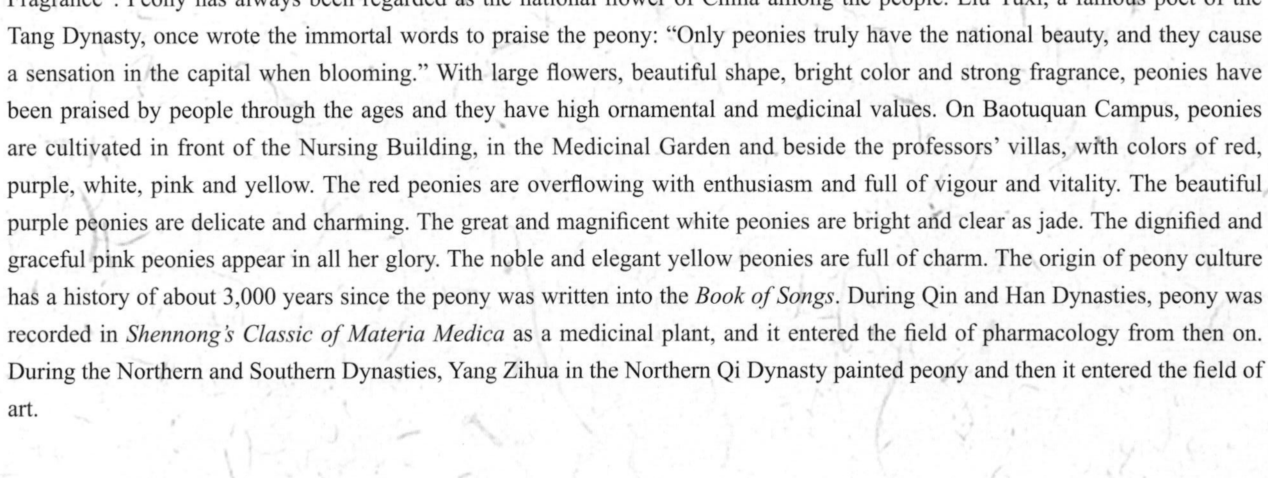

Peony is a kind of perennial deciduous shrub and is recognized as “King of Flowers” and “National Beauty and Heavenly Fragrance”. Peony has always been regarded as the national flower of China among the people. Liu Yuxi, a famous poet of the Tang Dynasty, once wrote the immortal words to praise the peony: “Only peonies truly have the national beauty, and they cause a sensation in the capital when blooming.” With large flowers, beautiful shape, bright color and strong fragrance, peonies have been praised by people through the ages and they have high ornamental and medicinal values. On Baotuquan Campus, peonies are cultivated in front of the Nursing Building, in the Medicinal Garden and beside the professors’ villas, with colors of red, purple, white, pink and yellow. The red peonies are overflowing with enthusiasm and full of vigour and vitality. The beautiful purple peonies are delicate and charming. The great and magnificent white peonies are bright and clear as jade. The dignified and graceful pink peonies appear in all her glory. The noble and elegant yellow peonies are full of charm. The origin of peony culture has a history of about 3,000 years since the peony was written into the *Book of Songs*. During Qin and Han Dynasties, peony was recorded in *Shennong's Classic of Materia Medica* as a medicinal plant, and it entered the field of pharmacology from then on. During the Northern and Southern Dynasties, Yang Zihua in the Northern Qi Dynasty painted peony and then it entered the field of art.

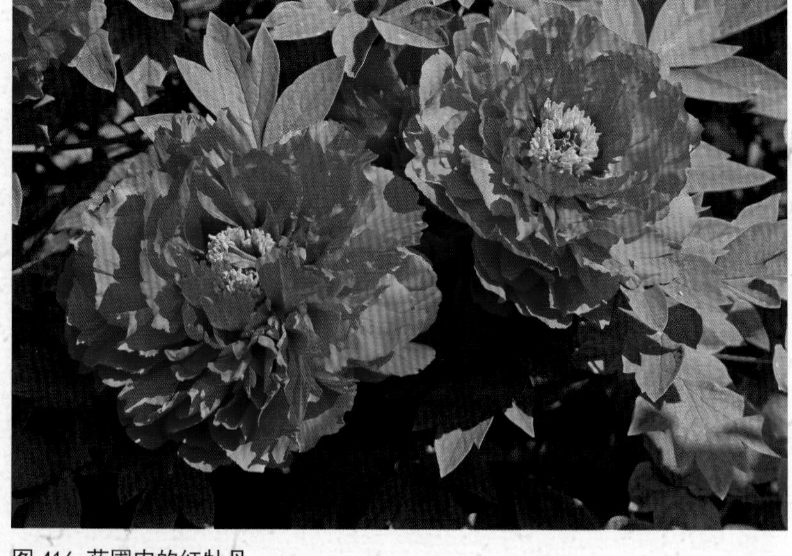

图 416 药圃内的红牡丹
Fig. 416 Red peonies in the Medicinal Garden

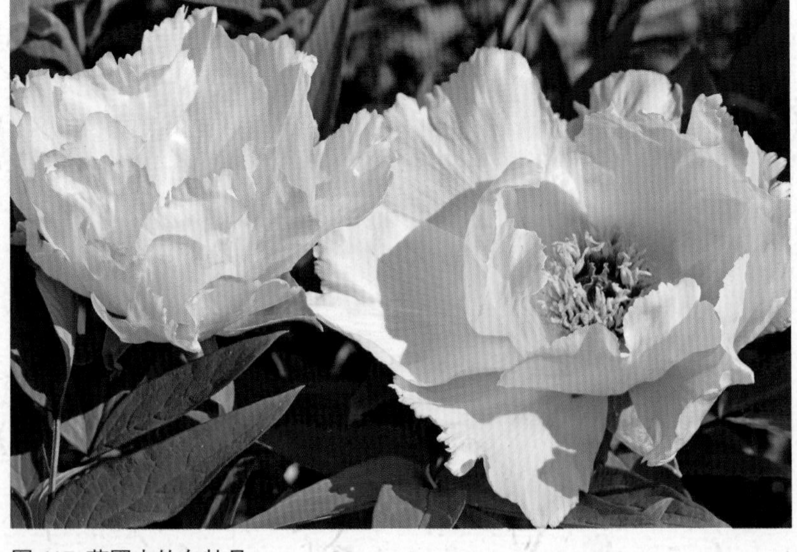

图 417 药圃内的白牡丹
Fig. 417 White peonies in the Medicinal Garden

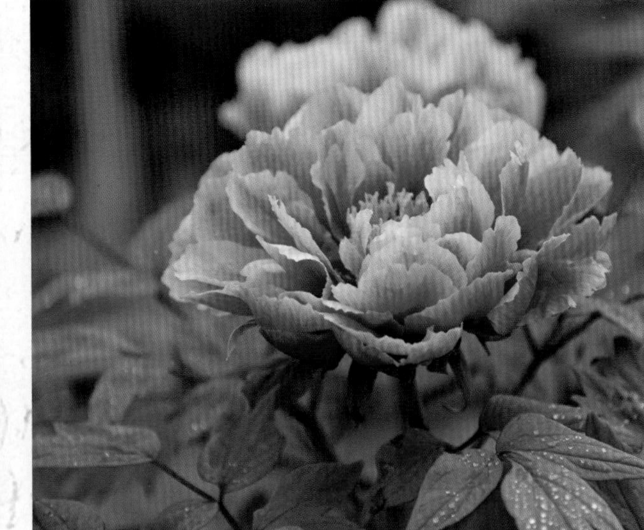

图 418 药圃内的粉色牡丹
Fig. 418 Pink peonies in the Medicinal Garden

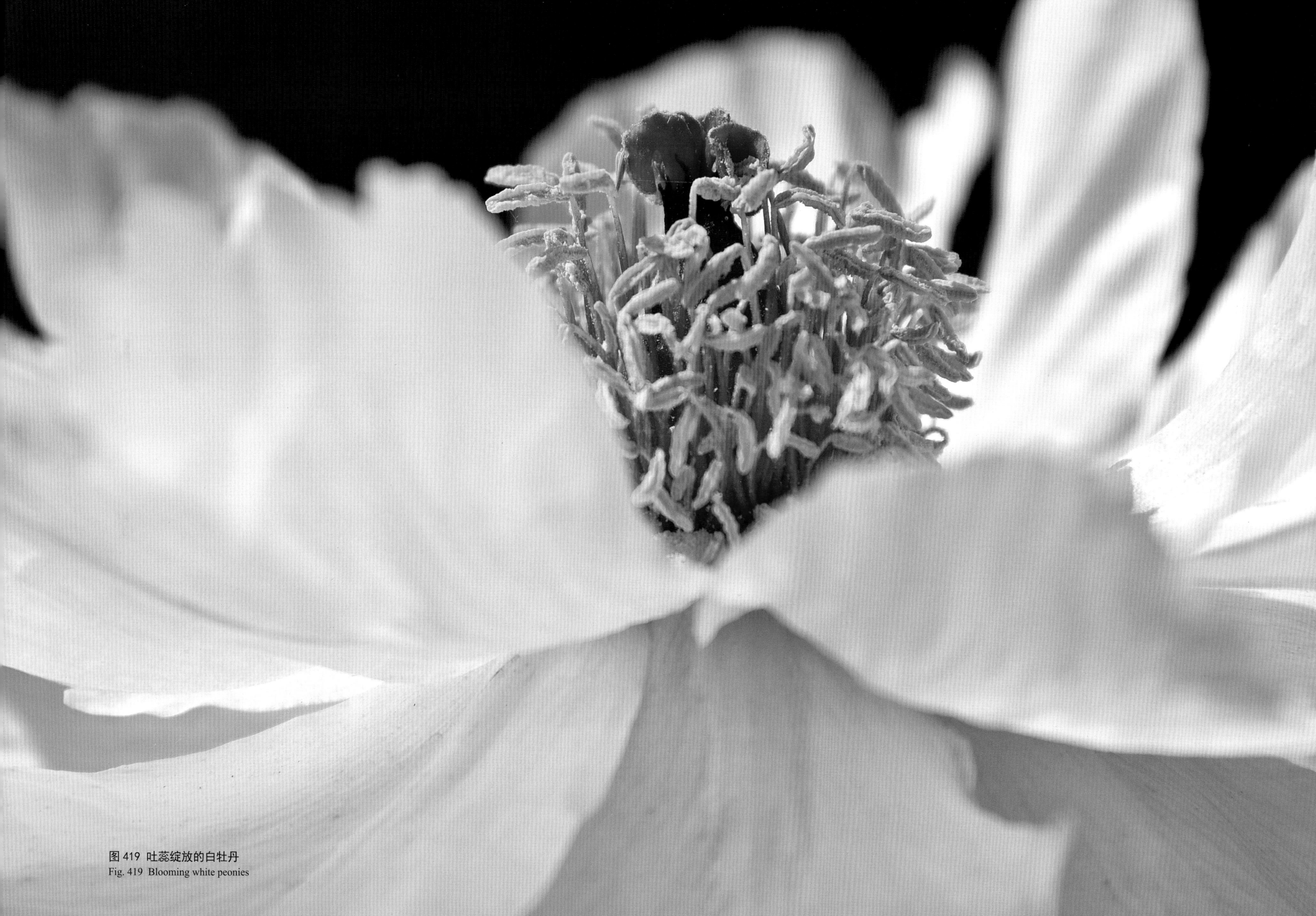

图 419 吐蕊绽放的白牡丹
Fig. 419 Blooming white peonies

51 春花烂漫（7）

Spring Flowers in Full Bloom (7)

据不完全统计，趵突泉校区内的树木花草约有 200 余种，本书只能选择具有代表性者予以介绍。在趵突泉校区内，种植最多的高大乔木恐怕就是国槐了，所以不能不说一说槐花。槐花一般在 4 ~ 5 月盛开，一串串洁白或红色的花朵挂在空中，随风摇曳，甚是赏心悦目。若有甜滋滋的香味袭来，则更沁人心脾。槐花的药用价值很高，其芦丁和三萜皂苷等成分，具有增强毛细血管韧性、防止冠状动脉硬化、降低血压、改善心肌循环的功效。在一排排的槐树中间，夹杂着几颗高大的楸树。平时过往的人们似乎对它们视而不见，只有某一天忽然间看到一片片美如小喇叭的花朵飘落在树下时，大家才抬头仰望那些高高在上、实际上也很难看清楚其“庐山”真面目的楸树花。这也许能给人以具有某种意义的人生启迪！

According to incomplete statistics, there are about 200 kinds of trees and flowers on Baotuquan Campus, and this book can only select the representative ones to introduce. On Baotuquan campus, the most planted tall trees are probably Chinese scholartrees, so we cannot but introduce sophora flowers. Sophora flowers generally bloom between April and May. Clusters of white or red flowers hanging in the air and swaying with the wind are very pleasant to the eye. If the sweet smell of sophora flowers strikes the nose, it is more refreshing. The sophora flower has high medicinal value, and its compositions such as rutin and triterpenoid saponin have the effects of enhancing capillary toughness, preventing coronary arteriosclerosis, reducing blood pressure and improving myocardial circulation. Among rows of Chinese scholartrees, there are several tall Catalpa bungei trees. Ordinarily people who pass by seem to turn a blind eye to them. Only one day when they suddenly see a sheet of flowers as beautiful as small horns falling under the tree, do they look up at those flowers of Catalpa bungei that are high above and actually difficult to be seen clearly. This may give people a sense of life enlightenment!

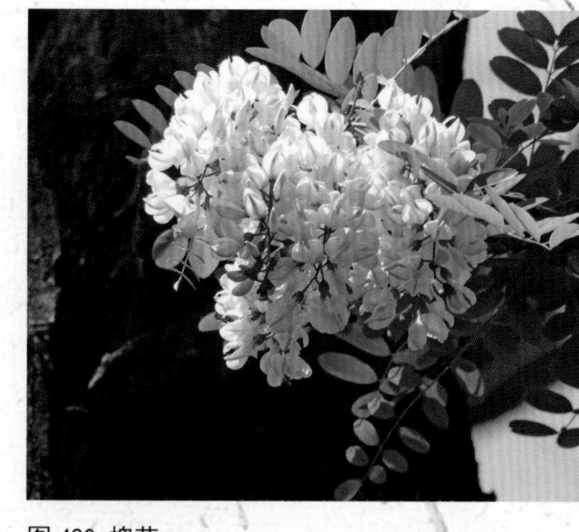

图 420 槐花
Fig. 420 Sophora flowers

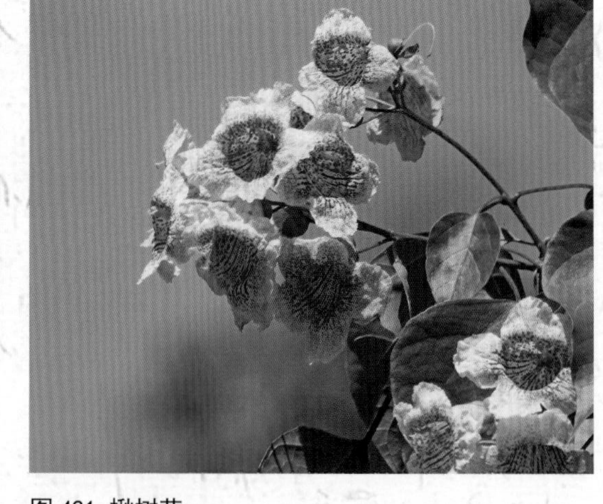

图 421 楸树花
Fig. 421 Flowers of catalpa bungei

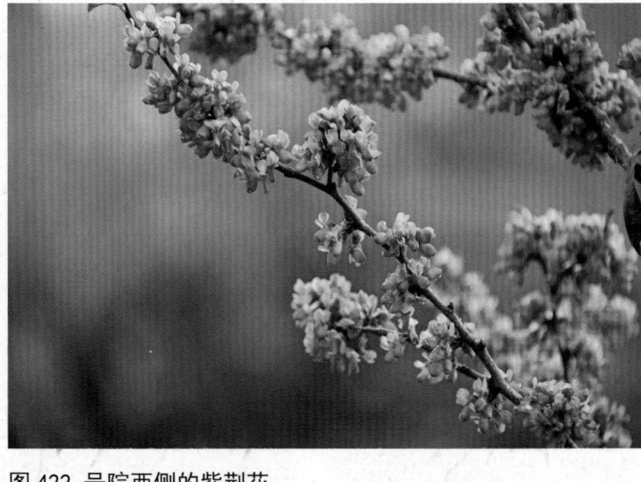

图 422 号院西侧的紫荆花
Fig. 422 Bauhinia flowers on the west side of the Courtyard

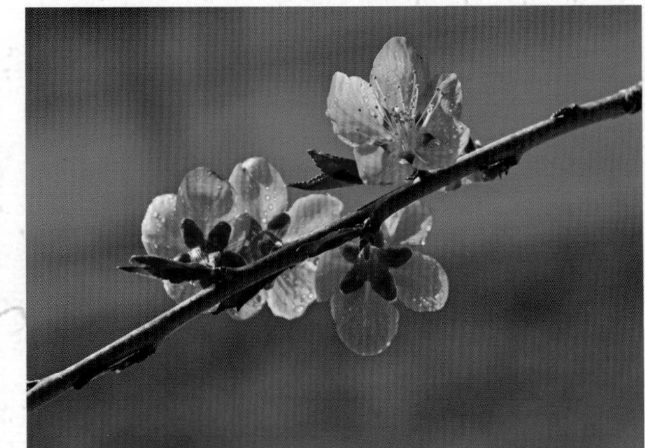

图 423 教学八楼北侧的红花碧桃
Fig. 423 Amygdalus persica f. rubro-plena on the north side of the Eight Teaching Building

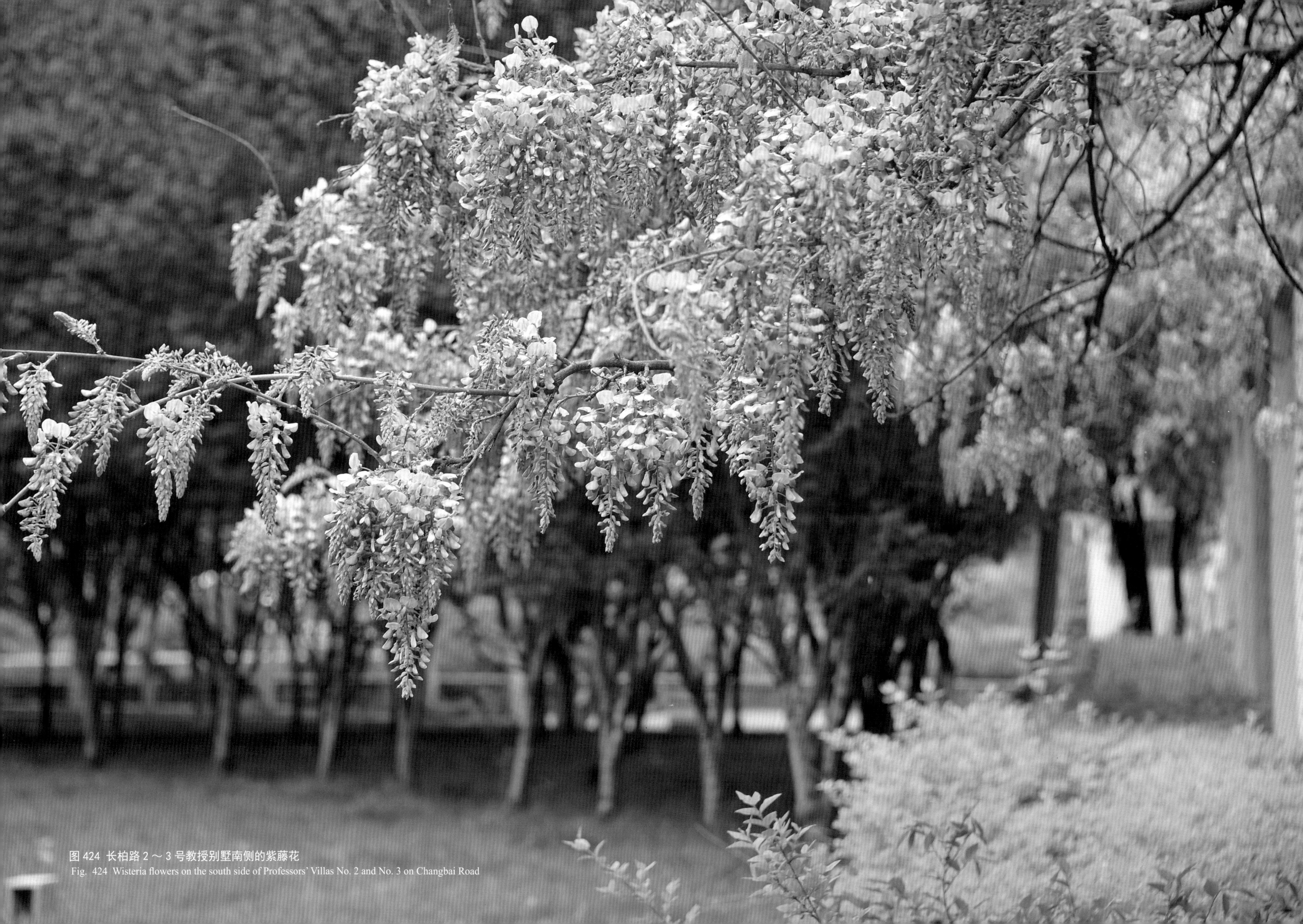

图 424 长柏路 2～3 号教授别墅南侧的紫藤花
Fig. 424 Wisteria flowers on the south side of Professors' Villas No. 2 and No. 3 on Changbai Road

51 春花烂漫（8）

Spring Flowers in Full Bloom (8)

鸢尾原产于欧洲，花大而姣美，叶茎碧绿如玉，甚为人们喜爱。鸢尾花色缤纷多彩，白色代表浪漫纯真，黄色表示热情开放，蓝色暗示赞赏对方，紫色则寓意爱意与吉祥。朱顶红又名红花莲，主要分布于巴西以及中国海南省等地。它花茎挺直，冠大色艳，给人以磅礴之势。又恰似指路明灯，无论在何时何地，只要人们看到它，总能驱散迷雾，向着正确的方向前进。

马兰花根系发达，抗旱，耐盐碱，在恶劣条件下也能生长，生命力十分顽强。马兰花不慕虚名，踏踏实实，花朵和长叶宛如展开的翅膀，就要飞向蓝天。所以有诗赞道：“不慕红花俏，无心碧树高。茁茁贴地草，展翅向云霄。” 紫花耧斗菜，又名鸽子花，多年生草本植物，叶子似芹菜，花形奇特，总是谦虚地低着头。它是那么地顽强，只要有些许泥土，点滴水分，便能茁壮成长。

The iris is native to Europe, with large and beautiful flowers and jade green leaves and stems, which is very popular. There is a great variety of colors: the white represents romance and innocence, the yellow represents enthusiasm and openness, the blue implies appreciation of other people, and the purple implies love and luck. Hippeastrum rutilum is mainly distributed in Brazil and Hainan Province of China. With upright flower stem and bright-colored large corolla, it gives people a feeling of tremendous momentum. It is also like a guiding light. Whenever and wherever people see it, they can always come through the fog and move in the right direction.

With well developed root system, Iris lactea is drought resisting and saline-alkaline tolerant. With tenacious vitality, it can grow under severe conditions. Iris lactea does not seek bubble reputation and stands on solid ground. Its flowers and long leaves like wings that will fly to the blue sky. Therefore, there is a poem to praise it: “Iris lactea neither envies the beauty of red flowers nor wants to be as tall as the green trees. It sticks to the grass when sprouting and then spreads its wings to the sky.” Aquilegia viridiflora f. atropurpurea is a perennial herb with celery-like leaves and flowers of strange shape that always lower the head modestly. It is so tenacious that it can thrive as long as there is a little soil and a little water.

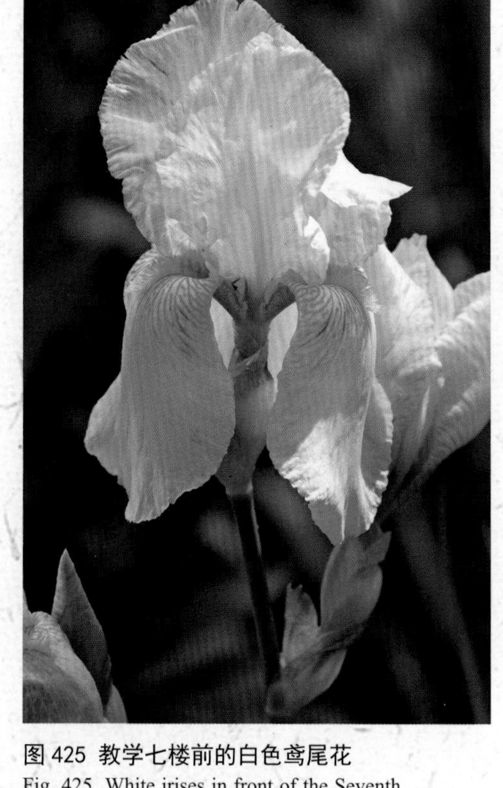

图 425 教学七楼前的白色鸢尾花

Fig. 425 White irises in front of the Seventh Teaching Building

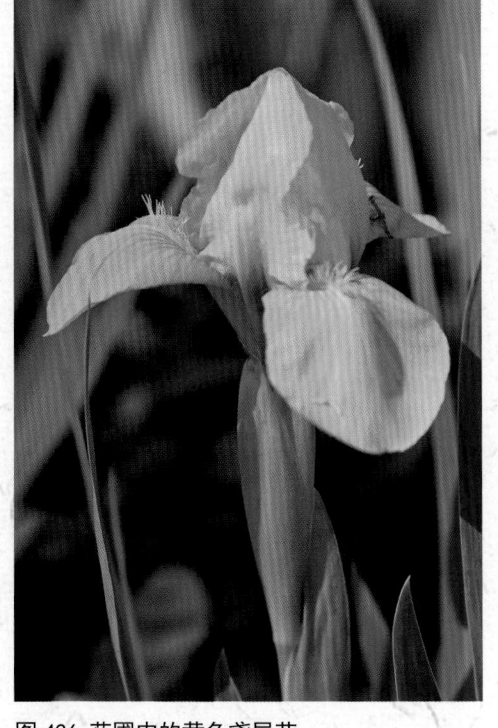

图 426 药圃内的黄色鸢尾花

Fig. 426 Yellow irises in the Medicinal Garden

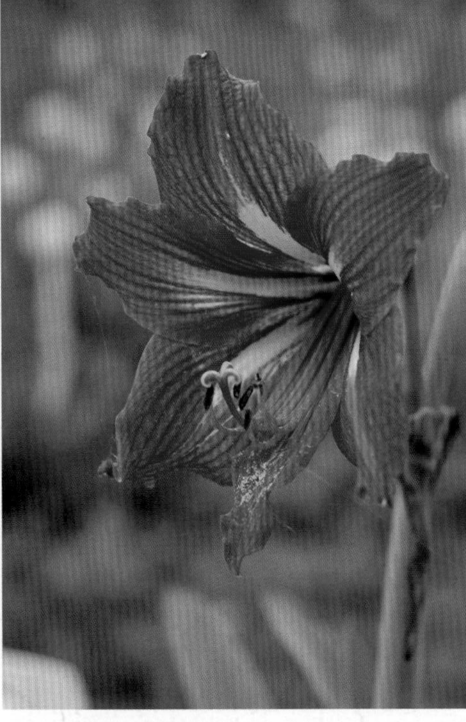

图 427 药圃内的朱顶红

Fig. 427 Hippeastrum rutilum in the Medicinal Garden

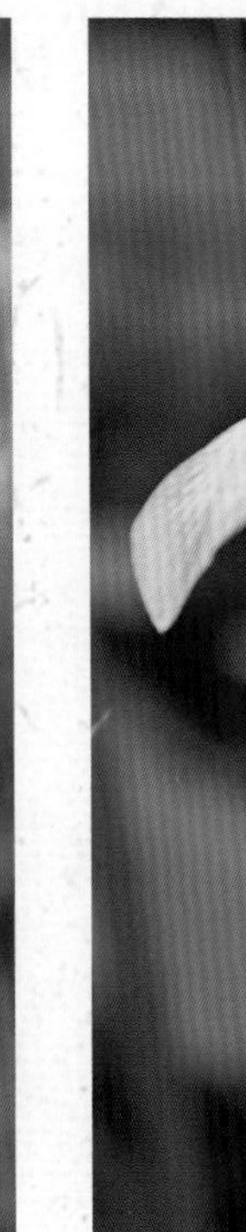

图 428 教学四楼前的马兰花

Fig. 428 Iris lactea in front of the Fourth Teaching Building

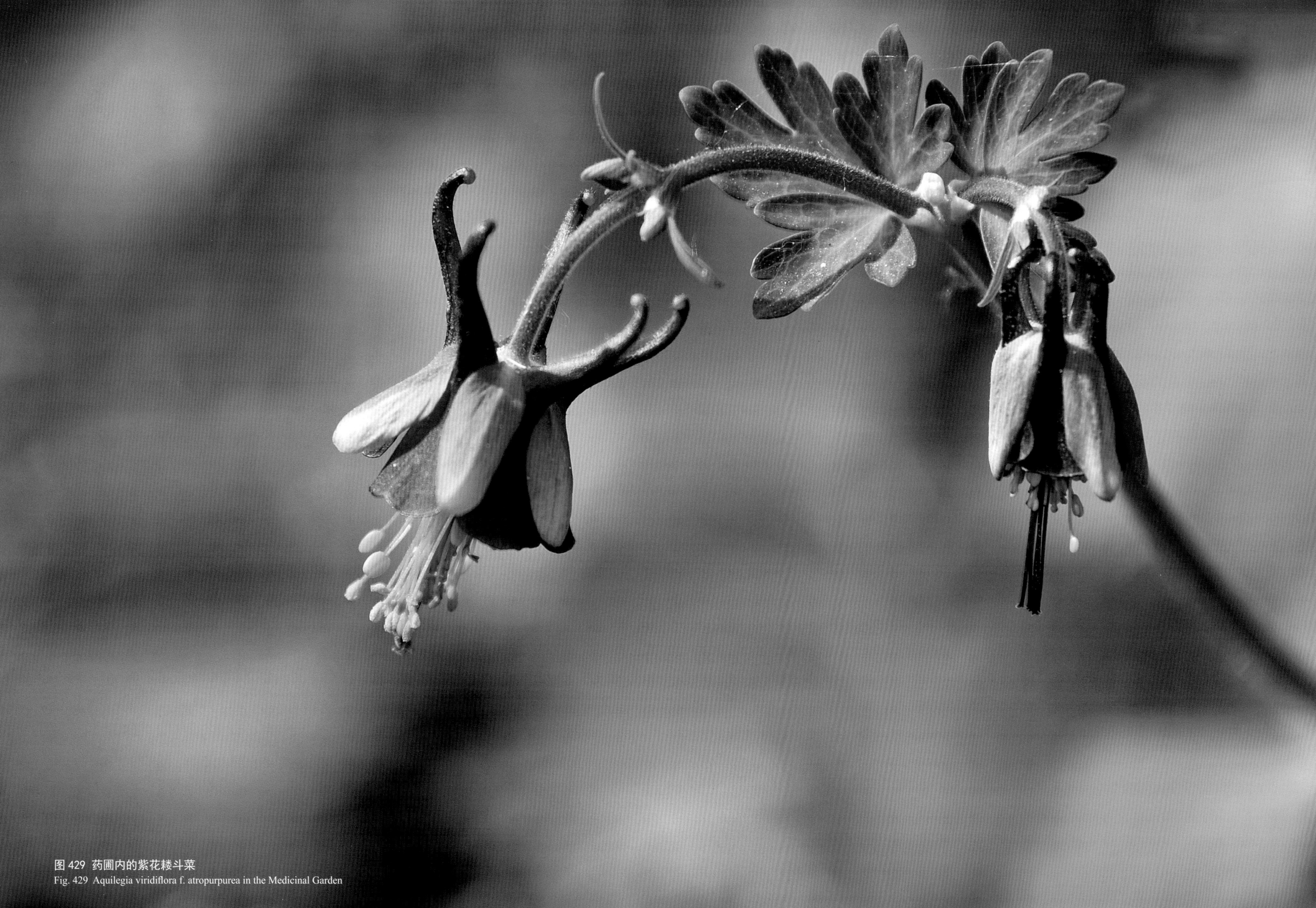
图 429 药圃内的紫花耧斗菜
Fig. 429 Aquilegia viridiflora f. atropurpurea in the Medicinal Garden

52 | 夏景宜人（1）

Attractive Scenery in Summer (1)

夏天，趵突泉校区笼罩在一片郁郁葱葱的树林之中。与车水马龙的闹市相比，虽显冷清宁静，然实则是“风声雨声读书声，声声入耳；家事国事天下事，事事关心”的内在繁忙。

校园内道路两旁绿树成荫，树干整齐排列，树冠两侧交织，形成了一条条林荫大道。有的林荫大道，两侧树木粗壮，遮天蔽日，则可称为绿色隧道。这些林荫大道多数由槐树构成，有的则由银杏、松柏、法桐或枫树织就，也有多树种的，如青杨路，东西两段路两侧为法桐，中段则由枫树、法桐和松树混合组成。在林荫大道上行走，定会有心旷神怡、疲劳尽释之感！

In summer, Baotuquan Campus is shrouded in a lush wood. Compared with the busy downtown area, it seems deserted and quiet. Actually it holds the busy inner which can be described as: “The sounds of the wind, of the rain, and of reading aloud all come to my ears; the affairs of the family, of the state and of the world are all my concerns.”

On campus, both sides of the roads are shaded by trees; the trunks are arranged in order and the crowns on both sides are interwoven to form tree-lined avenues. Some avenues, with strong trees on both sides that can blot out the sky and cover the sun, can be called green tunnels. Most of these avenues are flanked by pagoda trees, and some are flanked by ginkgo trees, pines and cypresses, plane trees or maple trees respectively. On Qingyang Road, there are plane trees on both sides of the east and west sections of the road, and there are maples, plane trees and pines in the middle section. Walking on the avenues, you will feel fresh and completely relaxed!

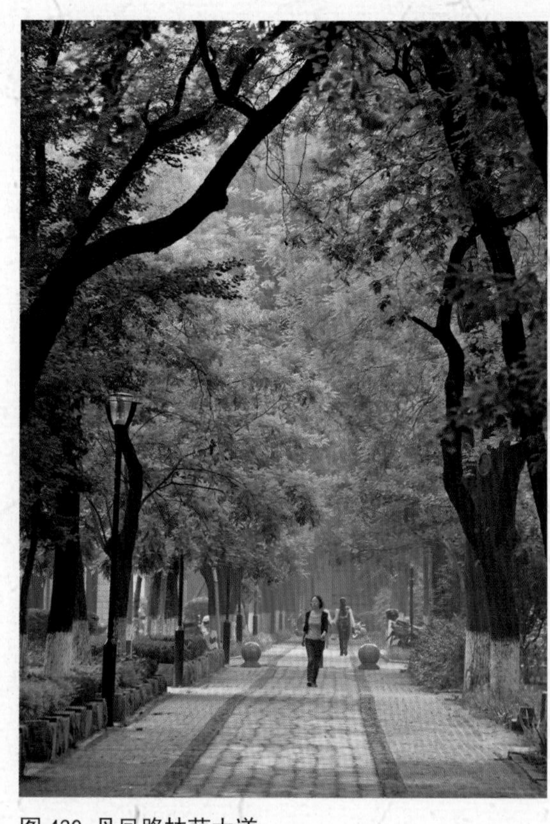

图 430 丹凤路林荫大道
Fig. 430 Avenue on Danfeng Road

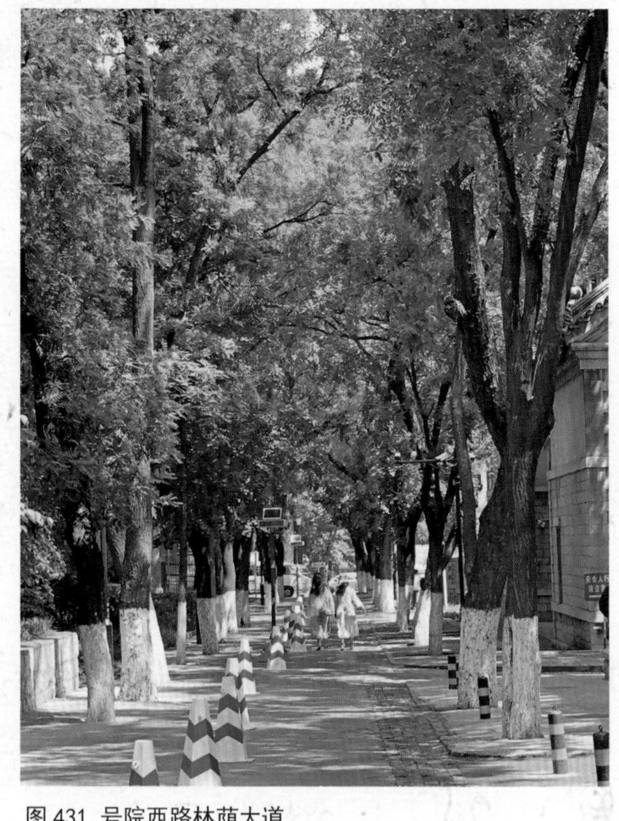

图 431 号院西路林荫大道
Fig. 431 Avenue on the west road of the Courtyard

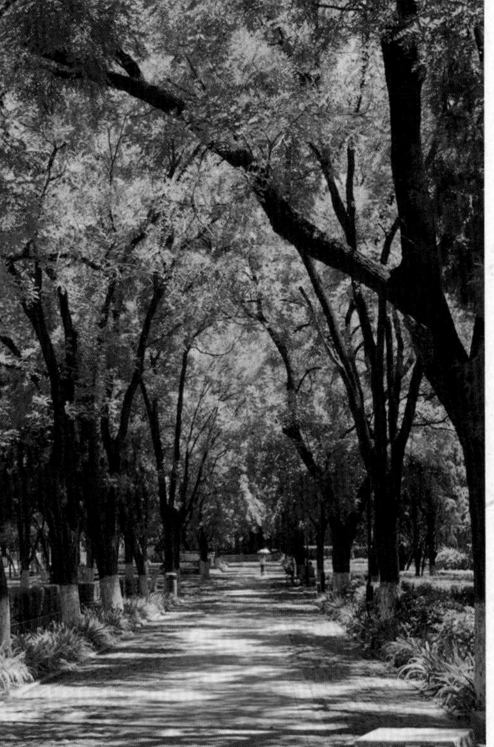

图 432 花园西路林荫大道
Fig. 432 Avenue on the west road of the garden

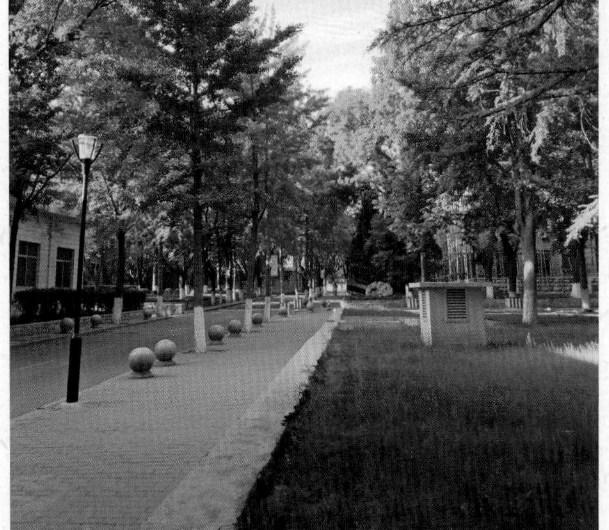

图 433 杏林路林荫大道
Fig. 433 Avenue on Xinglin Road

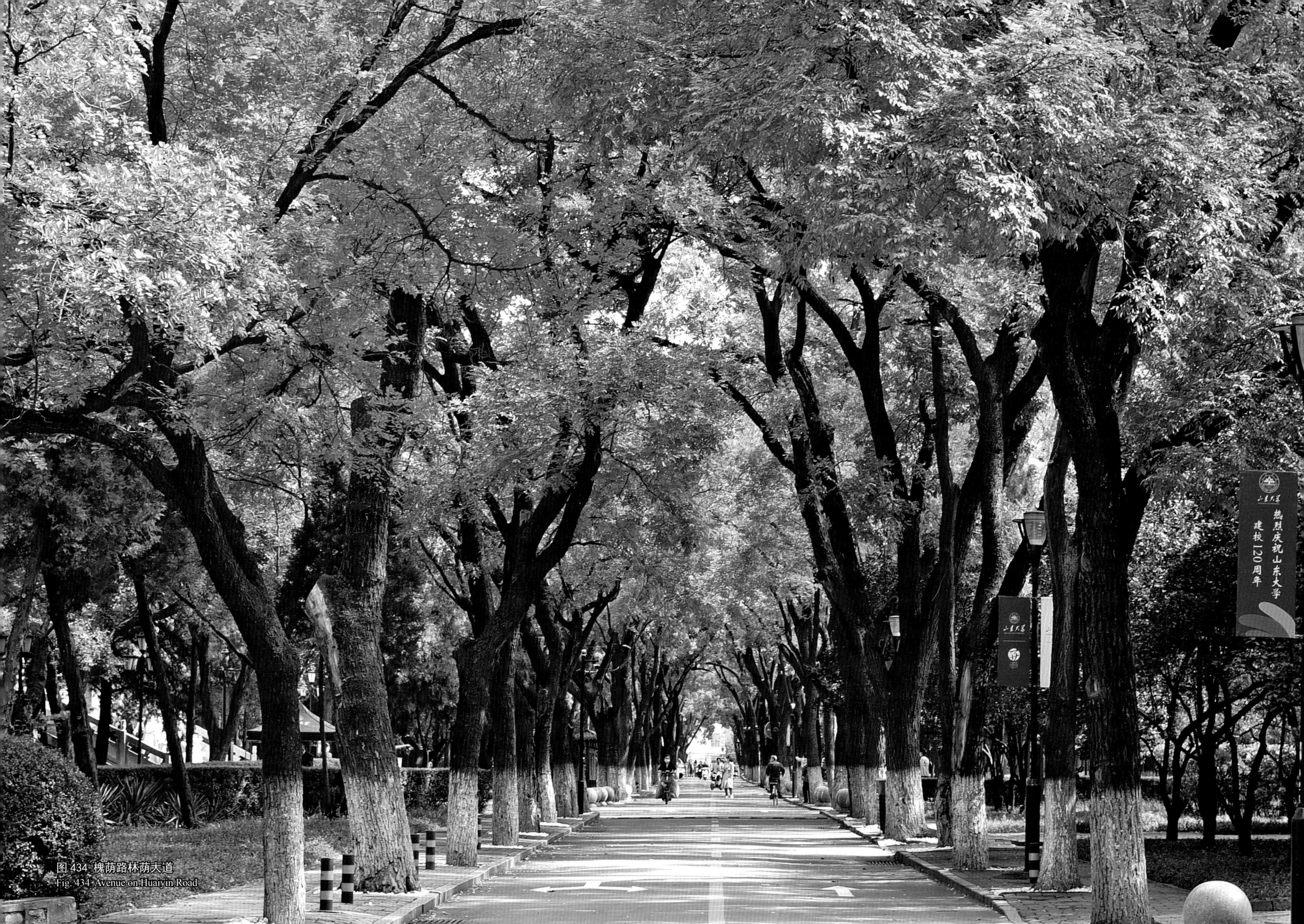

图 434 槐荫路林荫大道
Fig. 434 Avenue on Huaiyin Road

52 夏景宜人（2）

Attractive Scenery in Summer (2)

夏天的校园，碧树成林，密布于楼周或楼间。树上鸟虫合鸣，枝间松鼠跳跃。主要由高大乔木构成的小树林位于楼间，如中心花园的枫树林、教学四楼旁的梧桐林、教学一楼与教学二楼之间的银杏林、教学一楼与电镜楼之间的法桐林、电镜楼北侧的红杉林和考文楼西侧的白杨林等。主要由低矮乔木构成的小树林位于楼周，以花木居多。夏日里，于工作之余，白天可席地一卧，感受一下“树阴满地日当午，梦觉流莺时一声”的闲适；晚间可石凳一坐，领略一番“明月松间照”的清宁。最可期待的是，带着全班同学，每人一凳，在夏日清晨来林下授课研讨，我想教学效果一定陡涨十倍。

Green trees are densely distributed around or between the buildings on campus in summer. Birds and insects sing in the trees, and squirrels jump among the branches. The small woods mainly composed of tall trees are located between the buildings, such as the maple grove in the Central Garden, the grove of Chinese parasol trees beside the Fourth Teaching Building, the ginkgo grove between the First Teaching Building and the Second Teaching Building, the grove of plane trees between the First Teaching Building and the Building of Electron Microscopy, the redwood grove on the north side of the Building of Electron Microscopy and the grove of white poplars on the west side of Calvin Mateer Hall. The small woods mainly composed of low trees are located around the buildings, with flowering wood in the majority. On a summer day after work, you can lie on the ground to enjoy the leisure of “At midday trees spread their shade all over the ground; Wakened from a dream, I hear time and again orioles warbling.” At night, you can sit on a stone stool to enjoy the tranquility of “a silvery moon shining through the pines”. What to be expected most is that the teacher and the students, each one with a stool, come to the woods to teach and discuss on an early summer morning. I think the teaching effects must rise ten times.

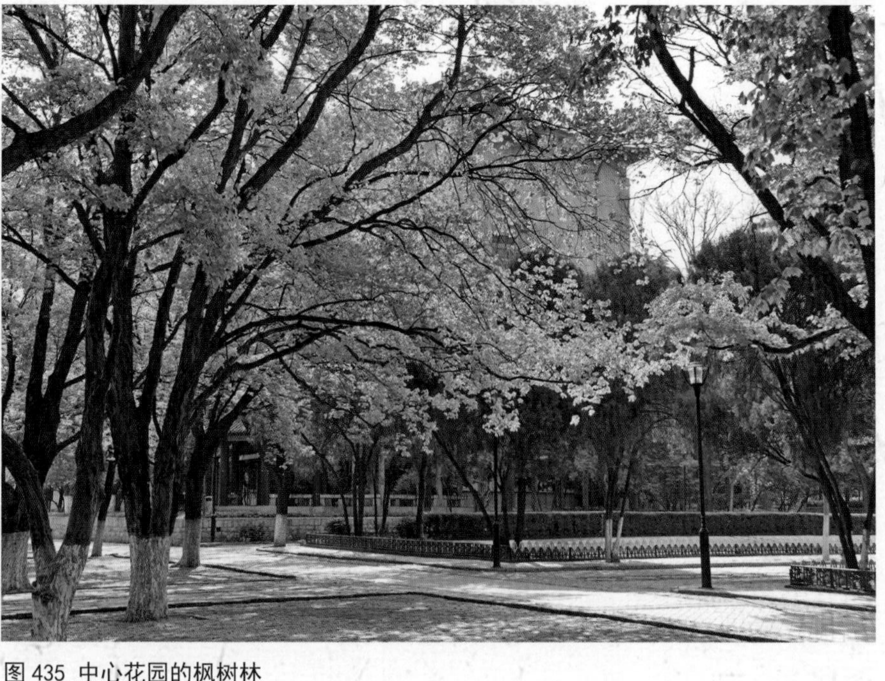

图 435 中心花园的枫树林

Fig. 435 Maple grove in the Central Garden

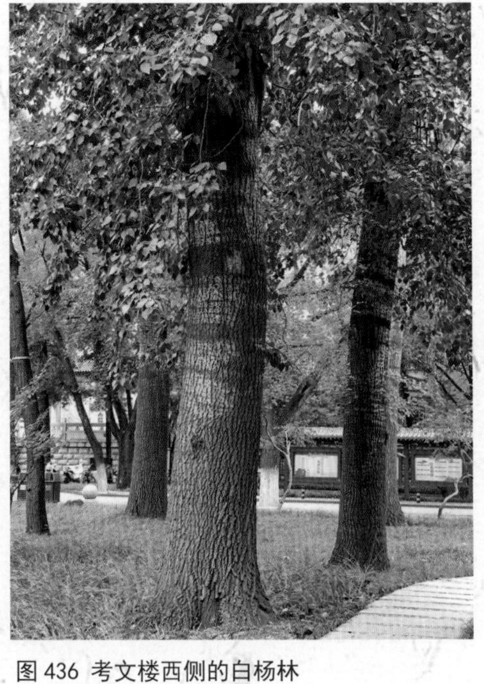

图 436 考文楼西侧的白杨林

Fig. 436 Grove of white poplars on the west side of Calvin Mateer Hall

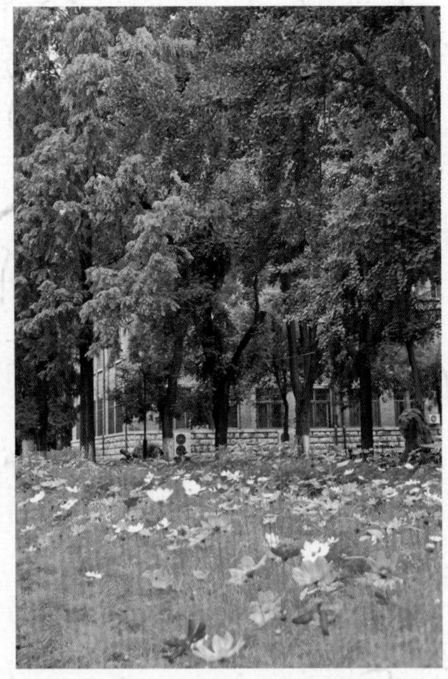

图 437 教学一、二楼之间的银杏林

Fig. 437 Grove of ginkgo trees between the First Teaching Building and the Second Teaching Building

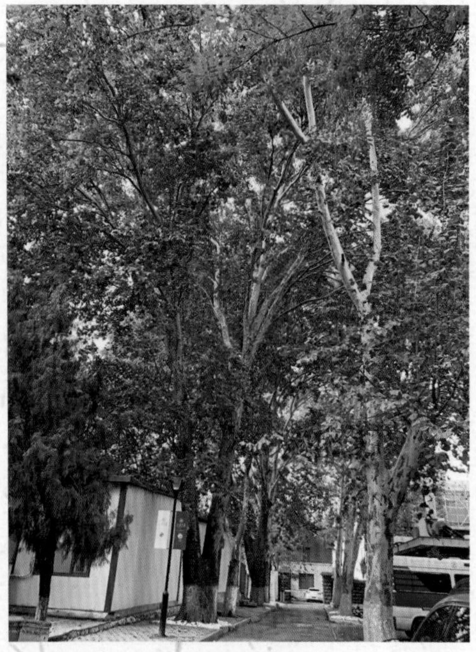

图 438 教学一楼北侧的法桐林

Fig. 438 Grove of plane trees on the north side of the First Teaching Building

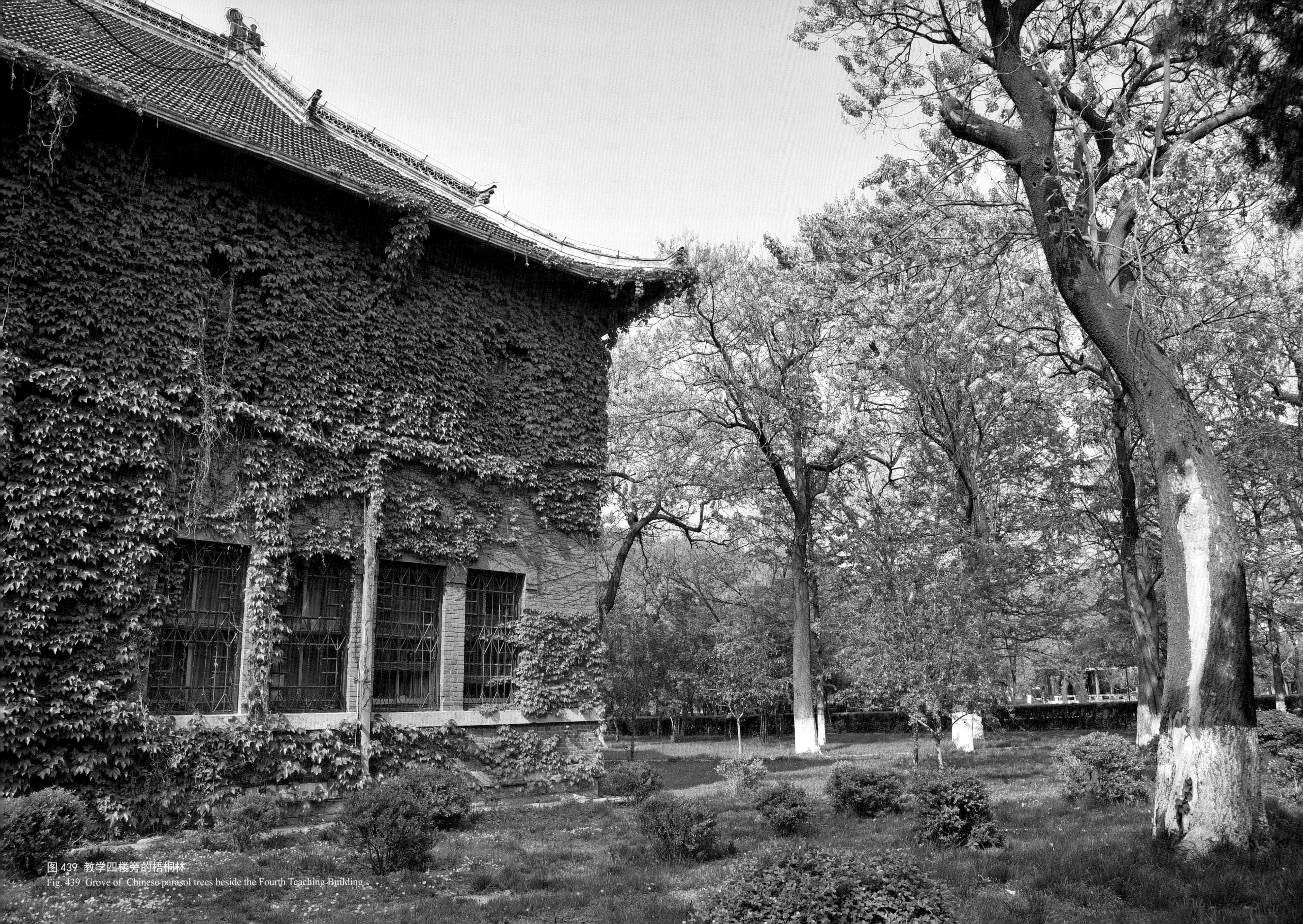

图 439 教学四楼旁的梧桐林
Fig. 439 Grove of Chinese parasol trees beside the Fourth Teaching Building

52 | 夏景宜人（3）

Attractive Scenery in Summer (3)

崇尚高大优美始终是人类审美的价值追求。婆娑多姿的大树总是给人一种壮美之感，令人心灵深处产生震撼，甚至敬畏。一进校门，便可见到一棵高大的迎客松，它树冠舒展，彬彬有礼，天天在那里欢迎来自五湖四海的宾朋。白杨树高耸入云，挺拔俊逸，显出一种无所畏惧的果敢。那一排排的国槐，比楼而生，树干上无数的裂纹，铭刻着岁月的沧桑。法桐树树冠茂密，童童如车盖，树干上老皮剥脱，裸露的青白色新皮昭示着其细胞分裂之迅速。俗语说：“十年树木，百年树人。”我想，树木也不必急功近利。看那些直上碧霄的松树，若不是历经风雨，怎能如此苍劲挺拔！看那棵百年老槐树，尽管佝偻的身躯几近干枯，但它的上部仍倔强地发出新枝！噫！“树犹如此”，可况人乎！

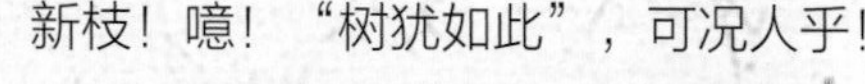

Advocating height and beauty is always the value pursuit of human appreciation. The spectacular trees always give people a sense of grandeur, and they are shocking and awe-inspiring in the deep heart of the people. As soon as you enter the school gate, you can see a tall guest-greeting pine. With stretched crown and politeness, it greets guests and friends from all over the world every day. The towering and upright white poplars give people a sense of fearless courage. Rows of pagoda trees are as tall as the buildings, and the countless cracks on the trunks have witnessed the years of vicissitudes. The dense crowns of the plane trees like the cover of a carriage; the fallen old bark and the exposed bluish white new bark on the trunks indicate the rapid division of their cells. As the saying goes, “It takes ten years to grow trees, but a hundred years to rear people.” I don't think trees have to rush for quick growing. If the soaring pines hadn’t gone through the wind and rain, how could they be so old and hardy! Although the bent body of that hundred-year-old pagoda tree is almost dry, new branches are still growing out from its upper part. Trees can still forge ahead against adversity, and humans should do more.

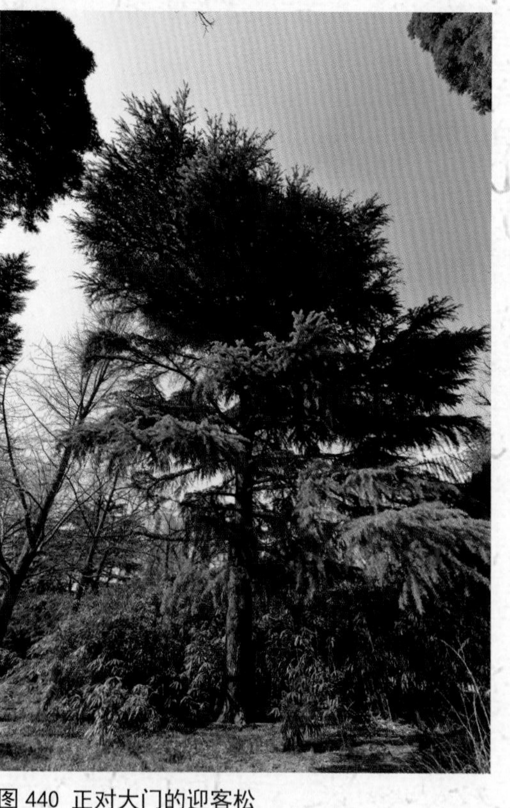

图 440 正对大门的迎客松
Fig. 440 A guest-greeting pine facing the gate

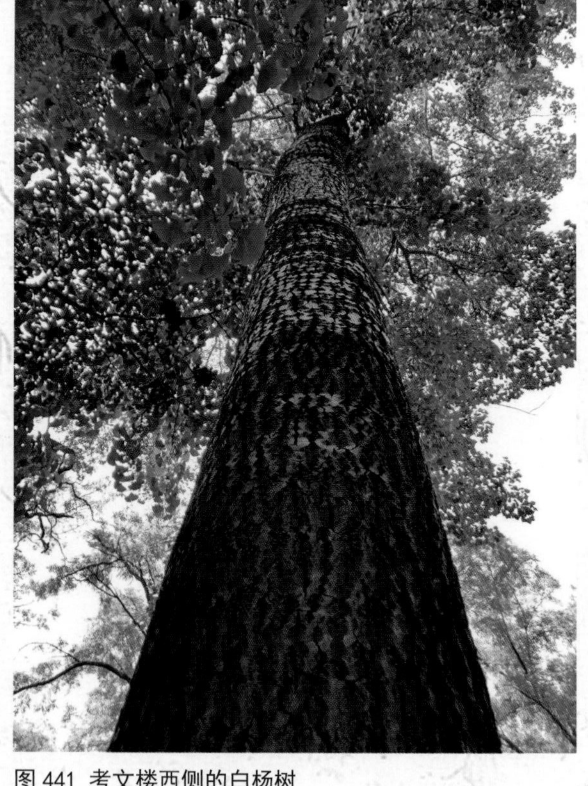

图 441 考文楼西侧的白杨树
Fig. 441 A white poplar on the west side of Calvin Mateer Hal

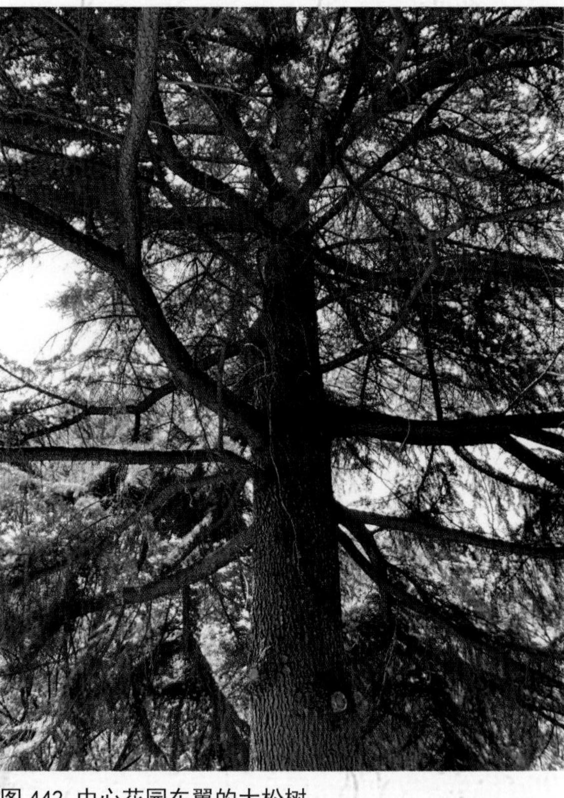

图 442 中心花园东翼的大松树
Fig. 442 A tall pine in the east wing of the Central Garden

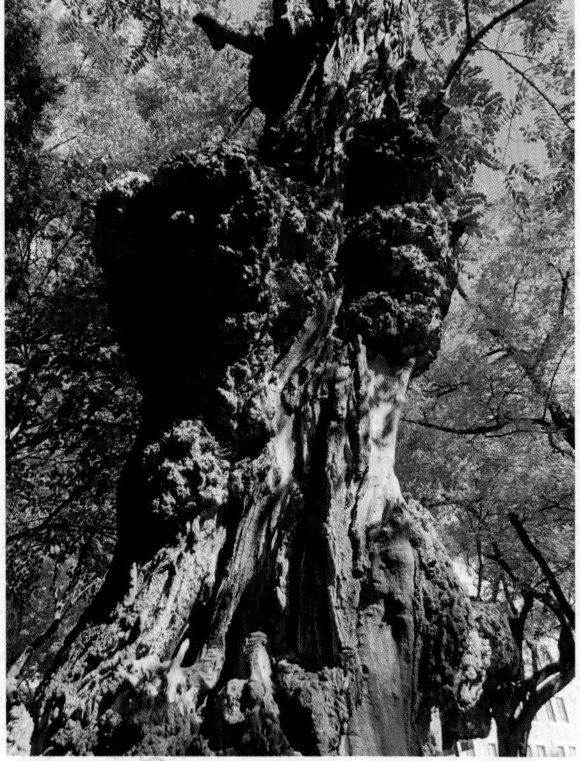

图 443 号院东北角处的老槐树
Fig. 443 An old pagoda tree in the northeast corner of the Courtyard

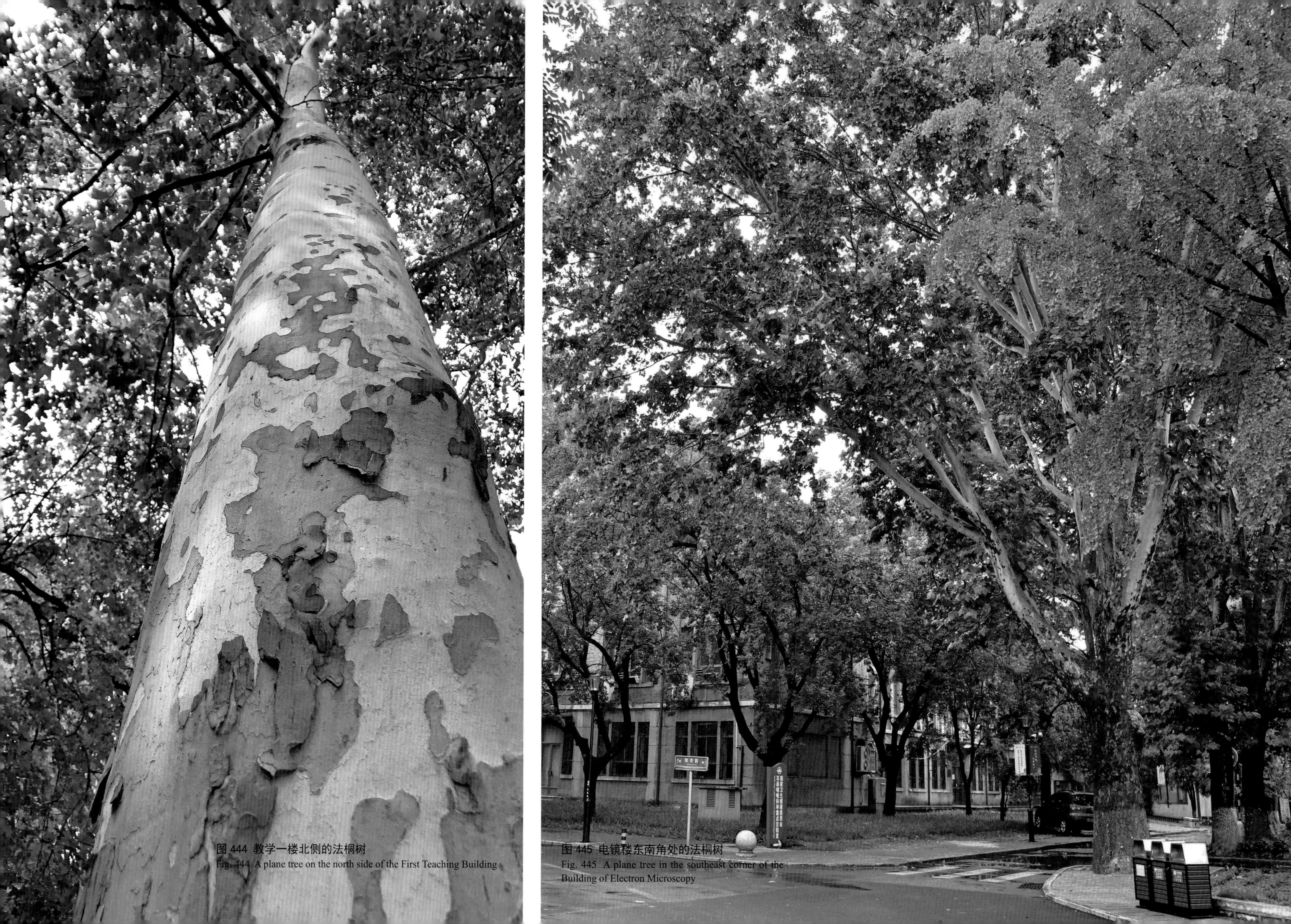

图 444 教学一楼北侧的法桐树
Fig. 444 A plane tree on the north side of the First Teaching Building

图 445 电镜楼东南角处的法桐树
Fig. 445 A plane tree in the southeast corner of the Building of Electron Microscopy

52 夏景宜人（4）

Attractive Scenery in Summer (4)

大多数花是要结果的。“花褪残红青杏小”，去年校园因疫情而封闭，让我看足了从青杏到黄杏的全过程，甚至连最惹人注目的石榴也长到了发红，最后回归到了大自然，实属不易。蜡梅也结出了纺锤形的果实，拥挤在枝头，连叶子都没处生长了。梅园内满树的梅子，青青的，太阳一照油光光发亮，不禁让人想起《三国演义》里曹操与刘备“青梅煮酒论英雄”的场景。与其他梅子由青变黄不同，榆叶梅的梅子由青变红，像玛瑙做成的珠子，三五成群地聚在一起，挂满了树枝。最令人惊奇的是紫荆果，一串串挂在树上，像碧玉做成的扁豆角，在阳光照耀下，晶莹剔透，发出绿色的荧光，在空中熠熠生辉。

Most flowers are meant to bear fruit. “Red flowers fade, and green apricots appear still small.” Last year, the campus was closed due to COVID-19, so that I saw the whole process of the apricots turning from green to yellow and the most eye-catching pomegranates growing to red and finally returning to nature. The wintersweet also bears spindle-shaped fruit that crowds in the branches, and even the leaves have no place to grow. The green plums shining in the sun in the Plum Garden can remind people of the scene of “Cao Cao Warms Wine and Rates the Heroes of the Realm”. Different from other plums turning from green to yellow, these of Prunus triloba turn from green to red, like beads made of agate, gathered in groups and hanging on branches. The most amazing is the fruit of Cercis chinensis, hanging on trees in strings like hyacinth beans made of jasper and emitting green fluorescence in the sun, glittering and translucent.

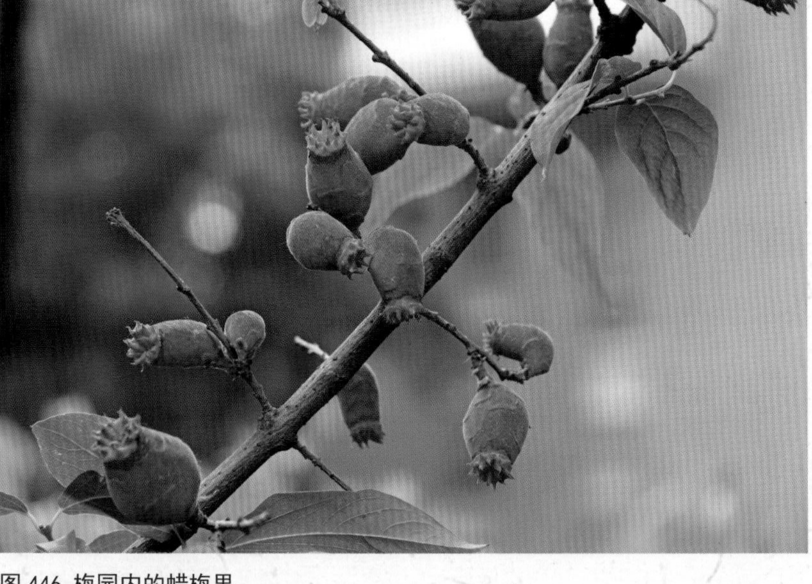

图 446 梅园内的蜡梅果
Fig. 446 Fruit of the wintersweet in the Plum Garden

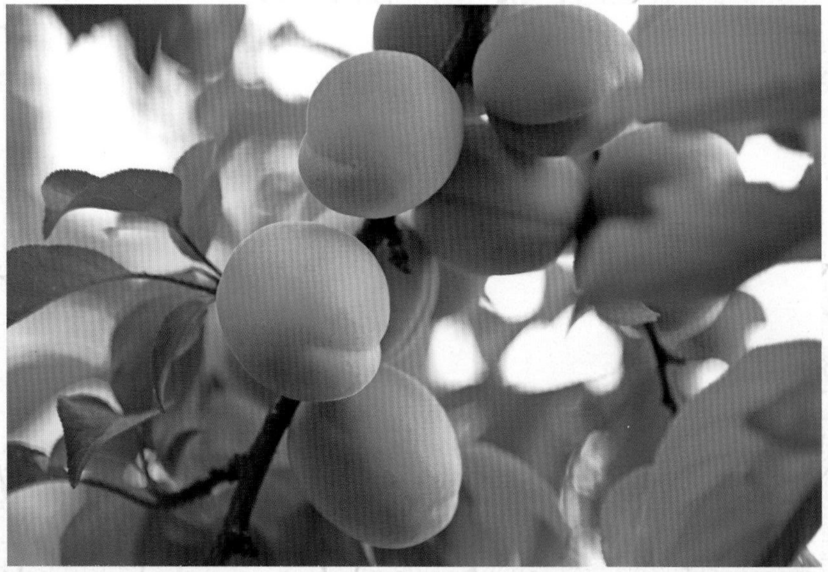

图 447 梅园内的杏
Fig. 447 Apricots in the Plum Garden

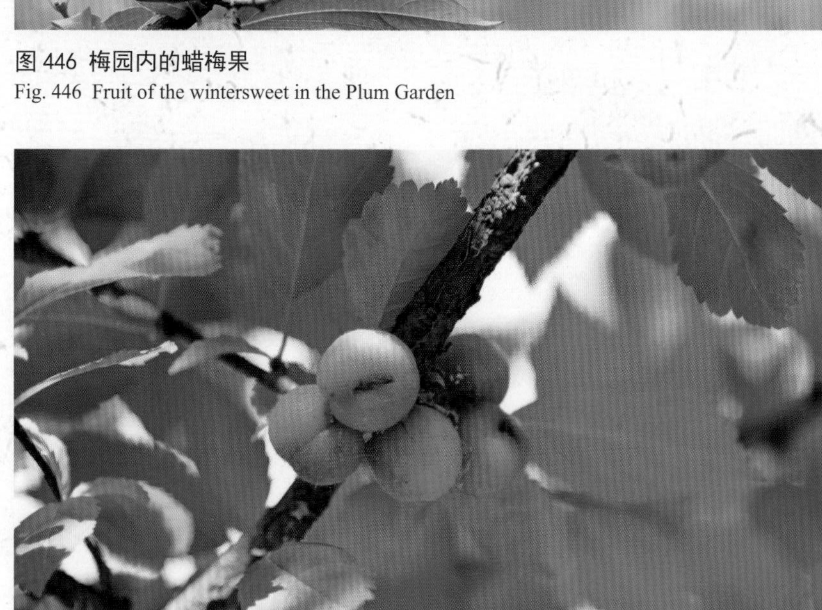

图 448 梅园内的榆叶梅果
Fig. 448 Fruit of Prunus triloba in the Plum Garden

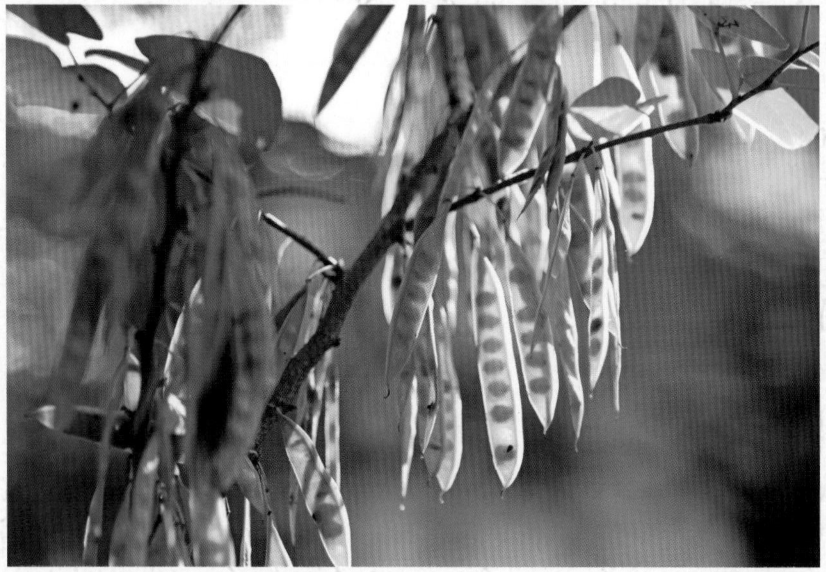

图 449 教学七楼北侧的紫荆果
Fig. 449 Fruit of Cercis chinensis on the north side of the Seventh Teaching Building

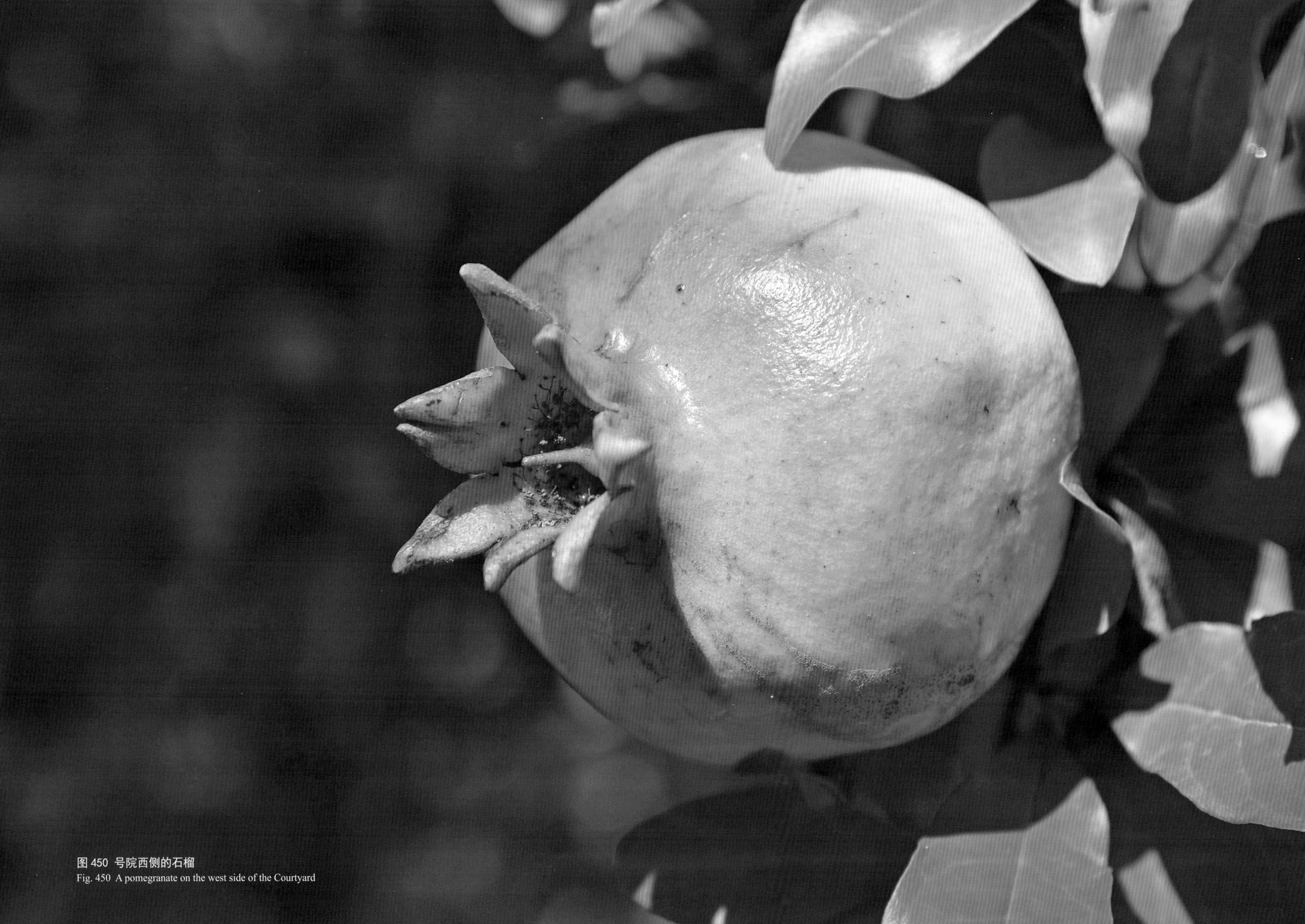

图 450 号院西侧的石榴
Fig. 450 A pomegranate on the west side of the Courtyard

52 夏景宜人（5）

Attractive Scenery in Summer (5)

“乌骓不逝项王穷，慷慨虞姬化草红。颔首图规籍志霸，舒腰为挺楚心雄。花如大纛迎风展，叶若千军陷阵冲。莫负美人捐碧血，挥戈再战起江东。”这篇七律由虞美人花联想到了垓下霸王别姬的壮烈场景，赞颂了项羽与虞姬的爱情故事，讴歌了虞姬的牺牲精神和慷慨胸襟，也对项王表达了不满和惋惜。每到春夏之交，虞美人花便迎风开放。它花叶碧绿，花茎颀长，花蕾总是娇羞地低着头，但一旦开放便昂首挺胸，激情迸发，常常连片齐放，给人一种勇不可挡、战无不胜的气势。所以，虞美人花是励志之花，它希望人们不畏艰险，百折不挠，敢于斗争，直至胜利。

“Xiang Yu lost his fighting spirit while his black steed stopped fighting; the generous Yu Ji turned into grass. The budding flowers inspire Xiang Yu to regain his aspiration; the blooming flowers inspire the State of Chu to regain the strength. The flowers are like banners against the wind; the leaves are like a thousand troops rushing into battle. Do not be unworthy of Yu Ji’s sacrifice; take up the weapons to fight again from the river.” This poem associates Papaver rhoeas with the heroic scene of “the Conqueror bids farewell to his concubine in Gaixia”. It praises the love story between Xiang Yu and Yu Ji, eulogizes Yu Ji’s spirit of sacrifice and generous mind, and also expresses dissatisfaction with Xiang Yu and a pity for him. At the turn of spring and summer, Papaver rhoeas blooms in the wind. It has green leaves, tall stems, and buds always lowering their heads shyly. But when they bloom, they hold their heads high with passion, and the flowers in full bloom give people a feeling of brave and invincible momentum. Therefore, Papaver rhoeas is a kind of flower of encouragement. It hopes that people will not fear difficulties and dangers, never yield in spite of reverses, and dare to fight until victory.

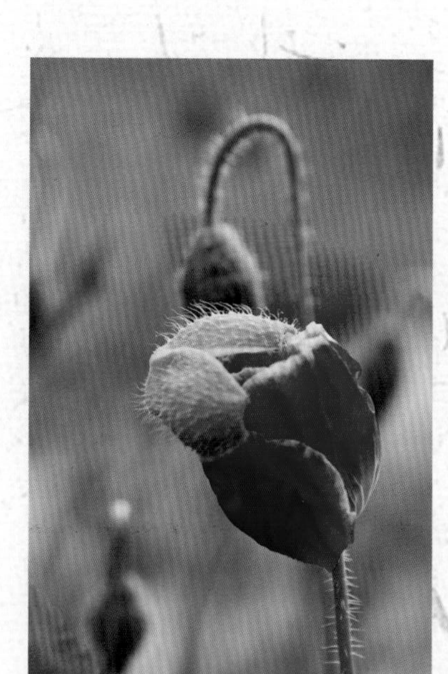

图 451 脱壳正出的红色虞美人花
Fig. 451 Red Papaver rhoeas in bud

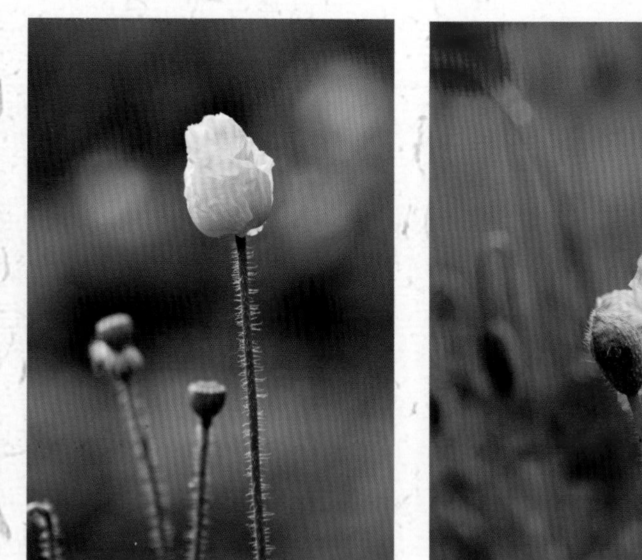

图 452 刚刚脱壳的白色虞美人花
Fig. 452 White Papaver rhoeas in bud

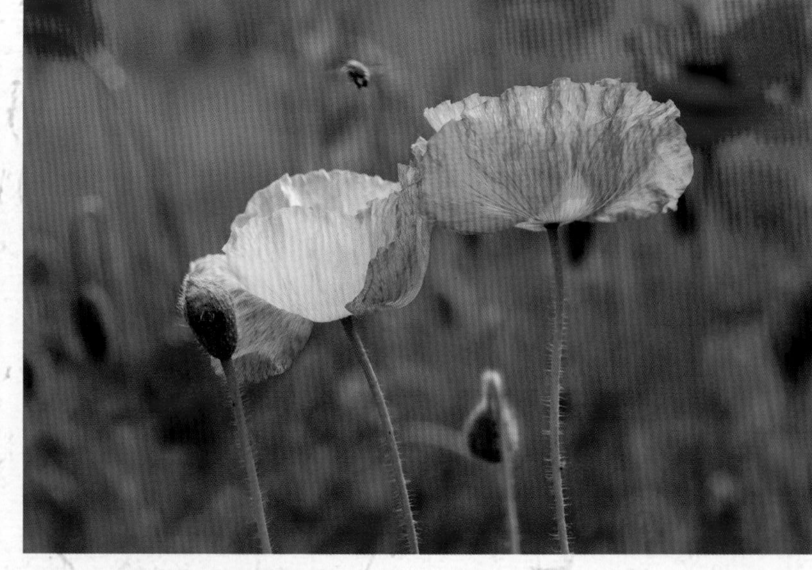

图 453 药圃内的粉色虞美人花
Fig. 453 Pink Papaver rhoeas in the Medicinal Garden

图 454 梦幻色彩的粉色虞美人花
Fig. 454 Pink Papaver rhoeas of dreamlike color

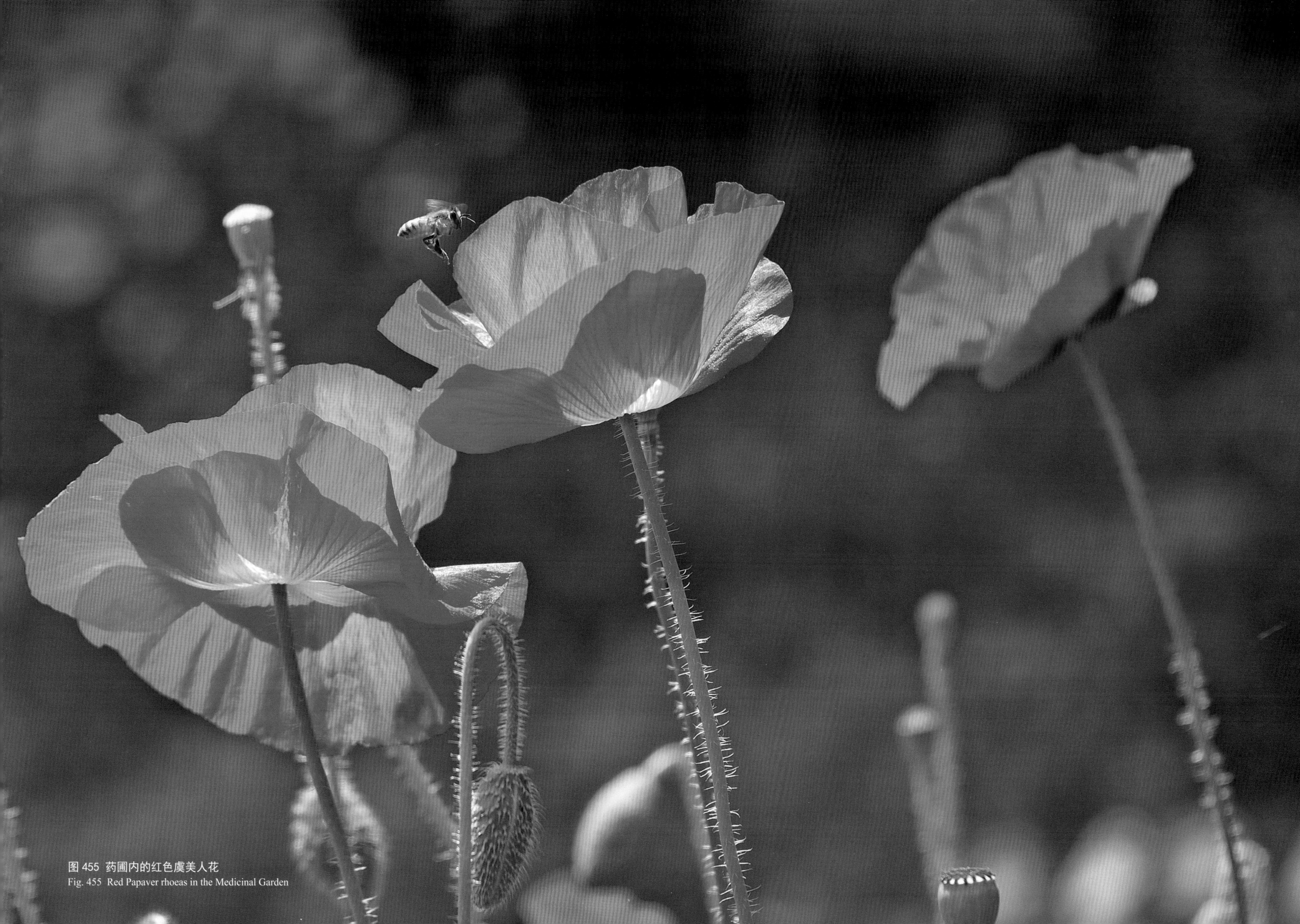

图 455 药圃内的红色虞美人花
Fig. 455 Red Papaver rhoeas in the Medicinal Garden

52 夏景宜人（6）

Attractive Scenery in Summer (6)

在藏语中，格桑花是“幸福花”之意，长期以来一直寄托着藏族人民期盼幸福吉祥的美好情感。格桑花在藏族人民心目中虽然具有很高的地位，但它具体为何种植物却存在着广泛争议，它极有可能是高原上生命力最顽强的一种野花的代名词。秋英（波斯菊）是目前认可度最高的格桑花，广泛存在于文艺与影视作品中。波斯菊原产墨西哥及南美其他地区，别名秋英、秋樱（学名：Cosmos bipinnata Cav.），为菊科秋英属一年生或多年生草本植物。秋英花呈“八瓣”形，美艳绝伦，适应高原环境，遍布雪域高原和全国各地，受到人民广泛喜爱。有诗赞曰：“秋英八瓣茎颀长，越近青天蕊愈香。只要芳心托雪域，凡花亦可作格桑。”

In Tibetan, Galsang flower means “flower of happiness”, which has been entrusted with the Tibetan people’s beautiful feelings of longing for happiness and luck for a long time. Although Galsang flower has a high status in the Tibetan people’s mind, there are widespread disputes about what kind of plant it is, and it is very likely to be the antonomasia of the most tenacious wild flower on the plateau. Cosmos bipinnatus is the most recognized Galsang flower at present, which widely exists in literary and artistic works and film and television works. Cosmos bipinnatus is native to Mexico and other parts of South America and it is an annual or perennial herbaceous plant in the daisy family Asteraceae. The beautiful flowers of Cosmos bipinnatus are in the shape of “eight petals”; they adapt to the plateau environment and spread all over the snowy plateau and other parts of the country, widely loved by the people. Here is a poem to praise Cosmos bipinnatus: “Cosmos bipinnatus has eight petals and tall stems; the closer to the sky, the more fragrant the petals are. As long as keeping the snowy plateau in the heart, regular flowers can also be Galsang flowers.”

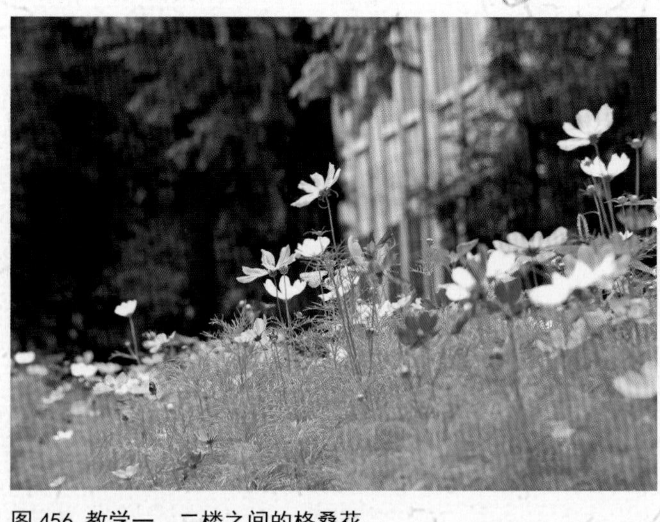

图 456 教学一、二楼之间的格桑花
Fig. 456 Galsang flowers between the First Teaching Building and the Second Teaching Building

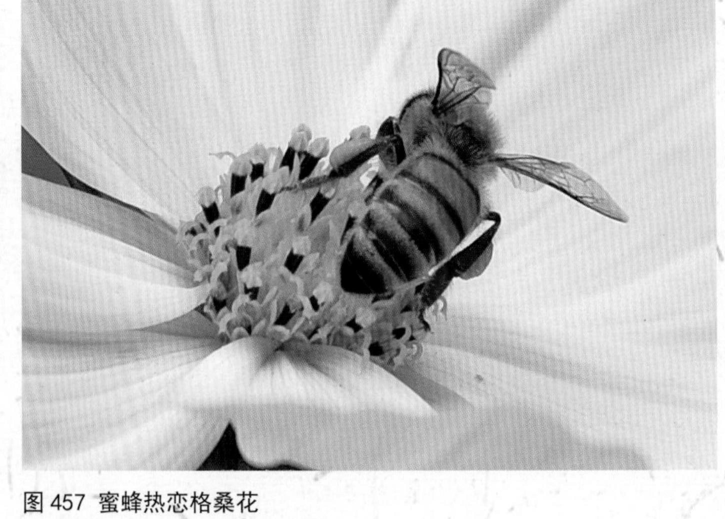

图 457 蜜蜂热恋格桑花
Fig. 457 A bee falling on a Galsang flower

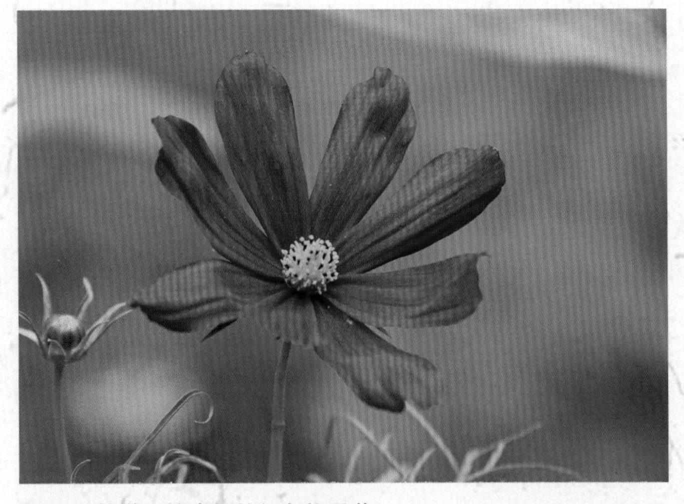

图 458 教学一楼南侧的红色格桑花
Fig. 458 Red Galsang flowers on the south side of the First Teaching Building

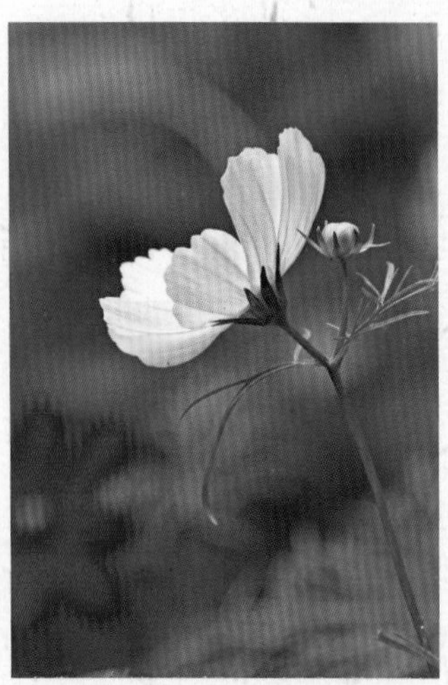

图 459 教学一楼南侧的白色格桑花
Fig. 459 White Galsang flowers on the south side of the First Teaching Building

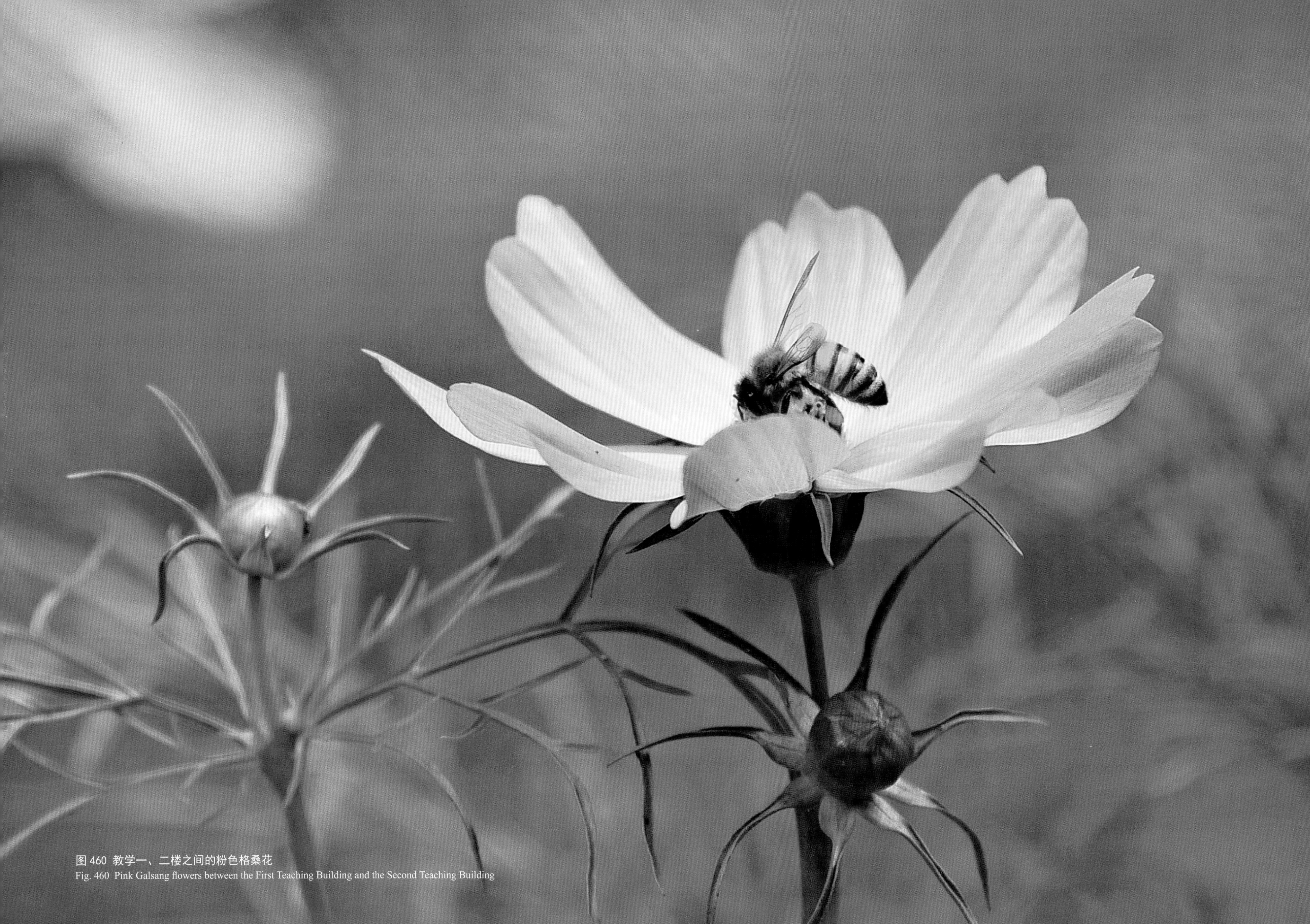

图 460 教学一、二楼之间的粉色格桑花
Fig. 460 Pink Galsang flowers between the First Teaching Building and the Second Teaching Building

52 夏景宜人（7）

Attractive Scenery in Summer (7)

百合的种头由鳞片抱合而成，取“百年好合”“百事合意”之意，中国自古为婚礼必不可少的吉祥花卉。百合花花丝细长，花色多样，高雅纯洁，素有“云裳仙子”之称。天主教以白百合花为圣母玛利亚的象征，而智利、梵蒂冈以百合花为国花。金光菊又名黑眼菊，花形似羽毛球，金黄色，在阳光下金碧辉煌。蒲公英种子上有白色冠毛结成的绒球，花开后随风飘洒，令人心生畅想。红花酢浆草又称夜合梅，喜阳光，昼开夜合，凡阴天或无阳光必合。复叶三片，呈倒心形，故又名三叶草。有诗赞道：“天生心叶伞花红，远似绯云近意浓。宁与阳光争艳丽，羞和月色比朦胧。”大花金鸡菊，别名大花波斯菊，花期长达四个多月，常成片开放，在绿叶衬托下，金光四射，绚丽夺目，犹如金鸡独立，赫然超群。

The lily's seed head is formed by the combination of scales. Implying the meaning of "a harmonious union lasting a hundred years" and "everything coming off satisfactorily", it is an indispensable auspicious flower for weddings since ancient times in China. The lily has tall and slender filaments and comes in a wide range of colors. Elegant and pure, it is known as the "fairy of cloud clothes". The Catholic Church takes the white lily as the symbol of Virgin Mary, and Chile and Vatican regard the lily as their national flower. Flowers of Rudbeckia laciniata are like badminton in shape, and the golden color looks brilliant in the sun. There are tomentum balls made of white pappus on the seeds of the dandelion. After the dandelions bloom, the balls float with the wind, which makes people think freely. Oxalis corymbosa likes the sun; it opens during the day and closes at night, but it does not open on cloudy days or days without sun. With three compound leaves in the shape of an inverted heart, it was also known as clover. Here is a poem to praise it: "With leaves in the shape of inverted heart and red flowers in the shape of umbrella, it looks like rosy clouds from afar but bears strong feelings nearby. It can compete with the bright sunshine, but is ashamed to compete with the dim moonlight." Coreopsis grandiflora has a flowering period of more than four months, and it often opens in clusters. The golden and gorgeous flowers against the green leaves stand out among others.

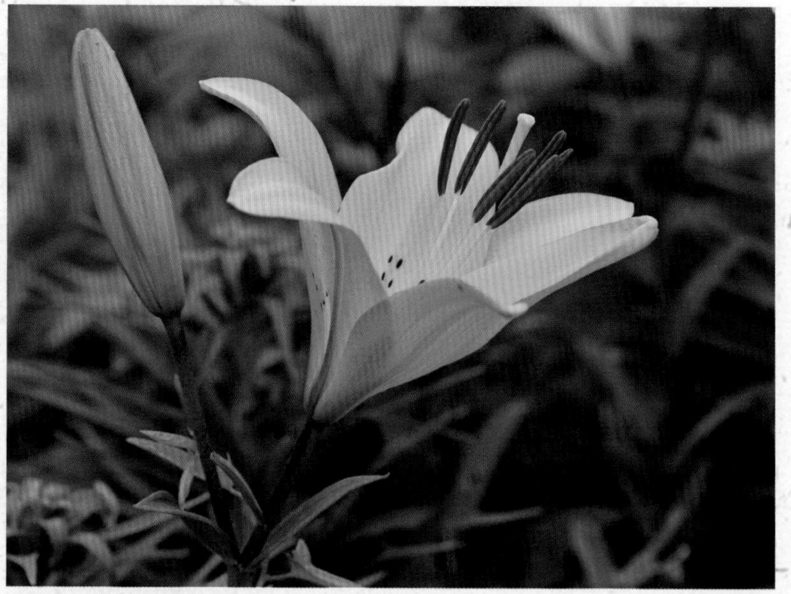

图 461 药圃内的黄色百合花
Fig. 461 Yellow lilies in the Medicinal Garden

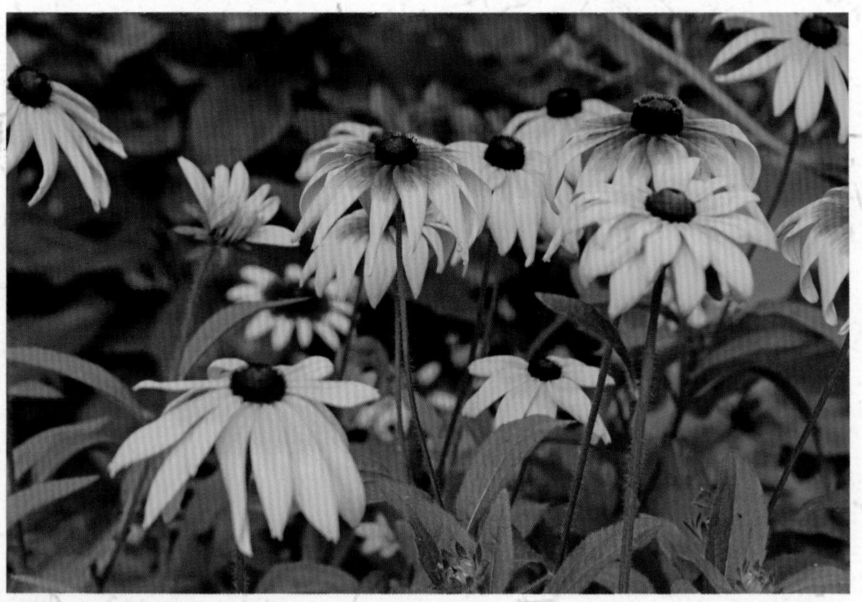

图 462 教学八楼西侧的金光菊
Fig. 462 Rudbeckia laciniata on the west side of the Eighth Teaching Building

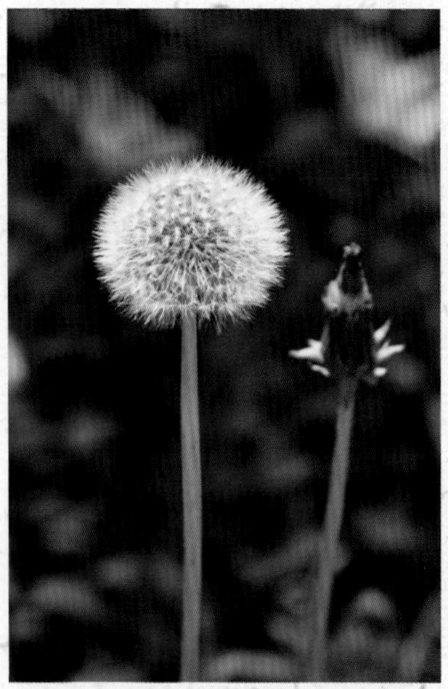

图 463 药圃内的蒲公英
Fig. 463 Dandelion in the Medicinal Garden

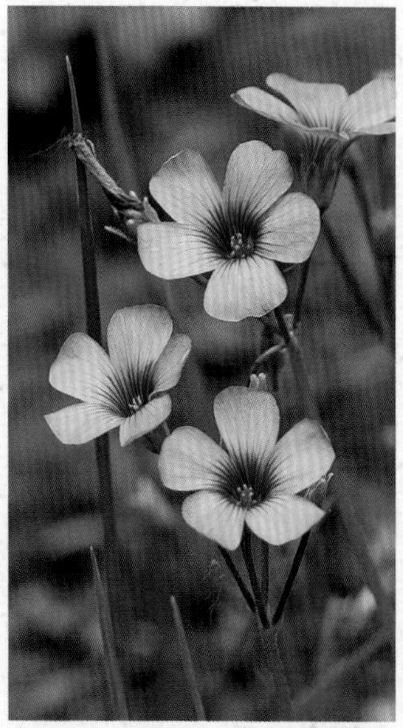

图 464 梅园内的红花酢浆草
Fig. 464 Oxalis corymbosa in the Plum Garden

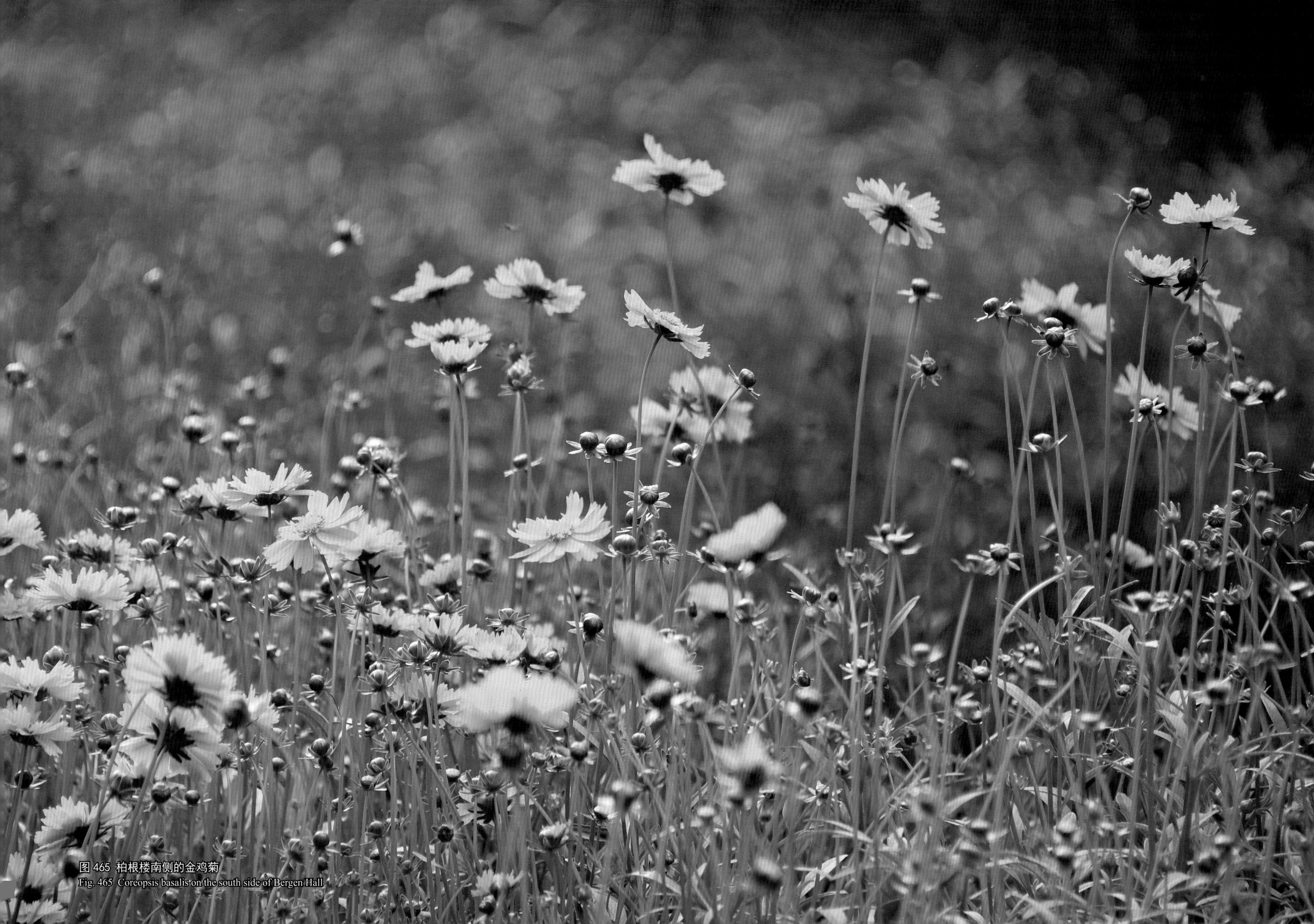

图 465 柏根楼南侧的金鸡菊
Fig. 465 Coreopsis basalis on the south side of Bergen Hall

52 夏景宜人（8）

Attractive Scenery in Summer (8)

桔梗为常用中草药，有止咳祛痰、宣肺、排脓等作用，其花十分漂亮，酷似五角星，暗蓝色，从很远处便能看到。在朝鲜半岛桔梗被用来制作泡菜，著名的《桔梗谣》轻快明朗，生动地塑造了朝鲜族姑娘勤劳活泼的形象。耧斗菜原产于欧洲和北美，花茎直立，花冠漏斗状、下垂，花瓣 5 枚，通常呈深蓝紫色或白色。大花耧斗菜花大而美丽，直径 6 ~ 9 厘米。宿根亚麻花茎丛生、直立而细长，花朵较小，花瓣 5 枚，淡蓝色，常生于干旱草原等艰苦的环境中。美丽月见草是月见草的一种，月见草见月开花，天亮即闭，而美丽月见草白天也会开放，花朵如杯盏状，常常丛生，一片粉色，别有园林风情。

Platycodon grandiflorus is a commonly used Chinese herbal medicine, and it has the effects of relieving cough and eliminating phlegm, dispersing lung, discharging pus and the like. The dark blue flowers are very beautiful; they resemble five-pointed stars and can be seen from a long distance. Platycodon grandiflorus is used to make kimchi in the Korean Peninsula. The famous light and clear “Ballad of Platycodon grandiflorus” vividly shapes the hard-working and lively image of Korean girls. Aquilegia viridiflora, native to Europe and North America, has the erect stem, pendulous funnel-shaped corolla and five petals which are usually dark blue-purple or white. The flowers of Aquilegia glandulosa are large and beautiful, which are 6 cm to 9 cm in diameter. The upright and slender stems of Linum perenne grow in clusters, and the pale blue flowers are small, with five petals. It often grows in arid grassland and other harsh environments. Oenothera speciosa is a kind of Oenothera biennis. Oenothera biennis opens at the sight of the moon and closes at dawn, while Oenothera speciosa also opens during the day and it bears its flowers in clusters. A wide range of pink cup-shaped flowers present a garden style.

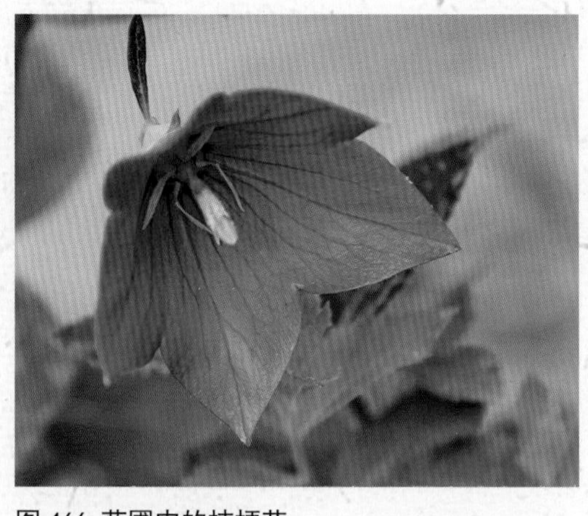

图 466 药圃内的桔梗花
Fig. 466 Platycodon grandiflorus in the Medicinal Garden

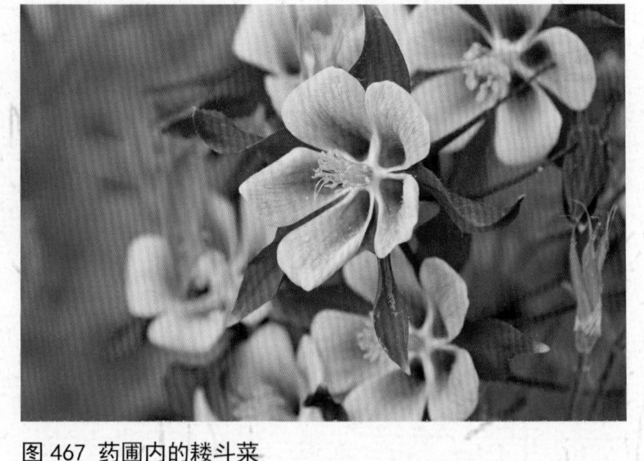

图 467 药圃内的耧斗菜
Fig. 467 Aquilegia viridiflora in the Medicinal Garden

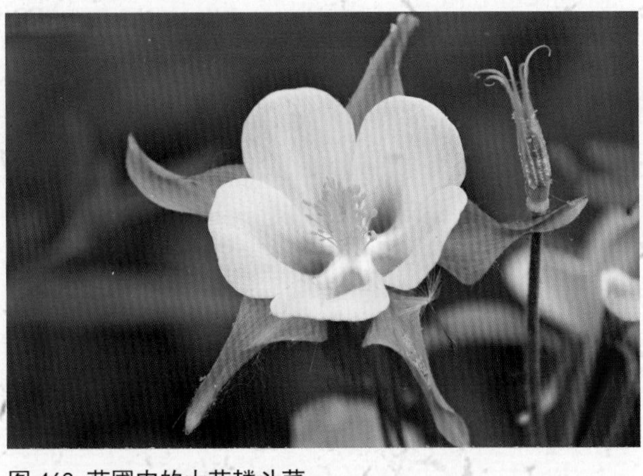

图 468 药圃内的大花耧斗菜
Fig. 468 Aquilegia glandulosa in the Medicinal Garden

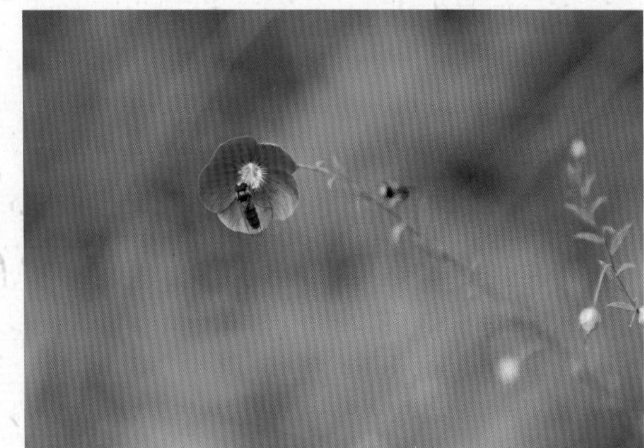

图 469 药圃内的宿根亚麻花
Fig. 469 Linum perenne in the Medicinal Garden

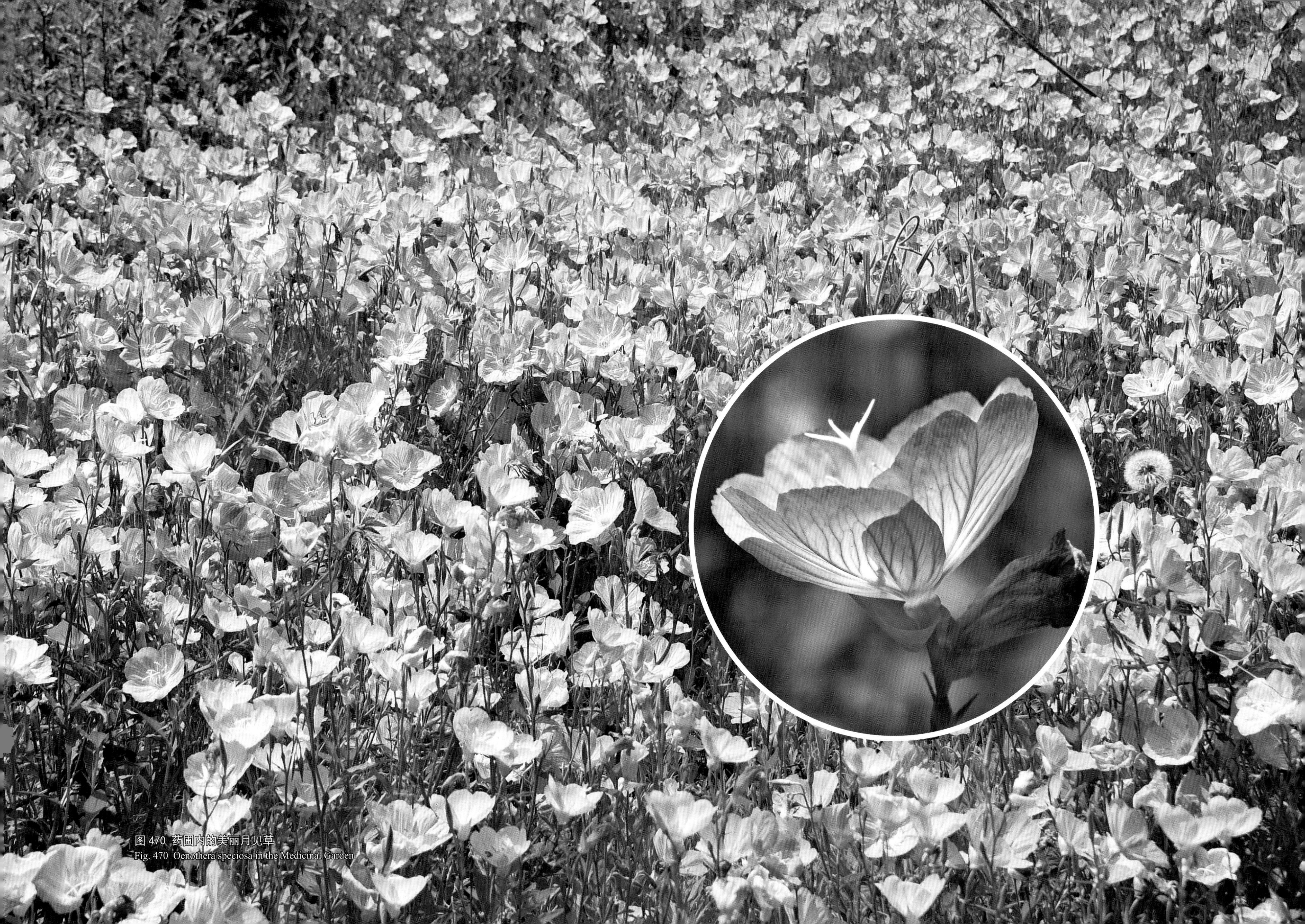

图 470 药圃内的美丽月见草
Fig. 470 Oenothera speciosa in the Medicinal Garden

53 秋叶金辉（1）

Golden Autumn Leaves (1)

每到仲秋时节，便能闻到桂花的清香。如果说梅花是报春者，那么桂花则是中秋节的信使。桂花虽贵为中国传统十大名花之一，号称仙树，但本身却十分低调，花小如米粒，常紧紧聚在一起。若不是它那扑鼻的香气，则常常被人忽视。出生于济南的著名词人李清照十分喜爱桂花，称赞道“何须浅碧深红色，自是花中第一流”。而另一位出生于济南的大词人辛弃疾似乎不太喜欢桂树，写道“斫去桂婆娑。人道是，清光更多”，则把桂树比喻成了奸佞小人。无论如何，古往今来，人们以画桂、咏桂和赏桂等各种形式来表达对桂花的热爱之情。趵突泉校区在护理楼前和景蓝斋院内栽有几棵桂树，太少。最好能多栽一些，让广大师生看一看桂树“揉破黄金万点轻，剪成碧玉叶层层”的风姿，闻一闻“桂花馥郁清无寐。觉身在，广寒宫里”的芬芳。

In August, you can smell the fragrance of the sweet-scented osmanthus. If the plum blossom is a harbinger of spring, then the sweet-scented osmanthus is a messenger of Mid-Autumn Festival. Although the sweet-scented osmanthus is one of the top ten famous flowers in China and is known as fairy tree, it is very low-key. The flowers are as small as rice grains and often gather together closely. If it wasn't for its strong aroma, it would have been ignored. Li Qingzhao, a famous poet born in Jinan, loves the sweet-scented osmanthus very much and once praised it in a poem: “There is no need to flaunt with light green and deep red colors; it is essentially among the first class in flowers.” Xin Qiji, another great poet born in Jinan, doesn't seem to like the laurel. He once wrote in a poem: “To cut off the swaying branches of the laurel in the moon, and this will make the moon sprinkle more glory on the world.” The laurel was likened to a treacherous villain. Throughout the ages, people have expressed their love for the sweet-scented osmanthus in various forms, such as painting it, chanting it and admiring it. On Baotuquan Campus, there are several laurels in front of the Nursing Building and in Jinglan Building. More laurels should be planted so that the teachers and students can enjoy the golden bright color and the knife-cut layers of dark green leaves of the laurel and smell the sweet-scented osmanthus whose strong fragrance makes people unable to sleep and feel they are in the Moon Palace.

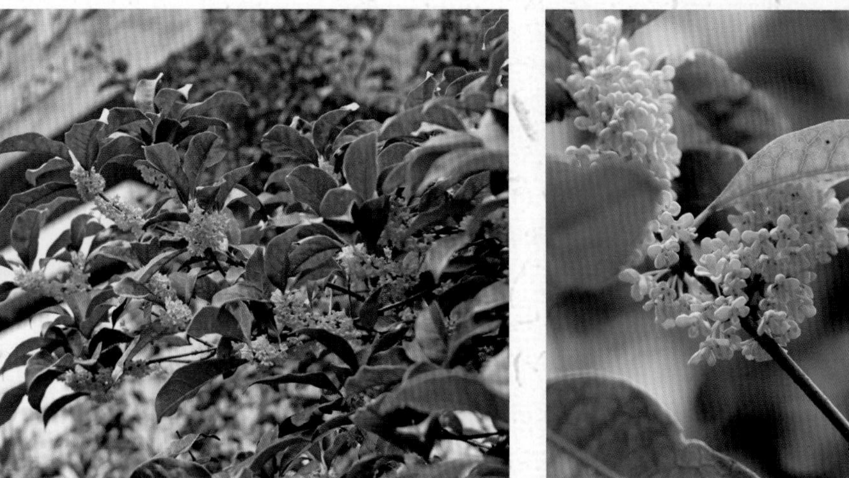

图 471 景蓝斋院内的桂花
Fig. 471 Sweet-scented osmanthus in Jinglan Building

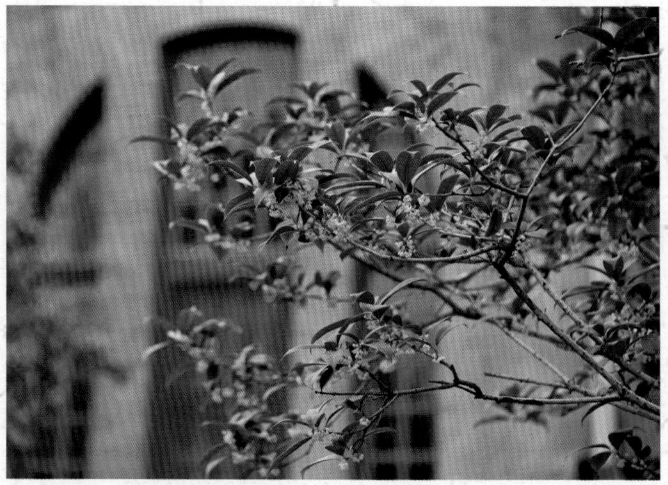

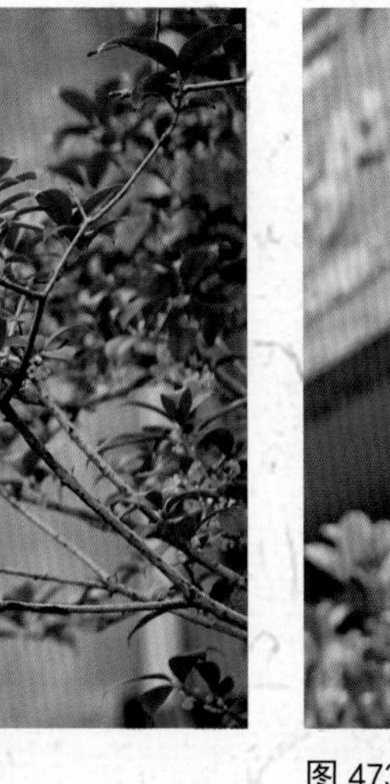

图 472 景蓝斋院内的金桂飘香
Fig. 472 Sweet-scented osmanthus giving off the fragrance in Jinglan Building

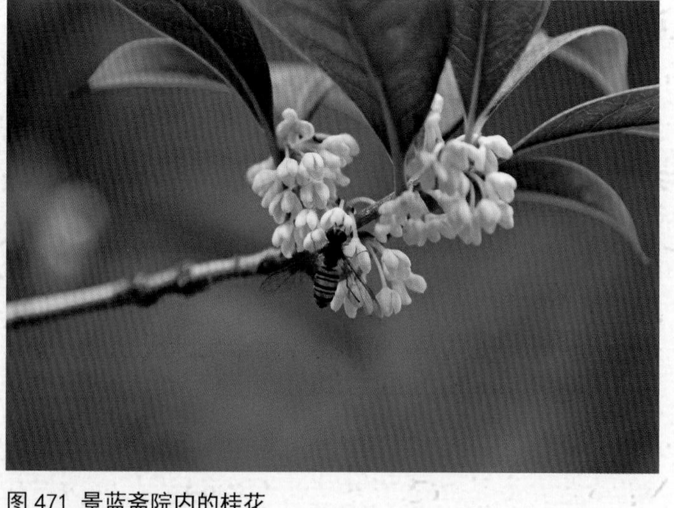

图 473 护理楼前盛开的金桂
Fig. 473 Sweet-scented osmanthus in full bloom in front of the Nursing Building

图 474 护理楼前金光四射的桂花
Fig. 474 Golden sweet-scented osmanthus in front of the Nursing Building

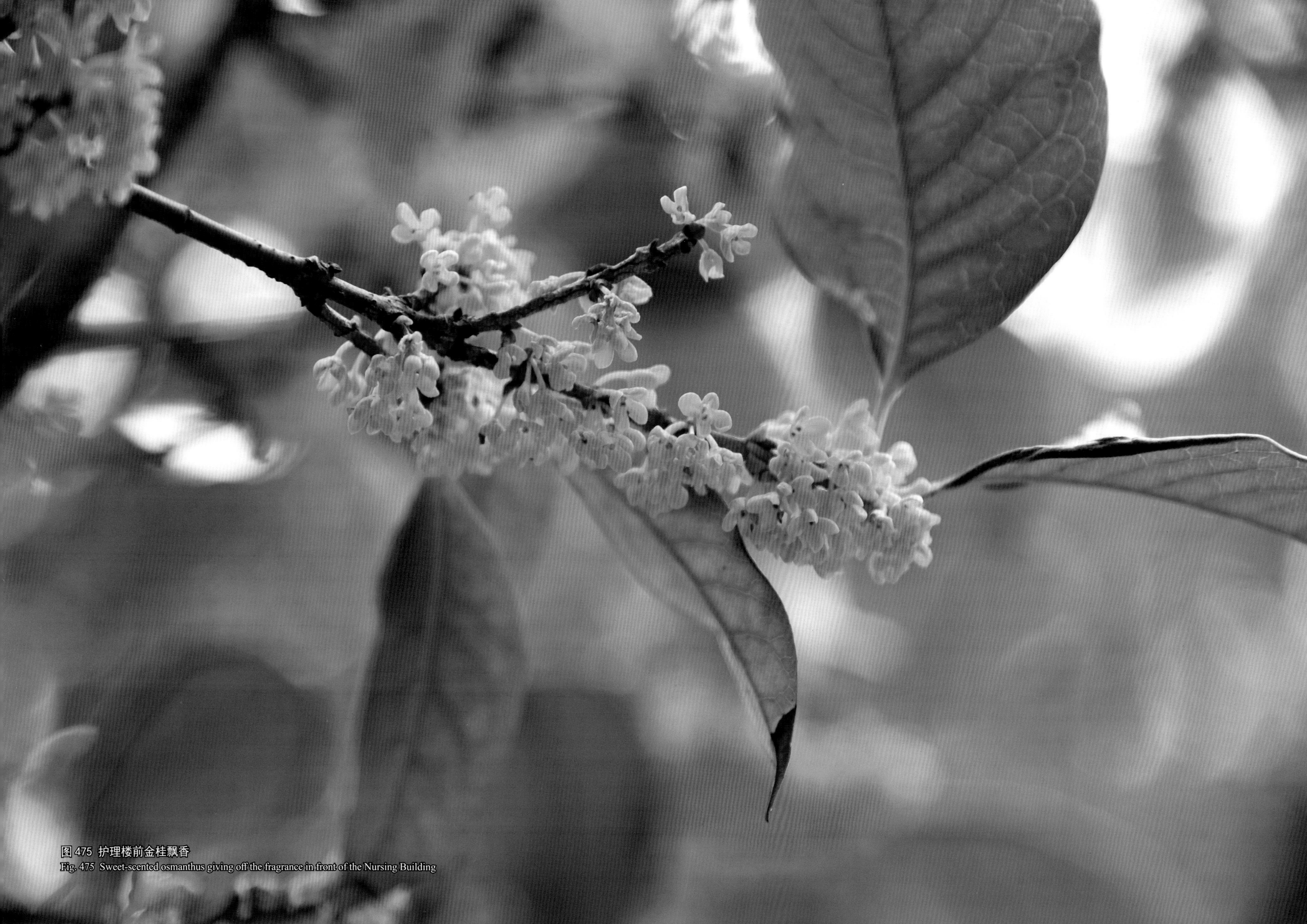

图 475 护理楼前金桂飘香

Fig. 475 Sweet-scented osmanthus giving off the fragrance in front of the Nursing Building

53 秋叶金辉（2）

Golden Autumn Leaves (2)

银杏为高大落叶乔木，躯干挺拔，树形优美，高度可达 40 米，胸径可达 4 米。银杏有数百年或千年以上的树龄，被誉为植物王国的“活化石”，是世界上现存最古老的树种之一。银杏树分为雌雄株，雄株不结果，而雌株一般要到 20 岁以后才开始结实。银杏浑身是宝，科学家已从其叶和果中提炼出多种化学物质，有益于心脑健康。但生白果含有氢氰酸等毒性成分，不宜多食。银杏树干多为栋梁之材，唐代大诗人王维曾咏曰：“文杏栽为梁，香茅结为宇。不知栋里云，去做人间雨。”趵突泉校区银杏树多，且与楼比高。每年十一月份，黄叶满树，随风飘金，此时在青瓦红窗的教学楼之间漫步，一种高贵与静雅的古今穿越感不禁油然而生。

The ginkgo is a tall deciduous tree, with straight trunk and beautiful shape. Its height can reach 40 meters and the diameter at breast can reach 4 meters. The ginkgo is hundreds or thousands years old and is one of the oldest existing tree species in the world, known as “the living fossil” in the plant kingdom. Ginkgo trees are divided into male and female plants; the male plants do not bear fruit, while the female plants generally begin to bear fruit after the age of 20. The ginkgo is full of treasure, and scientists have extracted a variety of chemicals from its leaves and fruits, which are good for heart and brain. But do not eat more raw ginkgo nuts because they contain hydrogen cyanide and other toxic ingredients. Trunks of the ginkgo are mostly the material of the beam, and the poet Wang Wei of the Tang Dynasty once praised it in a poem: “Of precious ginko wood are these graceful beams; the eaves are woven lemongrass so sweet. The lingering clouds between the purlins, it seems; would turn to downpour the human world to greet.” There are many ginkgo trees on Baotuquan Campus, and they are as tall as the buildings. Every November, the ginkgo trees are full of golden leaves floating in the wind. At this time, walking among the teaching buildings with blue tiles and red windows can give you a feeling of noble and elegant travel between ancient and modern times.

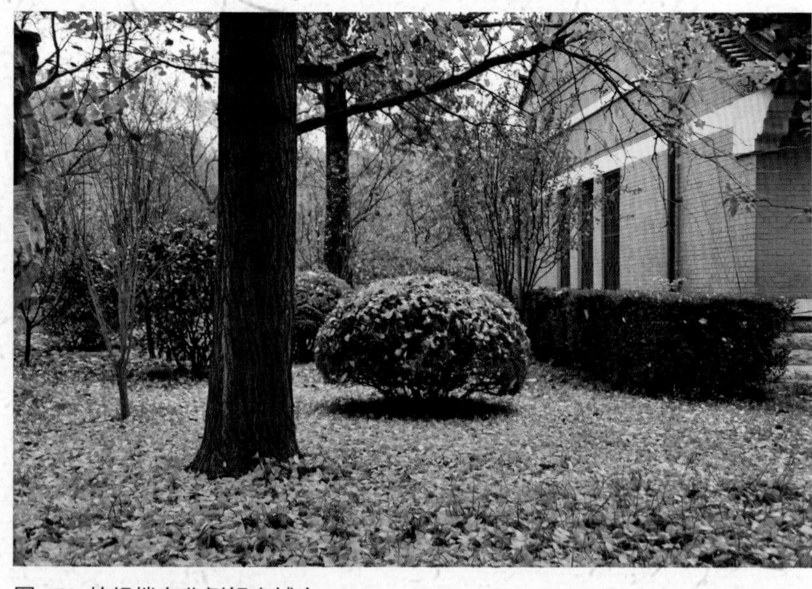

图 476 柏根楼东北侧银杏铺金
Fig. 476 Golden ginkgo leaves on the northeast side of Bergen Hall

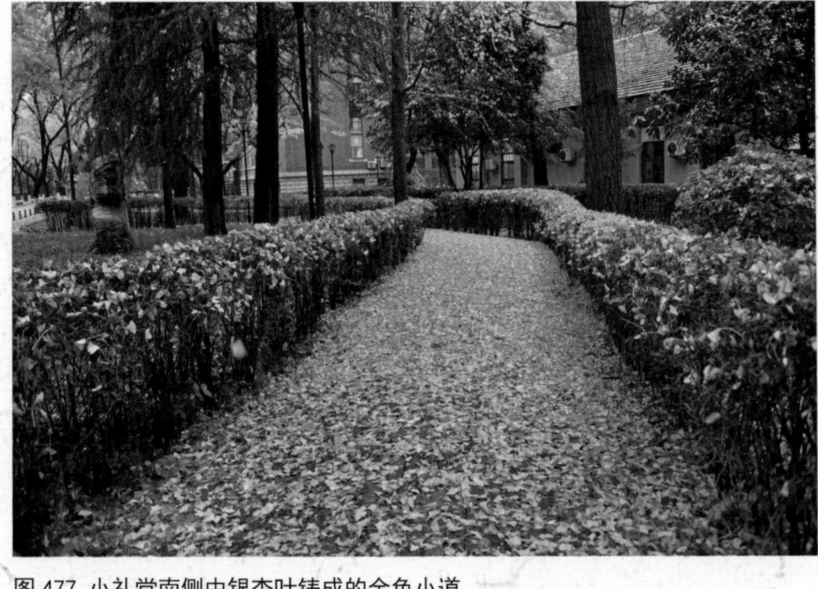

图 477 小礼堂南侧由银杏叶铸成的金色小道
Fig. 477 Golden path of ginkgo leaves on the south side of the chapel

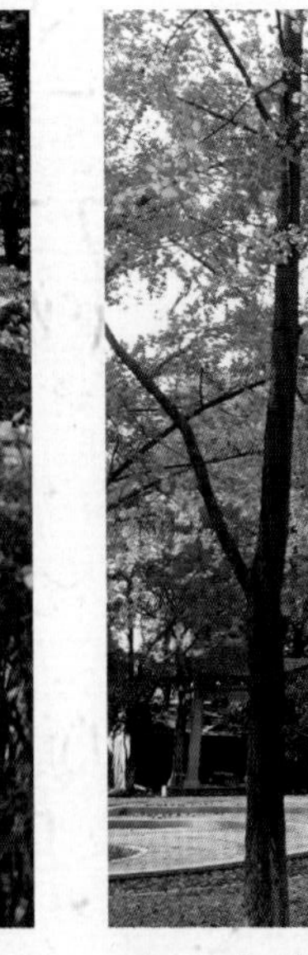

图 478 教学一、二楼之间的银杏林
Fig. 478 Grove of ginkgo trees between the First Teaching Building and the Second Teaching Building

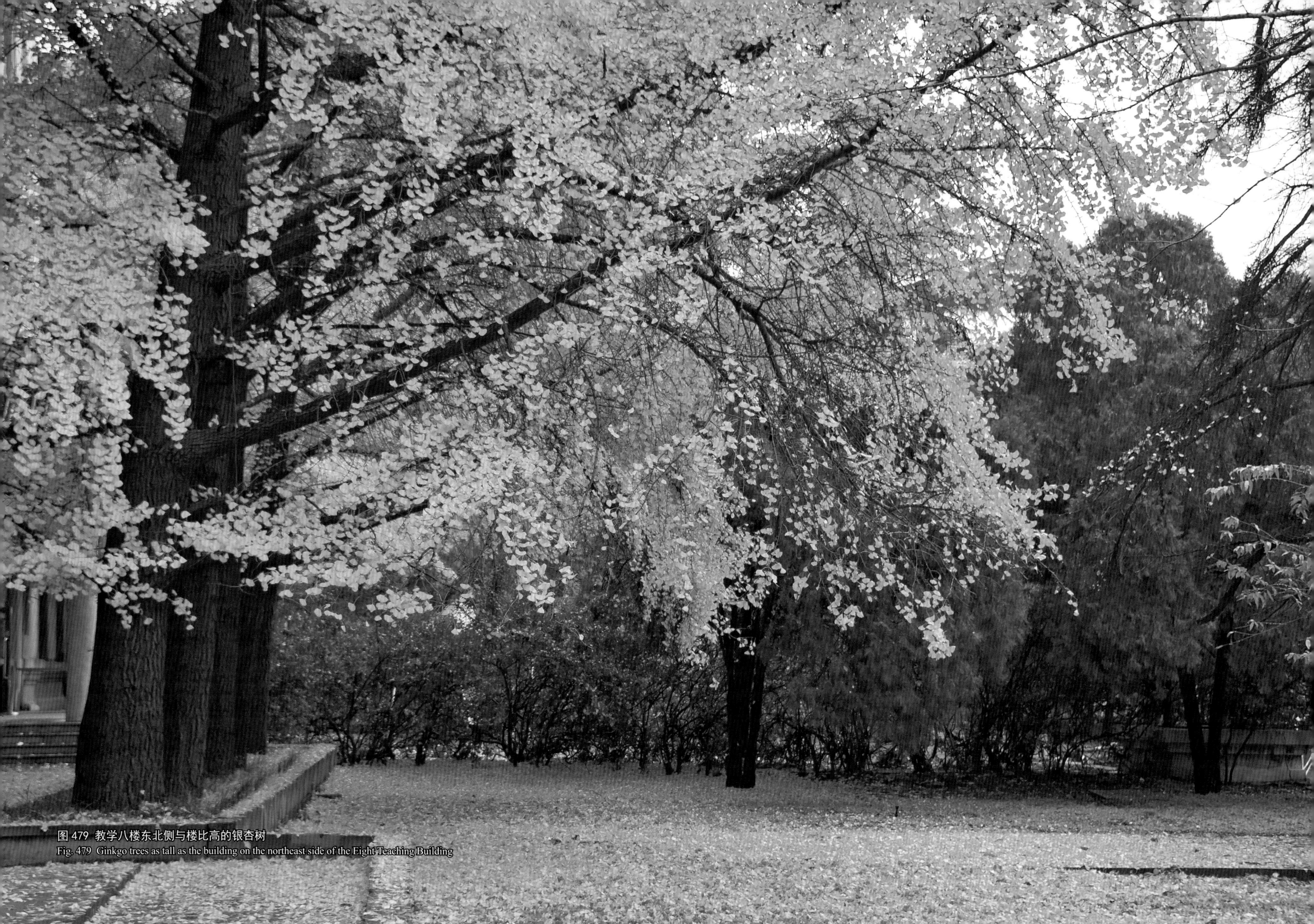

图 479 教学八楼东北侧与楼比高的银杏树
Fig. 479 Ginkgo trees as tall as the building on the northeast side of the Eight Teaching Building

53 秋叶金辉（3）

Golden Autumn Leaves (3)

“停车坐爱枫林晚，霜叶红于二月花。”这是唐代杰出诗人杜牧描写枫叶的千古名句。每年十一月，枫叶红了，银杏叶黄了，槐叶仍是绿的，这时校园变成了彩色的世界！无风且秋叶自落，若有微风袭来，彩叶则簌簌而下，斜飞于空中，令人兴奋不已。这彩色的树上、空中、地上的三维立体空间，只能用“此景只应天上有”来描述了。而下句却是“人间一年一回见”，正应验了毛泽东所写的“萧瑟秋风今又是，换了人间”的英明论断。校园内的枫树主要分布于中心花园、教学一楼西侧与南侧、青杨路中段和教授别墅周围，有鸡爪枫、三角枫、五角枫等品种。

The outstanding poet Du Mu of the Tang Dynasty once described the maple leaves in one of his poems: “I stop the coach to enjoy the late maple woods; Frosty leaves are redder than the February flowers.” In November every year, maple leaves turn red, ginkgo leaves turn yellow, and leaves of pagoda trees are still green, making the campus a colorful world. Even if there is no wind, leaves still fall down. If there is a breeze, the colorful rustling leaves fall from the trees and float in the air, which is very exciting. This colorful three-dimensional space of trees, air and ground can only be described as a scene that only belongs to the heaven. However, “this scene that can only be enjoyed once a year in the world” is the fulfillment of Mao Zedong’s wise judgment in his poem: “Today the autumn wind still sighs, but the world has changed!” The maple trees on campus are mainly distributed in the Central Garden, on the west and south sides of the First Teaching Building, in the middle section of Qingyang Road and around professors’ villas. There are Acer palmatum, Acer buergerianum, Acer mono and other varieties.

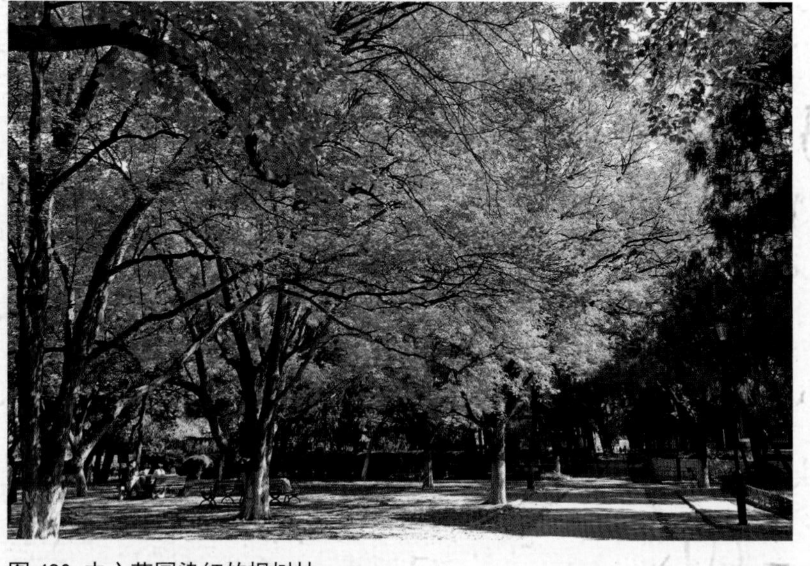

图 480 中心花园染红的枫树林
Fig. 480 Reddish maples in the Central Garden

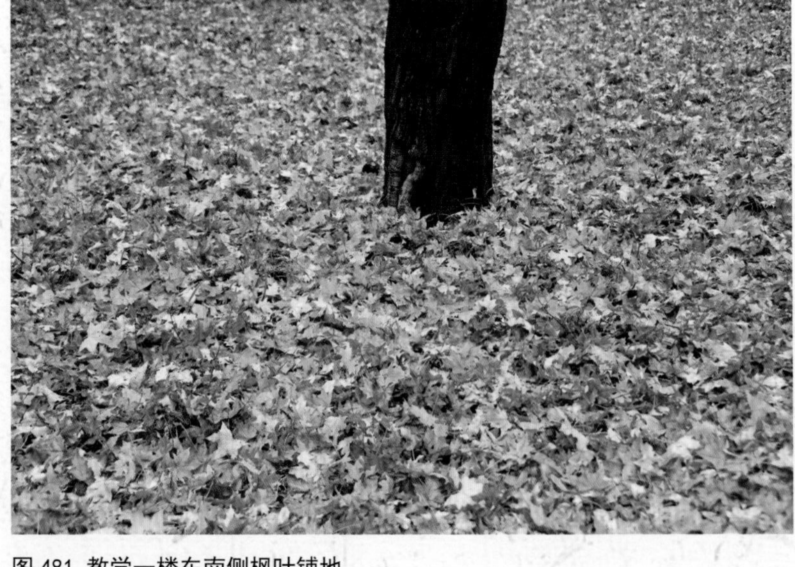

图 481 教学一楼东南侧枫叶铺地
Fig. 481 Maple leaves covering the ground on the southeast side of the First Teaching Building

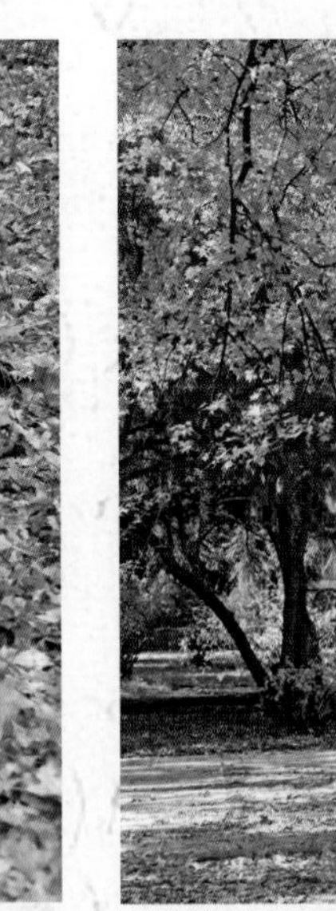

图 482 中心花园西翼枫叶秋染
Fig. 482 Maple leaves with autumn tints in the west wing of the Central Garden

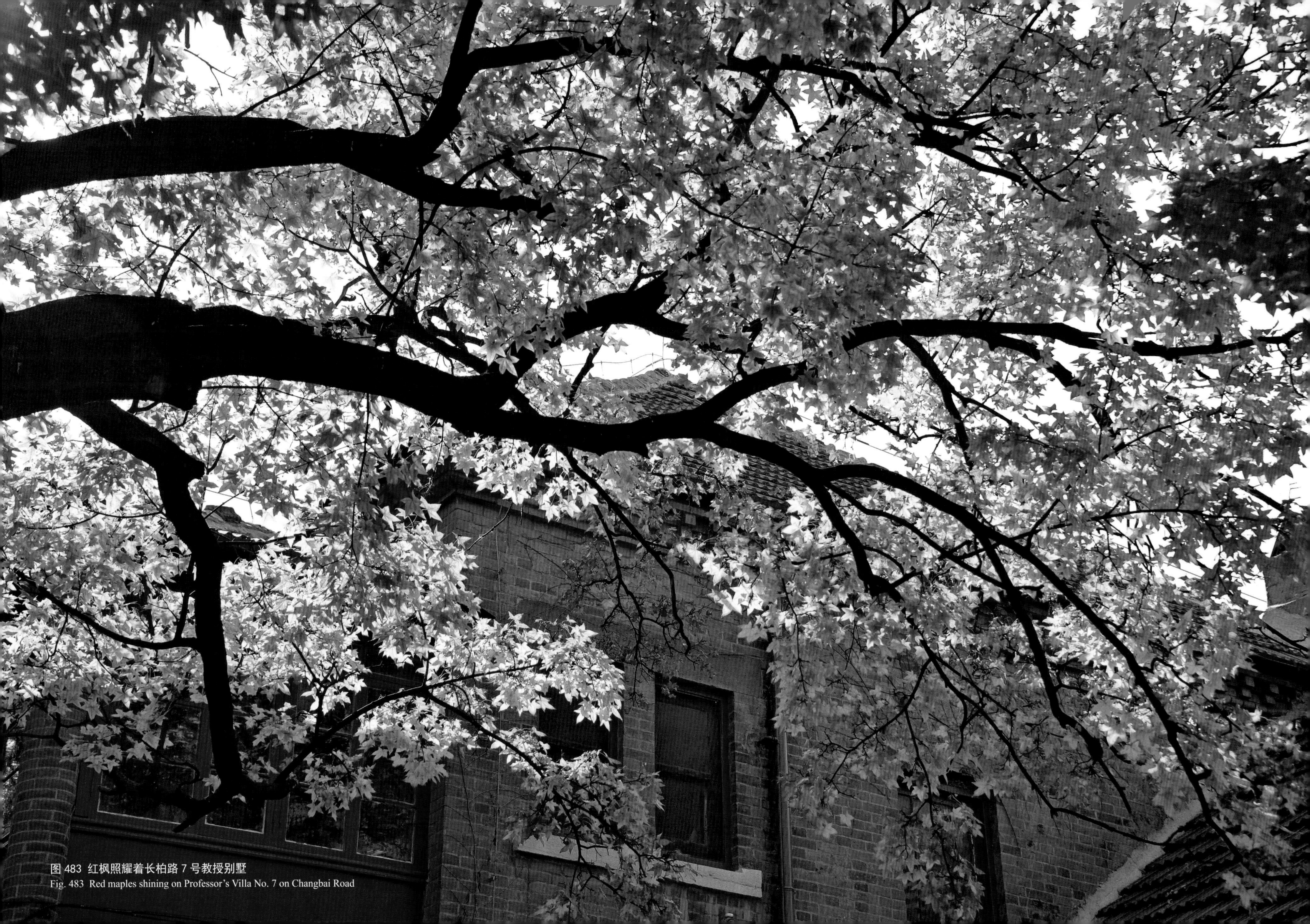
图 483 红枫照耀着长柏路 7 号教授别墅
Fig. 483 Red maples shining on Professor’s Villa No. 7 on Changbai Road

53 秋叶金辉（4）

Golden Autumn Leaves (4)

法桐树叶大荫浓，树姿优美，既高耸入云，给人以高大挺拔之感，又易整修成各种形状，创造出柔美宜人的氛围。它常被用作行道树和庭园绿化树，故有“世界行道树之王”的美誉。趵突泉校区的法桐树主要种植于教学一楼与电镜楼之间、翠桐路和青杨路等处，秋天来临，其绿叶渐变为黄色，最后定格为古铜色。

法桐的学名为法国桐，又称二球悬铃木。它实际上是美国梧桐的杂交种，1640 年在英国伦敦育成。20 世纪一二十年代，主要由法国人种植于上海的法租界内，故称之为“法国梧桐”，俗称“法桐”。法桐树体高大，可高达 30 多米，寿命也长，可达数百年，甚至上千年。

The large leaves of the plane trees provide large areas of shade. The beautiful tall and straight trees tower up towards the sky, and they can be trimmed into various shapes to create a soft and pleasant atmosphere. The plane tree is often used as street tree and garden greening tree, so it has gained the reputation of “king of street trees in the world”. The plane trees on Baotuquan Campus are mainly planted between the First Teaching Building and the Building of Electron Microscopy, and on Cuitong Road and Qingyang Road. When autumn comes, their green leaves gradually turn yellow, and finally turn to bronze.

The scientific name of the plane tree is Platanus acerifolia. It is actually a hybrid of American plane trees and was bred in London, United Kingdom in 1640. In the 1910s and 1920s, the plane trees were mainly planted by the French in French Concession in Shanghai. The body of the plane tree is so tall that it can be as high as more than 30 meters. Its life span is also long and it can be hundreds or even thousands of years old.

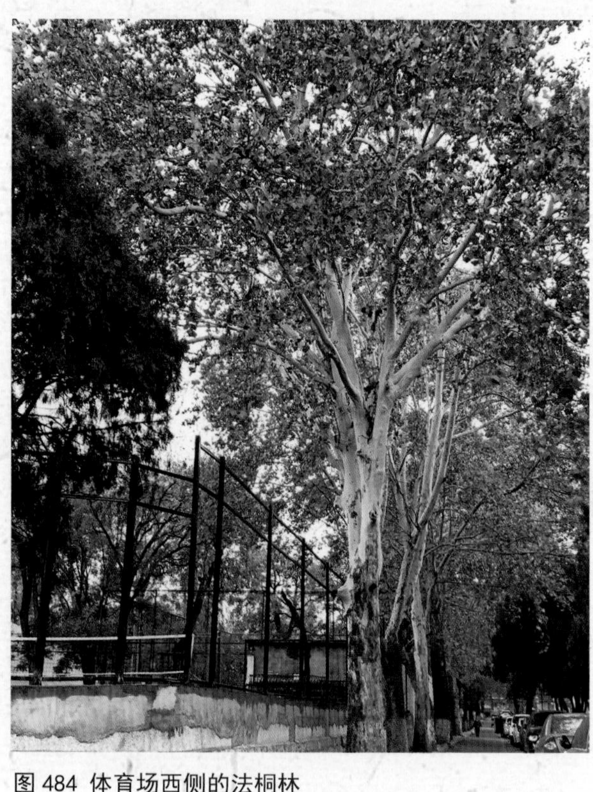

图 484 体育场西侧的法桐林
Fig. 484 Plane trees on the west side of the stadium

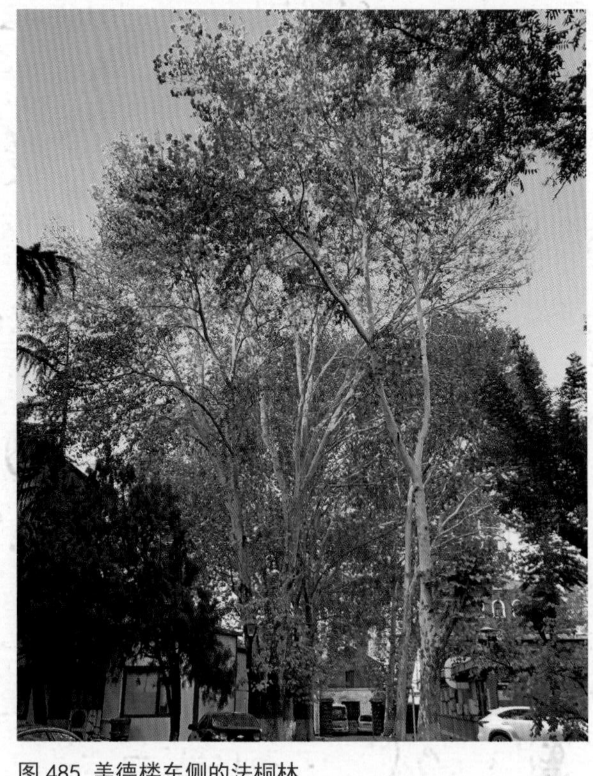

图 485 美德楼东侧的法桐林
Fig. 485 Plane trees on the east side of Miner Building

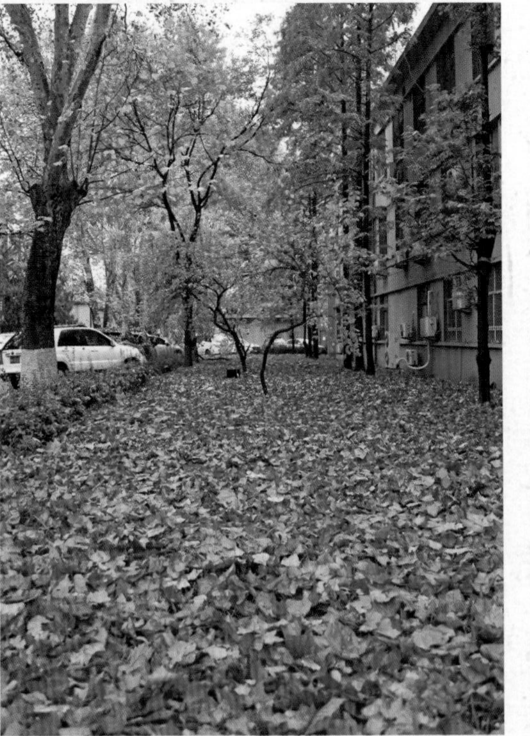

图 486 电镜楼南侧飘落的法桐叶
Fig. 486 Fallen leaves of the plane trees on the south side of the Building of Electron Microscopy

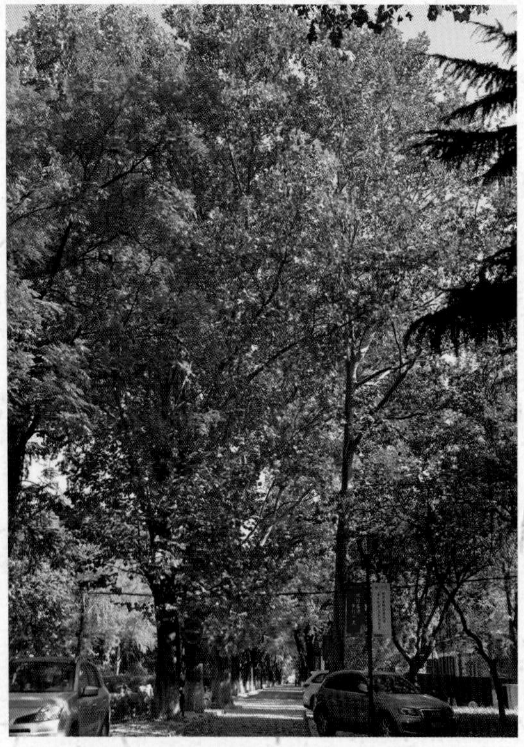

图 487 教学一楼与电镜楼之间的法桐林
Fig. 487 Plane trees between the First Teaching Building and the Building of Electron Microscopy

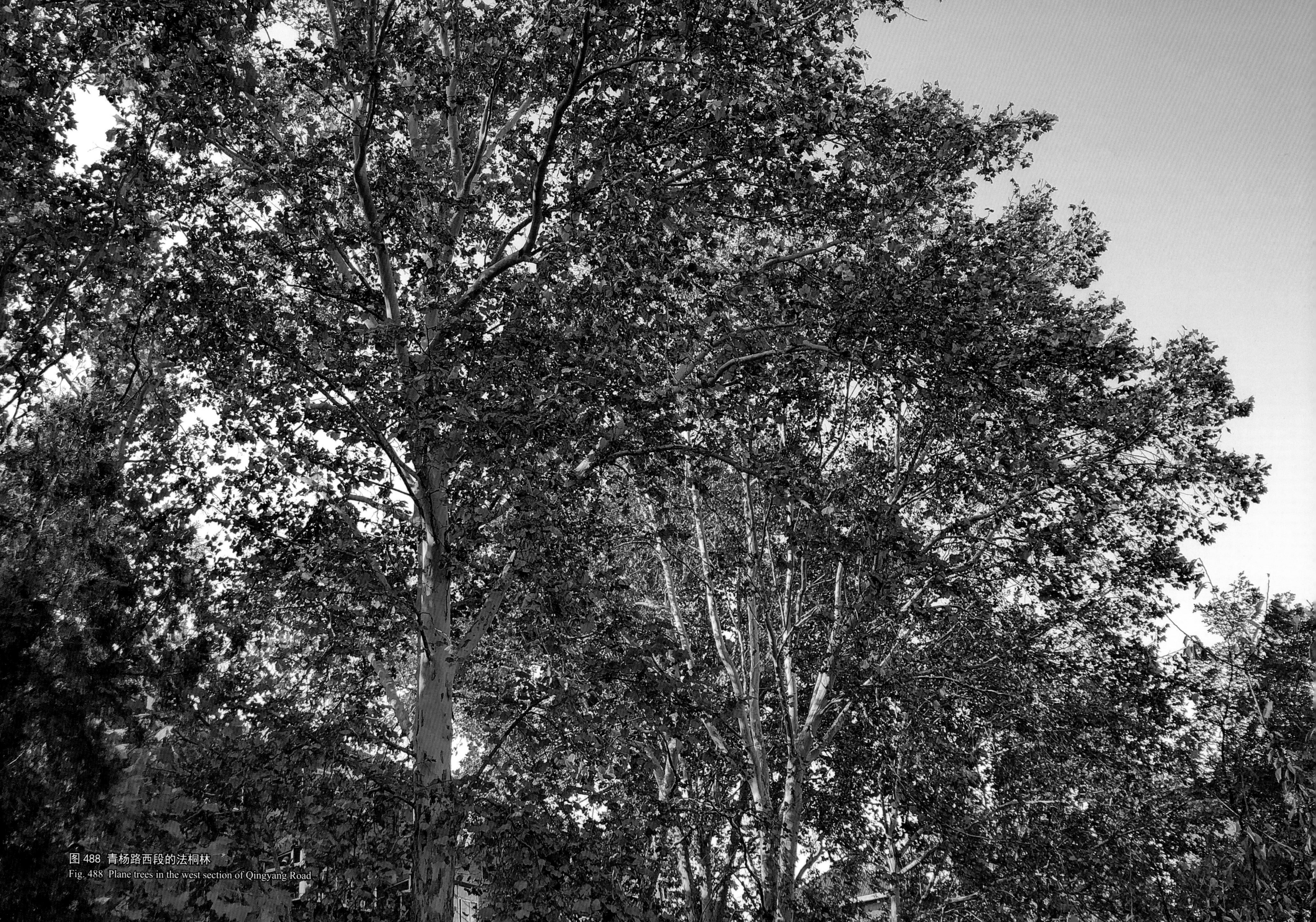

图 488 青杨路西段的法桐林
Fig. 488 Plane trees in the west section of Qingyang Road

53 秋叶金辉（5）

Golden Autumn Leaves (5)

“西山红叶好，霜重色愈浓。”这是陈毅元帅赞颂红叶的诗句。红叶是生命力旺盛的标志，是顽强斗志的象征。人们怀着不同的心境在红叶上寻找着不同的精神寄托，使红叶在秋天里独树一帜，极具魅力。秋天，校园内不仅枫叶会变红，紫薇树叶、爬山虎叶和樱花树叶等也会变红。红叶极其醒目，特别是在绿色背景下。爬山虎最富有毅力，攀登能力堪为人师，不论多高的大楼，它都能爬到顶上。夏天它们将楼染绿，秋天则将楼变红。考文楼的爬山虎最富有灵性，它爬上窗户，欲窥视一下室内的景物，不料却被满屋的书香熏醉了，通体泛红。

“The red leaves on the West Hill are beautiful; the color becomes more stronger with the heavy frost.” These are lines from Marshal Chen Yi’s poem praising red leaves. Red leaves are a sign of vigorous vitality and a symbol of tenacious fighting will. People with different states of mind look for different spiritual ballast in the red leaves, making the red leaves unique and attractive in autumn. On campus in autumn, not only the maple leaves will turn red, but also the leaves of crape myrtle, creepers and the flowering cherries will turn red. The red leaves strikingly stand out, especially against a green background. The most persistent are the creepers whose climbing ability is worthy of a teacher. No matter how high the building is, they can climb to the top. They dye the building green in summer and turn it red in autumn. The creepers of Calvin Mateer Hall are the most spiritual. They climb up the window to peep inside the room, but are drunk by the book fragrance and then turn red.

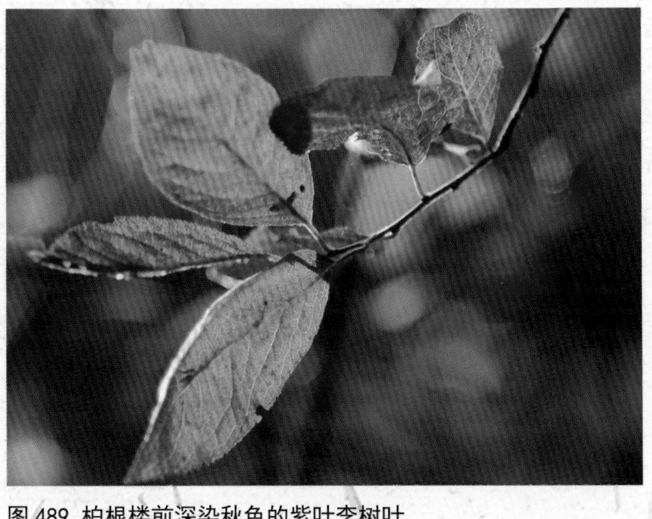

图 489 柏根楼前深染秋色的紫叶李树叶

Fig. 489 Leaves of Prunus cerasifera f. atropurpurea stained with autumn color

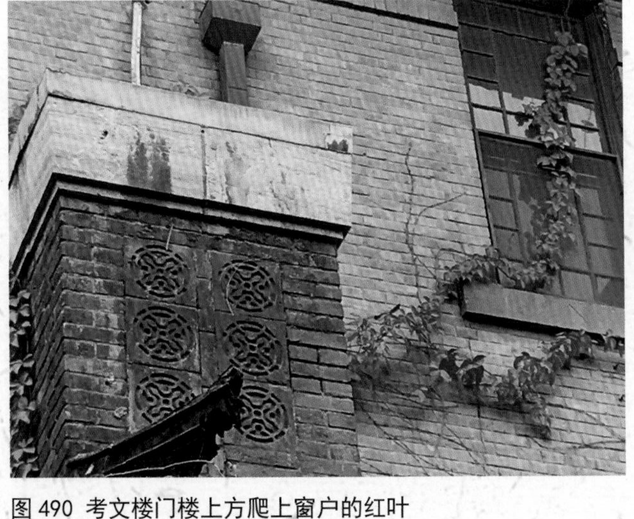

图 490 考文楼门楼上方爬上窗户的红叶

Fig. 490 Red leaves above the gatehouse climbing up the window of Calvin Mateer Hall

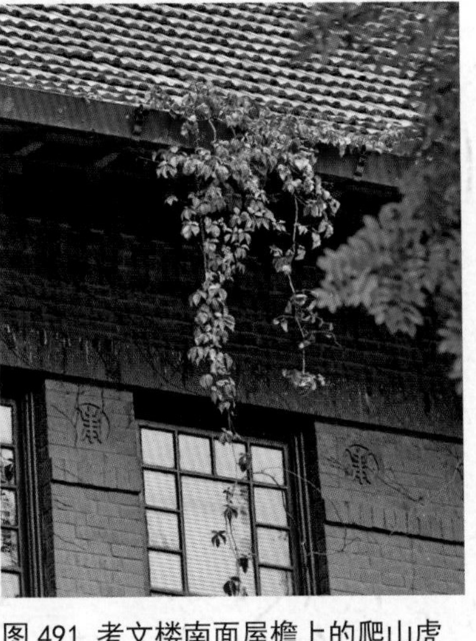

图 491 考文楼南面屋檐上的爬山虎

Fig. 491 Creepers on the south eaves of Calvin Mateer Hall

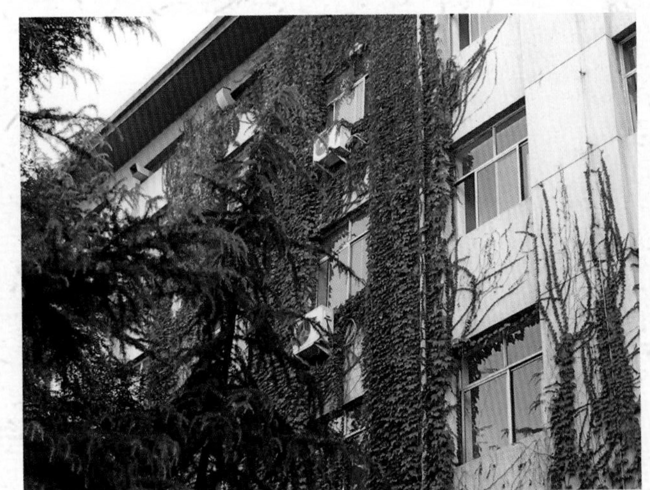

图 492 教学七楼北墙的红色爬山虎

Fig. 492 Red creepers on the north wall of the Seventh Teaching Building

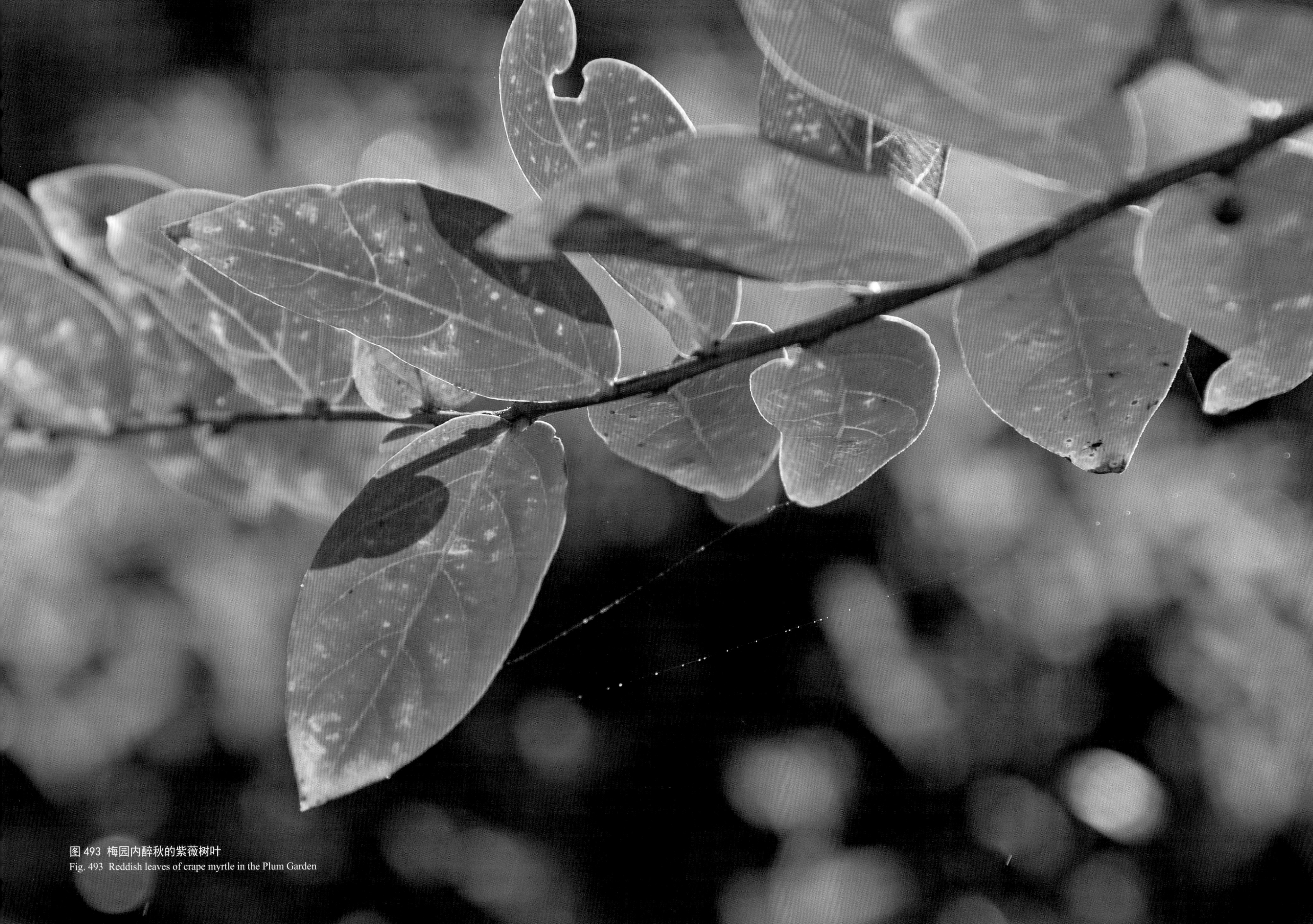

图 493 梅园内醉秋的紫薇树叶
Fig. 493 Reddish leaves of crape myrtle in the Plum Garden

53 秋叶金辉（6）

Golden Autumn Leaves (6)

“朝酌白露晚披霞，不是仙花更胜花。旭日焉知卑草志，乘风驭水蔓天涯。”这不就是描写狼尾草的吗？狼尾草又称大狗尾草，为多年生草本植物，因其穗酷似狼尾巴而得名。狼尾草适应性强，生命力旺盛，耐旱耐酸碱，不惧贫瘠，常萋萋生长于荒野或路边，颇有“野火烧不尽，春风吹又生。远芳侵古道，晴翠接荒城”的气质，故常被用作固堤防沙。在自然状态下，狼尾草的种子借风、水及收获物进行传播。狼尾草普普通通，默默无闻，无拘无束。虽常遭嫌弃，然朝饮白露，晚披彩霞，倒是活的逍遥自在，胜过那些招蜂引蝶的鲜花。每天早晨，高贵的旭日冉冉升起，然而它哪里知道这种地位卑微的大狗尾草的志向，它欲乘着秋风驾着秋水把种子洒向远方，来年蔓延至世界的各个角落。噫！狼尾草这种自由自在的生活态度，倔强不屈的性格，远大的理想抱负，是不是也值得我们学习呢？

“Drinking white dew in the morning and covered in rosy clouds in the evening, it is not but better than the flower. How can the rising sun know the ambition of the humble grass! It rides wind and water to spread all over the world.” These lines are to describe Pennisetum alopecuroides. Pennisetum alopecuroides is a perennial herb and it is so named because its ears resemble the tail of a wolf. With strong adaptability, vigorous vitality, drought endurance, acid and alkali resistance, and no fear of barrenness, it often grows in wilderness or roadside, embodying the temperament described in the poem: “Wildfire can not burn it out; Spring breeze blows it back to life. Distant scent invades the ancient path; Sunny green joi ns the arid towns.” Therefore, it is often used to strengthen embankments and prevent sand. In the natural state, seeds of Pennisetum alopecuroides are spread by wind, water and harvest. Pennisetum alopecuroides is ordinary, unknown and unrestrained. Although often cold-shouldered, it lives at ease, drinking white dew in the morning and covered in rosy clouds in the evening, and is better than those flowers that attract bees and butterflies. Every morning, the noble sun rises slowly, but how does it know the ambition of this humble Pennisetum alopecuroides? This grass wants to ride the autumn wind and water to sprinkle the seeds far away in order to spread all over the world next year. The free and unrestrained attitude towards life, the unyielding character, and lofty ideals and aspirations of Pennisetum alopecuroides are of great worth for us to learn.

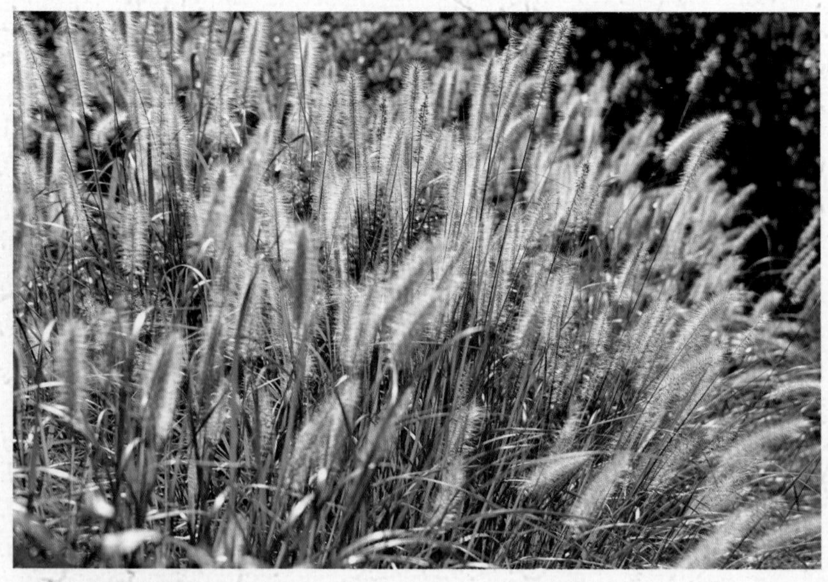

图 494 梅园内成片的狼尾草
Fig. 494 A patch of Pennisetum alopecuroides in the Plum Garden

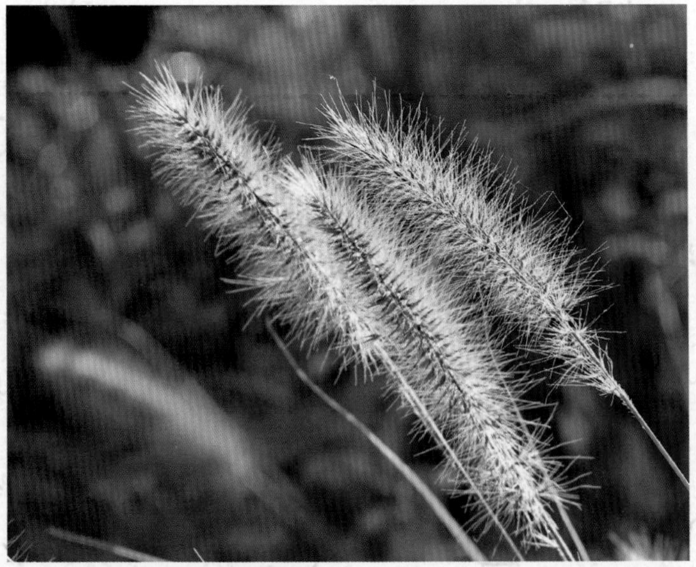

图 495 梅园内发黄的狼尾草
Fig. 495 Yellowish Pennisetum alopecuroides in the Plum Garden

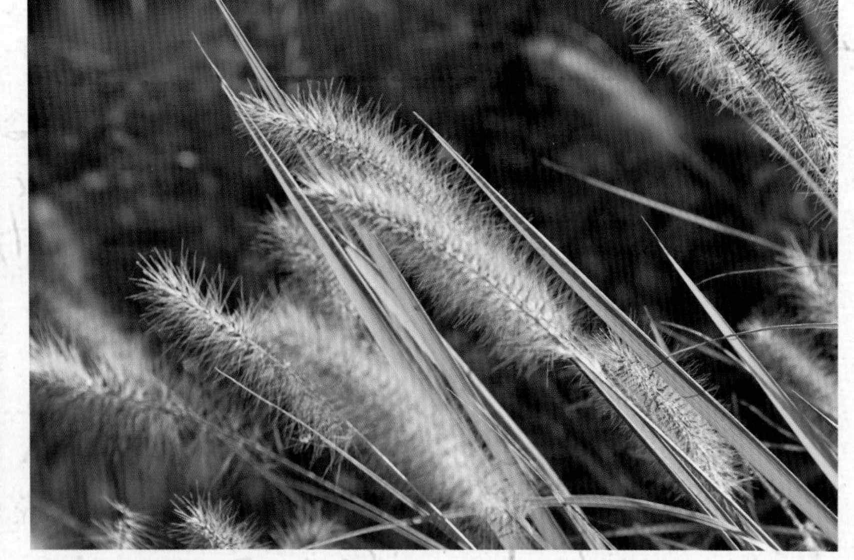

图 496 梅园内狼尾草在秋风中摇曳
Fig. 496 Pennisetum alopecuroides swaying in the autumn wind in the Plum Garden

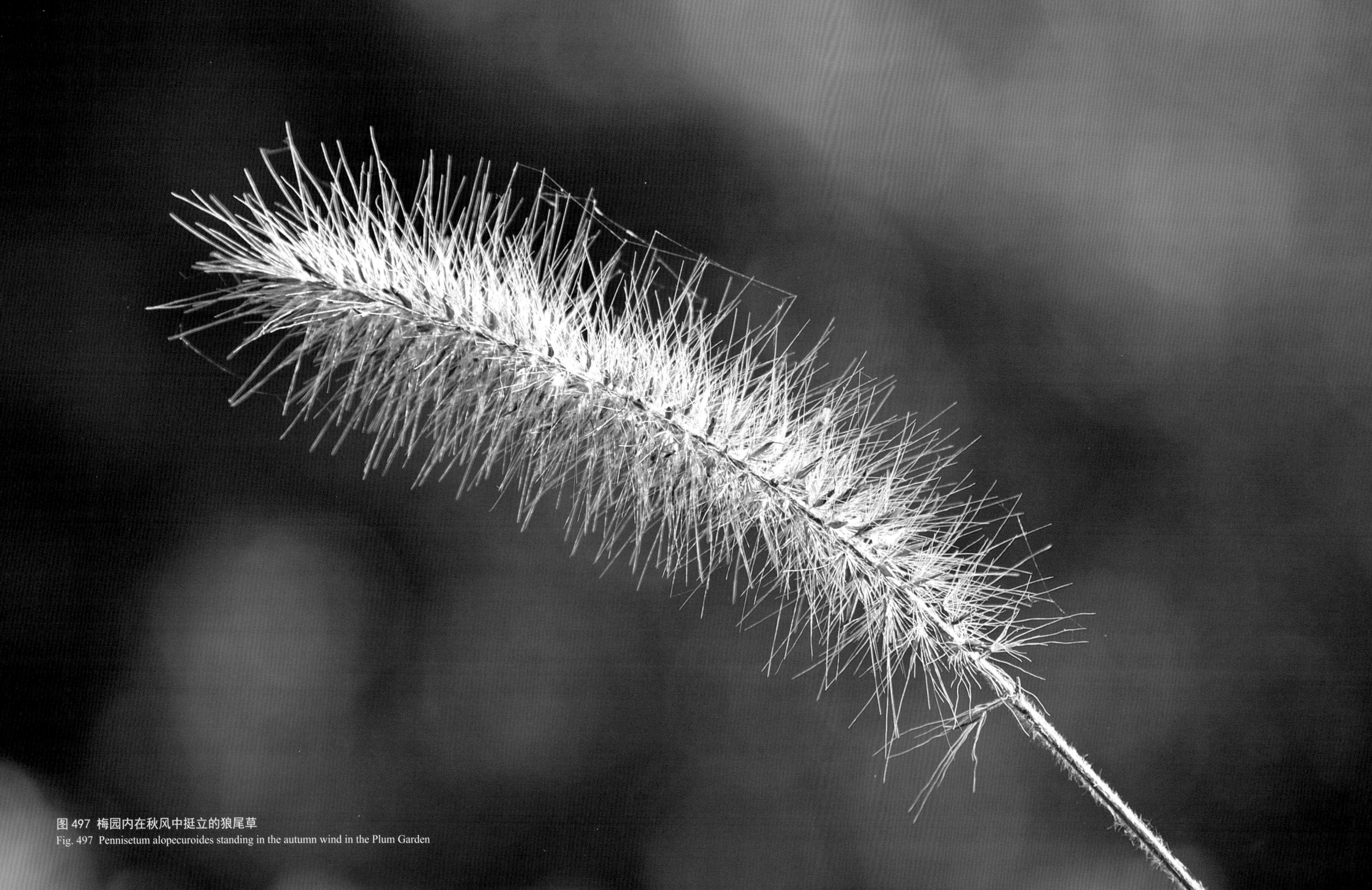

图 497 梅园内在秋风中挺立的狼尾草
Fig. 497 Pennisetum alopecuroides standing in the autumn wind in the Plum Garden

53 秋叶金辉（7）

Golden Autumn Leaves (7)

“满树红灯照古庐，游人不济露枫殊。谁知万点黄金蕊，今日方成赤玉珠。”秋天来临，人们特别关注红艳艳的枫叶，而冷落了红如灯笼的满树山茱萸果。茱萸实际上是非常有名的，王维“遥知兄弟登高处，遍插茱萸少一人”的诗句想必每个人都耳熟能详。山茱萸开花时如黄金万点立在枝上，今日的山茱萸果更像赤玉做成的珠子，在阳光下发出红色荧光，韵味十足。

秋天校园内的果实确实还有不少。山麦冬果恰如绿莹莹的玛瑙珠子，一串串地立在草丛中，只有慧眼识珠的人才能看到它们。山麦冬开花时也煞是好看，一片片，一行行，阵势一点不输浪漫的薰衣草。西府海棠的果实近似球形，黄里泛红，在枝头摇曳，令人望而生津。教学一楼西南侧的大皂角树更是孩子们经常光顾的地方，他们手持杆子或石块，非要弄到盆满钵满才肯罢休。形如灯笼的栾树果高高地挂在树上，十分醒目，春天满树的黄花竟然变成了红得发紫的棱果。

“The trees full of red lantern-shaped fruits of Cornus officinalis shine on the ancient house, but the tourists pay special attention to maple leaves. The branches are dotted with golden flowers when Cornus officinalis blooms, and the fruits are like beads made of red jade.” When autumn comes, people usually pay special attention to the red maple leaves while neglecting the red lantern-shaped fruits of Cornus officinalis. Cornus officinalis is actually very famous which has once been written in Wang Wei’s poem familiar to us: “When brothers carry Cornus officinalis up the mountain, each of them a branch—and my branch missing.” When Cornus officinalis blooms, the branches are dotted with golden flowers. The frtuits of Cornus officinalis are more like beads made of red jade, emitting red fluorescence in the sun and with lingering charm.

There are indeed many fruits on campus in autumn. The fruits of Liriope spicata are like green glittering beads made of agate which stand in the grass in strings and can only be viewed by the appreciative people. Liriope spicata also looks beautiful when blooming, and patches of flowers are not inferior to the romantic lavender. The spherical fruits of Malus micromalus which are yellow touched with red sway in the branches, making people run at the mouth. The big Gleditsia sinensis on the southwest side of the First Teaching Building is a frequent place for children. They use poles or stones to collect the fruits and only stop when they get a full pot. The lantern-shaped fruits of Koelreuteria paniculata hang high on the trees strikingly; the trees full of yellow flowers in spring now bear the crimson prismatic fruits.

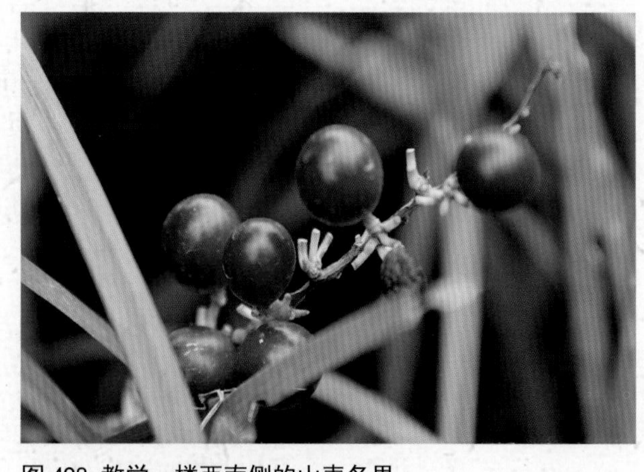

图 498 教学一楼西南侧的山麦冬果

Fig. 498 Fruits of Liriope spicata on the southwest side of the First Teaching Building

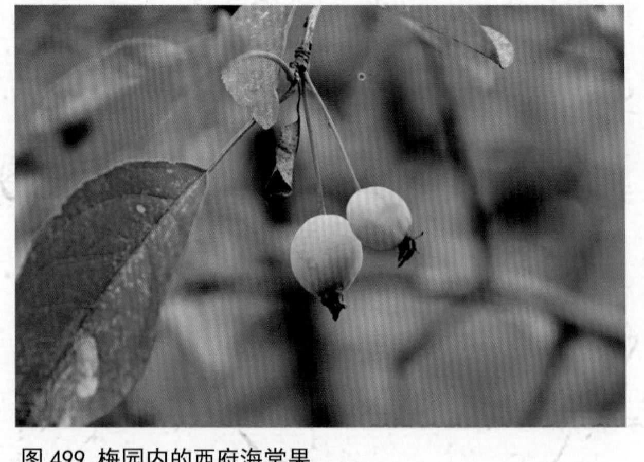

图 499 梅园内的西府海棠果

Fig. 499 Fruits of Malus micromalus in the Plum Garden

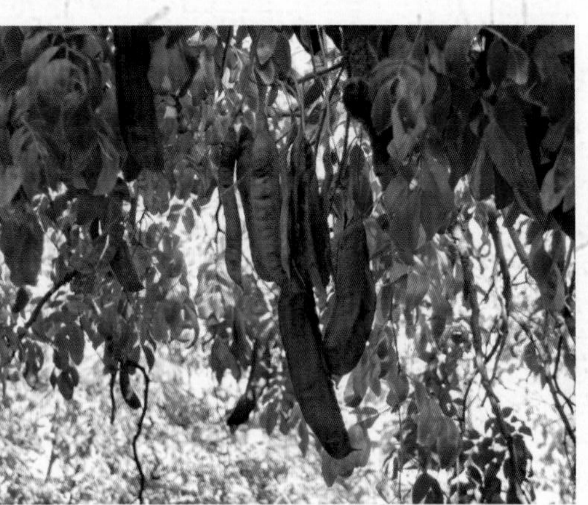

图 500 教学一楼西南侧的皂角

Fig. 500 Gleditsia sinensis on the southwest side of the First Teaching Building

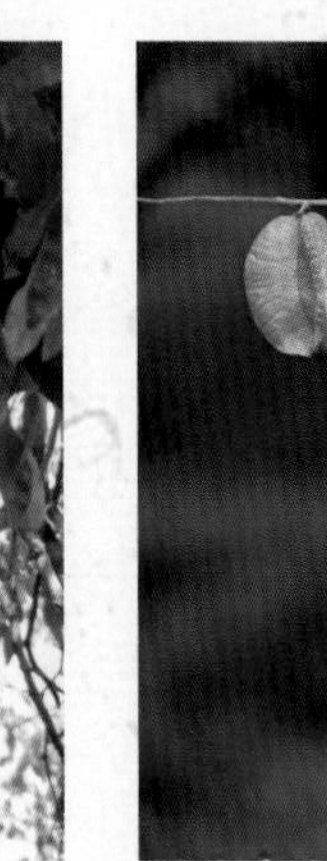

图 501 柏根楼东侧的栾树果

Fig. 501 Fruits of Koelreuteria paniculata on the east side of Bergen Hall

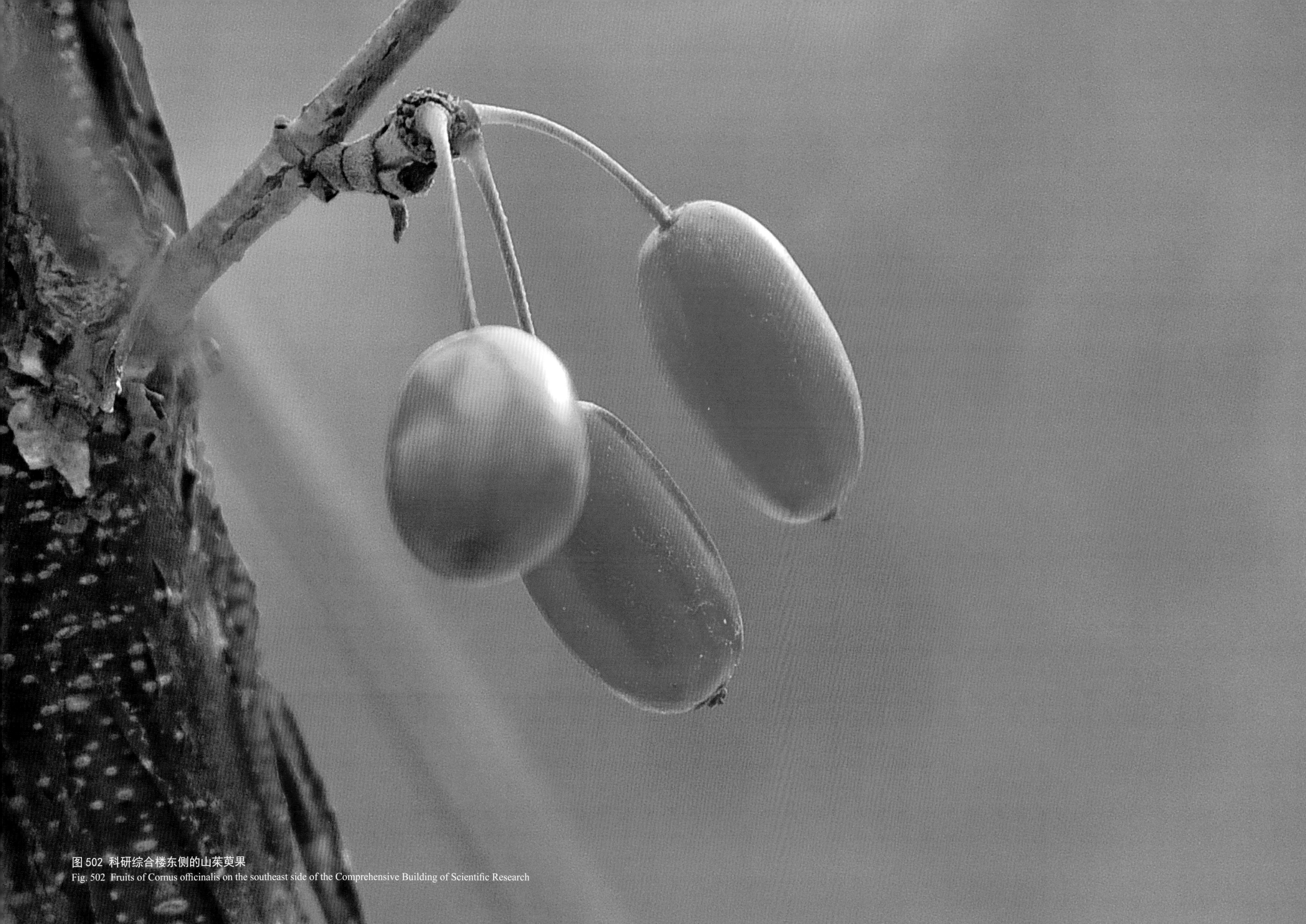

图 502 科研综合楼东侧的山茱萸果
Fig. 502 Fruits of Cornus officinalis on the southeast side of the Comprehensive Building of Scientific Research

53 秋叶金辉（8）

Golden Autumn Leaves (8)

秋天亦是花的季节。牵牛花俗称喇叭花，为一年生缠绕草本植物。牵牛花一般春天播种，夏秋开花，品种众多，花色有蓝、绯红、桃红、紫色等，亦有混色的。鸭跖草亦称碧竹子、翠蝴蝶，属一年生披散草本植物。鸭跖草茎为匍匐茎，花朵为聚花序，雌雄同株，花瓣上面两瓣为蓝色，下面一瓣为白色。马兰属多年生草本植物，菊科，花托呈圆锥形，舌状花，舌片浅紫色。美人蕉是亚热带和热带常见植物，花色多样，花大而柔软，花形别致，极具观赏价值。天人菊为菊科一年生草本植物，黄色舌状花，基部带紫色。天人菊色彩艳丽，花期长，常常成片种植，远远望去如一片黄云，异常壮观，给人以同心协力的团队精神，是秋天里难得的一道风景线。有诗赞曰：“绿茵冉冉黄烟升，气质不与众菊同。长醉蝴蝶红蕊上，秋花香比夏花浓。”

Autumn is also the season for flowers. Morning glory, commonly known as trumpet flower, is an annual winding herb. Morning glory is generally sown in spring and flowers in summer and autumn. There are many varieties of the morning glory; the flowers are blue, crimson, peach and purple, and some others are of mixed colors. Commelina communis is an annual herb. Stems of Commelina communis are typically decumbent and flowers are arranged on inflorescences. Commelina communis is monoecious, with two blue petals on the top and one white petal on the bottom. Aster indicus is a perennial herb of the Asteraceae family, with conical receptacles and tongue-shaped flowers which are light purple. Canna indica is a common plant in subtropical and tropical regions, with large and soft flowers that are of various colors. The unique shape of flowers has high ornamental value. Gaillardia pulchella is an annual herb of Asteraceae family, with yellow tongue-shaped flowers and purple base. Gaillardia pulchella is bright-colored and has long flowering period; it is often planted in patches, looking like a patch of yellow cloud from afar. Such rare spectacular scenery in autumn gives people a feeling of the team spirit to unite in a concerted effort. Here is a poem to praise it: “The yellow Gaillardia pulchella rises from the green grass; its temperament is different from that of other chrysanthemums. The butterflies indulge in the red stamens; the autumn flowers are more fragrant than the summer flowers.”

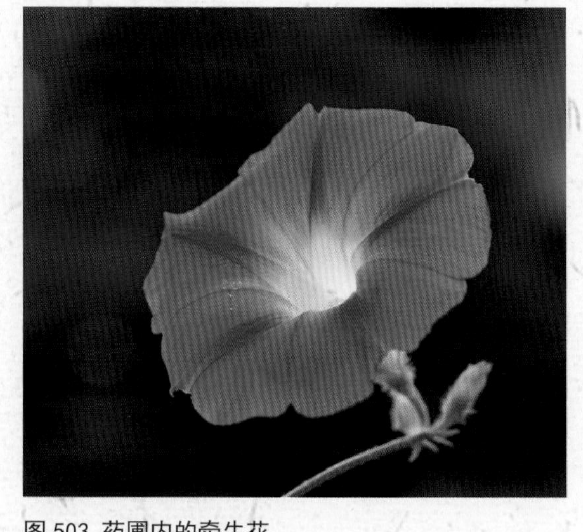

图 503 药圃内的牵牛花
Fig. 503 Morning glory in the Medicinal Garden

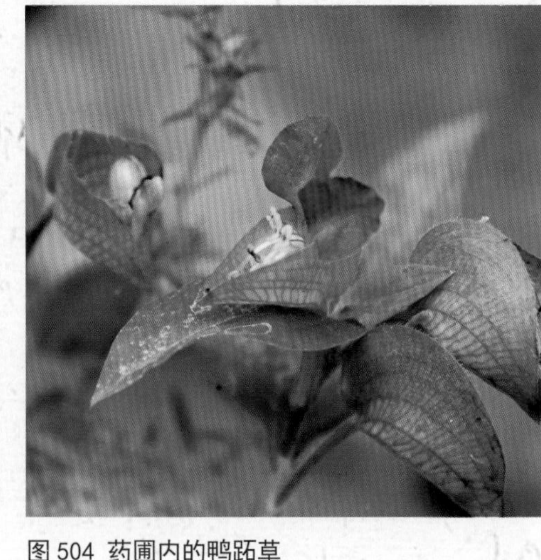

图 504 药圃内的鸭跖草
Fig. 504 Commelina communis in the Medicinal Garden

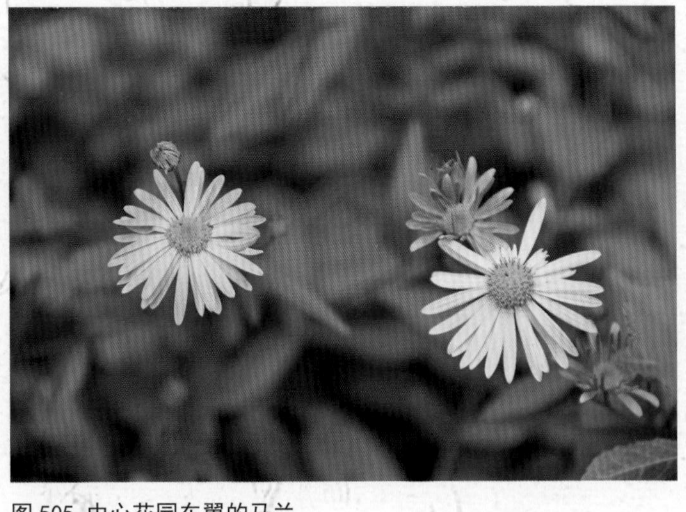

图 505 中心花园东翼的马兰
Fig. 505 Aster indicus in the east wing of the Central Garden

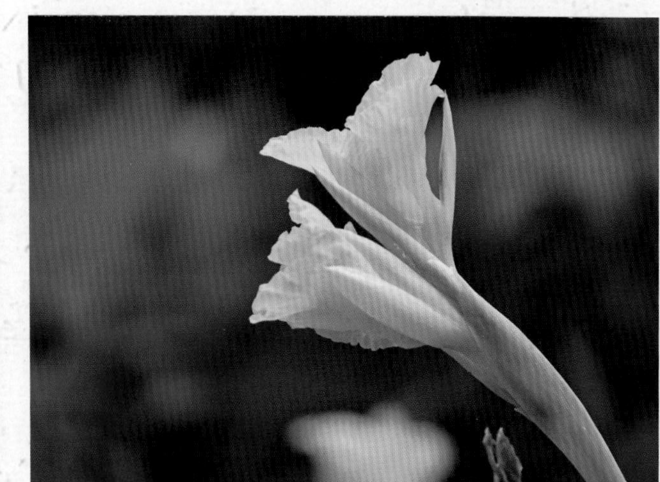

图 506 柏根楼南侧的美人蕉
Fig. 506 Canna indica on the south side of Bergen Hall

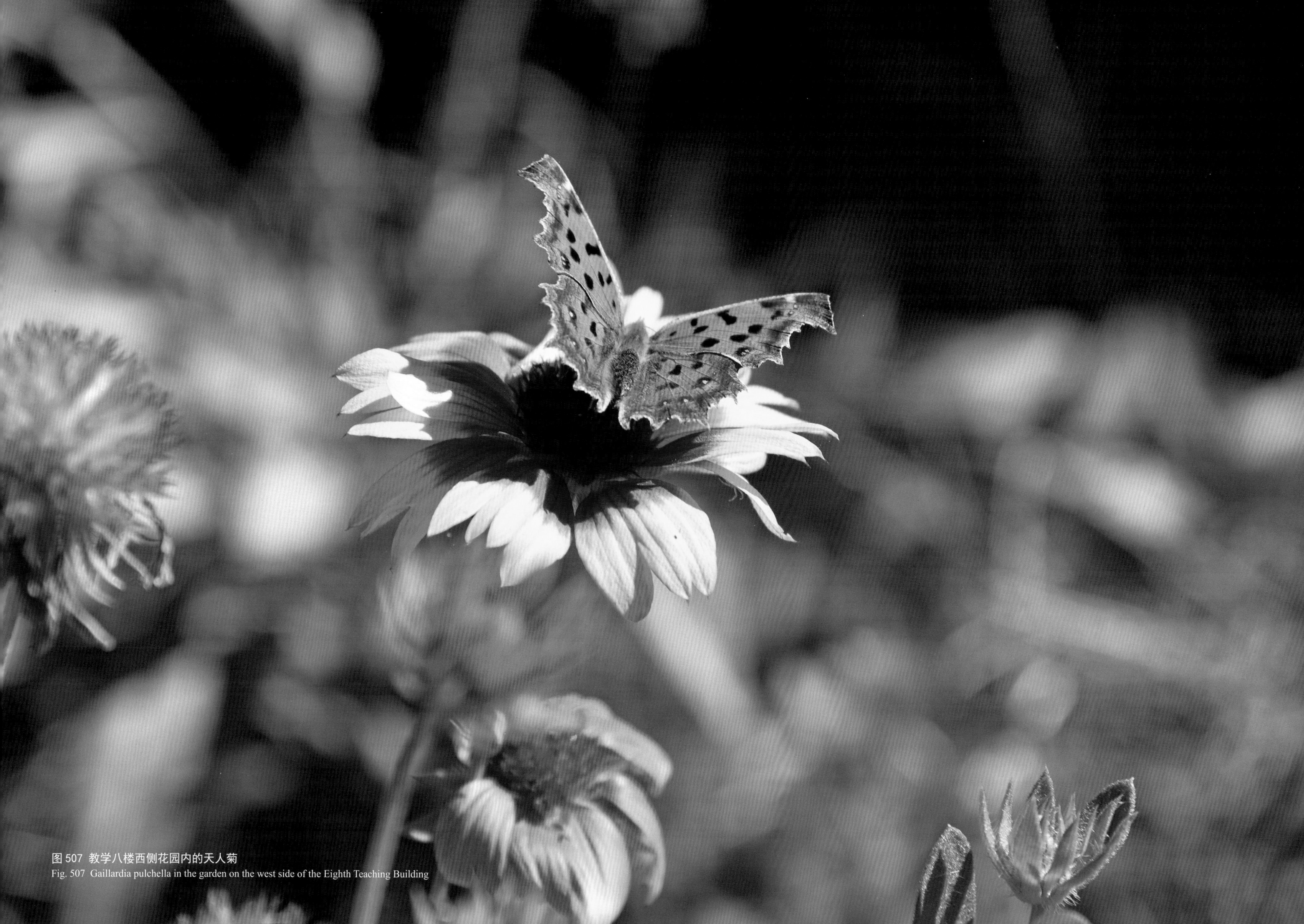

图 507 教学八楼西侧花园内的天人菊
Fig. 507 Gaillardia pulchella in the garden on the west side of the Eighth Teaching Building

54 冬雪映梅（1）

Wintersweet in the Winter Snow (1)

“玉瓣晶黄，朱芯碧透，丝丝香郁薰双袖。群蜂上下闹春枝，芳亭隐隐花间露。月移窗前，楼明继昼，挑灯伏案催白首。晨来出户问朝阳，吾身可比梅花瘦？”这首《踏莎行》对校园蜡梅进行了传神描写。蜡梅是校园冬季里唯一的花朵，它傲寒斗雪，谦虚勤奋，默默地日夜散发着幽香。这幽香激励着师生为攀登科学高峰而努力奋斗，不惜身瘦如梅。

蜡梅原称黄梅，一般在 11 月至翌年 3 月开花，性喜阳光，耐寒，耐旱，有“旱不死的蜡梅”之说。趵突泉校区内的蜡梅有数个品种。最好认的是狗牙蜡梅，亦称九英蜡梅，花瓣小而尖，外轮浅黄色，内轮有紫色条纹。第二种为素心蜡梅，为蜡梅中最为名贵的品种，花瓣长椭圆形，向后反卷，淡黄色，也叫荷花梅。第三种为磬口蜡梅，花瓣圆润，芯紫瓣黄，香气浓郁，又叫檀香梅。第四种为金钟蜡梅，花瓣椭圆，复瓣，形似倒挂金钟而得名。

“The petal is crystal yellow, the core is red and translucent, and my sleeves are perfumed by the fragrance. The bees dance around the spring twigs; the pavilion is dimly seen among flowers. The moonlight shines on the window, the building is still bright at night, and bending over the desk by lamplight makes people look old. I go out in the morning to ask the rising run, ‘Am I thinner than a plum blossom?’” This poem entitled “Treading on Grass” vividly describes the wintersweet on campus. The wintersweet is the only flower in winter on campus. Standing proudly against the cold in the snow, the modest and diligent wintersweet silently emits fragrance day and night. This fragrance encourages teachers and students to strive hard to climb the peak of science, regardless of the body as thin as the wintersweet.

The wintersweet usually flowers from November to the next March. Being cold-resistant and drought-resistant, the sunshine-loving wintersweet is considered to survive the drought. There are several varieties of the wintersweet on Baotuquan Campus. Chimonanthus praecox var. intermedius is the easiest to be recognized. Its petals are small and pointed; the outer layer is light yellow and the inner layer has purple stripes. The second is Chimonanthus praecox var. concolor, the most precious variety of the wintersweet. The light yellow petals are long oval and roll backward. The third is Chimonanthus praecox var. grandiflorus. The round yellow petals have purple core and emit strong fragrance. The fourth is the Golden Bell of Chimonanthus praecox. With oval and double petals, it is named for its shape similar to an inverted golden bell.

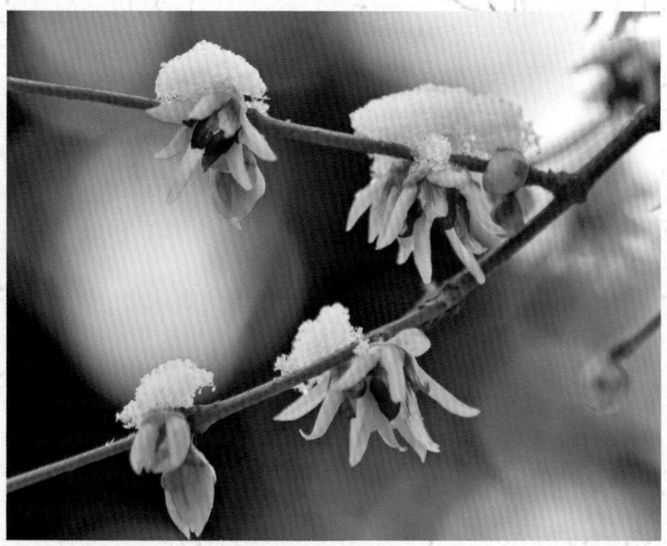

图 508 梅园内的狗牙蜡梅
Fig. 508 Chimonanthus praecox var. intermedius in the Plum Garden

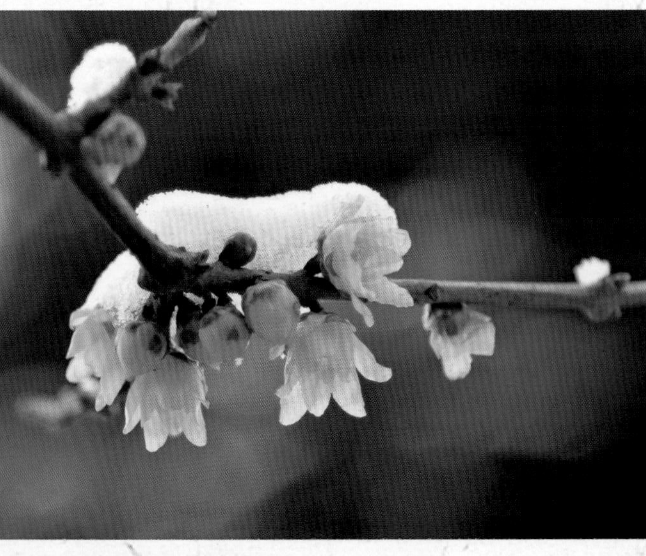

图 509 梅园内的素心蜡梅
Fig. 509 Chimonanthus praecox var. concolor in the Plum Garden

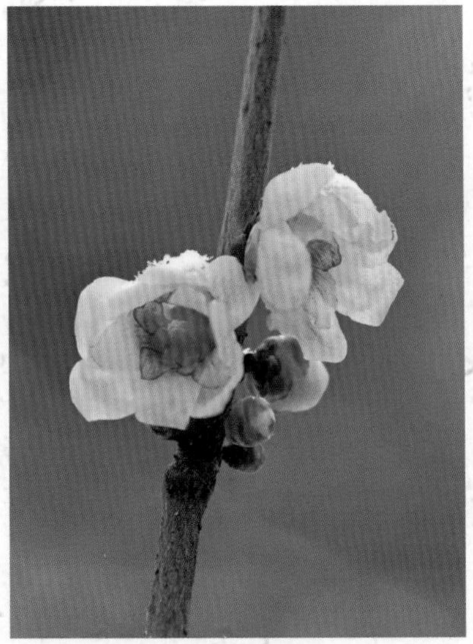

图 510 梅园内的磬口蜡梅
Fig. 510 Chimonanthus praecox var. grandiflorus in the Plum Garden

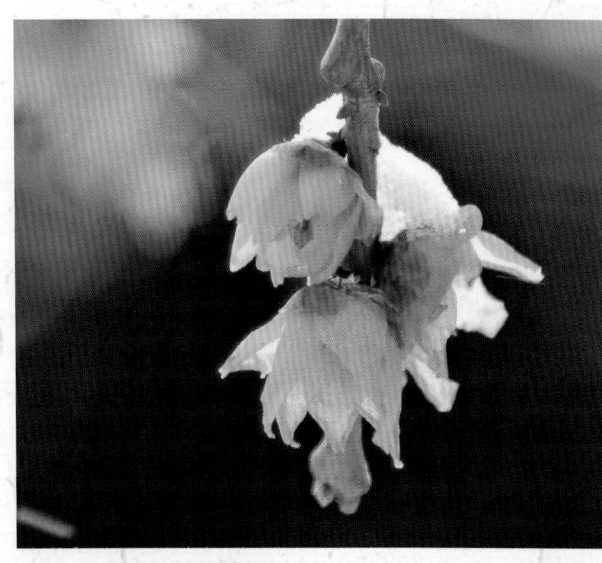

图 511 梅园内的金钟蜡梅
Fig. 511 Golden Bell of Chimonanthus praecox in the Plum Garden

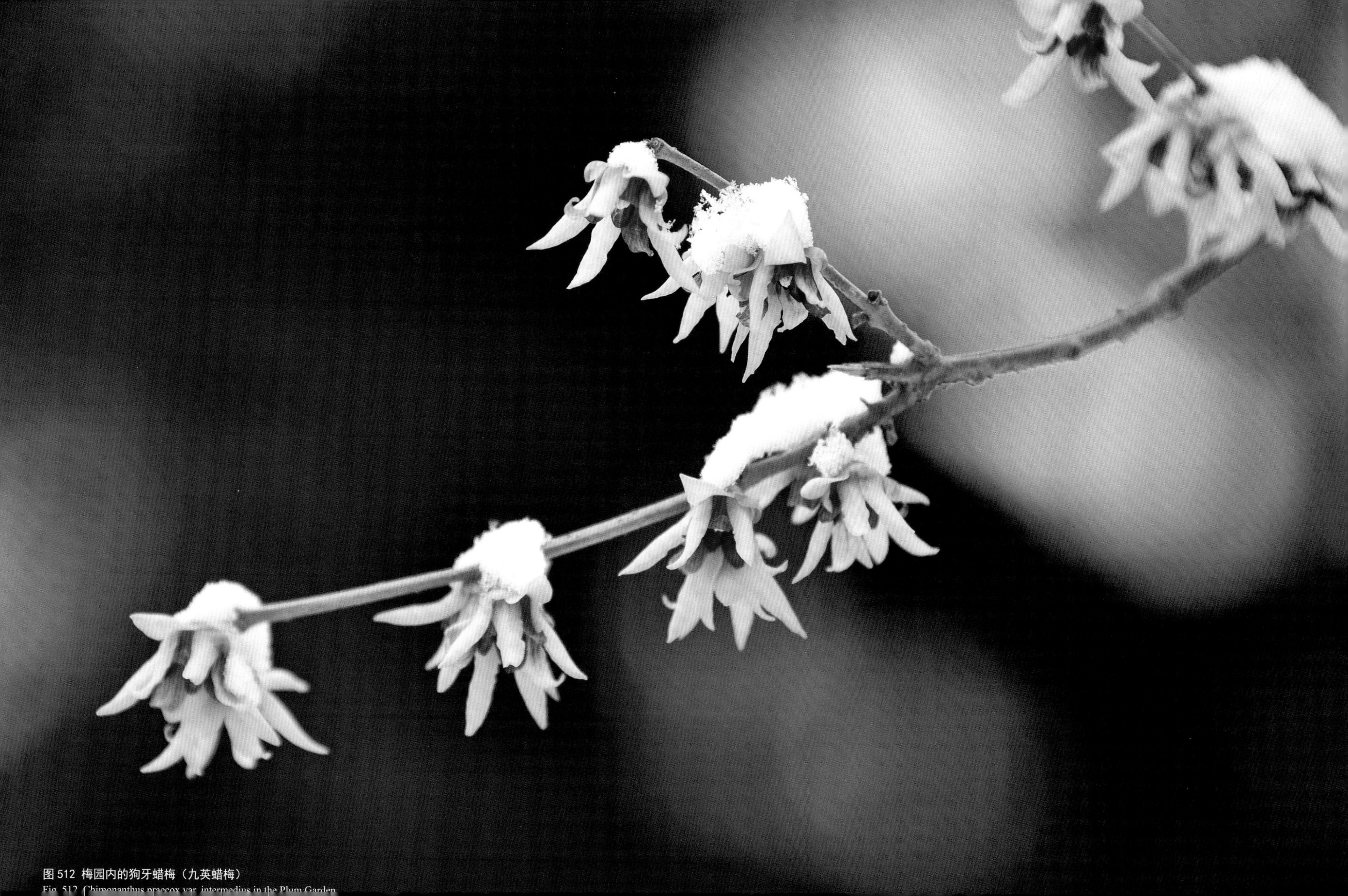

图 512 梅园内的狗牙蜡梅（九英蜡梅）

Fig. 512 Chimonanthus praecox var. intermedius in the Plum Garden

54 冬雪映梅（2）

Wintersweet in the Winter Snow (2)

老舍在他那篇著名的散文《济南的冬天》里描写道：“最妙的是下点小雪呀。看吧，山上的矮松越发的青黑，树尖上顶着一髻儿白花，好像日本看护妇。山尖全白了，给蓝天镶上一道银边。……等到快日落的时候，微黄的阳光斜射在山腰上，那点薄雪好像忽然害了羞，微微露出点粉色。就是下小雪吧，济南是受不住大雪的，那些小山太秀气！”实际上，在冬春两季，济南也经常下中到大雪。这时你若站在校园高处，便可看到南面连绵的群山似乎离我们更近了，左边是千佛山，右边为英雄山。校园的屋顶和地面全白了，树枝被沉甸甸的白雪压弯了，只有雪松还傲然挺立。

Lao She once wrote in his famous essay “Winter in Jinan”: “A light snow makes the scene even prettier. Look at the short dark pine tress crowned with white nurse caps. Or the line of white etching the hilltops like a silver hemline on the azure sky. ... As the sun sets, the golden rays slant on to the light snow that suddenly blushes a shy pink. Just a light snowfall, nothing heavier, turns those low hills into real beauties.”In fact, in winter and spring, Jinan often has moderate to heavy snow. At this time, if you stand high on the campus, you can see that the continuous mountains in the south seem to be closer to us; Qianfo Hill is on the left and Hero Mountain is on the right. The roofs and ground of the campus are all white, the branches have been bent by the heavy snow, and only the cedars stand proudly.

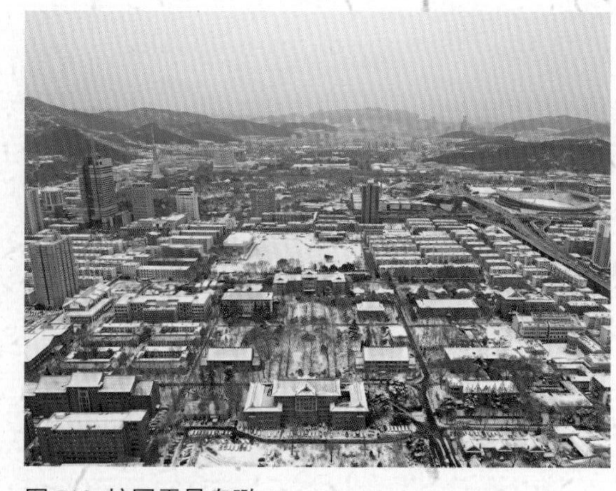

图 513 校园雪景鸟瞰

Fig. 513 A bird’s-eye view of the snow-covered campus

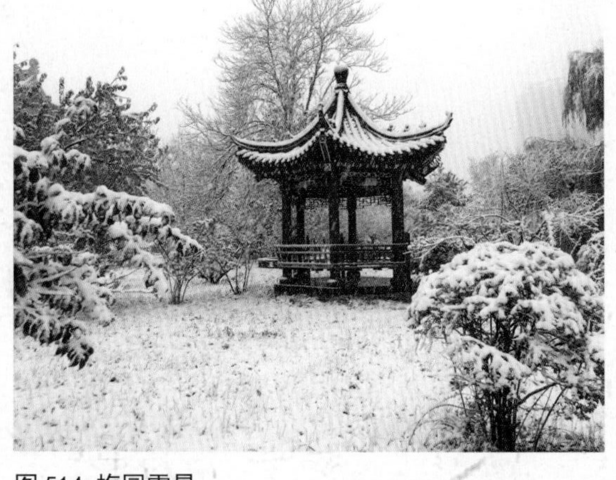

图 514 梅园雪景

Fig. 514 Snow view of the Plum Garden

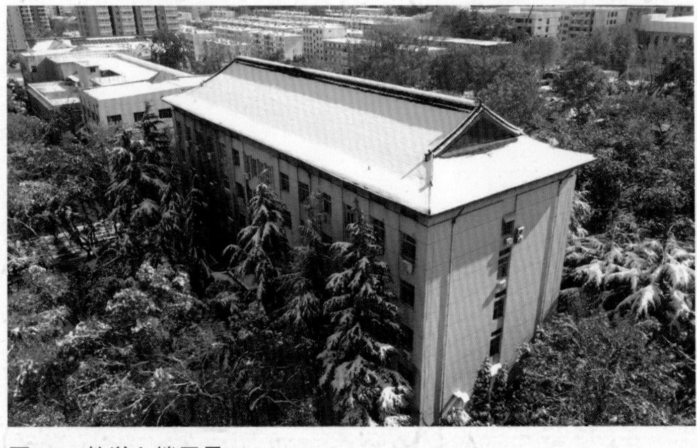

图 515 教学七楼雪景

Fig. 515 Snow view of the Seventh Teaching Building

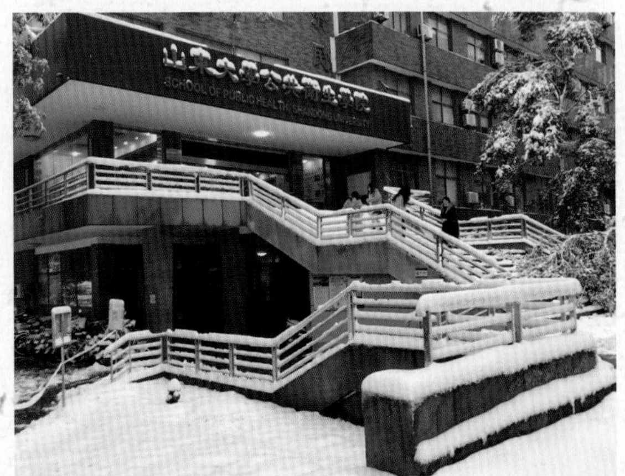

图 516 教学九楼雪景

Fig. 516 Snow view of the Ninth Teaching Building

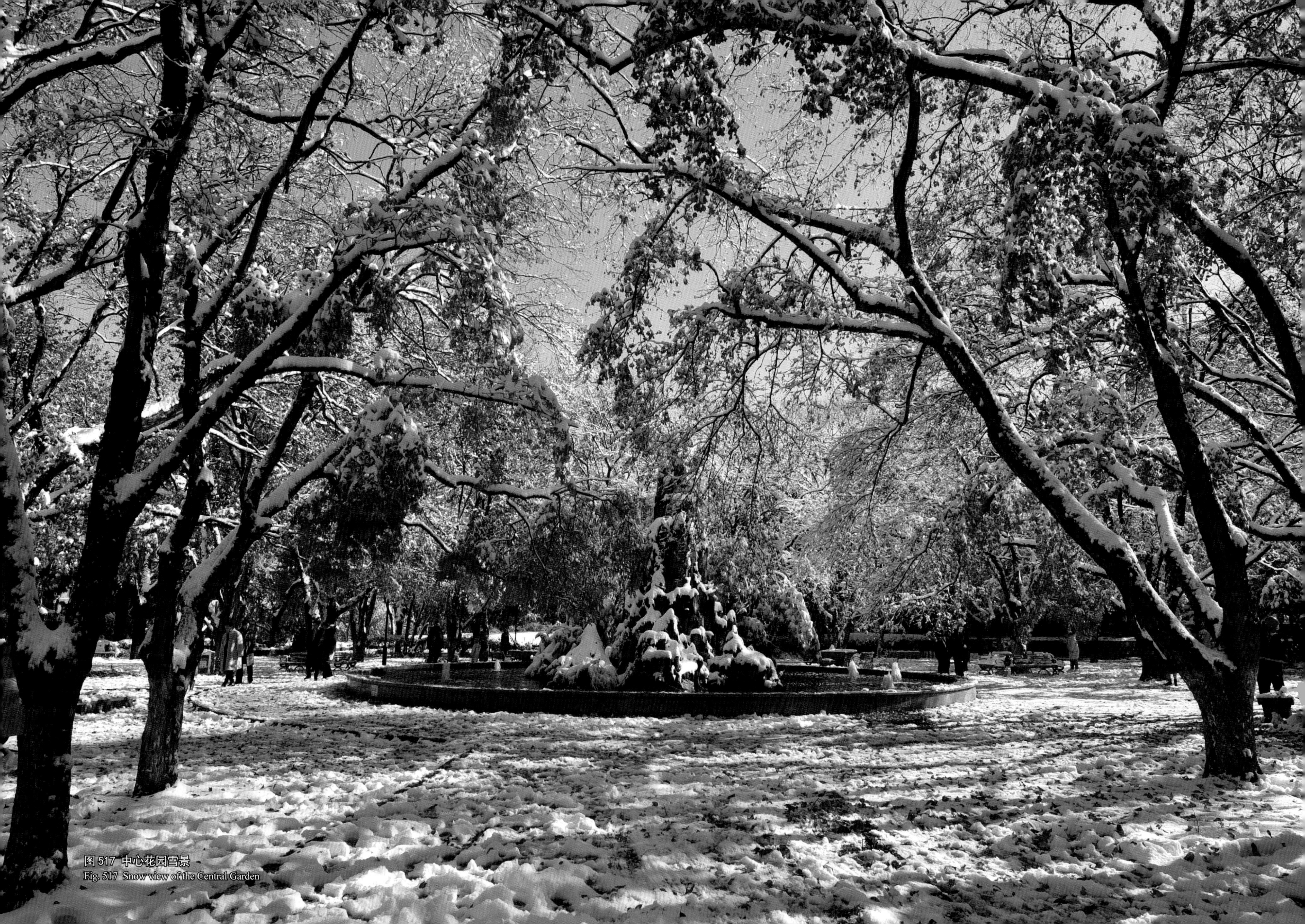

图 517 中心花园雪景
Fig. 517 Snow view of the Central Garden

54 冬雪映梅（3）

Wintersweet in the Winter Snow (3)

在白雪茫茫、天地一色的校园内，忽然看到鲜亮的红色是令人倍感惊艳的！那是晶莹剔透、红如玛瑙的山茱萸果，在寒风中虽摇不落。那是粉红色或红色的月季花，在初雪中仍然笑吐芬芳。那是红胜春花的枫叶，在洁如白云的雪花映衬下更加鲜艳夺目。那是诱人相思的南天竹，在冰天雪地里祈盼着春天的到来。“血虐风号愈凛然，花中气节最高坚”的岂止梅花，还有这么多红色的花果。红色是寒风中的顽强不屈，红色是白雪里的豪迈情怀。正如毛泽东在《沁园春·雪》中所描写的那样：“须晴日，看红妆素裹，分外妖娆。”

In the snow-covered campus, it is amazing to see the bright red suddenly. They are the fruits of Cornus officinalis that are crystal clear and as red as agate, shaking but not falling in the cold wind. They are pink or red roses that still give off fragrance smilingly in the first snow. They are the maple leaves that are redder than spring flowers, looking attractively bright-colored against the snowflakes that are as white as clouds. It is the lovesickness-evoking nandina domestica, praying for the arrival of spring in a world of ice and snow. The wintersweet is not the only to proudly stand against the raging snow and howling wind; there are many red flowers and fruits. Red shows the iron-willed and unyielding spirit in the cold wind, and it shows the heroic spirit in the snow, just as Mao Zedong once described in “Snow—To the Tune of Qin Yuan Chun”: “On a fine day, the land, clad in white, adorned in red, grows more enchanting.”

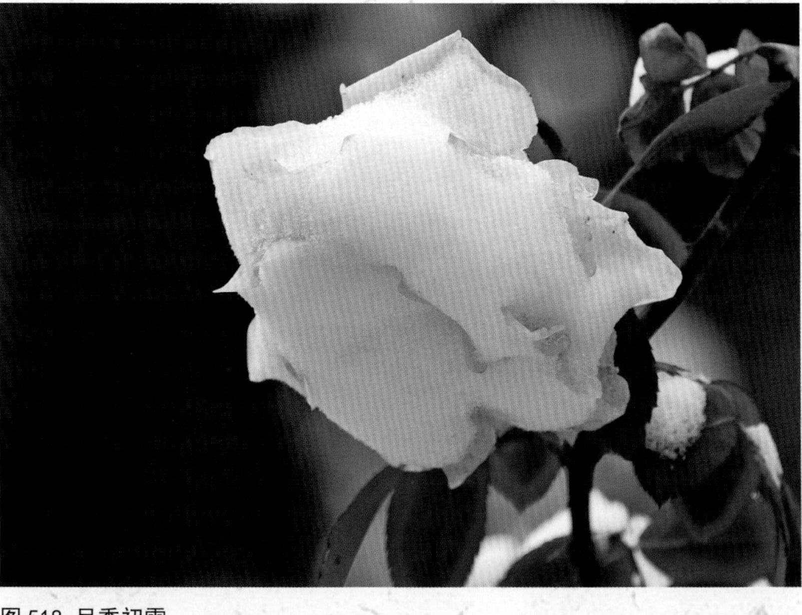

图 518 月季初雪

Fig. 518 Chinese rose covered with the first snow

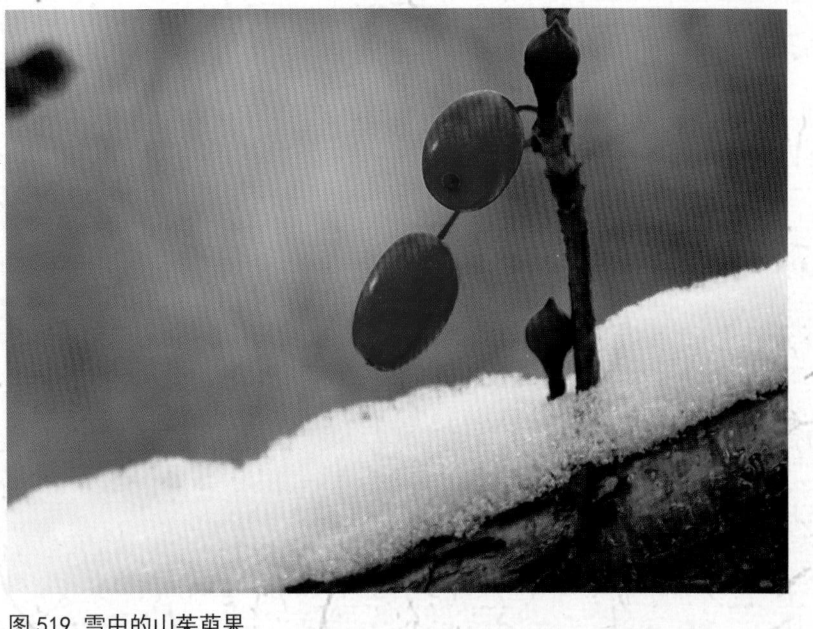

图 519 雪中的山茱萸果

Fig. 519 Fruits of Cornus officinalis in the snow

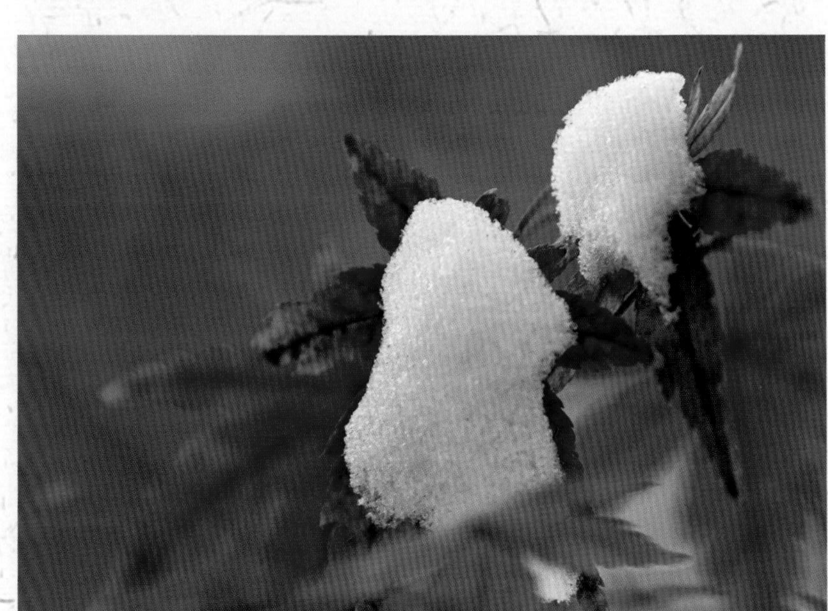

图 520 红枫映雪

Fig. 520 Red maple leaves in the snow

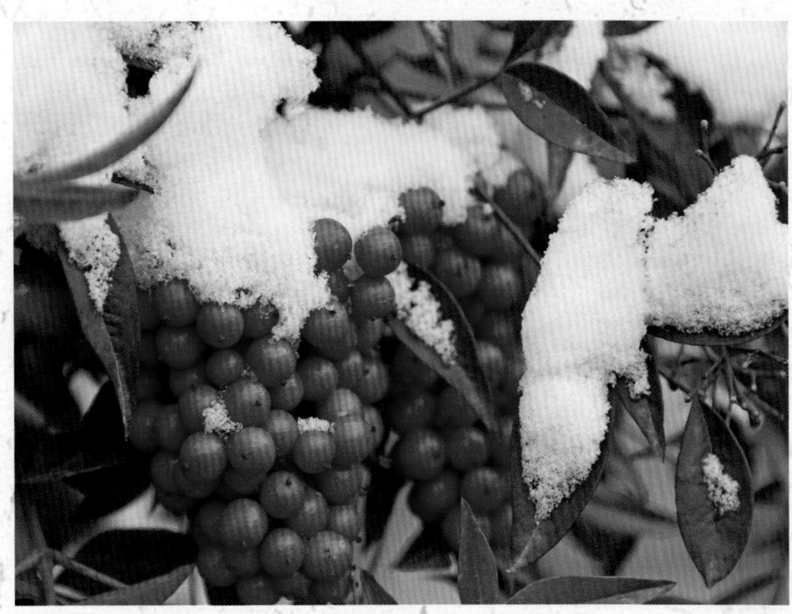

图 521 令人相思的南天竹

Fig. 521 Lovesickness-evoking nandina domestica

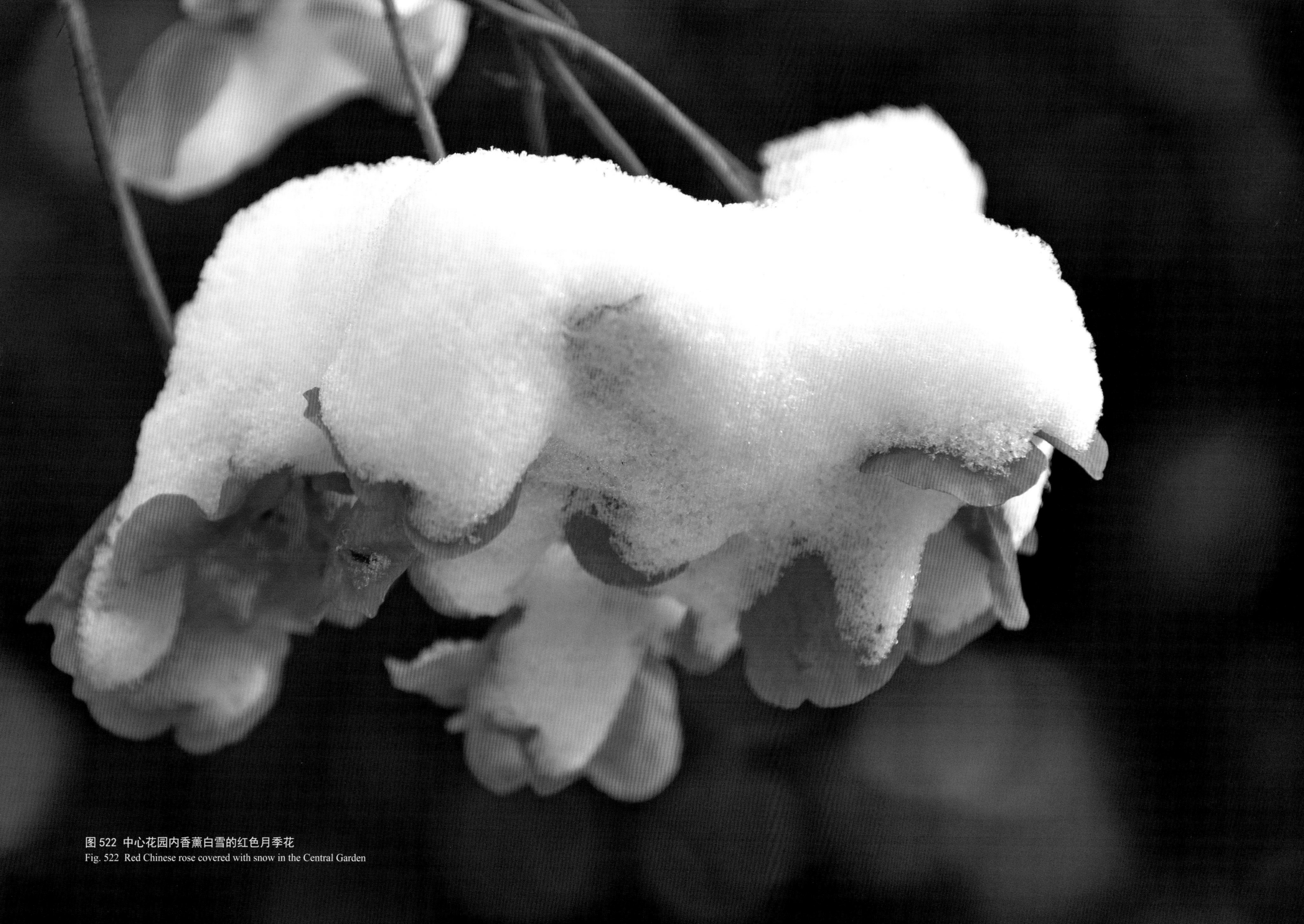

图 522 中心花园内香薰白雪的红色月季花
Fig. 522 Red Chinese rose covered with snow in the Central Garden

54 冬雪映梅（4）

Wintersweet in the Winter Snow (4)

松、竹经冬不凋，梅花耐寒开放，因此有“岁寒三友”之称。校园内的松树主要位于长柏路两侧、教学一楼北门两侧、柏根楼北侧、青杨路中段和中心花园东西两翼，竹林主要位于柏根楼北侧和长柏路 6 号教授别墅内，梅花主要位于校友门东侧的梅园内。

鲁迅在他著名的散文《雪》里描写的“七八个一齐来塑雪罗汉”的故事十分生动幽默。在中心花园里，不知谁也塑起了一尊雪人，引来了不少观赏者。由于地球气候变暖，冰溜子也不像小时候见过的那样长了，但总是能见到。由于齐鲁医学院校园内缺少一条小溪，也没有一汪湖水，所以冬天只能在中心花园中央的喷水池内见到冰了。就这一点点冰，也让孩子们兴奋不已，爬进去溜上一番。

The pine and bamboo have not withered through winter, and the plum blossom flowers against the cold, so they are called “three durable plants of winter”. The pine trees on campus are mainly located on both sides of Changbai Road, on both sides of the north gate of the First Teaching Building, on the north side of Bergen Hall, in the middle section of Qingyang Road, and on the east and west wings of the Central Garden. The bamboo forest is mainly located on the north side of Bergen Hall and in professor’s villa No. 6 on Changbai Road. The plum blossoms are mainly located in the Plum Garden on the east side of the Alumni Gate.

The story of “seven or eight children have gathered to build a snowman” described by Lu Xun in his famous prose “Snow” is very vivid and humorous. In the Central Garden, someone also made a snowman, attracting a lot of viewers. The are also some icicles, but they are not as long as they used to be due to the warming of the climate on earth. Due to the lack of a creek or a pool of water on the campus of Cheeloo College of Medicine, the ice can only be seen in the fountain in the middle of the Central Garden in winter, which makes the children excited to slide on the ice.

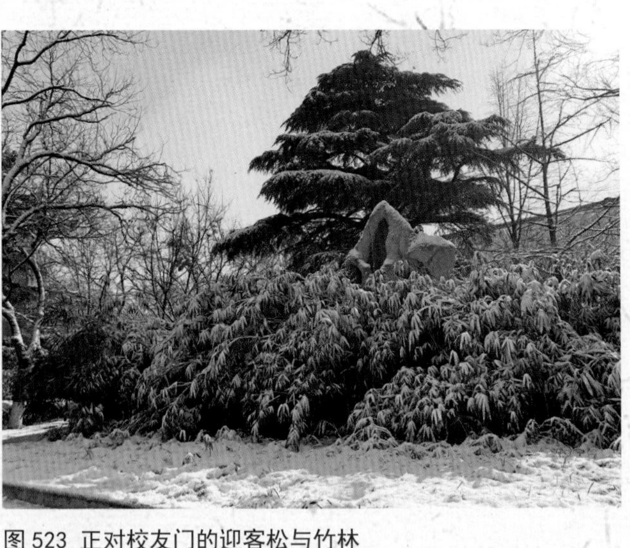

图 523 正对校友门的迎客松与竹林
Fig. 523 Guest-greeting pine and bamboo forest facing the Alumni Gate

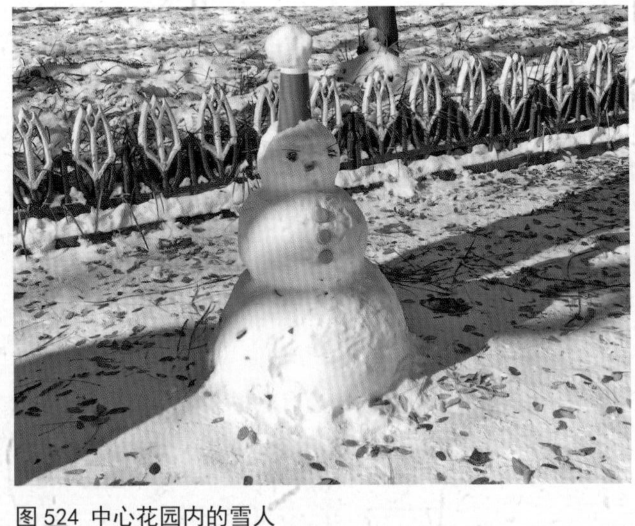

图 524 中心花园内的雪人
Fig. 524 Snowman in the Central Garden

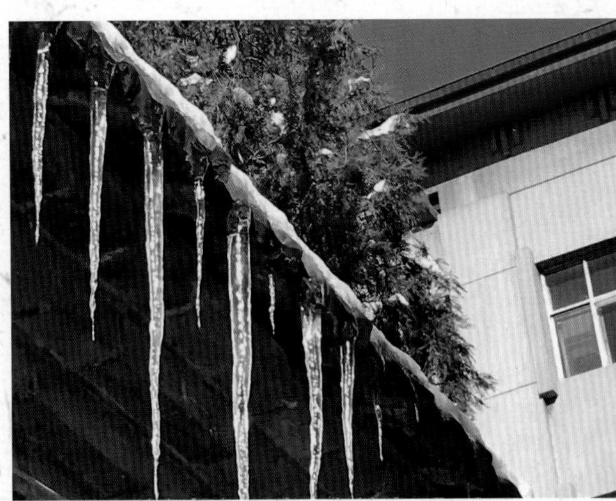

图 525 长柏路 5 号教授别墅的冰溜子
Fig. 525 Icicles in professor’s villa at No. 5 Changbai Road

图 526 冰封雪盖的中心花园中央喷水池
Fig. 526 Fountain in the middle of the snow-covered Central Garden

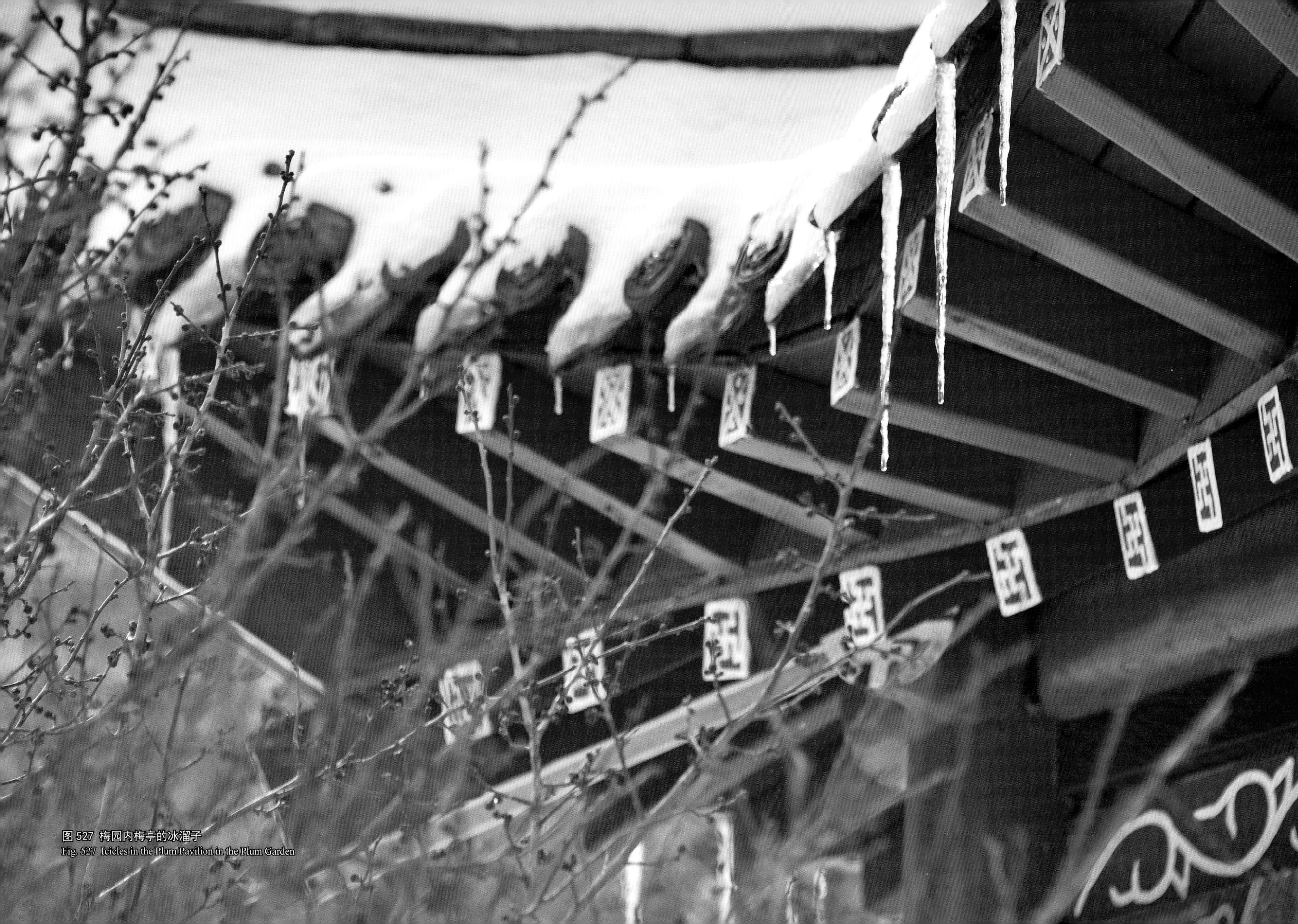

图 527 梅园内梅亭的冰溜子
Fig. 527 Icicles in the Plum Pavilion in the Plum Garden

55 林间魅影（1）

Glamour of the Woodland (1)

心亭位于教学一、二楼之间杏林广场的西侧。坐于此亭内，东可尽览杏林广场和银杏林的四季变化，南可眺望教学二楼，西能欣赏药学科研楼、新建的实验动物中心、齐鲁大学水塔、美德楼和卫生部耳鼻咽喉科重点实验室，北能近观教学一楼。心亭建于2012年5月，由山东医学院医学系七七级二班全体同学毕业三十周年时捐建并题联。亭顶四角卷翘向上，有凌空欲飞之感，东西边均刻有“心亭”二字。底座四方形，东西边各设一门，南北边各建一条坐板，可坐或卧于其上。体部为四根四面体立柱，立柱四面均刻有对联，共有八幅对联，以各种字体镌刻。这些对联是：苑秀育芳菲桃李馨香飘域外，坛真求善美春辉和煦暖心中；日起意飞扬医海泛舟行未尽，月临思转辗校园寻梦断还留；辞妙镌石新小亭玉立风趁雅，心灵逢地秀学子常临趣近幽；学子亭间多勤奋，众生世上少苦疾；五载同窗手足诚挚曾感慨情怀似梦，卅年聚首师长谊深更细陈往事如烟；青春伴明月正是少年读书夜，光阴随流水常思恩师教诲时；十五月圆时水逝流光寻旧地，三十人聚日岁积风采照新天；五年捧卷何觉苦，半世行医终晓难。

The Heart Pavilion is located on the west side of Xinglin Square between the First Teaching Building and the Second Teaching Building. Sitting in this pavilion, you can appreciate the four seasons of Xinglin Square and the ginkgo forest in the east, overlook the Second Teaching Building in the south, enjoy the Pharmaceutical Research Building, the newly built Laboratory Animal Center, the Water Tower of Cheeloo University, the Miner Building and the Key Laboratory of Otorhinolaryngology of the National Health Commission (former Ministry of Health) in the west, and have a close look at the First Teaching Building in the north. The Heart Pavilion was built in May 2012, funded by all the students of Class 2 of 1977 from the Medical Department of Shandong Medical College on the 30th anniversary of graduation. The four corners on the top of the pavilion are upturned, high up in the air. The east and west sides are both engraved with the Chinese characters “Xin Ting”. The base is square, the east and west sides are respectively provided with an entrance, and the north and south sides are respectively provided with a sitting board on which you can sit or lie. The body part is four tetrahedral upright pillars, and the four sides of the pillars are all engraved with couplets. There are eight couplets in total, which are engraved in various fonts.

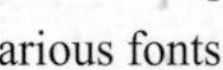

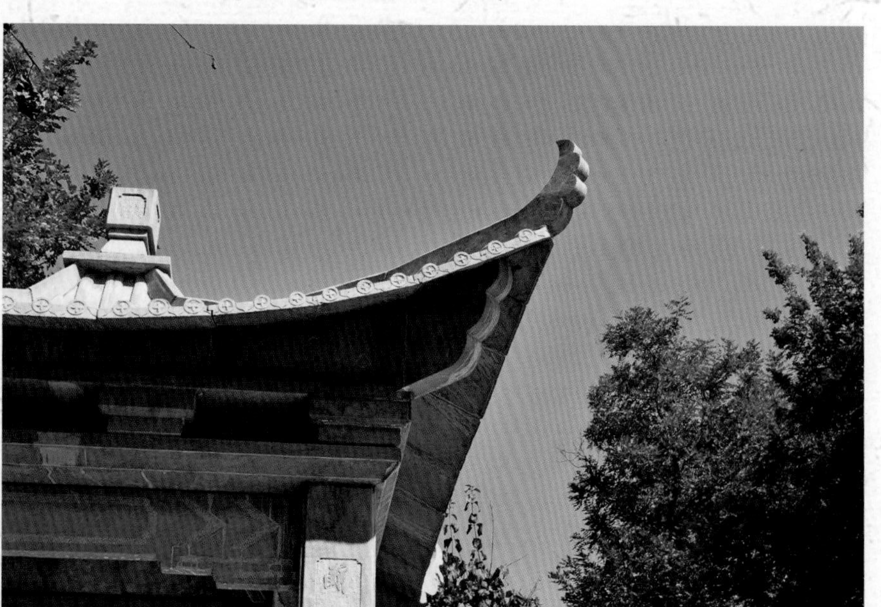

图528 心亭的顶和飞檐

Fig. 528 Roof and cornice of the Heart Pavilion

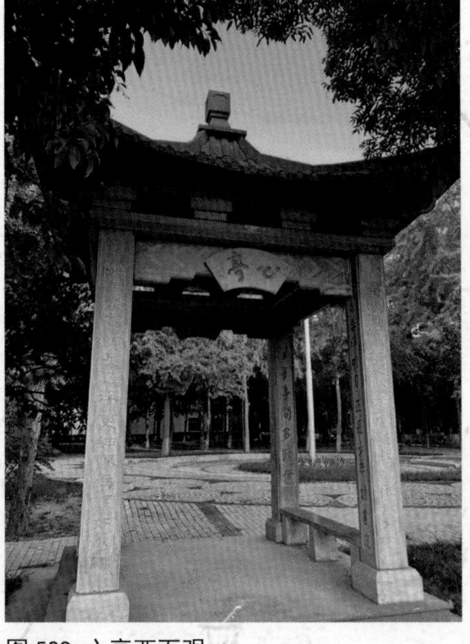

图529 心亭西面观

Fig. 529 The west view of the Heart Pavilion

图530 心亭的立柱

Fig. 530 Upright columns of the Heart Pavilion

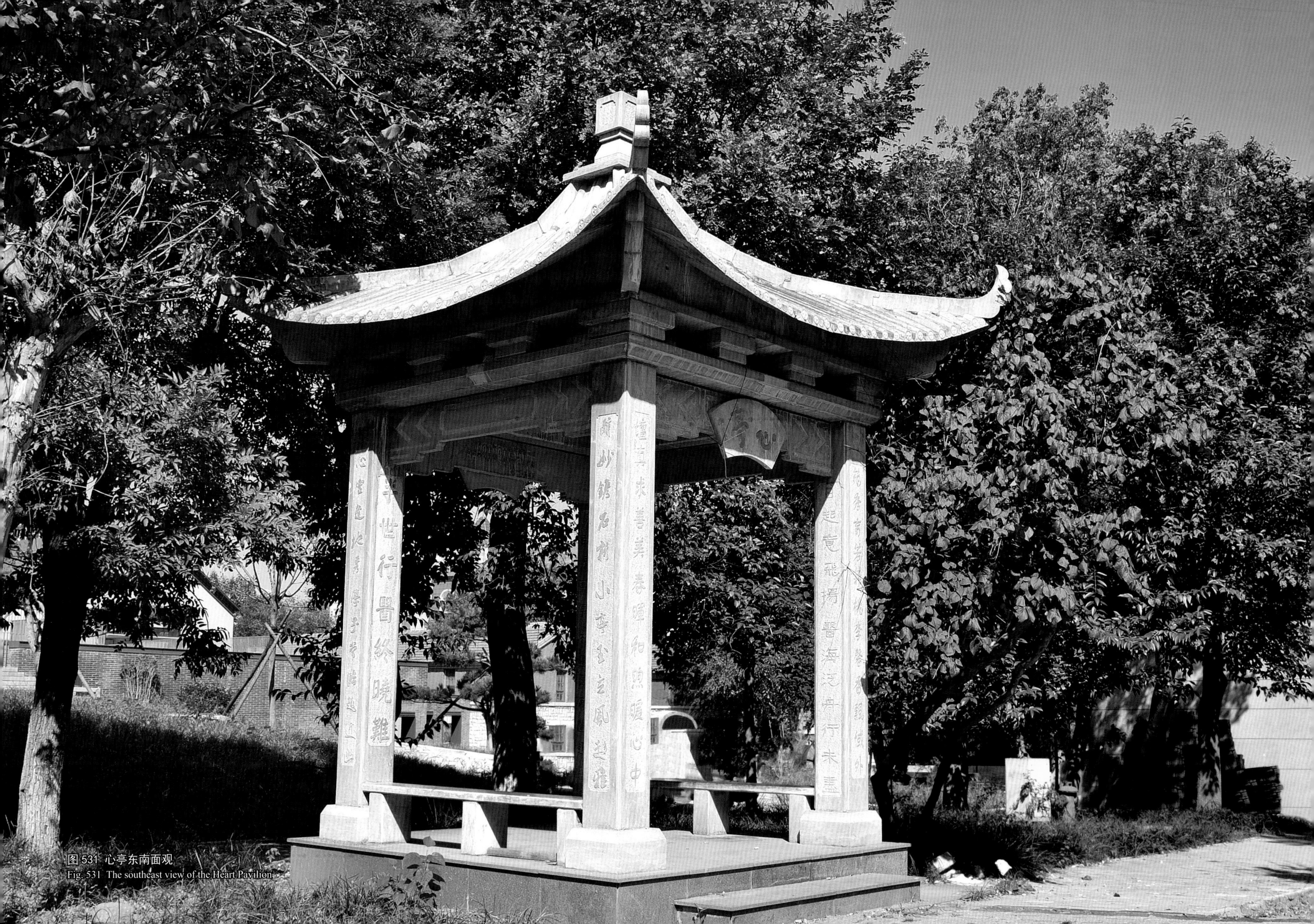

图 531 心亭东南面观
Fig. 531 The southeast view of the Heart Pavilion

55 林间魅影（2）

Glamour of the Woodland (2)

梅亭位于梅园东部，建于 2001 年左右，木质结构。此亭通体红色，在四周绿树的衬托下，格外显眼。顶部六角凌空，亭脊上方立有三尊脊兽。体为六根红色圆木立柱，下方为扁球形垫柱石，上方六边外面绘有四季自然风景、内面画有花中四君子等图案。底座在北部和西部各开有一门，其余四边为带有护栏的木板座位。闲来亭内一坐，微风拂面，清香沁脾，春可饮梅花之坠露，秋可观海棠之落叶，真可起醒脑去疲之神效。梅亭四周高楼林立，景色变幻莫测。东可遥望教学九楼与教学六楼之朝晖，西能远眺校友门与圣保罗楼之夕阴。南近临新麦考密可楼之日月，可感一流学府立德树人之律动。北紧贴齐鲁医院群厦之风云，能知百年老院悬壶济世之仁心。梅亭一憩，仿佛穿越古今时空，诚可常临也！

Located in the east of the Plum Garden, Plum Pavilion was built around 2003, of wooden structure. The pavilion looks red and stands out against green trees around it. The hexagonal top is high up in the air, and above the ridge of the pavilion stand three animal ornaments. The body part is six red upright columns of wood, and the lower part is flat ball-shaped cushion stones. The outer surface of the upper six sides is painted with the natural scenery of the four seasons, and the inner surface is painted with the patterns of the Four Noble Ones, that is, the plum blossom, the orchid, the bamboo and the chrysanthemum. The north and west sides are respectively provided with an entrance, and the left four sides are respectively provided with a wooden seat with guardrails. Come and sit in the pavilion in your spare time, you can enjoy the breeze and the refreshing fragrance. In spring, you can appreciate the dew from plum blossoms; in autumn, you can view the falling leaves of begonia. All of these can make you mentally refreshing and physically relaxed. Plum Pavilion is surrounded by high-rise buildings and the scenery is unpredictable. You can look up into the morning sunlight on the Ninth Teaching Building and the Sixth Teaching Building in the east, and look far into the afterglow on the Alumni Gate and St. Paul's Building in the west. The new McCormick Building is in the south and you can feel the rhythm of the establishment of morality and cultivation of people in the first-class university. The buildings of Qilu Hospital are in the north and you can learn the benevolence of the century-old hospital. It feels like passing through the ancient and modern times to rest in Plum Pavilion, so you can really come here frequently.

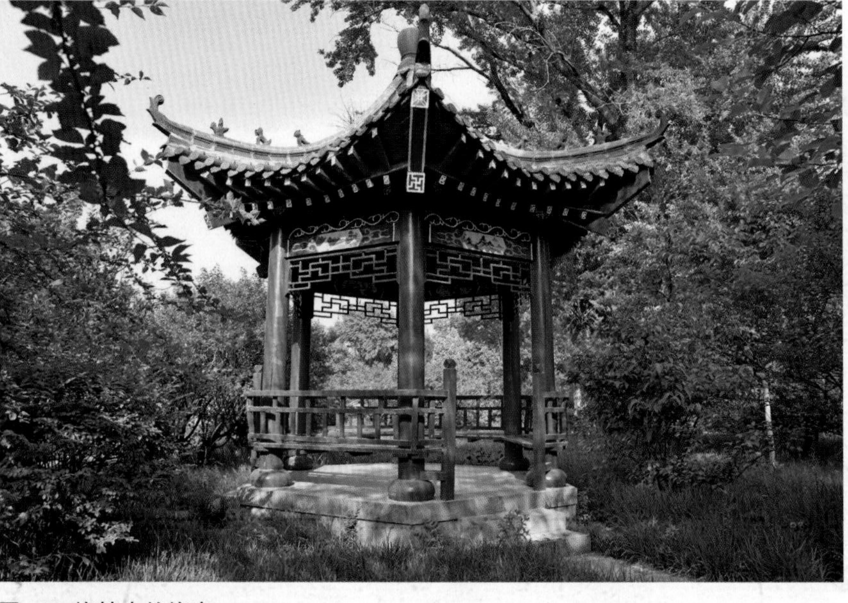

图 532 梅林中的梅亭
Fig. 532 Plum Pavilion in the plum forest

图 533 梅花盛开时的梅亭
Fig. 533 Plum Pavilion surrounded by plum blossoms

图 534 春雪覆盖的梅亭
Fig. 534 Plum Pavilion covered with spring snow

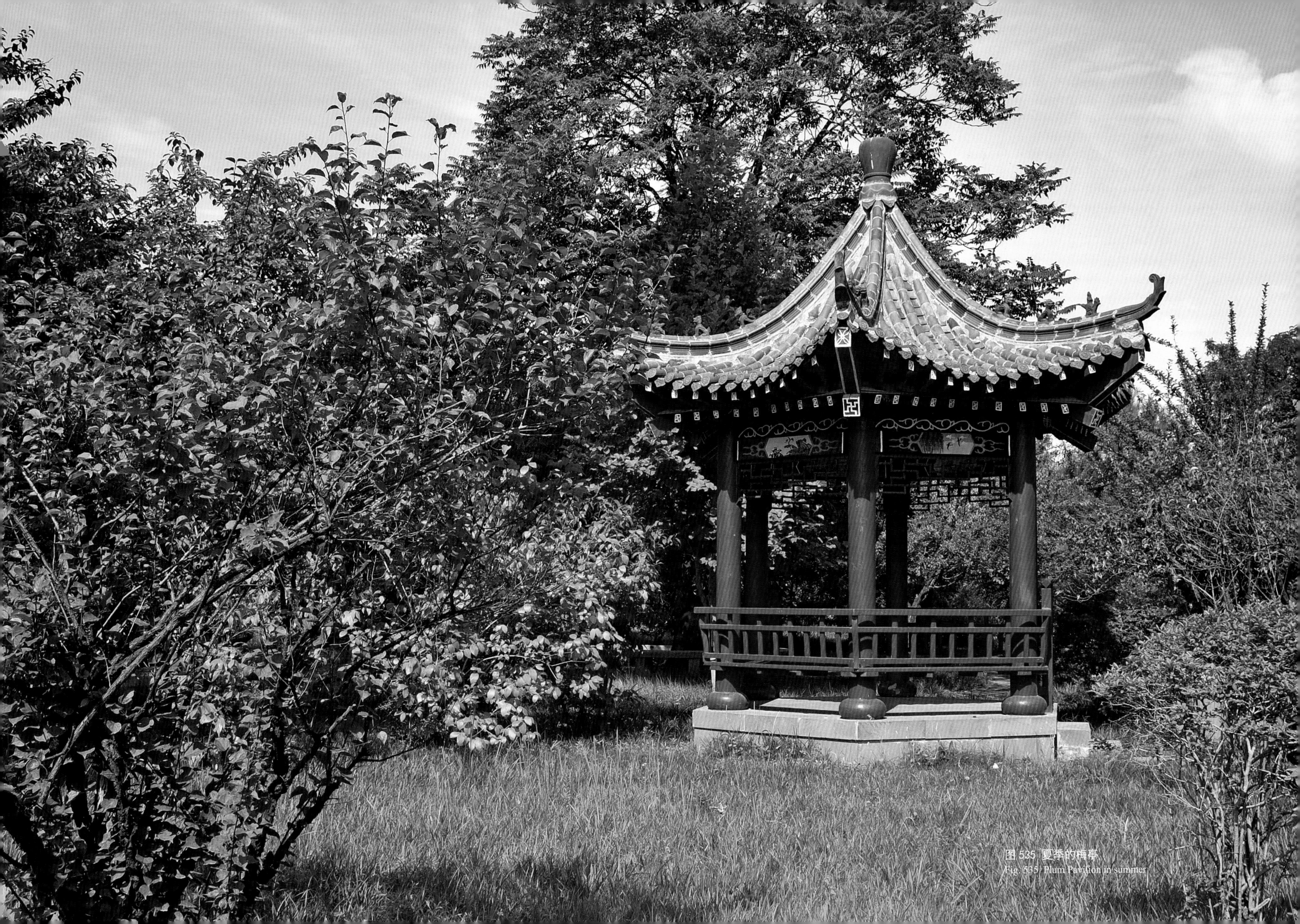

图 535 夏季的梅亭

Fig. 535 Plum Pavilion in summer

55 林间魅影（3）

Glamour of the Woodland (3)

药圣亭建于20世纪80年代，位于教学七楼西北角的高台上，混合结构，六根红柒圆形水泥立柱粗壮有力，六角形木质顶盖内面涂以红色，上覆黄色琉璃瓦，亭脊上立有六尊神兽。此亭位置绝佳，须调动所有眼球外肌的功能，上下左右转动眼球，方能尽览周围风景。信步拾级而上，头转东南可仰视教学七楼红色大柒屋山，面向西北中心花园的四季变化尽收眼帘。北望，呈“品”字形排列的新麦考密可楼、柏根楼与考文楼古色古香，彰显着齐鲁医学的百年底蕴；南观，教学八楼巍然耸立云端，其前面白求恩像银光闪烁，北门两侧参天的松树和银杏树青黄杂糅；西眺，葛罗神学院楼安坐在一片花木之中，它那布满爬山虎的东墙时隐时现；东看，号院鳞次栉比，药圣李时珍表情严肃，好似在告诉我们，你已环视中心花园一周，该去用功了。

Built in the 1980s, Pavilion of Pharmacological Sage is located on a high platform in the northwest corner of the Seventh Teaching Building, of mixed structure. Six red cement columns are thick and strong. The inner surface of the hexagonal wooden top is painted with red and the outer surface is covered with yellow glazed tiles, with six animal ornaments standing on the ridge of the pavilion. The excellent position of this pavilion makes you mobilize the functions of all extraocular muscles of the eyes to enjoy the surrounding scenery. Walking up the steps, you can look up at the red gable of the Seventh Teaching Building in the southeast, and have an overall view of the four seasons in the Central Garden in the northwest. The new McCormick Hall, Bergen Hall and Calvin Mateer Hall in ancient styles are arranged in the shape of the Chinese character “pin” in the north, demonstrating the century-old heritage of Qilu medicine. The Eighth Teaching Building towers up towards the sky in the south, in front of which is the glistening statue of Bethune, and the towering pines and ginkgo trees on both sides of the north gate present mixed colors of green and yellow. Gotch-Robinson Theological Building is located among flowers and trees in the west, and its east wall full of creepers appears and disappears from time to time. The buildings in the Courtyard are arranged in rows in the east. The serious look of Li Shizhen, the Pharmacological Sage, seems to tell us that you have already looked around the Central Garden and it is time to study hard.

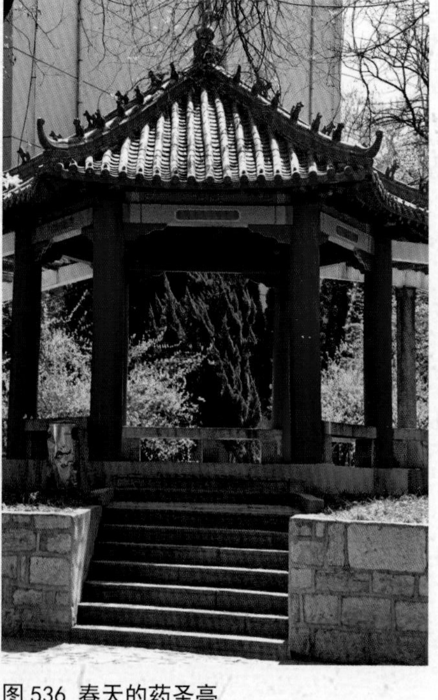

图 536 春天的药圣亭
Fig. 536 Pavilion of Pharmacological Sage in spring

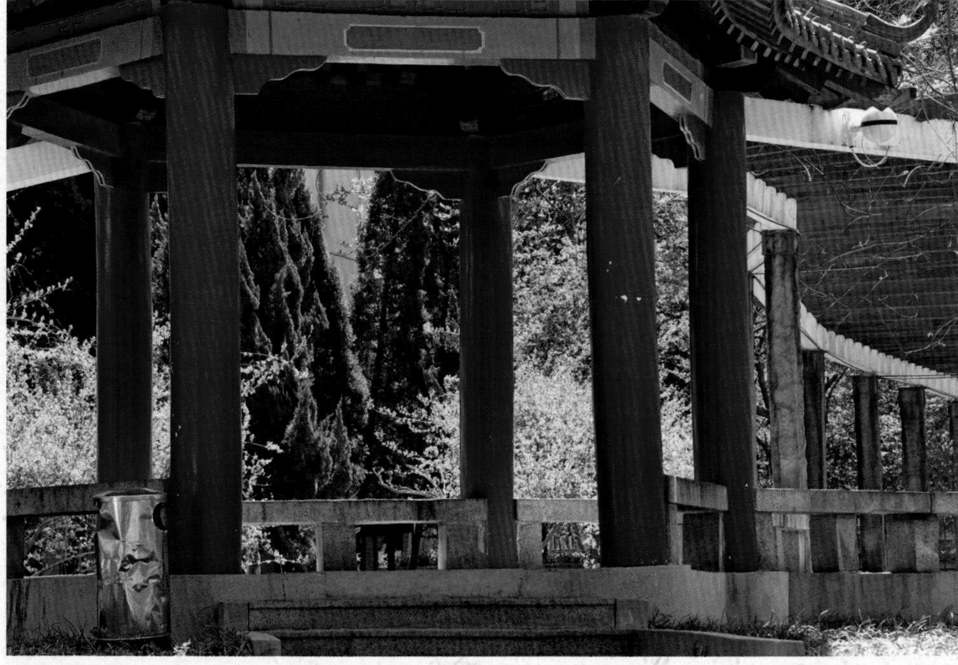

图 537 药圣亭的立柱
Fig. 537 Upright columns of Pavilion of Pharmacological Sage

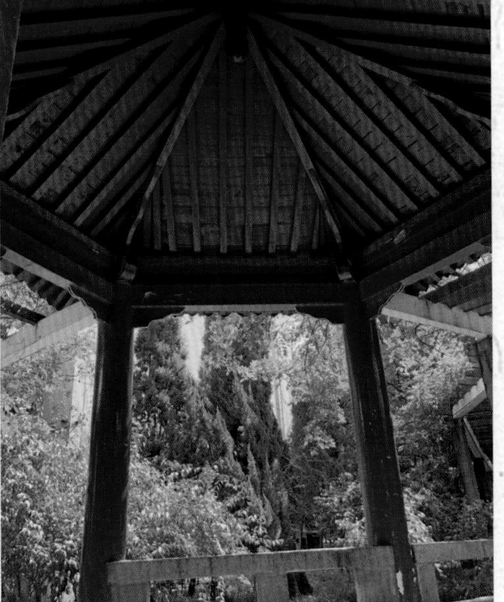

图 538 药圣亭内面观
Fig. 538 The interior view of Pavilion of Pharmacological Sage

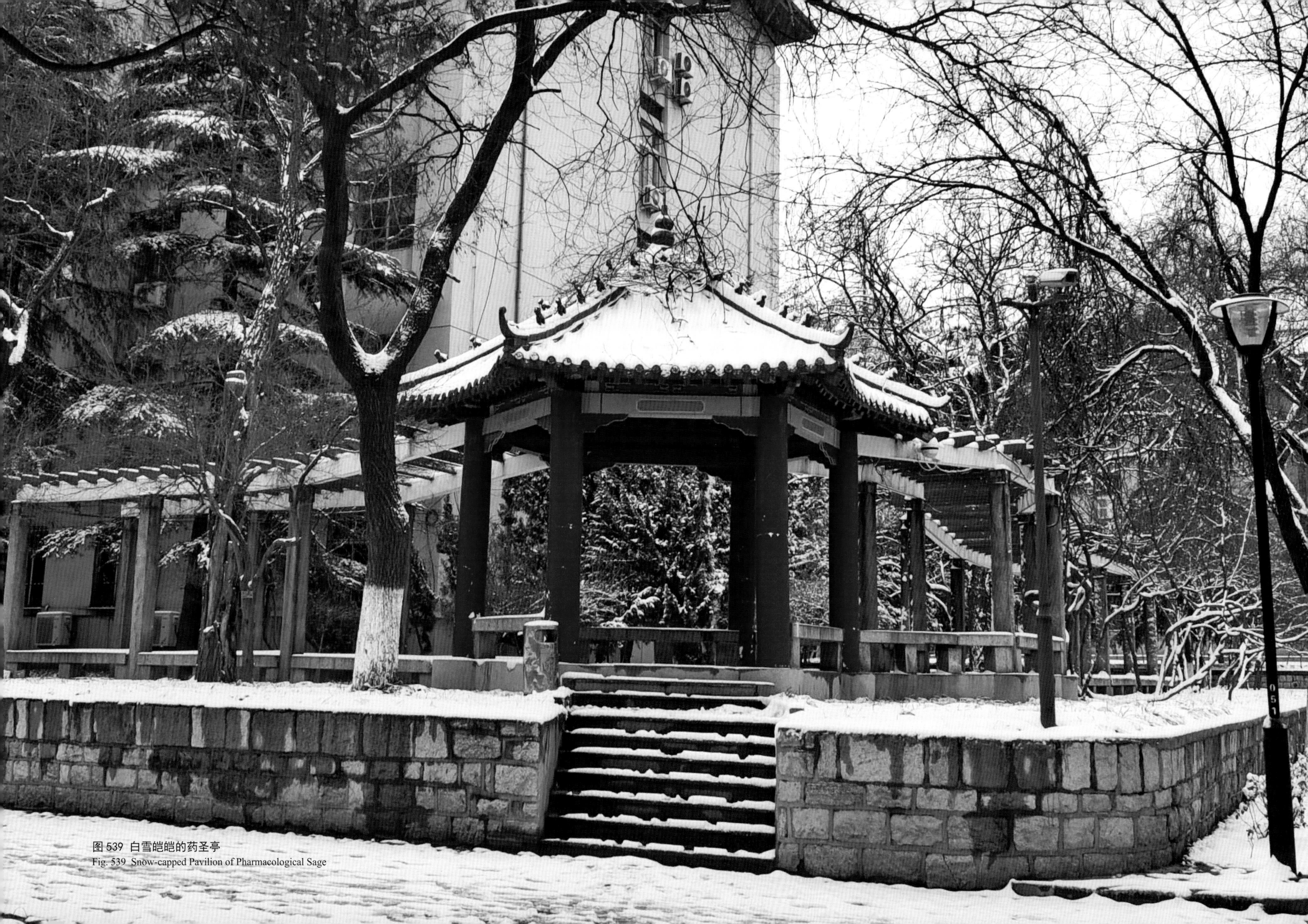

图 539 白雪皑皑的药圣亭
Fig. 539 Snow-capped Pavilion of Pharmacological Sage

55 林间魅影（4）

Glamour of the Woodland (4)

趵突泉校区建有三处花架长廊，主要供紫藤攀爬。第一处位于长柏路第 1 ～ 3 号教授别墅的南侧，钢筋水泥结构。每到春天，紫藤花盛开，远望若紫蓝色的云雾缭绕，近观一串串的紫花呈锥状下垂，上方的花已完全开放，中间的刚刚开了一半，下方的还含苞欲放。坐在花架下，清香阵阵，蜜蜂飞来飞去，嗡嗡作响。若是阳光明媚，透过光线，紫藤花串如无数的珍珠，晶莹透亮，光彩夺目。第二处位于教学七楼西侧，石质立柱，木质横梁，向北与药圣亭相连，周围的紫藤已十分粗壮，盘根错节。第三处位于校友门东侧、梅园西头，木质结构。春天紫藤花氤氲浪漫，夏天紫藤荚饱满垂空，秋天紫藤叶金辉璀璨。

On Baotuquan Campus there are three corridors of trellis for the wisteria. The first place is located on the south side of professors' villas Nos. 1-3 on Changbai Road, of reinforced concrete structure. The wisteria flowers in spring, like a haze of bluish violet mist from a distance. From a closer look, strings of purple flowers droop like cones; the upper parts have fully opened, the middle just half opened, and the lower still in bud. Sitting under the trellis, you will be met by a waft of fragrance and see the bees flying around and buzzing. Against the bright sunshine, strings of wisteria flowers look like countless pearls, crystal clear and dazzling. The second place is located on the west side of the Seventh Teaching Building, with stone columns and wooden beams, which is connected with Pavilion of Pharmacological Sage in the north. The wisterias around it have been very strong and intertwined. The third place is located on the east side of the Alumni Gate and at the west end of Plum Garden, of wooden structure. In spring, the wisteria flowers are dense and romantic; in summer, the wisteria pods hang fully in the air; and in autumn, the golden wisteria leaves are lustrous and brilliant.

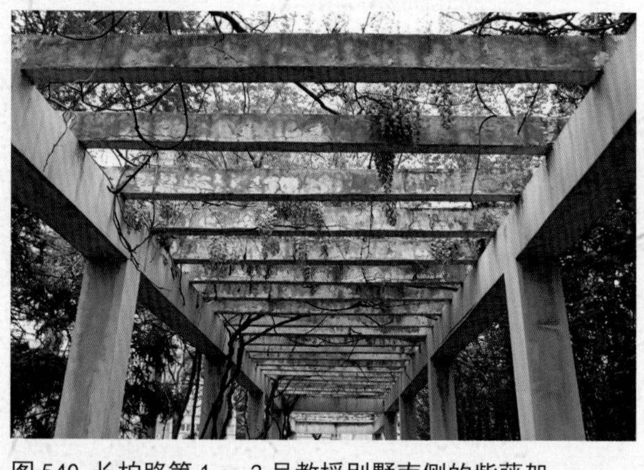

图 540 长柏路第 1 ～ 3 号教授别墅南侧的紫藤架

Fig. 540 Wisteria trellis on the south side of professors' villas Nos. 1-3 on Changbai Road

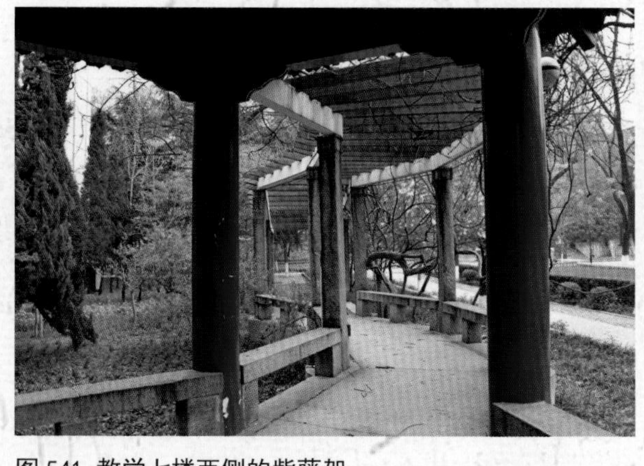

图 541 教学七楼西侧的紫藤架

Fig. 541 Wisteria trellis on the west side of the Seventh Teaching Building

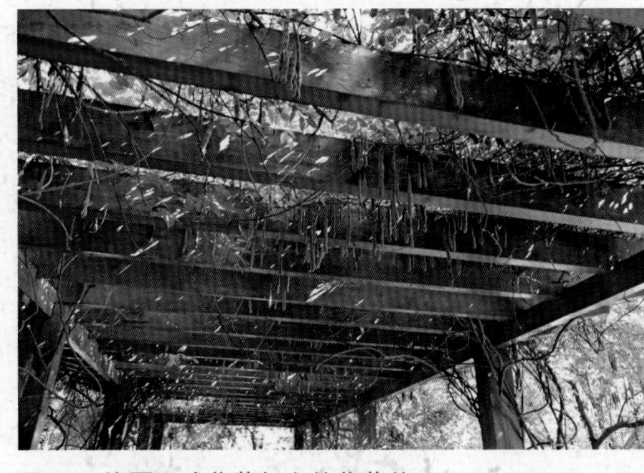

图 542 梅园西头紫藤架上的紫藤荚

Fig. 542 Wisteria pods on the wisteria trellis at the west end of the Plum Garden

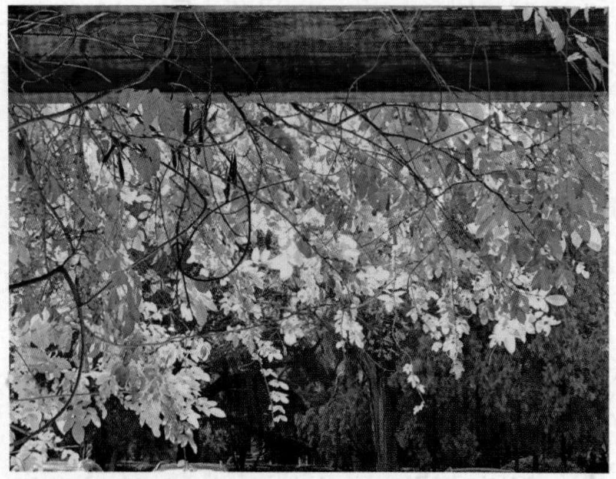

图 543 梅园西头紫藤架上的紫藤叶

Fig. 543 Wisteria leaves on the wisteria trellis at the west end of the Plum Garden

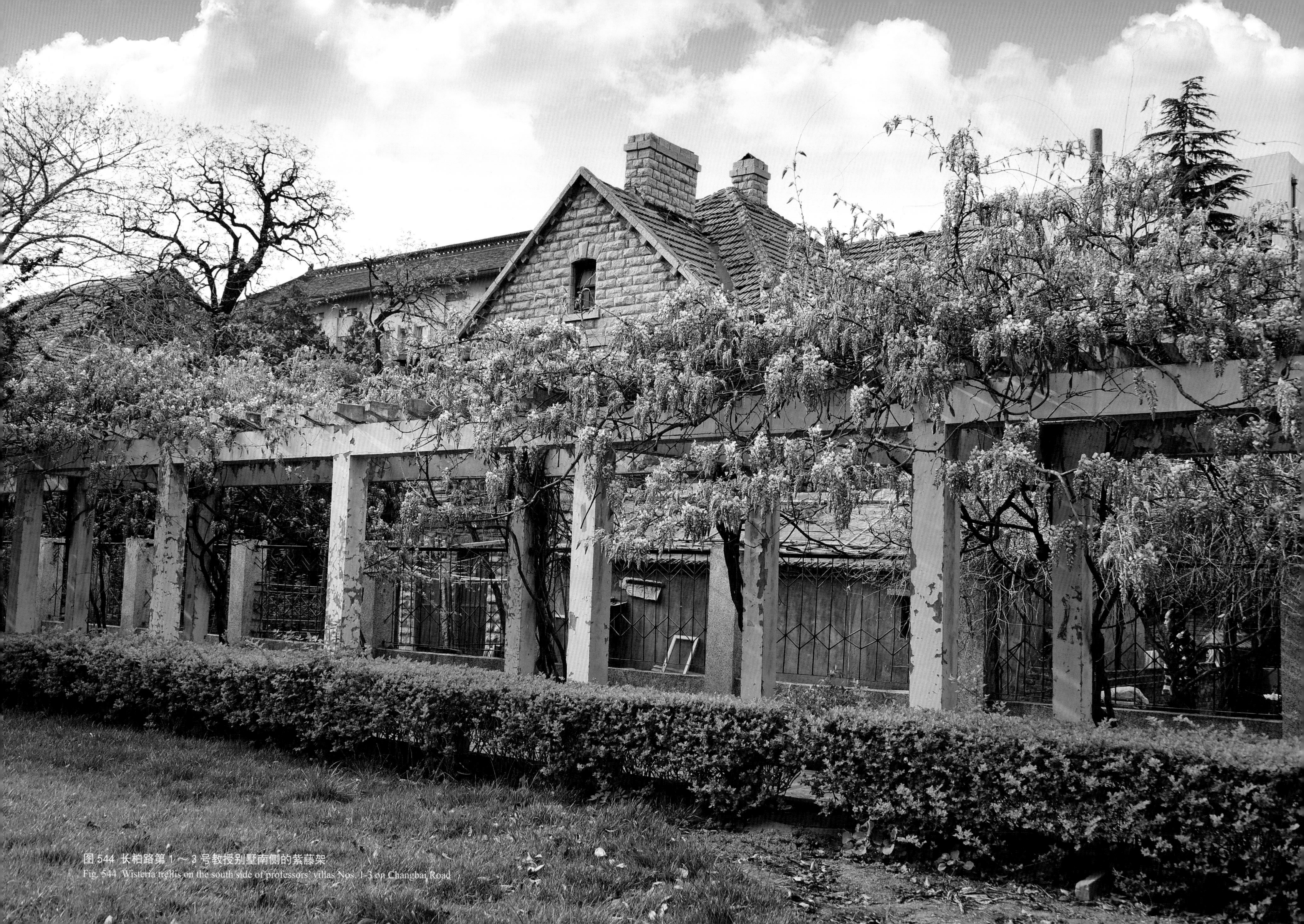

图 544 长柏路第 1～3 号教授别墅南侧的紫藤架
Fig. 544 Wisteria trellis on the south side of professors' villas Nos. 1-3 on Changbai Road

55 林间魅影（5）

Glamour of the Woodland (5)

从空中看来，趵突泉校区是济南市中心高楼大厦之中少有的几处大片绿地之一。常年身处这片绿林之中，林上、林间、树上和林下有很多令人心驰神往之处。

先说林上。万里晴空是单调的，若有几朵白云飘过则灵性倍增。若夫朝霞腾空，东方醉云满天，大地一切均处剪影之中，此时晨练，则朝气满胸，吐故纳新，定成蓬勃之势。至若日升中天，空朗气清，千顷薄絮飘浮于苍穹，此时漫步校园，则耳聪目明，思路大开，尽采宇宙之晟。若遇大雨之后，或红云抹空，轻绡淡染，或长云浩荡，清光万里，此时可端坐于心亭之中，饱赏水塔倩影，似游于梦境矣！

The aerial view shows that Baotuquan Campus is one of the few large green spaces among high-rise buildings in central Jinan. Staying in this green woodland all the year round, you will find many fascinating things.

Let's start with what is above the woodland. A few white clouds make the monotonous clear sky more lively. With the morning glow and cloud spreading all over the sky, the earth is like in silhouette. If you do morning exercises at this time, then you will be full of vitality, get rid of the stale and take in the fresh, presenting a vigorous momentum. With the sun high in the sky, the sky is clear and bright; and masses of light clouds float in the sky. When you take a stroll around the campus at this time, you will be quick at hearing and seeing and generous in thoughts, fully gathering the essence of the universe. After the heavy rain, a rainbow may appear in the sky or there will be a stretch of clear and cloudy skies. At this time, you can take a seat in Heart Pavilion, enjoying the beautiful image of Water Tower, just like in a dream.

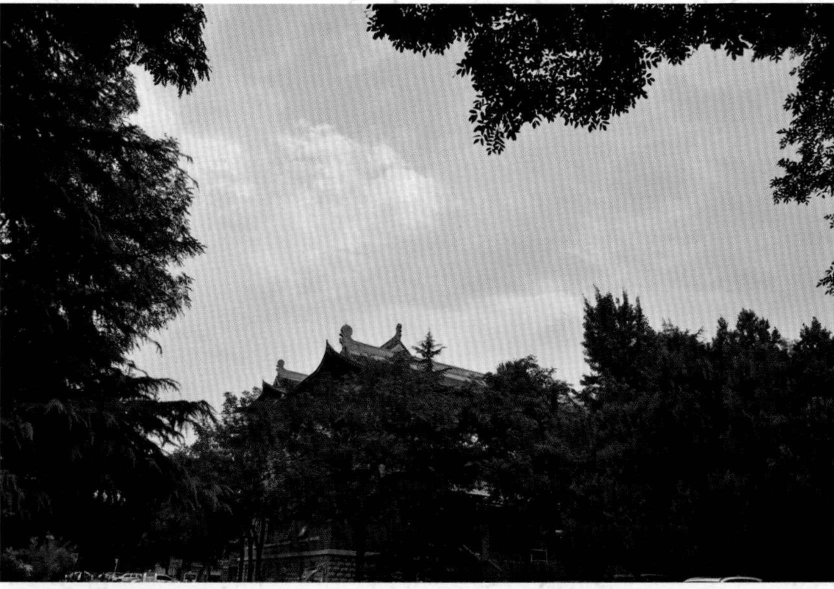

图 545 朝霞满天的校园
Fig. 545 Campus shrouded in morning glow

图 546 朝霞杉影
Fig. 546 Spruce shrouded in morning glow

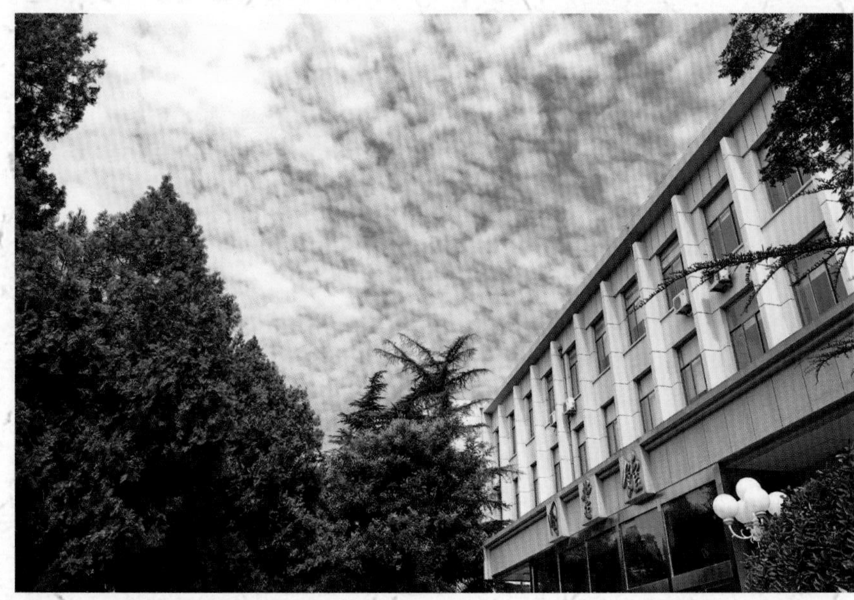

图 547 校园上空白云飘飞
Fig. 547 White clouds floating above the campus

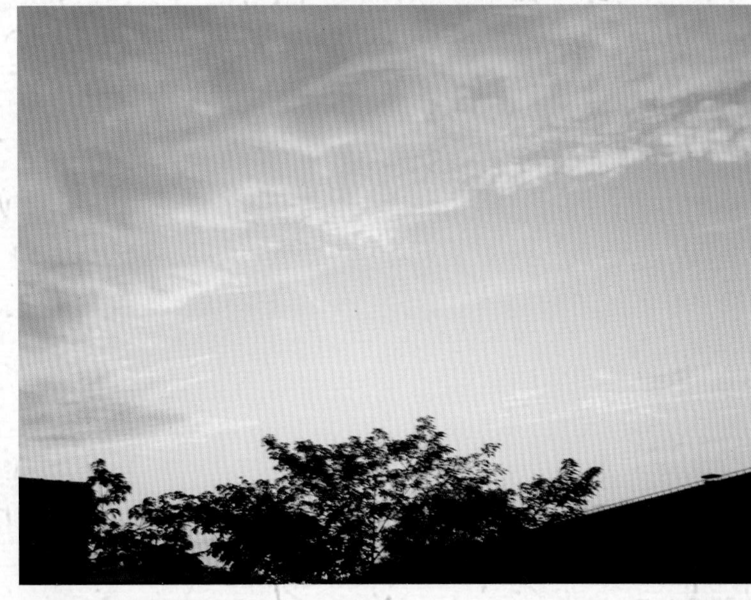

图 548 校园上空的晚霞
Fig. 548 Afterglow above the campus

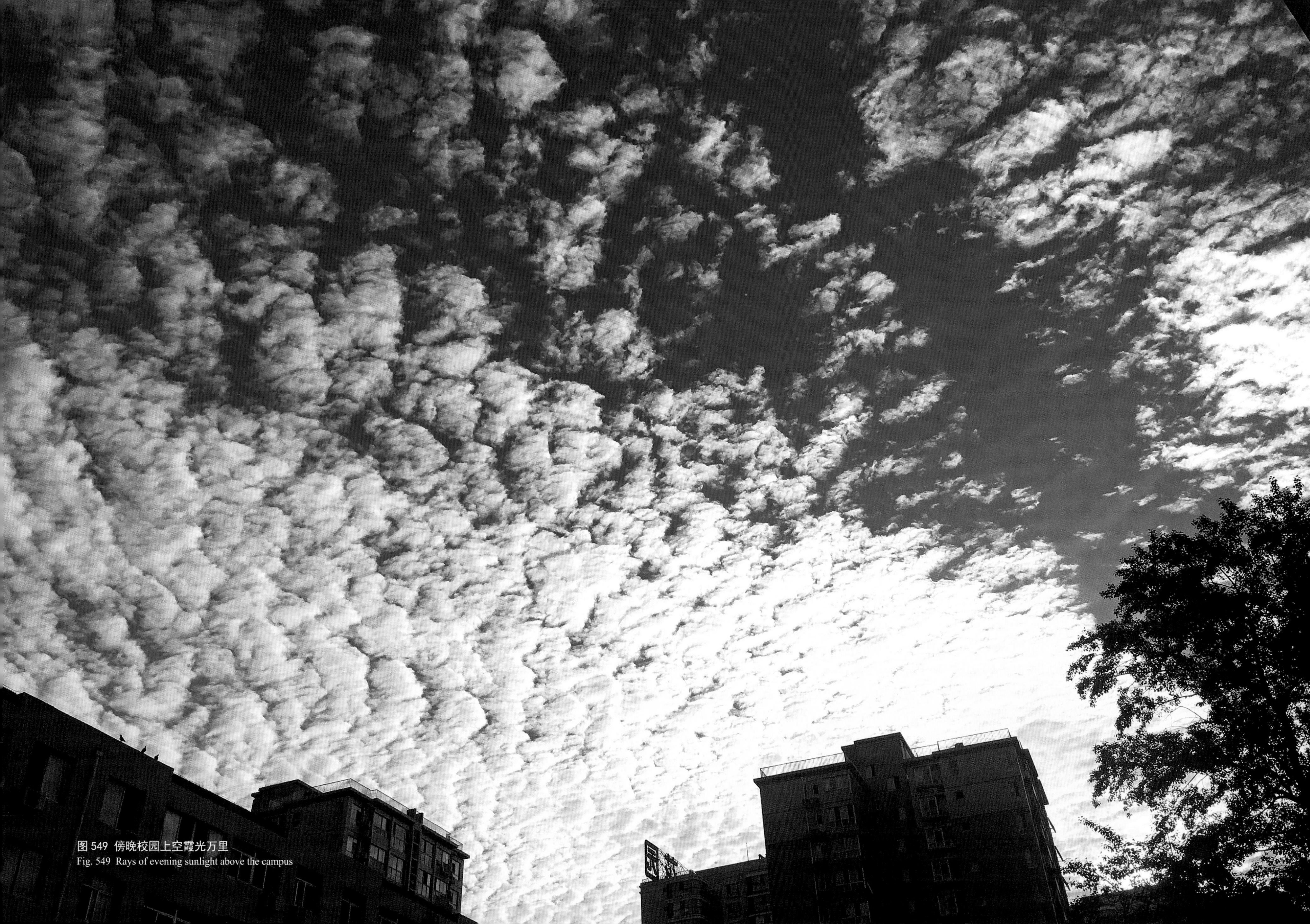

图 549 傍晚校园上空霞光万里
Fig. 549 Rays of evening sunlight above the campus

55 林间魅影（6）

Glamour of the Woodland (6)

林间更是妙趣横生。早醒入园，晨曦初露，则可见云杉或塔松亭亭玉立之身姿。继而，红日喷薄而出，光线穿过树叶，映照在林荫小道上，橘光环生，如梦如幻。待日高而白，上班路上，仰望天空，于树梢之间，或月影徘徊，或白云飘飞，或红楼半露，或鸱吻飞扬……下班路上，夕阳洒在林间，更是幻影丛生，连教授别墅上的烟囱都变得金壁辉煌，魅力四射。

The woodland is even more fabulous. When you wake up early to go to the garden, you can see the spruce or cedar standing gracefully erect against the light of the early morning sun. Then, the red sun spurts out, and the orange light shines on the tree-lined path through the leaves, as if being in a dream. On the way to work, looking up at the sky with the sun riding high through the treetops, you can see the moving moonlight, the floating clouds, the half-exposed red building or the flying *chiwen*... On the way home from work, you can see that the sunset makes the woodland full of phantoms, and even the chimneys of the professors' villas become glorious and charming.

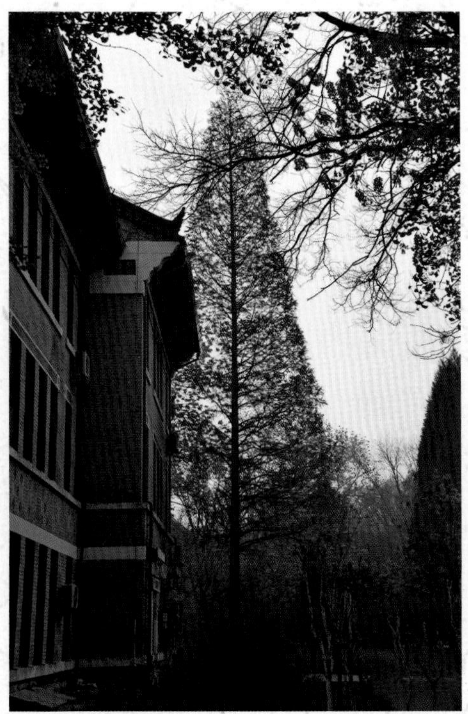
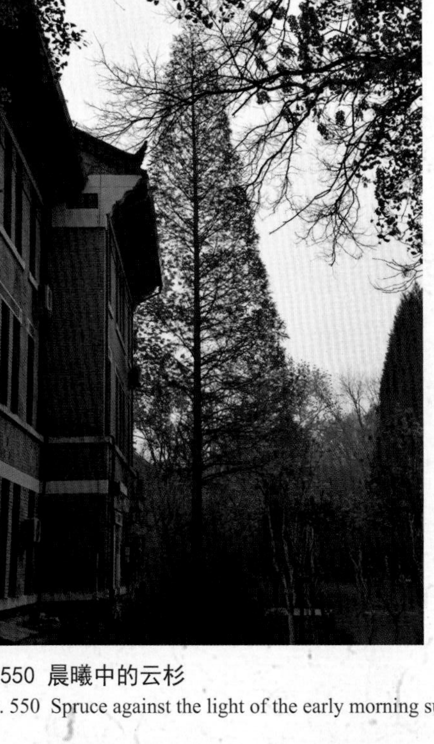

图 550 晨曦中的云杉

Fig. 550 Spruce against the light of the early morning sun

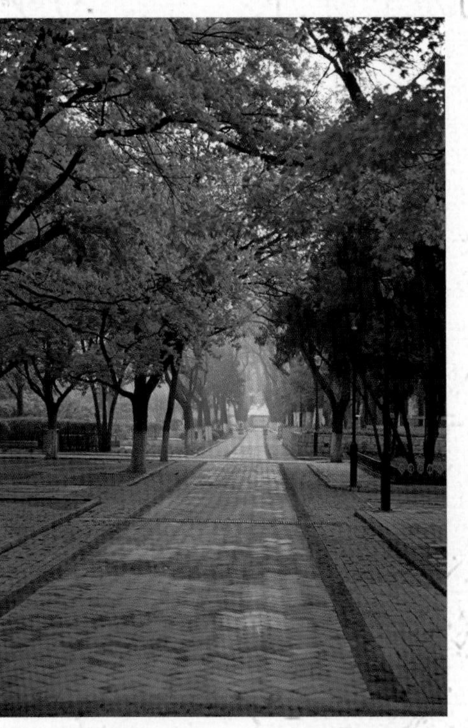

图 551 初升的阳光洒在林间小道上

Fig. 551 The rising sun shining on the tree-lined path

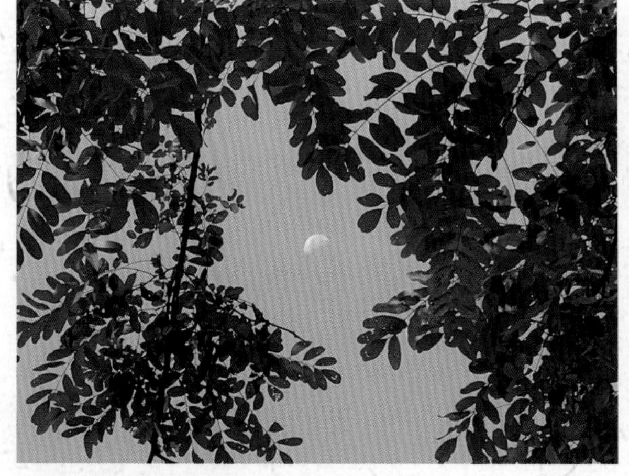

图 552 树梢间的月亮

Fig. 552 Moon between the treetops

图 553 林间云影

Fig. 553 White clouds floating over the woodland

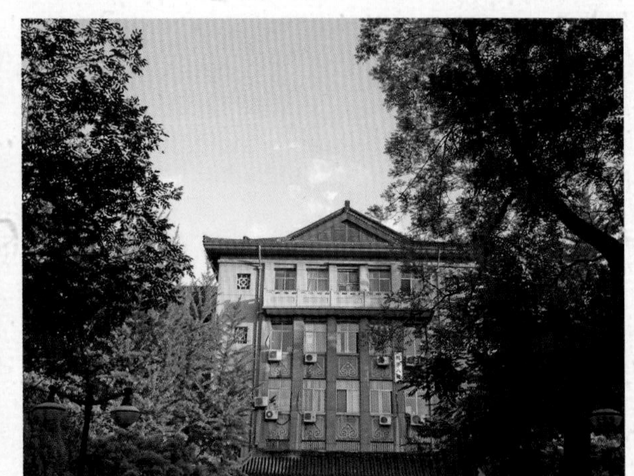

图 554 林间半露的教学八楼

Fig. 554 The Eighth Teaching Building half-exposed in the woodland

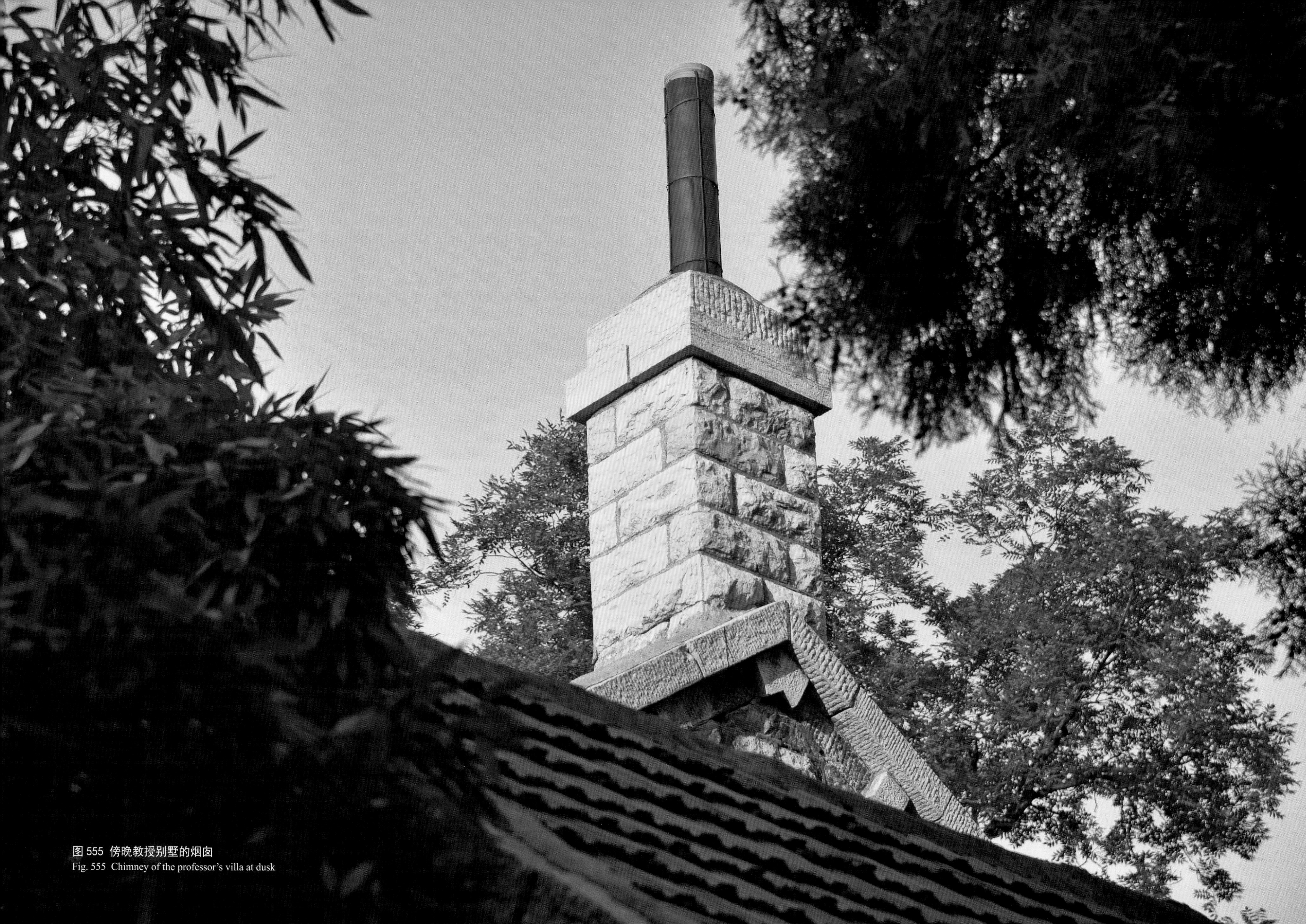

图 555 傍晚教授别墅的烟囱
Fig. 555 Chimney of the professor's villa at dusk

55 林间魅影（7）

Glamour of the Woodland (7)

树上的鸟儿是幸运的，在大学校园里耳濡目染，似乎也变得学究气十足。校园里喜鹊很多，有的灰色羽毛长尾巴，有的黑白搭配短尾巴，在林间地上飞来飞去，鸣叫不绝。有一种黄喙乌鸦也是常见的，三五成群地在草坪里觅食。乌鸦的名声好像不好，但今天我要给它正名。一是乌鸦智力超群，具有制造和运用工具的能力以及逻辑推理能力，是人类之外具有第一流智商的动物；二是乌鸦具有高度的组织性，社会性极强；三是乌鸦反哺老鸟，是有名的孝鸟，儒学经典中就有“乌鸦反哺，羔羊跪乳”的说法。麻雀也很多，常成群地栖息于树上，颇有树上结麻雀的效果。这几年树上的松鼠也多了起来，它们不太怕人，我行我素，任你拍照。

The birds in the trees are so lucky that they seem to have become pedantic when they are exposed to the university campus. There are many magpies on campus, some with grey feathers and long tails, and some with black and white feathers and short tails. They fly around in the woods and tweet endlessly. There's a kind of yellow-billed crows which are a common sight, and they always forage on the lawn in small groups. It seems that crows have a bad reputation, but today I'm going to rectify this. First, in addition to humans, crows are animals with first-class intelligence; they have the ability to make and use tools and logical reasoning ability. Second, crows have a high degree of organization and strong sociality. Third, crows feed their mother birds and are famous filial birds. There is such a saying in Confucian classics: “The crow feeds its parents and the lamb kneels down to suckle.” There are also many sparrows, often perching on trees in groups, as if borne by the trees. In recent years, there have been more squirrels in the trees. They are not afraid of people and go their own way; you can take pictures of them at will.

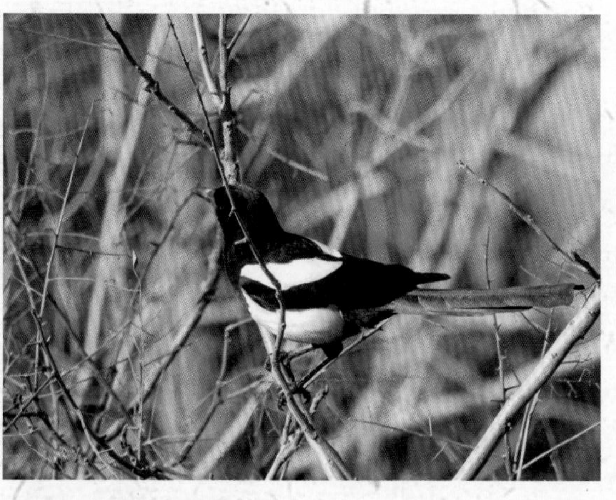

图 556 冬天树上的喜鹊
Fig. 556 Amagpie in the tree in winter

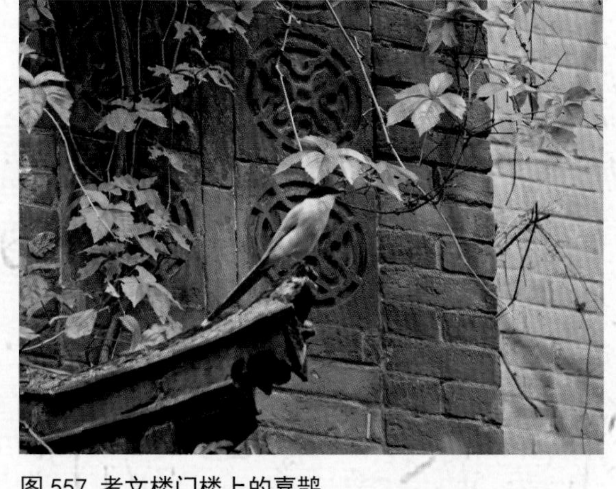

图 557 考文楼门楼上的喜鹊
Fig. 557 A magpie on the gatehouse of Calvin Mateer Hall

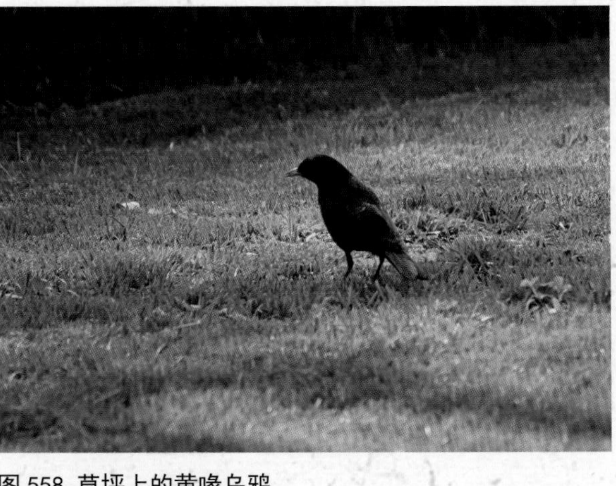

图 558 草坪上的黄喙乌鸦
Fig. 558 A yellow-billed crow on the lawn

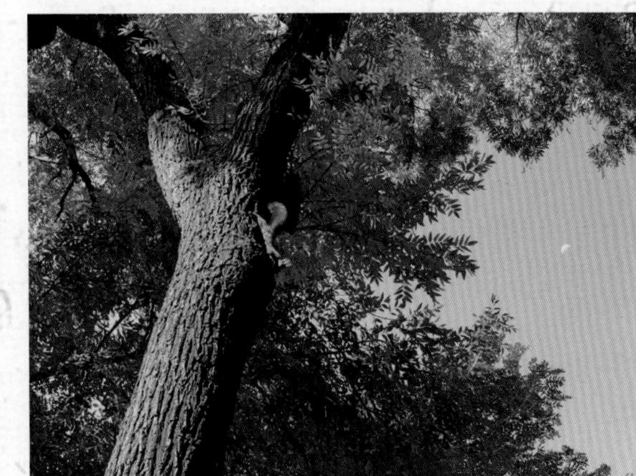

图 559 树上的松鼠
Fig. 559 A squirrel in the tree

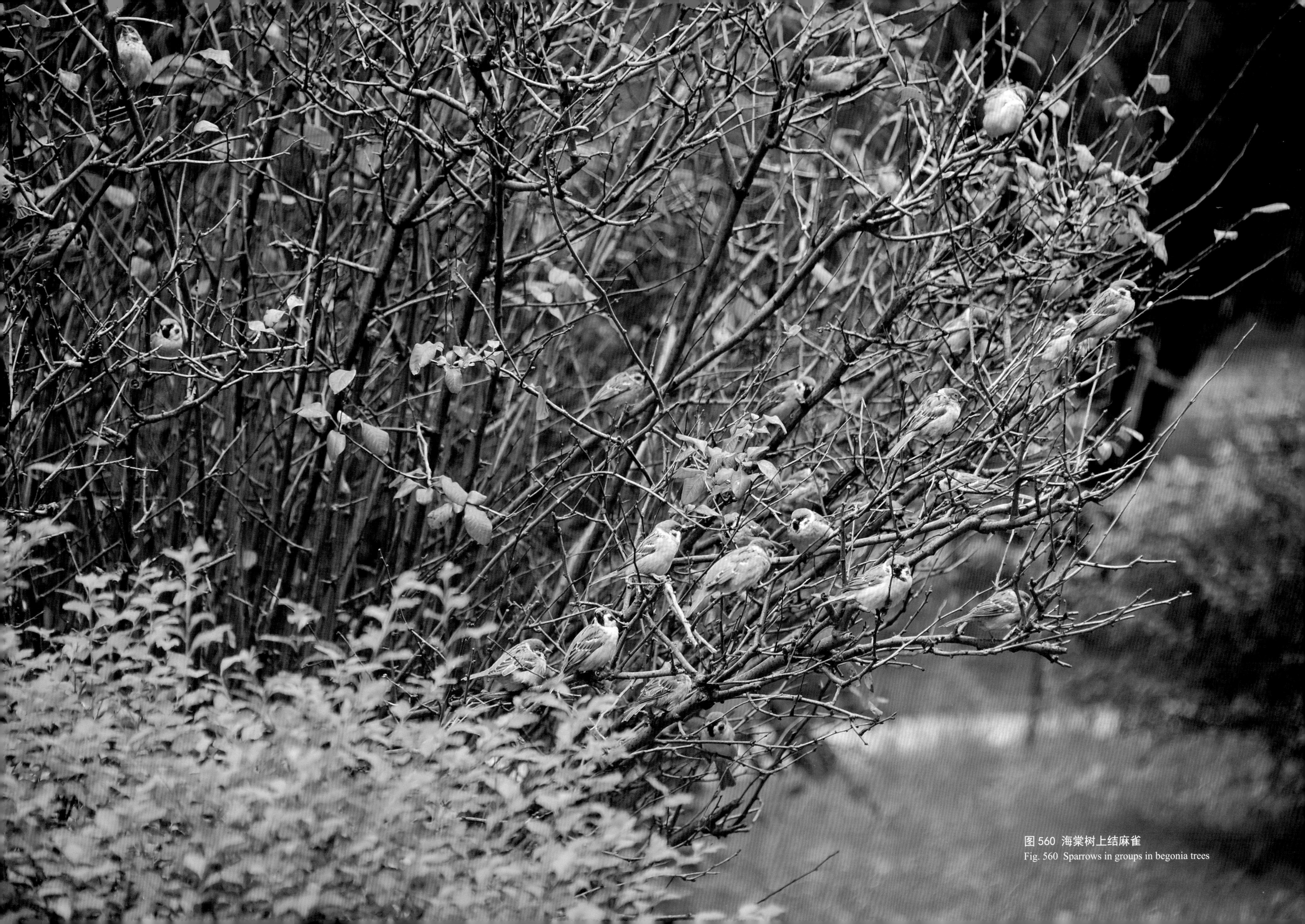

图 560 海棠树上结麻雀
Fig. 560 Sparrows in groups in begonia trees

55 | 林间魅影（8）

Glamour of the Woodland (8)

林下的小道很多，但那些弯弯曲曲的羊肠阡陌更富有曲径通幽的魅力。教学一楼东南侧的斜曲小道，春可闻丁香，秋可赏枫叶，夏天其两侧绿油油的、开着蓝花的山麦冬也韵味无穷。教学二楼北侧的小路两侧萋萋芳草丛生，还有满地的各色小花，恨不得每天来回走上几遍。梅园内的小道纵横交错，有的圆形环绕，路旁还有石板可坐，梅花还是要慢慢品味的。考文楼北侧的小路呈波浪状，在丁香味里欣赏石鼓，还真是不错的选择。最有魅力的还应是葛罗神学院楼东侧的斜行石径，既曲且长，穿行于云杉与梧桐林下，春闻桐花之香，夏看茵茵绿草，秋赏红叶绣壁，冬踏白雪寻梅。夏日炎炎，若悬一吊床于斯，临风高卧，什么功名利禄之类，早已如过眼云烟，飞到九霄天外了。

There are many woodland paths, but those crisscross footpaths are more full of the charm of the winding path leading to a secluded spot. Walking along the slanting and winding trail on the southeast side of the First Teaching Building, you can smell the lilac flowers in spring and enjoy maple leaves in autumn. In summer, green Liriope spicata with blue flowers on both sides of the trail also has a lasting appeal. Both sides of the path on the north side of the Second Teaching Building are overgrown with luxuriant grass, and there are also many small flowers of various colors all over the ground. I wish I could walk back and forth several times a day. In the Plum Garden, you can sit on the stone benches along the criss-cross paths or circular walks to enjoy the plum blossoms slowly. The path on the north side of Calvin Mateer Hall is wavy and it is a good place to enjoy the drum-shaped stone blocks with the fragrance of lilac flowers. The most attractive should be the long winding and slanting stone path on the east side of Gotch-Robinson Theological College. Walking along this path through the spruces and plane trees, you can smell the tung flowers in spring, view the green grass in summer, enjoy the red leaves that embellish the walls, and tread on snow to look for plum flowers in winter. On a blistering summer day, you can hang a hammock and lie on it in the wind, and then the high official positions and riches are like passing clouds and have been thrown to the winds.

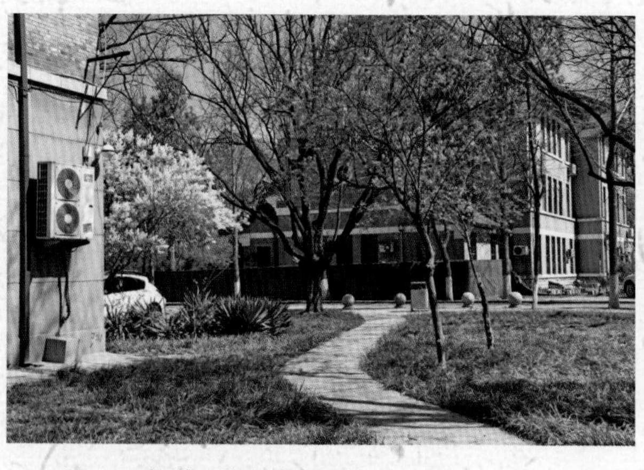

图 561 教学一楼东南侧的林下小道
Fig. 561 A woodland path on the southeast side of the First Teaching Building

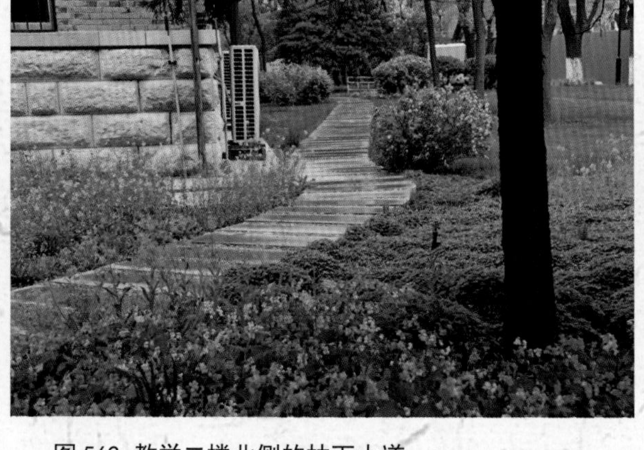

图 562 教学二楼北侧的林下小道
Fig. 562 A woodland path on the north side of the Second Teaching Building

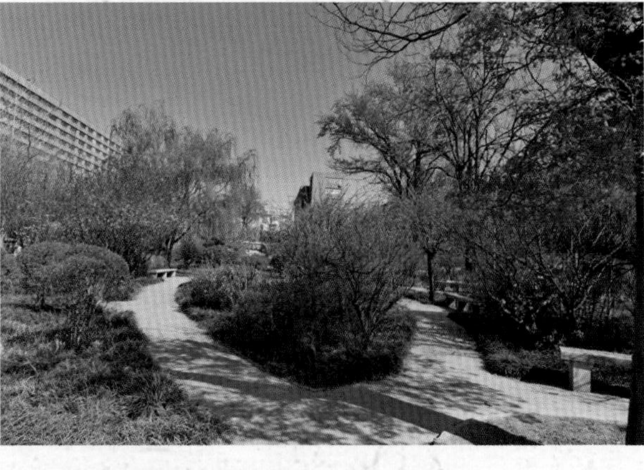

图 563 梅园内的羊肠小道
Fig. 563 A meandering footpath in the Plum Garden

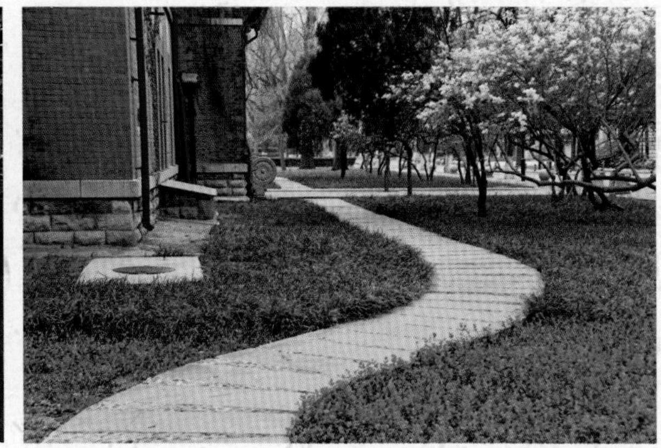

图 564 考文楼北侧的林下小道
Fig. 564 A woodland path on the north side of Calvin Mateer Hall

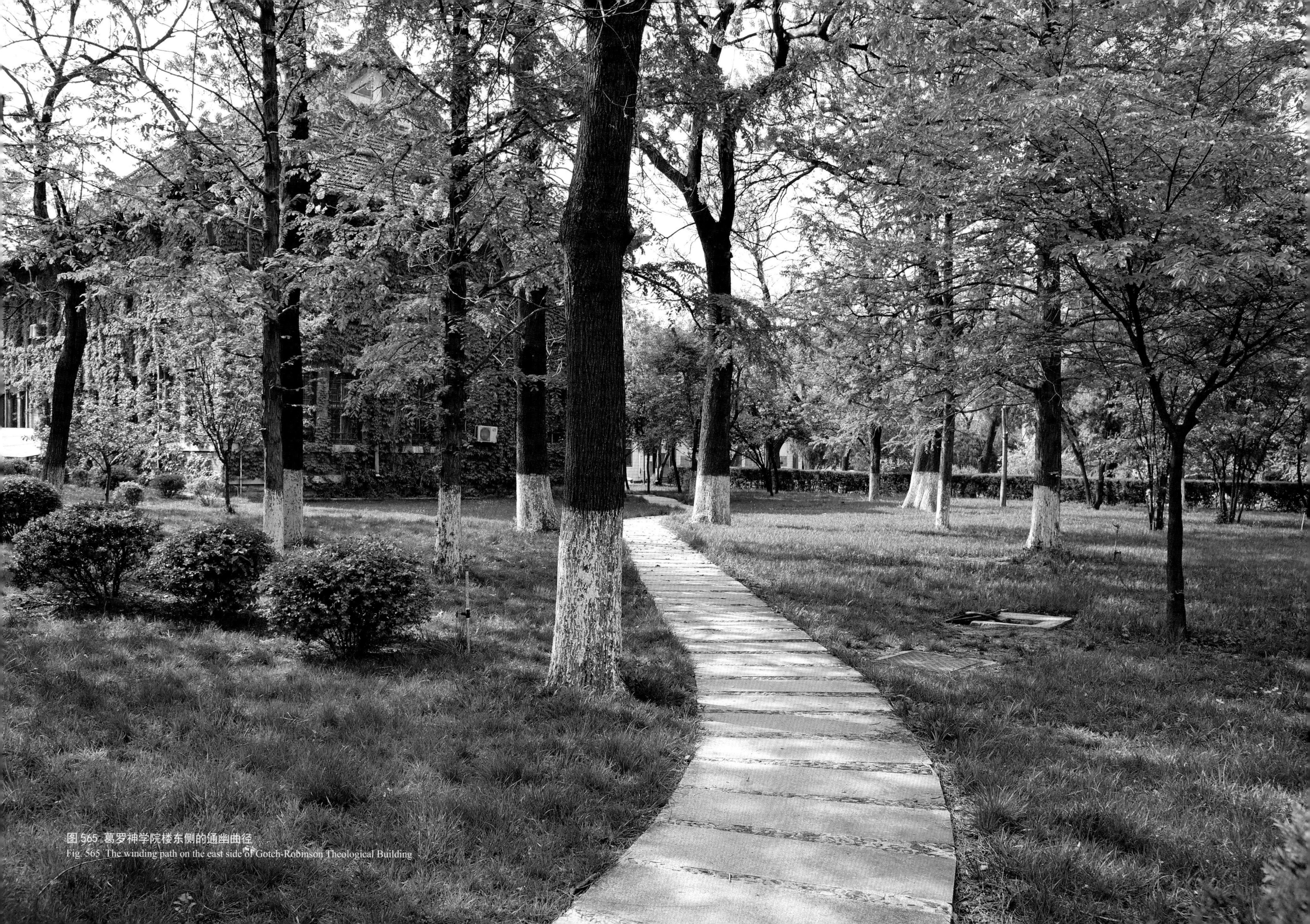

图 565 葛罗神学院楼东侧的通幽曲径
Fig. 565 The winding path on the east side of Gotch-Robinson Theological Building

56 大教无声（1）

Great Teaching in Silence (1)

白求恩医生塑像坐落于教学八楼北侧，由华东白求恩医学院校友联谊会于1998年10月捐建。

白求恩，全名亨利·诺尔曼·白求恩（Henry Norman Bethune，1890年3月4日~1939年11月12日），加拿大共产党员，国际主义战士，著名胸外科医师。1890年白求恩出生于加拿大安大略省格雷文赫斯特镇，1916年毕业于多伦多大学医学院，1922年成为英国皇家外科医学会会员，1928年初在麦吉尔大学皇家维多利亚医院作胸外科医生。他发明和改进了12种医疗手术器械，发表学术论文14篇。1935年被选为美国胸外科学会会员、理事，同年加入加拿大共产党。1938年来到中国参与抗日革命，因手术中感染转为败血症，于1939年11月12日凌晨逝世。毛泽东在其著名的《纪念白求恩》一文中称白求恩医生为“一个高尚的人，一个纯粹的人，一个有道德的人，一个脱离了低级趣味的人，一个有益于人民的人”。

The statue of Dr. Bethune is located on the north side of the Eighth Teaching Building. It was donated by the Alumni Association of East China Bethune Medical College in October 1998.

The full name of Bethune is Henry Norman Bethune (4 March 1890-12 November 1939). He is a Canadian Communist, an internationalist fighter and a famous thoracic surgeon. Bethune was born in Gravenhurst, Ontario, Canada in 1890. He graduated from the Medical School of University of Toronto in 1916 and became a member of the Royal College of Surgeons of England in 1922. He worked as a thoracic surgeon at the Royal Victoria Hospital of McGill University in early 1928. He invented and improved 12 kinds of medical surgical instruments and published 14 academic papers. In 1935, he was elected member and director of the American Association of Thoracic Surgery and joined the Communist Party of Canada in the same year. In 1938, he came to China to participate in the War of Resistance against Japanese Aggression. He died in the early morning of 12 November 1939 due to infection during surgery which turned to septicemia. In his famous "In Memory of Norman Bethune", Mao Zedong praised Dr. Bethune as: "He is already noble-minded and pure, a man of moral integrity and above vulgar interests, a man who is of value to the people."

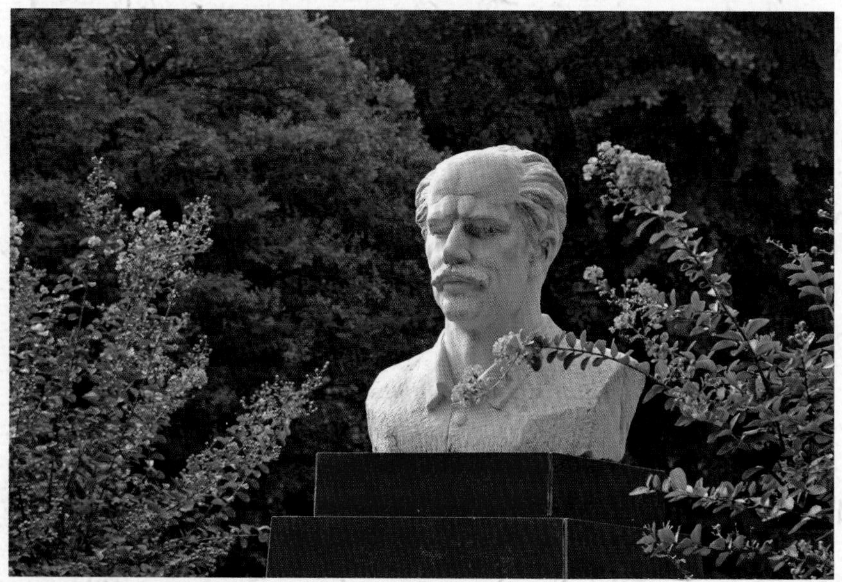

图566 白求恩医生塑像
Fig. 566 Statue of Dr. Bethune

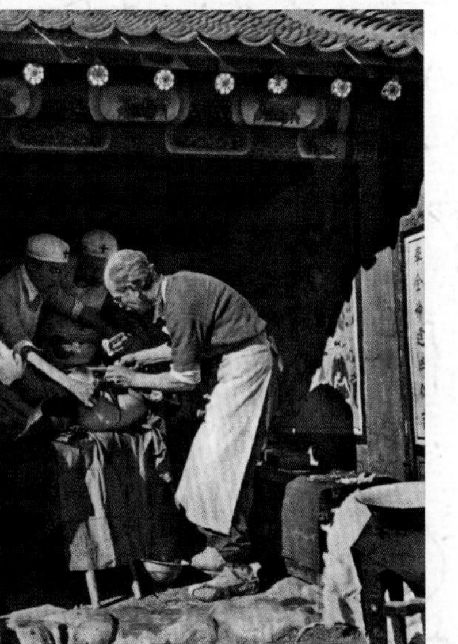

图567 白求恩医生在救治伤员
Fig. 567 Dr. Bethune treating the wounded

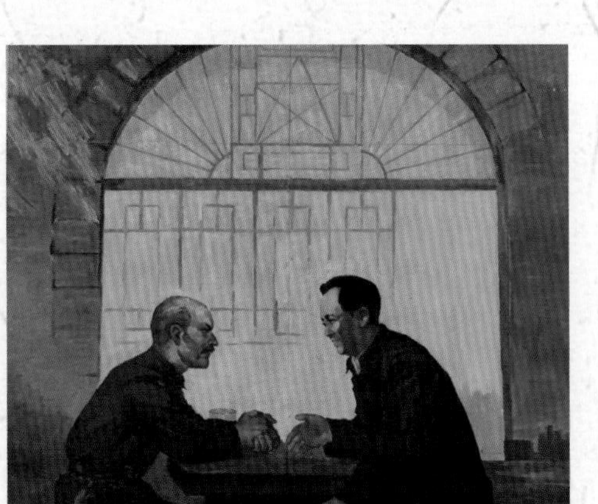

图568 教学八楼内的油画《毛主席会见白求恩》
Fig. 568 Oil painting "Chairman Mao meeting Bethune" in the Eighth Teaching Building

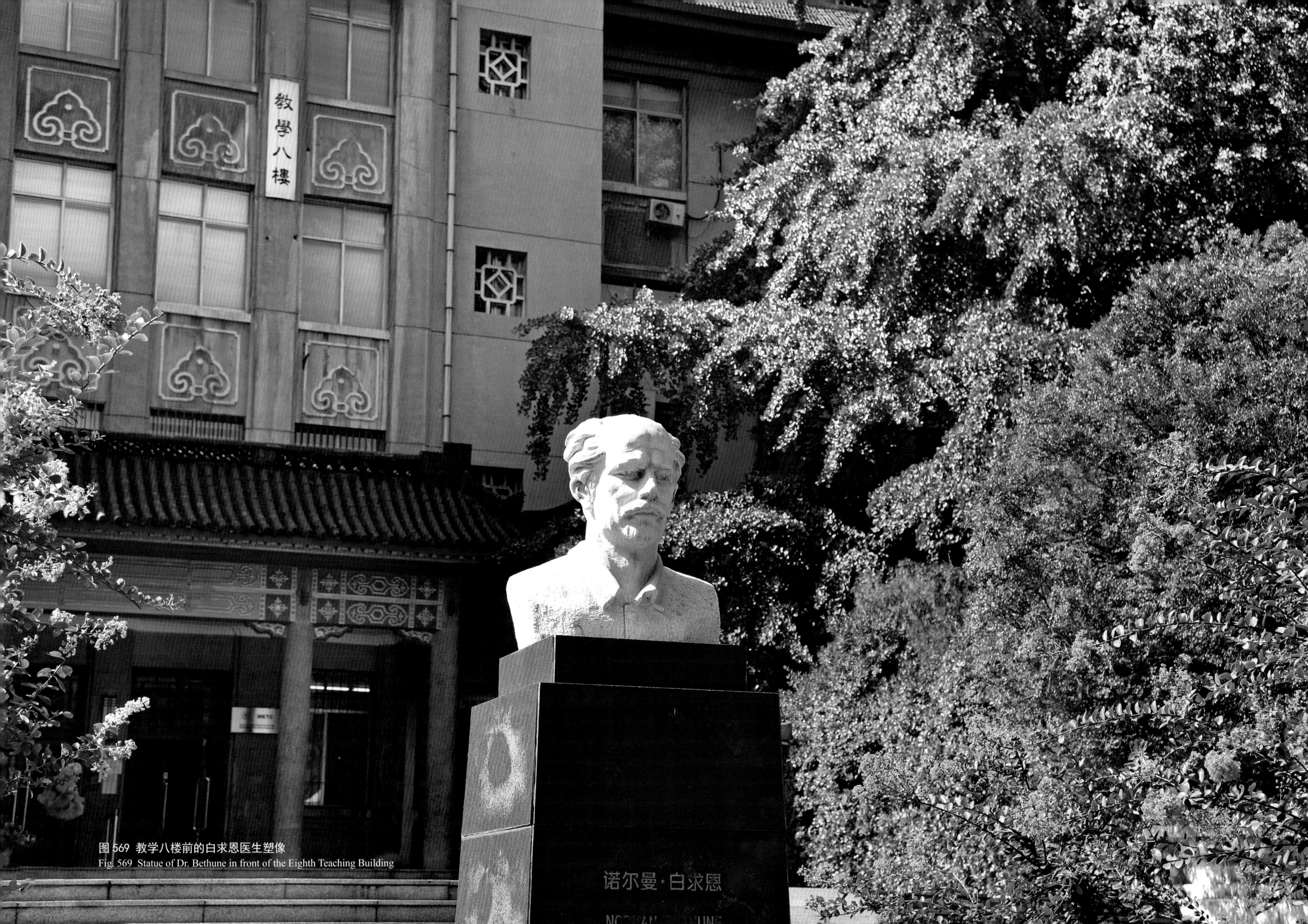

图 569 教学八楼前的白求恩医生塑像
Fig. 569 Statue of Dr. Bethune in front of the Eighth Teaching Building

56 大教无声（2）

Great Teaching in Silence (2)

华东白求恩医学院为齐鲁医学院的源头之一，红色基因的根源，其前身为新四军军医学校。1944 年 10 月 16 日，新四军军部决定建立新四军军医学校，目标是培养政治坚定、技术优良、身体健康的白求恩式的医务工作者。1945 年 5 月 12 日，新四军军医学校在安徽省天长县长庄开学。此后，随军辗转办学于临沂、沂水、胶东等地，1947 年 1 月更名为华东白求恩医学院。1948 年 9 月济南解放，学校由益都县进驻济南市经五路纬九路。不久，山东省立医学院并入，原附属医院华东国际和平医院与山东省立医院合并，继续作为附属医院。1950 年 12 月，学校改名为山东医学院。1952 年 9 月，全国高等学校院系调整，山东医学院与齐鲁大学医学院合并仍称山东医学院，并迁入原齐鲁大学校园。1985 年 5 月改称山东医科大学。2000 年 7 月，山东大学、山东医科大学和山东工业大学合并为新的山东大学，原山东医科大学成为山东大学齐鲁医学院。

East China Bethune Medical College is one of the sources of Cheeloo College of Medicine and the root of red gene. Its predecessor was the Military Medical School of the New Fourth Army. On 16 October 1944, the army headquarters of the New Fourth Army decided to establish the Military Medical School of the New Fourth Army, with the goal of training Bethune-style medical workers with political firmness, excellent skills and good health. On 12 May 1945, the Military Medical School of the New Fourth Army opened in Changzhuang, Tianchang County, Anhui Province. Since then, it went along with the army to run schools in Linyi, Yishui, Jiaodong and other places. In January 1947, it was renamed East China Bethune Medical College. In September 1948, Jinan was liberated, and the college entered and was stationed on Jingwu Road, Weijiu Road of Jinan City from Yidu County. Later, Shandong Provincial Hospital was merged into East China Bethune Medical College and then merged with East China International Peace Hospital, the former Affiliated Hospital, to continue to be an affiliated hospital. In December 1950, the college was renamed Shandong Medical College. In September 1952, the schools and departments of colleges and universities across the country were adjusted. Shandong Medical College and Medical School of Cheeloo University merged to form new Shandong Medical College, and moved to the campus of Cheeloo University. In May 1985, it was renamed Shandong Medical University. In July 2000, Shandong University, Shandong Medical University and Shandong University of Technology merged into a new Shandong University, and the former Shandong Medical University became Cheeloo College of Medicine of Shandong University.

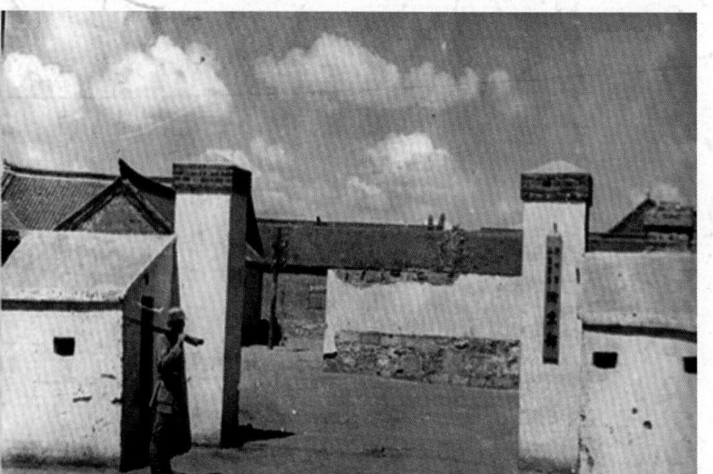
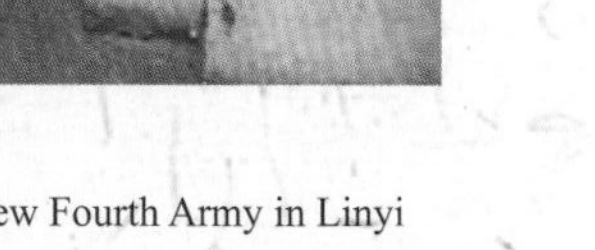

图 570 新四军军医学校临沂旧址
Fig. 570 Old site of the Military Medical School of the New Fourth Army in Linyi

图 571 华东白求恩医学院的附属医院
Fig. 571 Affiliated Hospital of East China Bethune Medical College

图 572 华东白求恩医学院院长宫乃泉（1910 ～ 1975），山东莱阳人，奉天医科大学毕业，曾任军事医学科学院首任院长，1955 年被授予少将军衔。
Fig. 572 Gong Naiquan (1910-1975), president of East China Bethune Medical College, was born in Laiyang, Shandong Province. He graduated from Mukden Medical College and once worked as the first president of the Academy of Military Medical Sciences. He was awarded the rank of Major General in 1955.

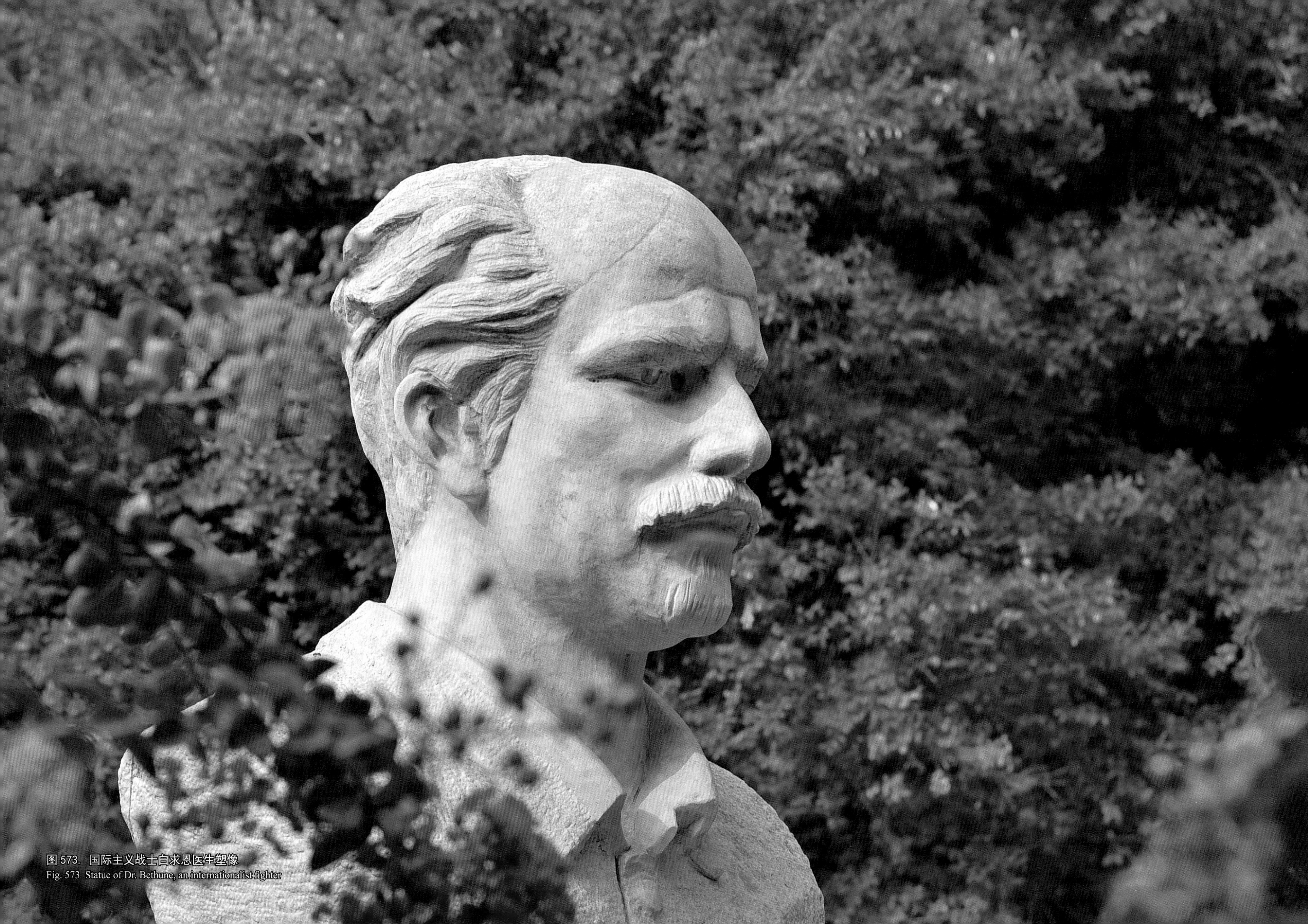

图 573. 国际主义战士白求恩医生塑像
Fig. 573 Statue of Dr. Bethune, an internationalist fighter

56 大教无声（3）

Great Teaching in Silence (3)

趵突泉校区内的人物雕像较少，除白求恩医生头像外，仅有药圣李时珍全身像、南丁格尔女士全身像及半身像、孙鸿泉教授半身像和徐荣祥先生头部浮雕像等几尊。黑色的李时珍全身像坐落于中心花园东端、教学七楼（药学院楼）北侧的小广场上。李时珍面向西侧的中心花园，手持《本草纲目》，表情呈沉思状，目视远方。南丁格尔全身像立于附属卫校院内，半身像位于护理楼大厅内。孙鸿泉教授半身像座落在中心花园东翼北侧，立于2011年，周围花木繁茂，四季风光优美。徐荣祥先生头部浮雕像安放于2018年，位于教学二楼北门东侧，整个作品由四本叠放于一起的汉白玉书组成，最上方的一本敞开，上有先生事迹简介及头像。另外，还有齐鲁大学医学院创始人之一的武成献先生墓碑。

There are few statues of people on Baotuquan Campus. In addition to the head sculpture of Dr. Bethune, there are only a whole-length sculpture of the Pharmacological Sage Li Shizhen, a whole-length sculpture and a bust of Ms. Nightingale, a bust of Professor Sun Hongquan and a head sculpture in relief of Mr. Xu Rongxiang. The black whole-length sculpture of Li Shizhen is located in the small square at the east end of the Central Garden and on the north side of the Seventh Teaching Building (Building of School of Pharmaceutical Sciences). Holding *Compendium of Materia Medica*, the statue of Li Shizhen faces the Central Garden on the west side, looking into the distance with thoughtfulness. The whole-length sculpture of Nightingale stands in the yard of the affiliated health school, and the bust is located in the hall of the Nursing Building. The bust of Professor Sun Hongquan stood on the north side of the east wing of the Central Garden in 2011, surrounded by lush flowers and trees and beautiful scenery during the four seasons. The head relief of Mr. Xu Rongxiang was placed on the east side of the north gate of the Second Teaching Building in 2018. The whole work consists of four white marble books stacked together, the top one being open, with a brief introduction to Mr. Xu Rongxiang's deeds and his head sculpture. In addition, there is a tombstone for Mr. James Russell Watson, one of the founders of the Medical School of Cheeloo University.

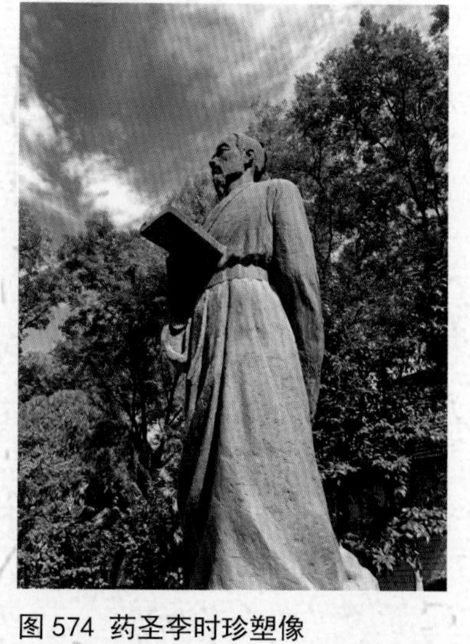

图 574 药圣李时珍塑像
Fig.574 Statue of Li Shizhen, the Pharmacological Sage

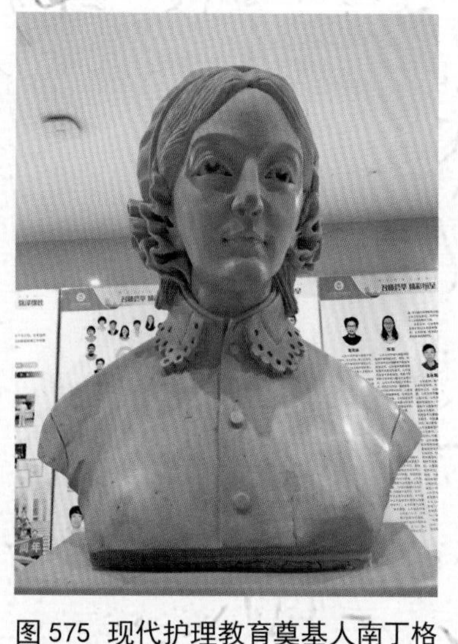

图 575 现代护理教育奠基人南丁格尔塑像
Fig. 575 Statue of Nightingale, founder of modern nursing education

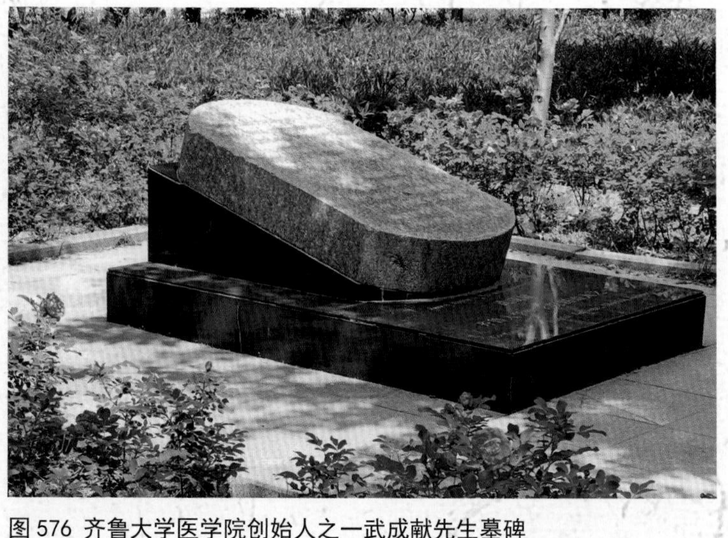

图 576 齐鲁大学医学院创始人之一武成献先生墓碑
Fig. 576 Tombstone of Mr. James Russell Watson, one of the founders of Medical School of Cheeloo University

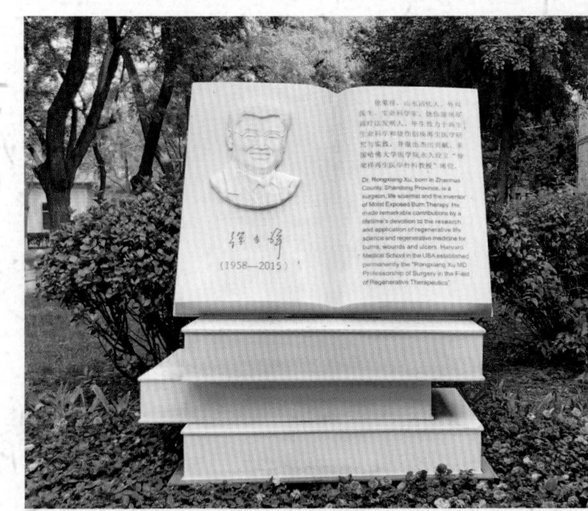

图 577 烧伤湿润暴露疗法创始人徐荣祥先生浮雕像
Fig. 577 Relief image of Mr. Xu Rongxiang, founder of moist exposed burn therapy

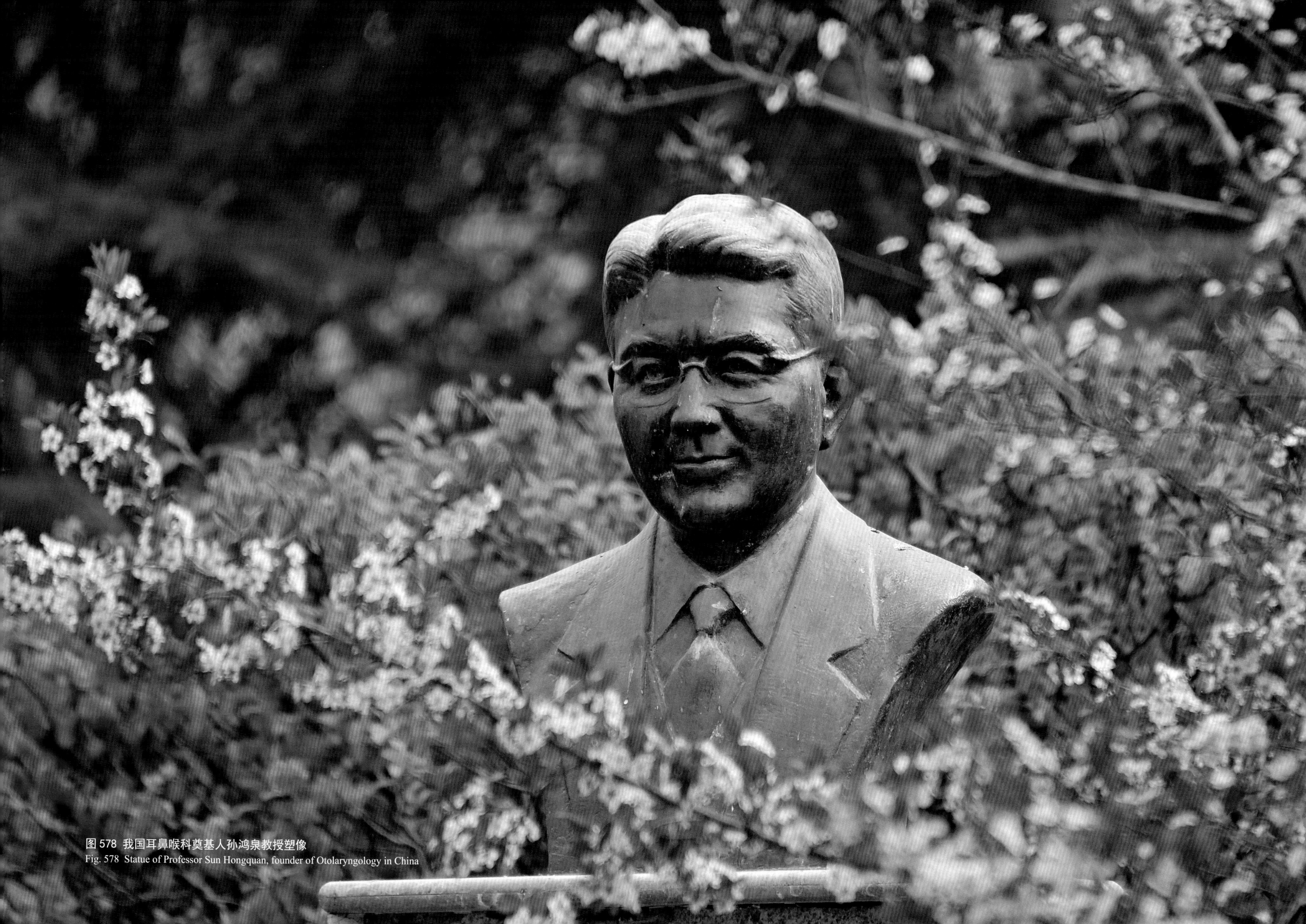

图 578 我国耳鼻喉科奠基人孙鸿泉教授塑像
Fig. 578 Statue of Professor Sun Hongquan, founder of Otolaryngology in China

56 大教无声（4）

Great Teaching in Silence (4)

趵突泉校区内石刻、巨石或怪石约有 19 块，分布于各教学楼前或树林中。依设立者身份不同，可将这些石刻艺术品分为三类。第一类，最多，由本校毕业生捐建，往往建立于捐建者就读学院所在教学楼前；第二类，由学校设立，往往立于树林内或宿舍旁，上面无字或未刻设立者名字；第三类，由政府或友好单位赠送。

未体现专业或医学系毕业生捐赠的石刻或巨石座落于综合楼、柏根楼、教学六楼、教学七楼和电镜楼前，约 5 块。

There are about 19 stone carvings and rocks on Baotuquan Campus which are distributed in front of the teaching buildings or in the woods. According to the identity of the founders, these stone carvings can be divided into three categories. The first category, with the largest number of rocks, is donated by the graduates; they were always built in front of the teaching buildings where the donors once studied. The second category is set up by the university, and they often stand in the woods or beside dormitories with no words or names of the founders. The third category is presented by the government or friendly units as gifts.

The stone carvings or rocks donated by medical graduates or other graduates with unknown specialities are located in front of the Comprehensive Building, Bergen Hall, the Sixth Teaching Building, the Seventh Teaching Building and the Building of Electron Microscopy, about 5 pieces.

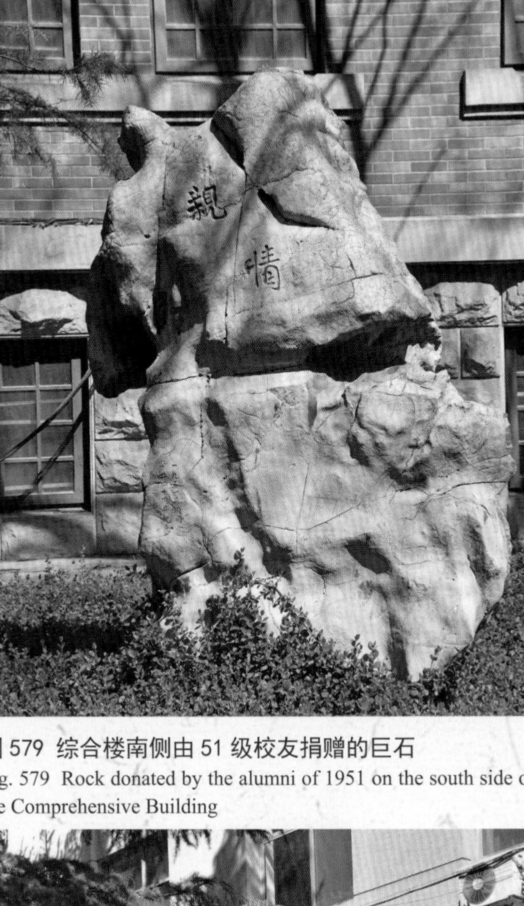

图 579 综合楼南侧由 51 级校友捐赠的巨石

Fig. 579 Rock donated by the alumni of 1951 on the south side of the Comprehensive Building

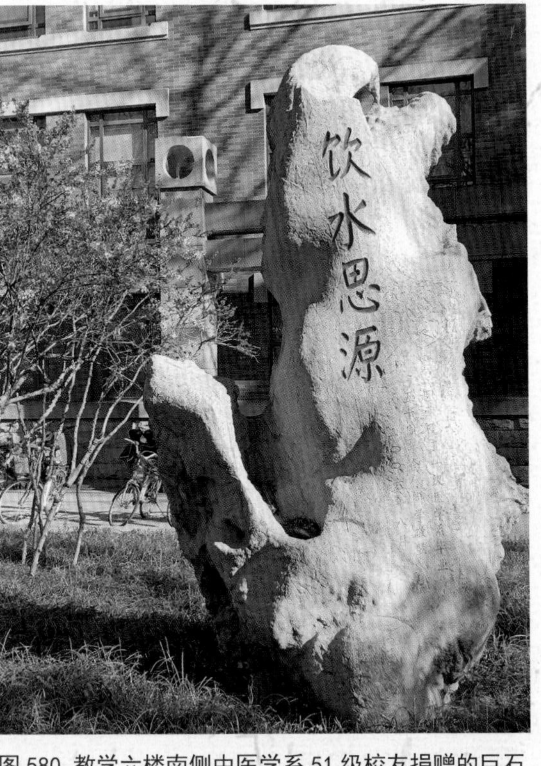

图 580 教学六楼南侧由医学系 51 级校友捐赠的巨石

Fig. 580 Rock donated by the alumni of 1951 of the Medical Department on the south side of the Sixth Teaching Building

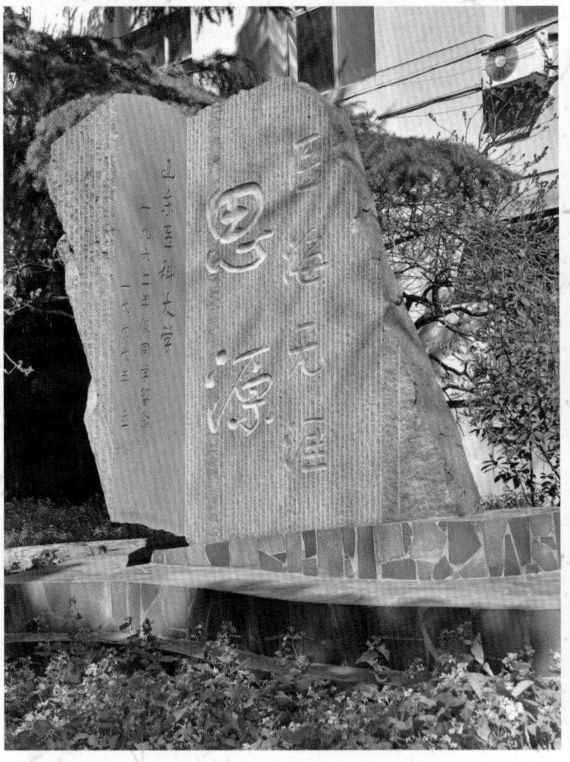

图 581 教学七楼南侧由 62 级校友捐赠的石刻

Fig. 581 Stone carving donated by the alumni of 1962 on the south side of the Seventh Teaching Building

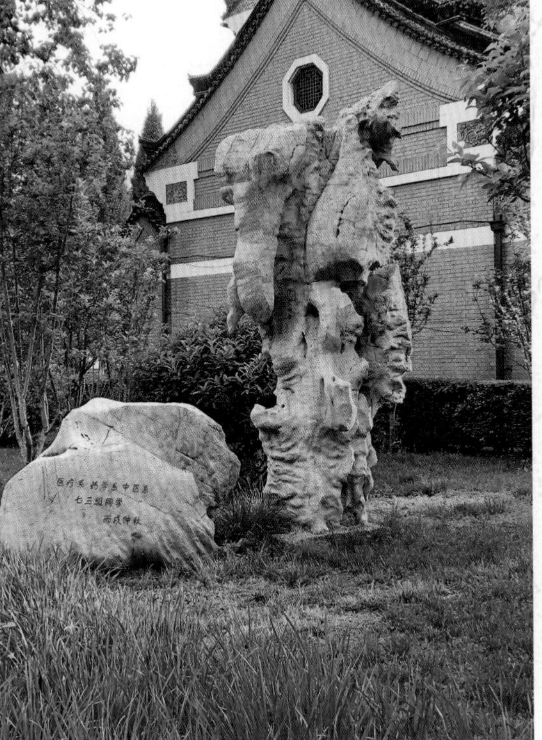

图 582 柏根楼东侧由医疗系、药学系和中医系 73 级校友捐赠的巨石

Fig. 582 Rock donated by the alumni of 1973 of the Medical Department, the Department of Pharmacy and the Department of Traditional Chinese Medicine on the east side of Bergen Hall

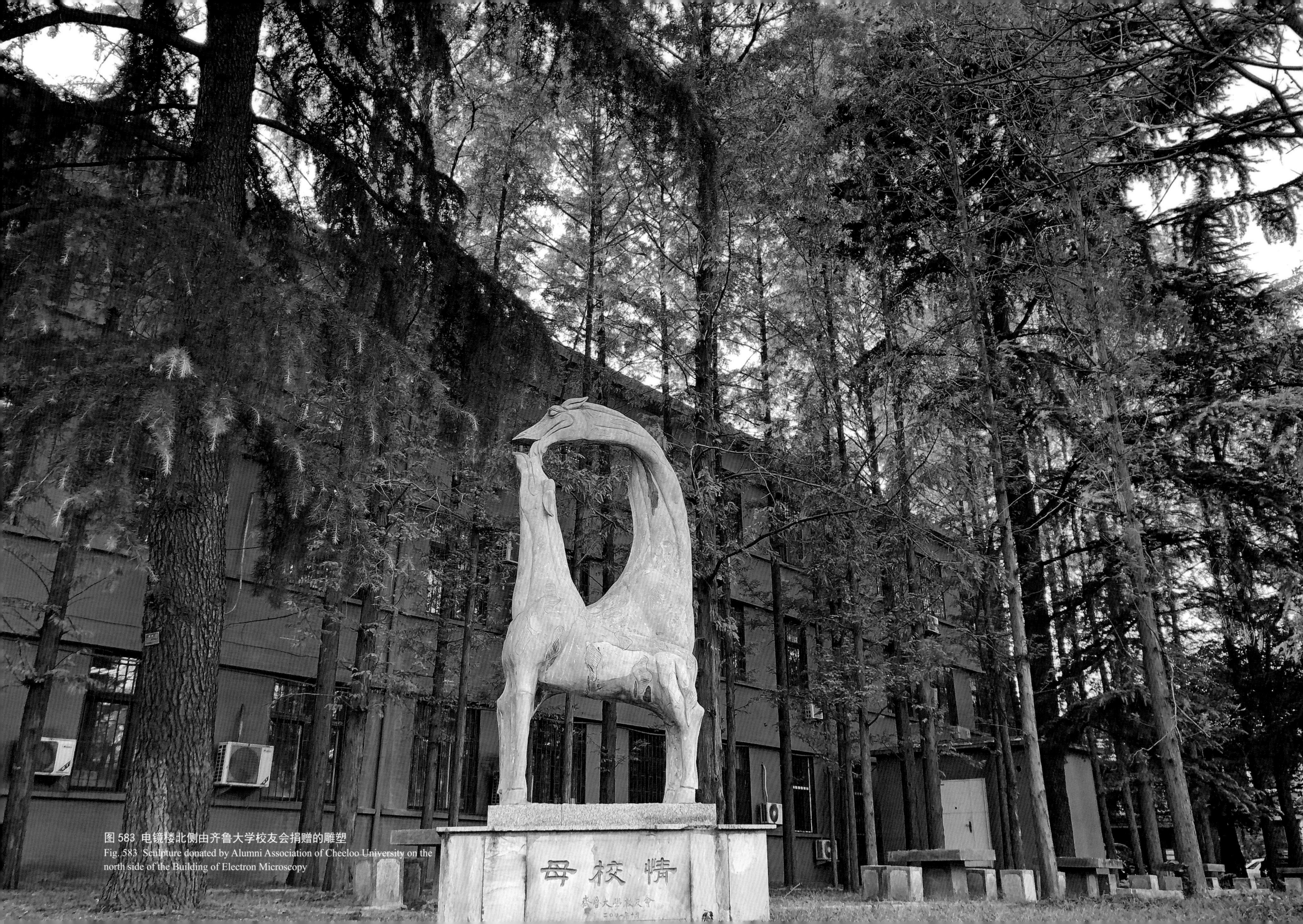

图 583 电镜楼北侧由齐鲁大学校友会捐赠的雕塑

Fig. 583 Sculpture donated by Alumni Association of Cheeloo University on the north side of the Building of Electron Microscopy

56 | 大教无声（5）

Great Teaching in Silence (5)

由公共卫生学院毕业生赠送的石刻艺术品共 3 块，立于教学九楼南侧，东西方向上一字排开。口腔医学院楼南侧立有石刻 1 块，由 78 级口腔医学系学生毕业廿周年时设立。药学专业毕业生设立的石刻艺术品 2 块，立于综合楼、药学科研楼前。

A total of three stone carvings presented by graduates of the School of Public Health stand on the south side of the Ninth Teaching Building and line up in the east-west direction. There is a stone carving standing on the south side of the Building of the School of Stomatology, which is set up by students of 1978 of the Department of Stomatology on the 20th anniversary of graduation. Two stone carvings are set up by pharmaceutical graduates and they stand in front of the Administration Building and the Pharmaceutical Research Building.

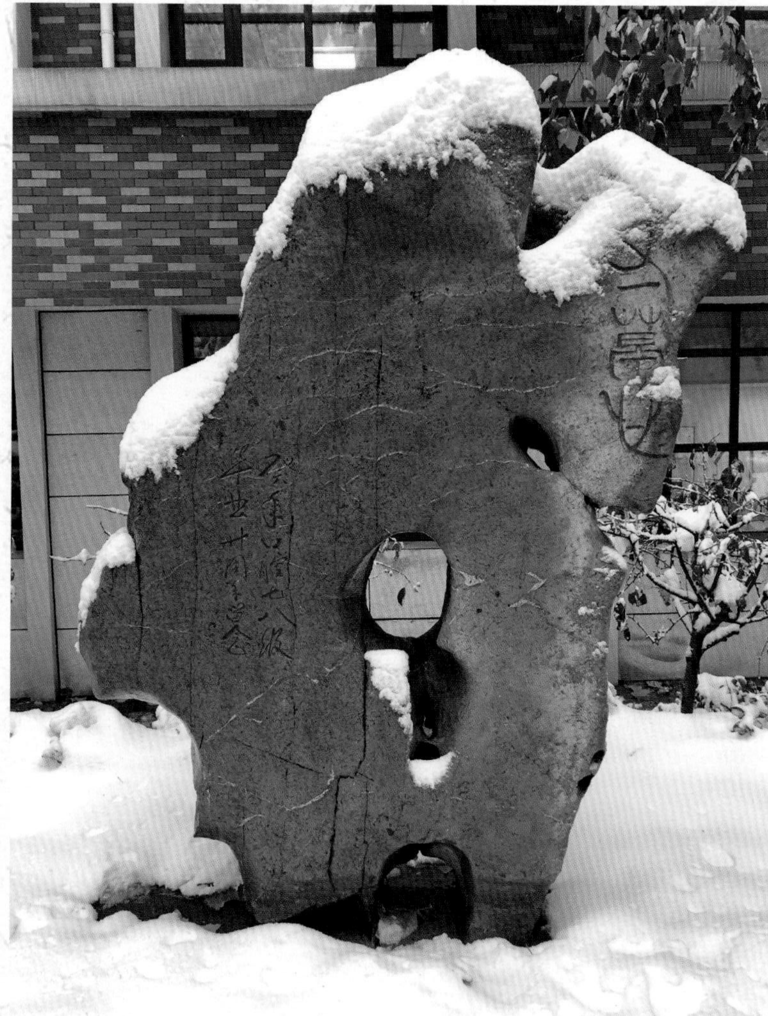

图 584 口腔楼南侧由 78 级口腔医学系校友捐赠的巨石
Fig. 584 Rock donated by the alumni of 1978 of the Department of Stomatology on the south side of the Building of Stomatology

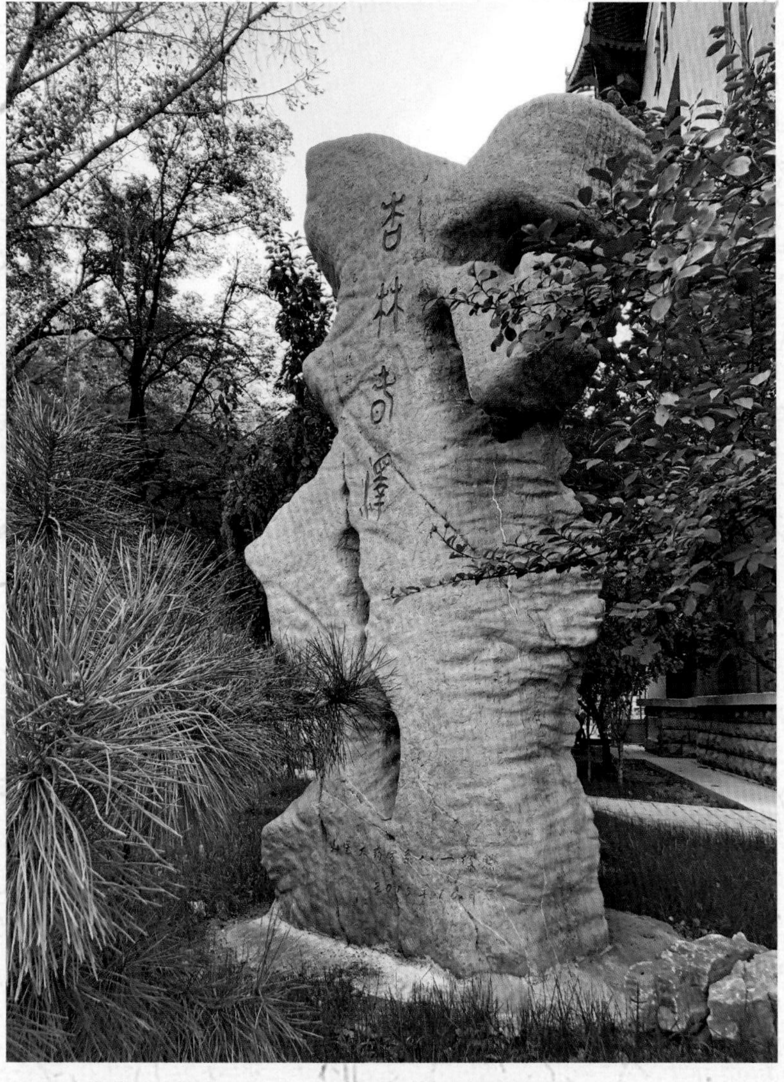

图 585 药学科研楼东北侧由 81 级药学系校友捐赠的巨石
Fig. 585 Rock donated by the alumni of 1981 of the Department of Pharmacy on the northeast side of the Pharmaceutical Research Building

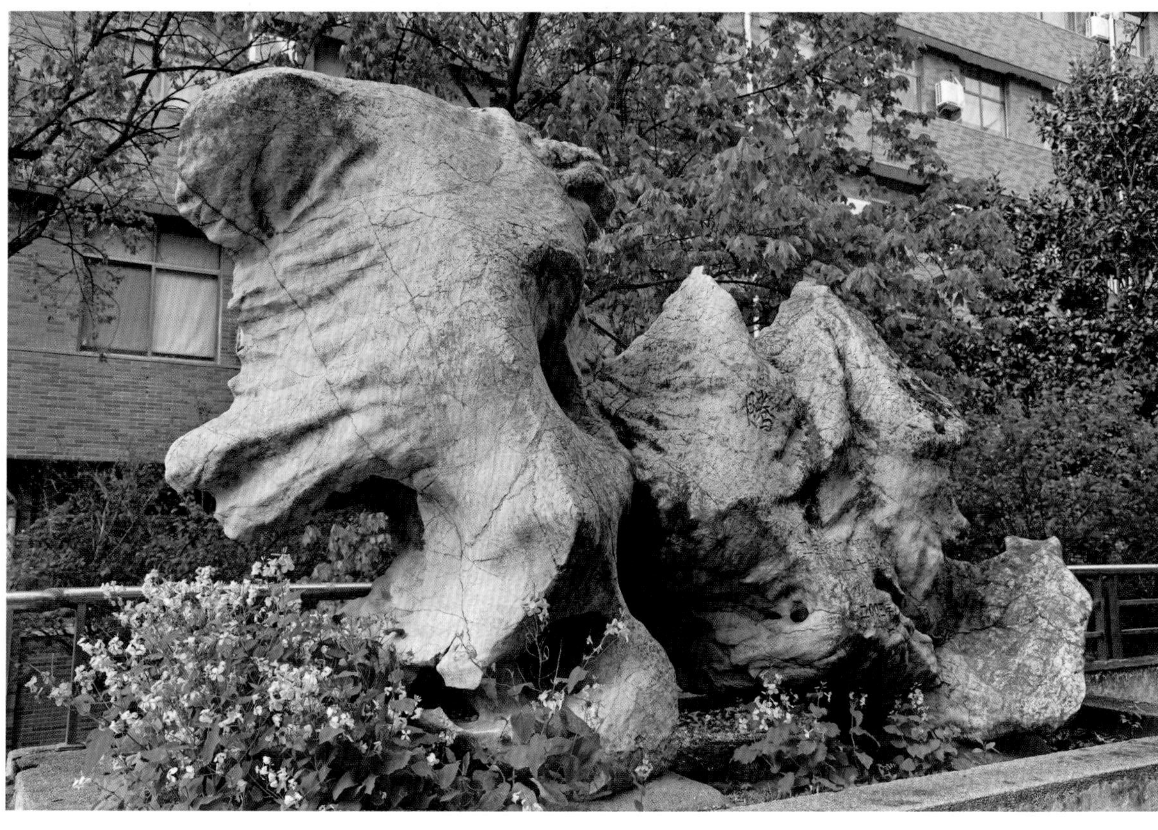

图 586 教学九楼南侧由卫生系 78 级校友捐赠的巨石

Fig. 586 Rock donated by the alumni of 1978 of the Department of Health on the south side of the Ninth Teaching Building

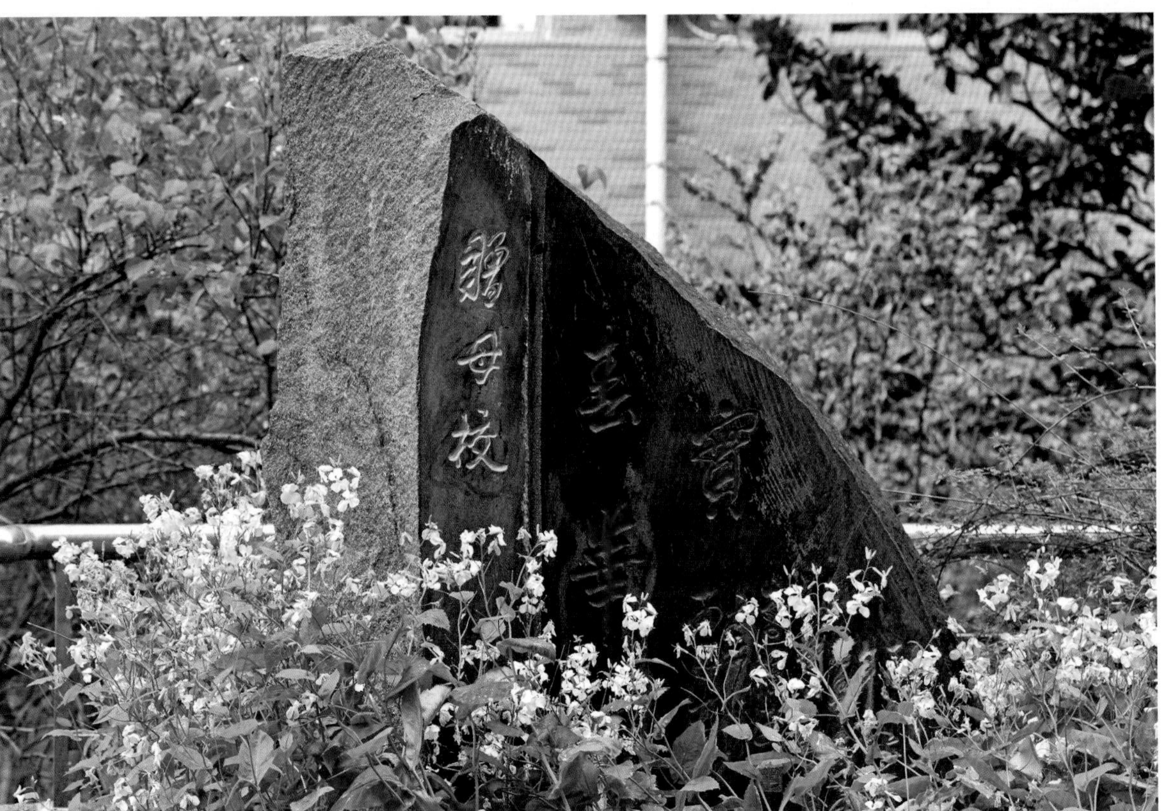

图 587 教学九楼南侧由卫生系 81 级校友捐赠的石刻

Fig. 587 Stone carving donated by the alumni of 1981 of the Department of Health on the south side of the Ninth Teaching Building

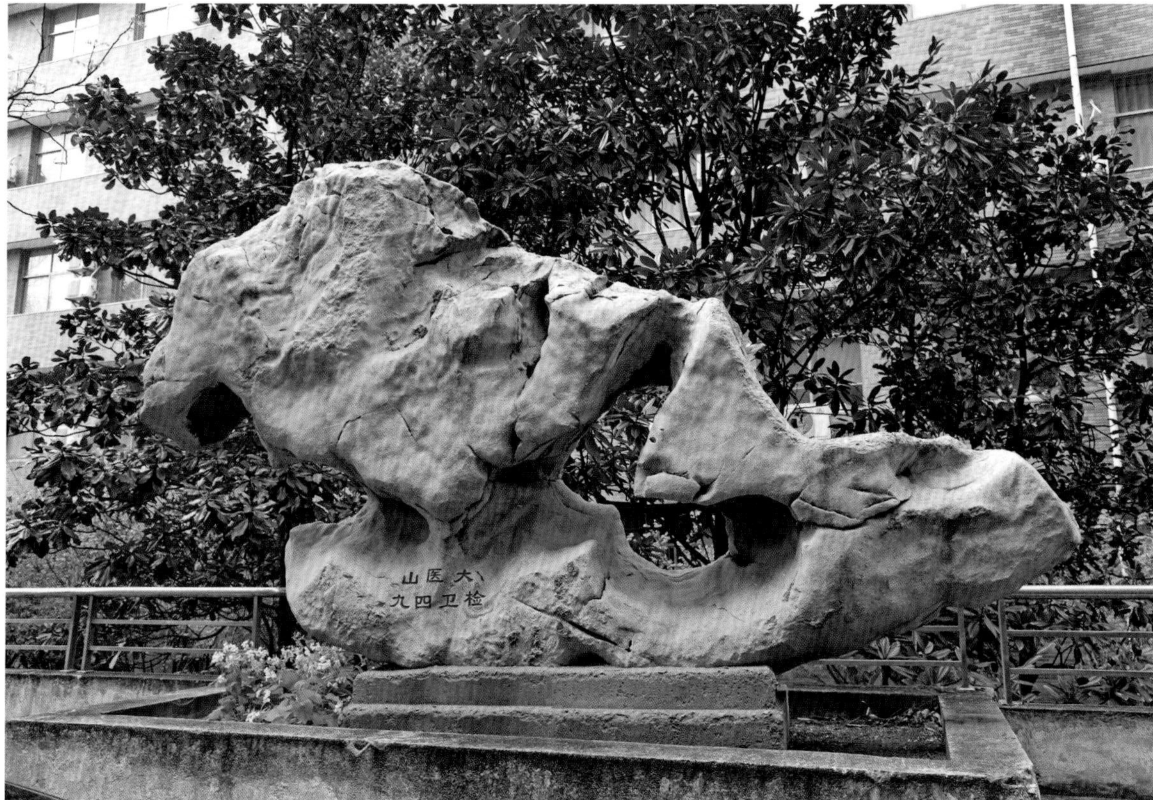

图 588 教学九楼南侧由 94 级卫检校友捐赠的巨石

Fig. 588 Rock donated by the alumni of 1994 of the Department of Health Inspection and Quarantine on the south side of the Ninth Teaching Building

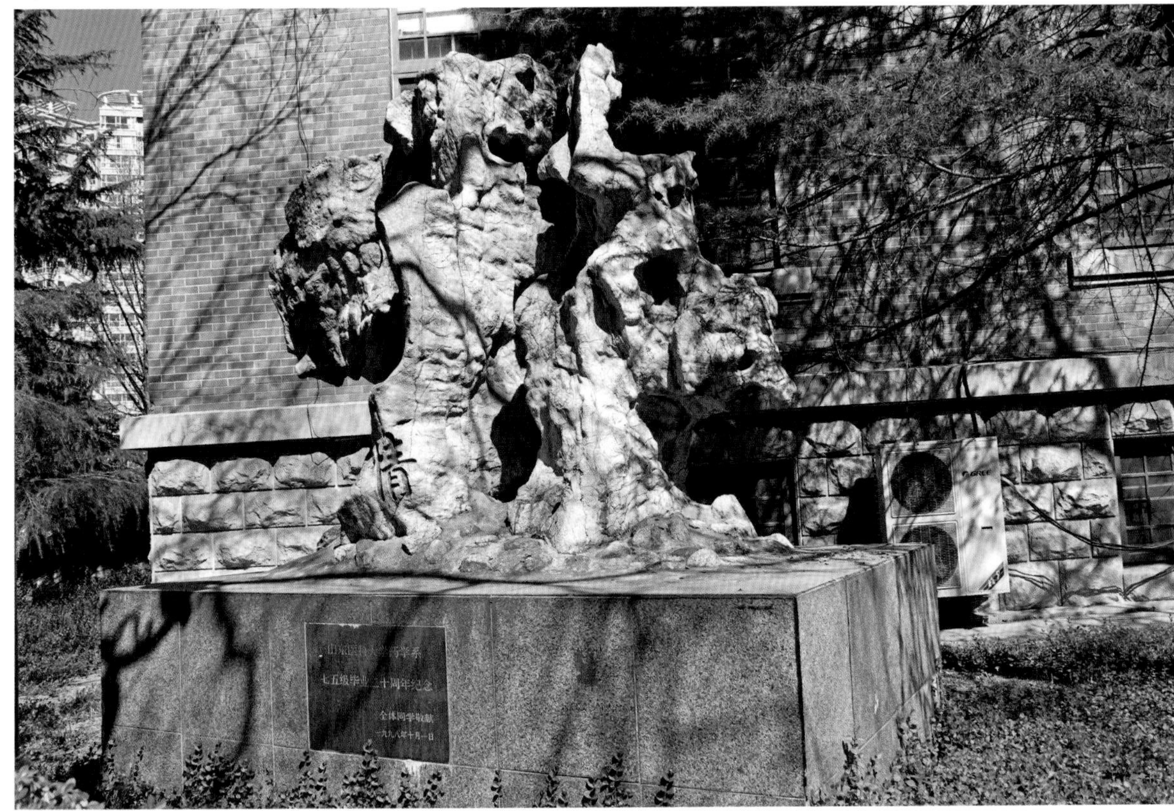

图 589 综合楼南侧由药学系 75 级校友捐赠的太湖石

Fig. 589 Taihu Lake stone donated by the alumni of 1975 of the Department of Pharmacy on the south side of the Comprehensive Building

56 | 大教无声（6）

Great Teaching in Silence (6)

由学校或友好单位设立的巨石或怪石 8 块，位于柏根楼旁、广场或树林内。尤其需要指出的是中共临沂市委和临沂市人民政府在山东大学建校 110 周年时，赠送了一块巨石，颇像一位负重远行的智者，立于长柏路第 1 ~ 3 号教授别墅前方的草坪上，体现了沂蒙老区人民与山东大学特别是华东白求恩医学院的战斗情谊、血肉联系和深厚感情。

Eight rocks are set up by the university or friendly units, and they are located next to Bergen Hall, on the square or in the wood. In particular, it should be pointed out that on the 110th anniversary of the founding of Shandong University, Linyi Municipal Committee of the Communist Party of China and Linyi Municipal People's Government presented a rock as a gift which is quite like a wise man traveling with a heavy load. It stands on the lawn in front of professors' villas Nos. 1-3 on Changbai Road, reflecting the fighting friendship, flesh-and-blood ties and deep feelings between the people of Yimeng old revolutionary base areas and Shandong University, especially East China Bethune Medical College.

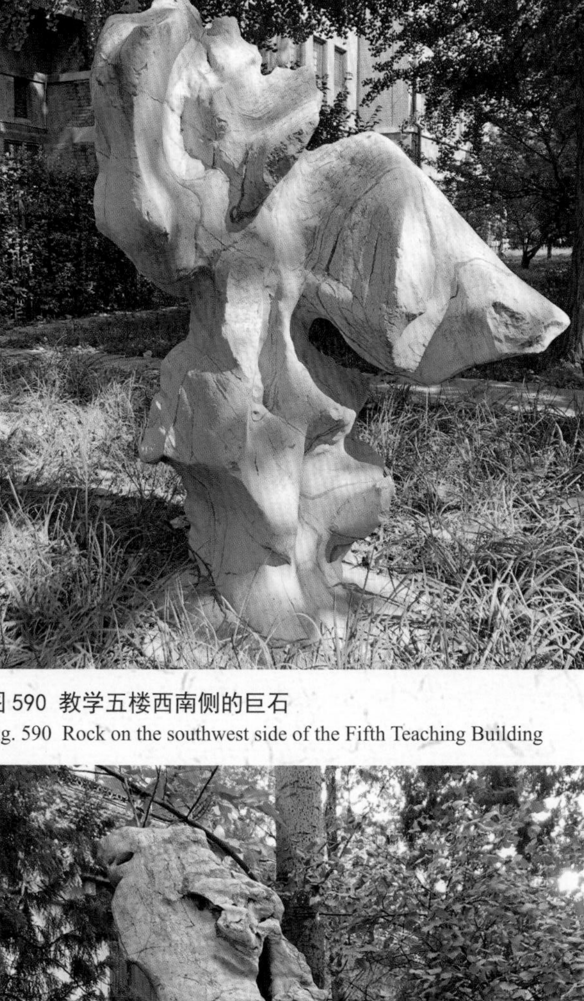

图 590 教学五楼西南侧的巨石
Fig. 590 Rock on the southwest side of the Fifth Teaching Building

图 591 教学二楼北侧的太湖石
Fig. 591 Taihu Lake stone on the north side of the Second Teaching Building

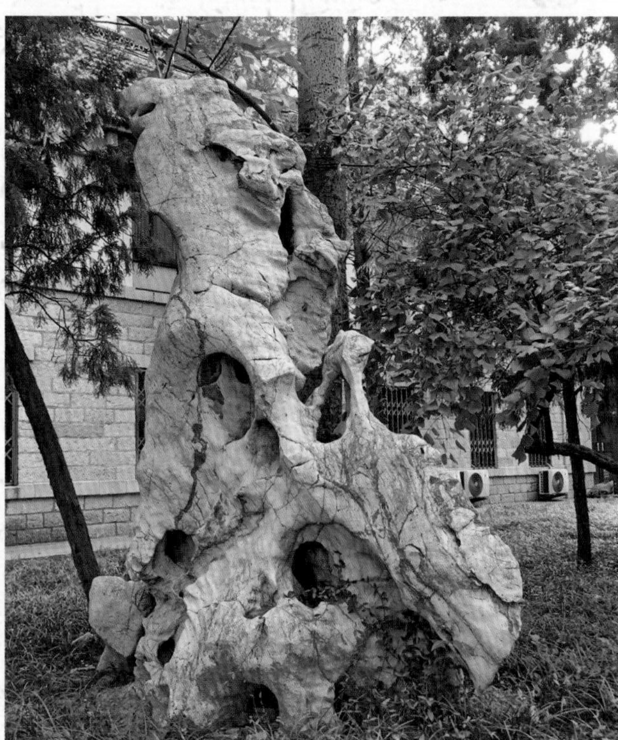

图 592 号院东北侧的太湖石
Fig. 592 Taihu Lake stone on the northeast side of the Courtyard

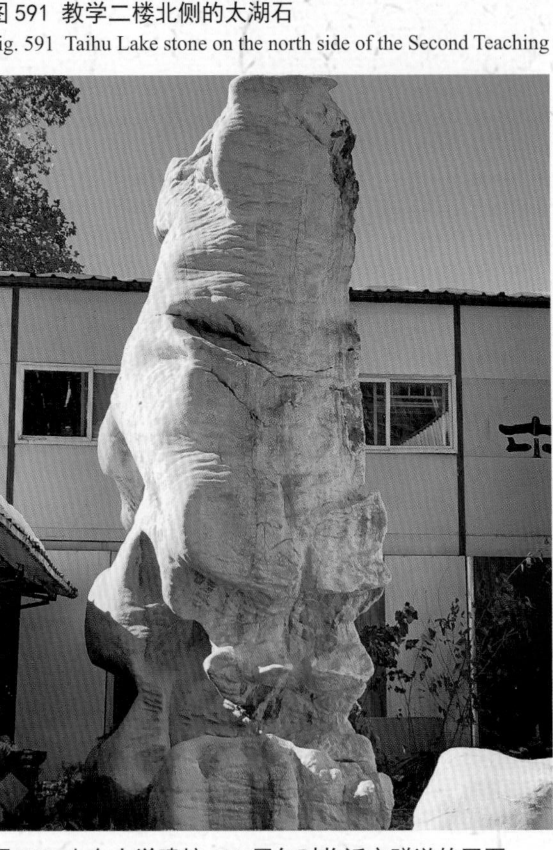

图 593 山东大学建校 110 周年时临沂市赠送的巨石
Fig. 593 Rock presented by Linyi City on the 110th anniversary of the founding of Shandong University

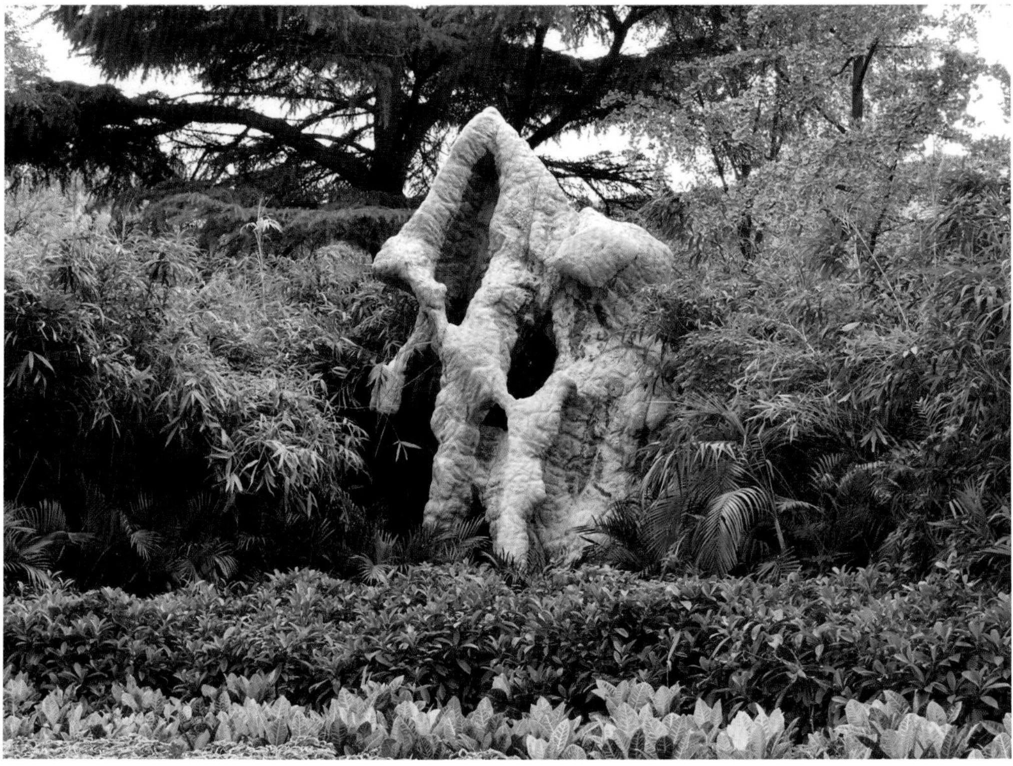

图 594 校门内三角区的太湖石
Fig. 594 Taihu Lake stone in the triangle area of the Alumni Gate

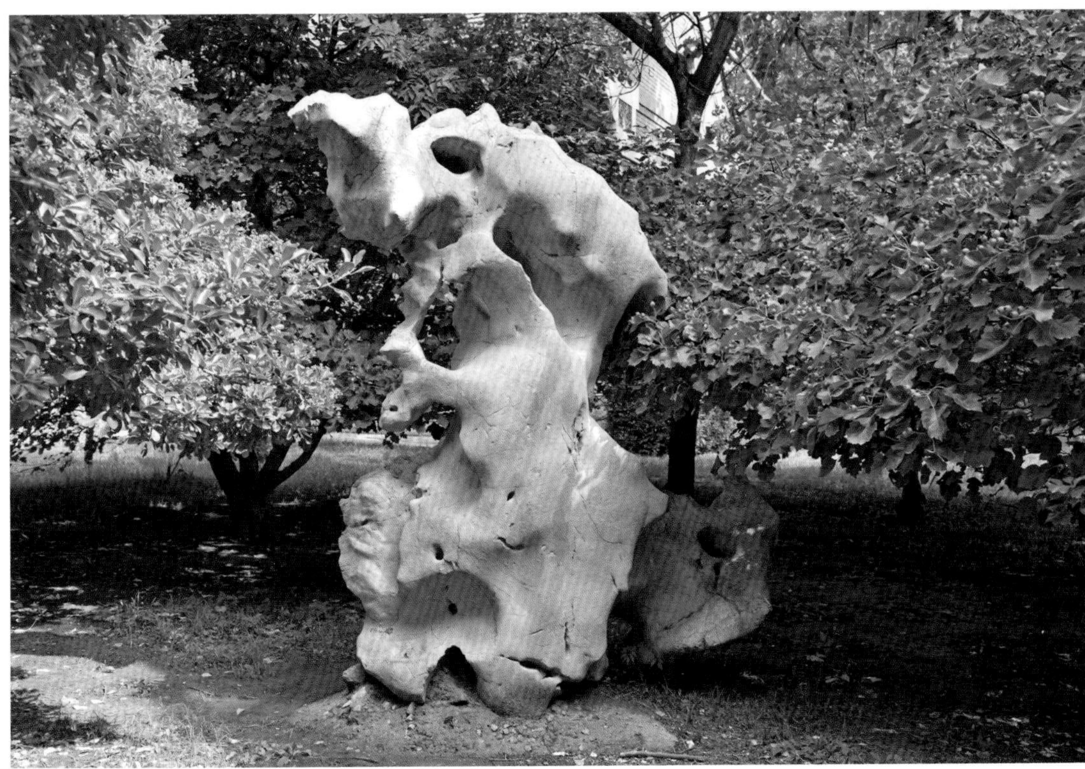

图 595 教学三楼东南侧的太湖石
Fig. 595 Taihu Lake stone on the southeast side of the Third Teaching Building

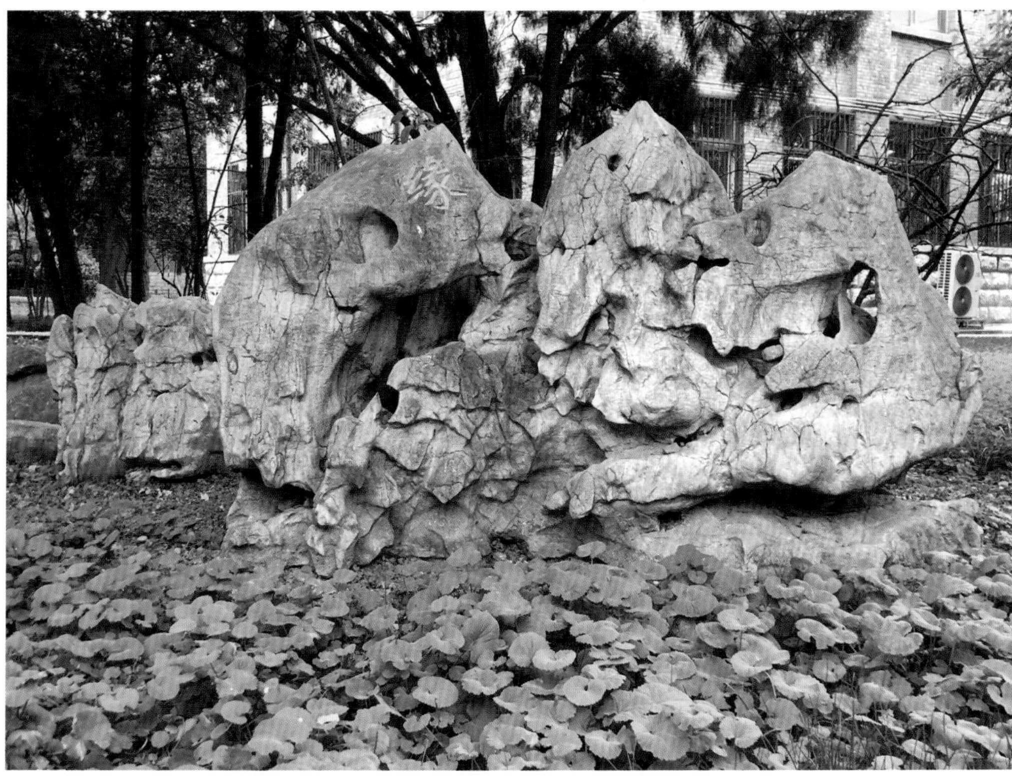

图 596 教学二楼东北处的太湖石
Fig. 596 Taihu Lake stone on the northeast side of the Second Teaching Building

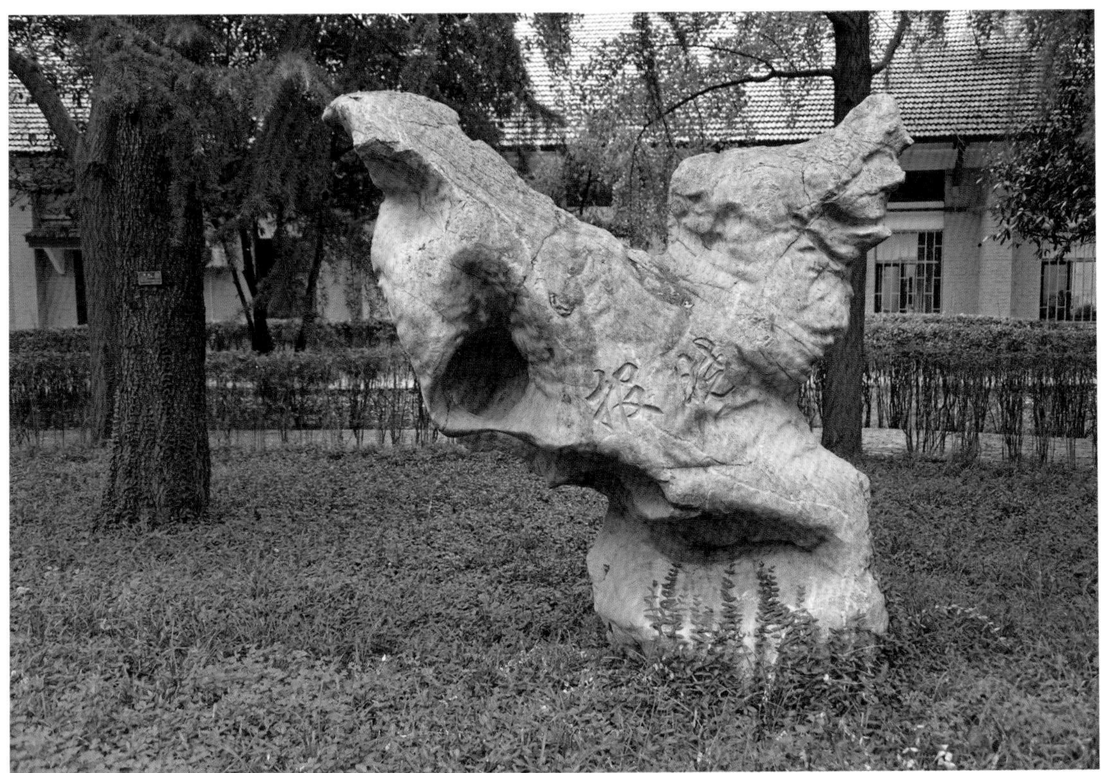

图 597 小礼堂南侧的景观石
Fig. 597 Landscape stone on the south side of the auditorium

第十章 Chapter Ten

直属附属医院
Directly Affiliated Hospitals

57 齐鲁医院（1）
Qilu Hospital (1)

齐鲁医院是国家卫生健康委委属（管）医院，首批委省共建国家区域医疗中心（综合类）牵头和主体建设单位。医院始建于 1890 年，先后称华美医院、共合医院、齐鲁医院、山东医科大学附属医院等，2000 年 10 月更名为山东大学齐鲁医院。现有包括中国工程院院士在内的国家级高层次人才 13 人、泰山学者 49 人。目前在济南、青岛形成了两地多院区发展格局，实际开放床位 5100 余张，门诊量年均近 400 万人次，在神经复合手术、心脏介入手术、内镜治疗等多个领域处于国内领先水平。现有临床医技科室 66 个，其中国家重点学科和国家临床重点专科 18 个。作为世界一流大学建设高校（A 类）的直属附属医院，齐鲁医院十分重视临床教学的创新与改革，为国家培养了包括冯兰洲院士、张运院士、谢立信院士、于金明院士和宁光院士等在内的一批又一批高级医务人才。

Qilu Hospital is a hospital under the administration of the National Health Commission. It is among the first batch of leading and main units to construct the national regional medical centers (comprehensive category) jointly built by the commission and the provincial governments. Founded in 1890, the hospital was successively called Sino-American Hospital, Union Hospital, Cheeloo Hospital and Affiliated Hospital of Shandong Medical University. In October 2000, it was renamed Qilu Hospital of Shandong University. Now there are 13 national high-level talents including academicians of Chinese Academy of Engineering and 49 Taishan scholars. At present, based in Jinan and Qingdao, the hospital has formed a development pattern of "multiple districts in two cities", with more than 5,100 beds and an average annual number of 4 million outpatient visits. The hospital is at the leading level in China in many fields such as neurorestorative procedure, cardiac interventional surgery and endoscopic treatment. Now there are 66 clinical and supportive departments, including 18 national key disciplines and National key clinical specialties. As a hospital directly affiliated to Shandong University aiming to become a first-class university of the world (Class A), Qilu Hospital attaches great importance to the innovation and reform of clinical teaching, and has cultivated a batch of senior medical talents for the country, including the academicians Feng Lanzhou, Zhang Yun, Xie Lixin, Yu Jinming and Ning Guang.

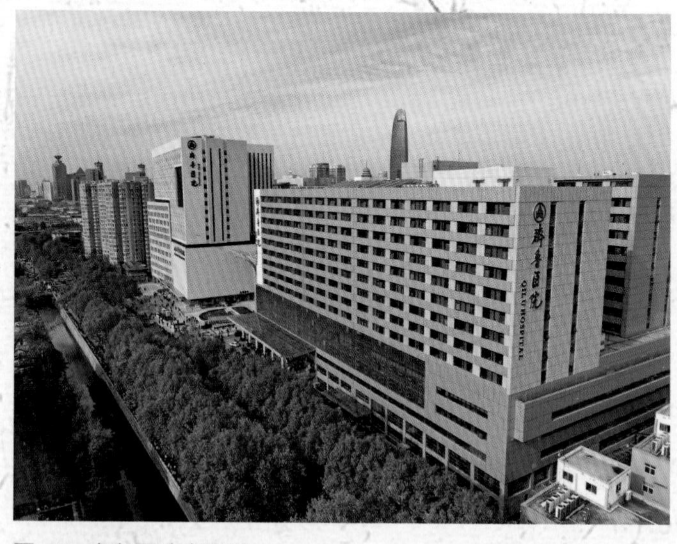

图 598 齐鲁医院南面观
Fig. 598 The south view of Qilu Hospital

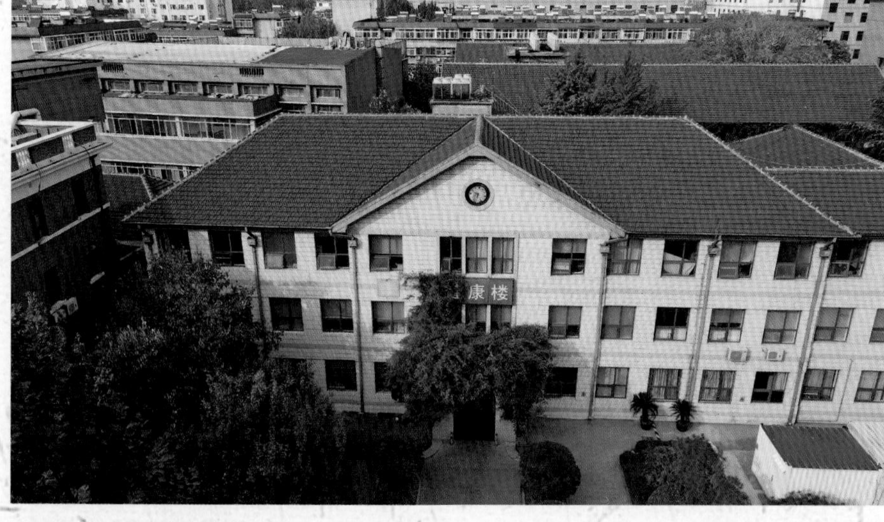

图 599 齐鲁医院健康楼
Fig. 599 Health Building of Qilu Hospital

图 600 齐鲁医院外景
Fig. 600 The exterior view of Qilu Hospital

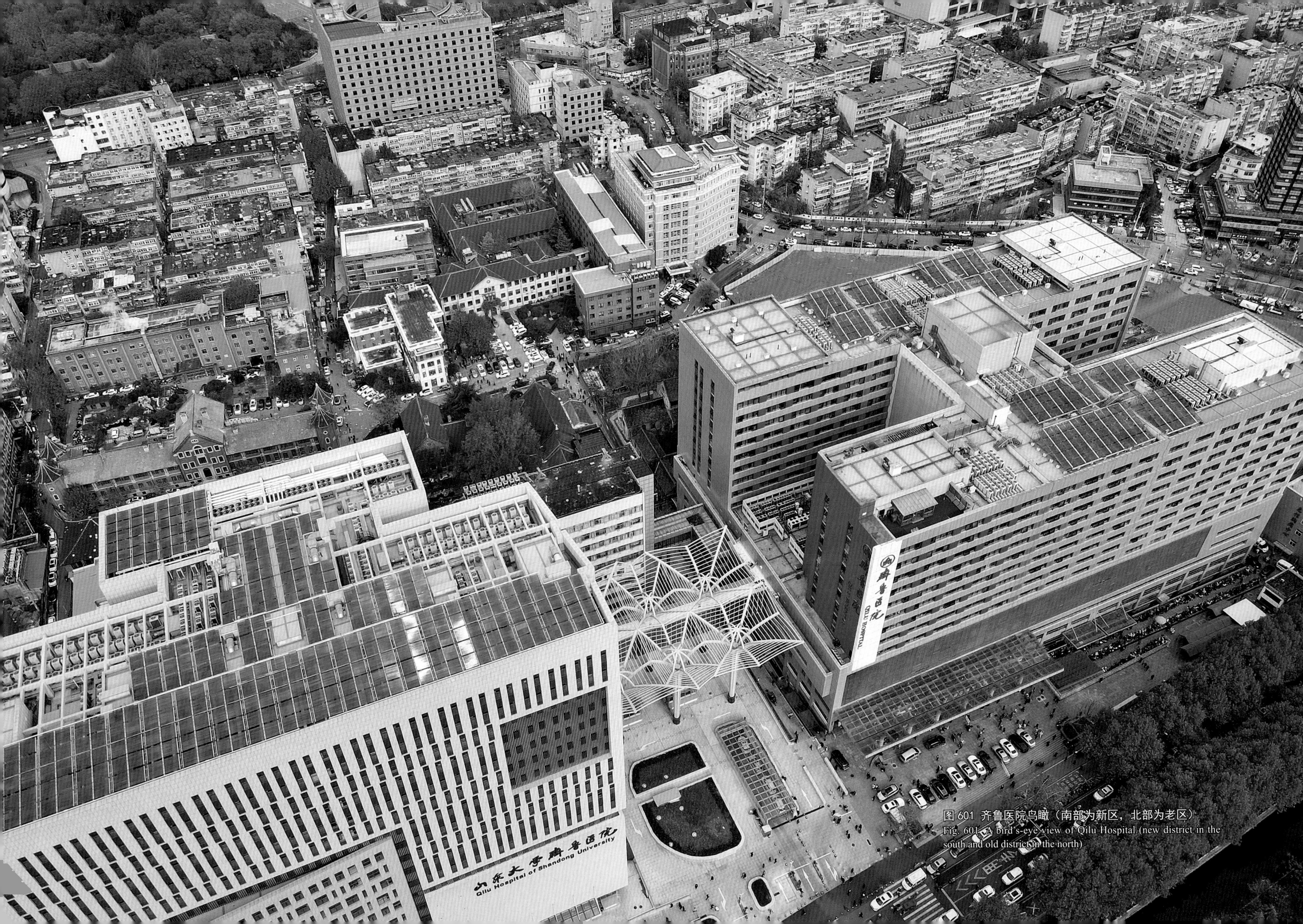

图 601 齐鲁医院鸟瞰（南部为新区，北部为老区）

Fig. 601 A bird's-eye view of Qilu Hospital (new district in the south and old district in the north)

57 齐鲁医院（2）

Qilu Hospital (2)

博施楼建于 1934 年，原为门诊病房楼、科研楼，现主要供科研使用。此楼东南角的奠基石上刻有“博施济众”四个篆字，为时任国民政府卫生部部长刘瑞恒手书。“博施济众”来源于《论语·雍也》篇“博施于民而能济众”一语，现已成为山东大学齐鲁医学院院训“博施济众，广智求真”的一部分。

齐鲁医院科研实力突出。现有各级科研平台 44 个（其中教育部重点实验室 1 个、国家卫生健康委重点实验室 2 个、国家中医药管理局实验室 1 个、国家药品监督管理局重点实验室 1 个、省部共建国家重点实验室培育基地 1 个、山东省重点实验室 4 个）。“十三五”期间，共获得国家重点研发计划项目和课题 21 项，国家自然科学基金 357 项，获得国家自然科学奖二等奖 1 项，“何梁何利基金 2020 年度科学与技术创新奖”1 项，省部级一等奖 9 项。

Built in 1934, Boshi Building was originally a building of outpatient service and scientific research and now it is mainly used for scientific research. The foundation stone in the southeast corner of the building is engraved with four seal characters of “Bo Shi Ji Zhong” which were written by Liu Ruiheng, then Health Minister of the National Government of the Republic of China. “Extensively conferring benefits on the people and able to assist all” comes from the saying in the chapter of “Yong Ye” of The Analects of Confucius and now has become a part of the motto of Cheeloo College of Medicine of Shandong University, that is, “We practice medicine for the welfare of all the people; we do research to pursue truth and enlightenment.”

Qilu Hospital has outstanding scientific research strength. At present, there are 44 scientific research platforms at all levels (including one key laboratory of the Ministry of Education, two key laboratories of the National Health Commission, one laboratory of the National Administration of Traditional Chinese Medicine, one key laboratory of the National Medical Products Administration, one breeding base of the national key laboratory jointly built by the provincial and ministerial departments, and four key laboratories of Shandong Province). During the “13th Five-Year Plan” period, the hospital has won a total of 21 projects and topics of national key research and development plan, 357 programs of National Natural Science Foundation of China, one second prize of the National Natural Science Award, one award for science and technology innovation of Ho Leung Ho Lee Foundation in 2020 and nine first prizes at the provincial and ministerial levels.

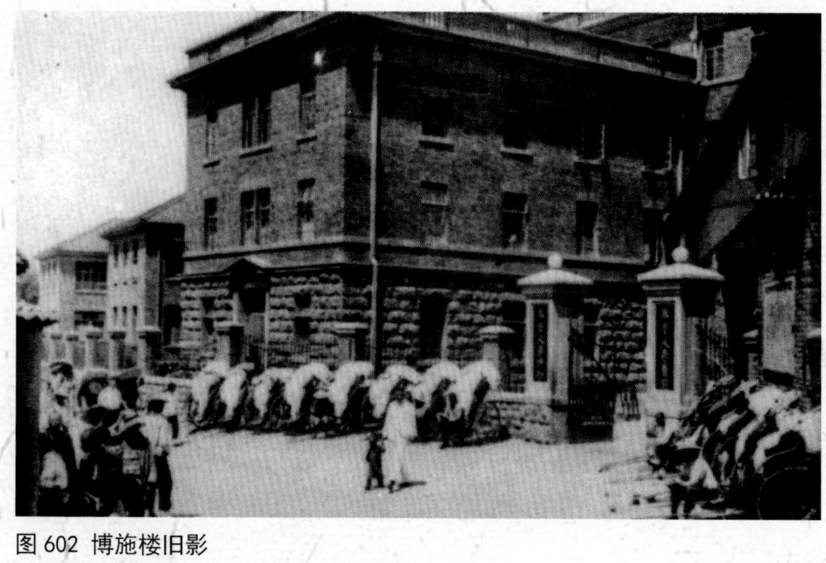

图 602 博施楼旧影

Fig. 602 An old photo of Boshi Building

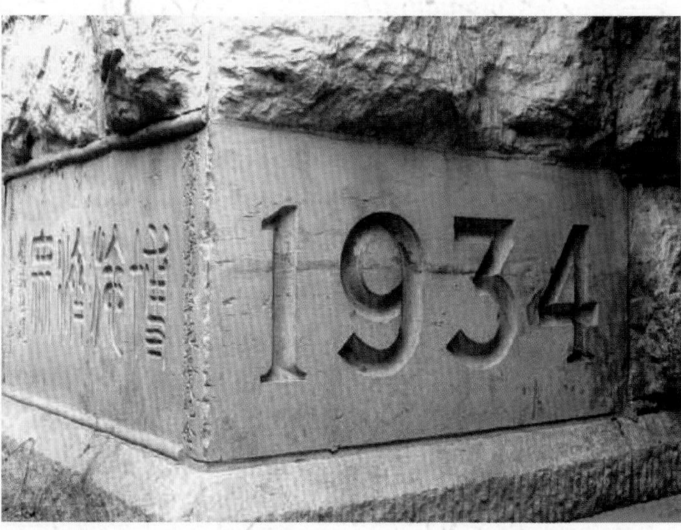

图 603 博施楼东南角的奠基石

Fig. 603 Foundation stone in the southeast corner of Boshi Building

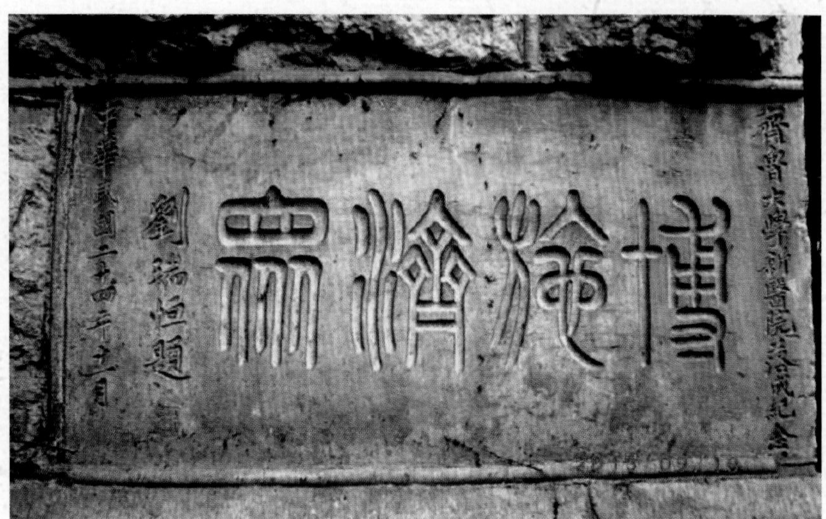

图 604 刘瑞恒题写的“博施济众”四字

Fig. 604 Four characters of “Bo Shi Ji Zhong” inscribed by Liu Ruiheng

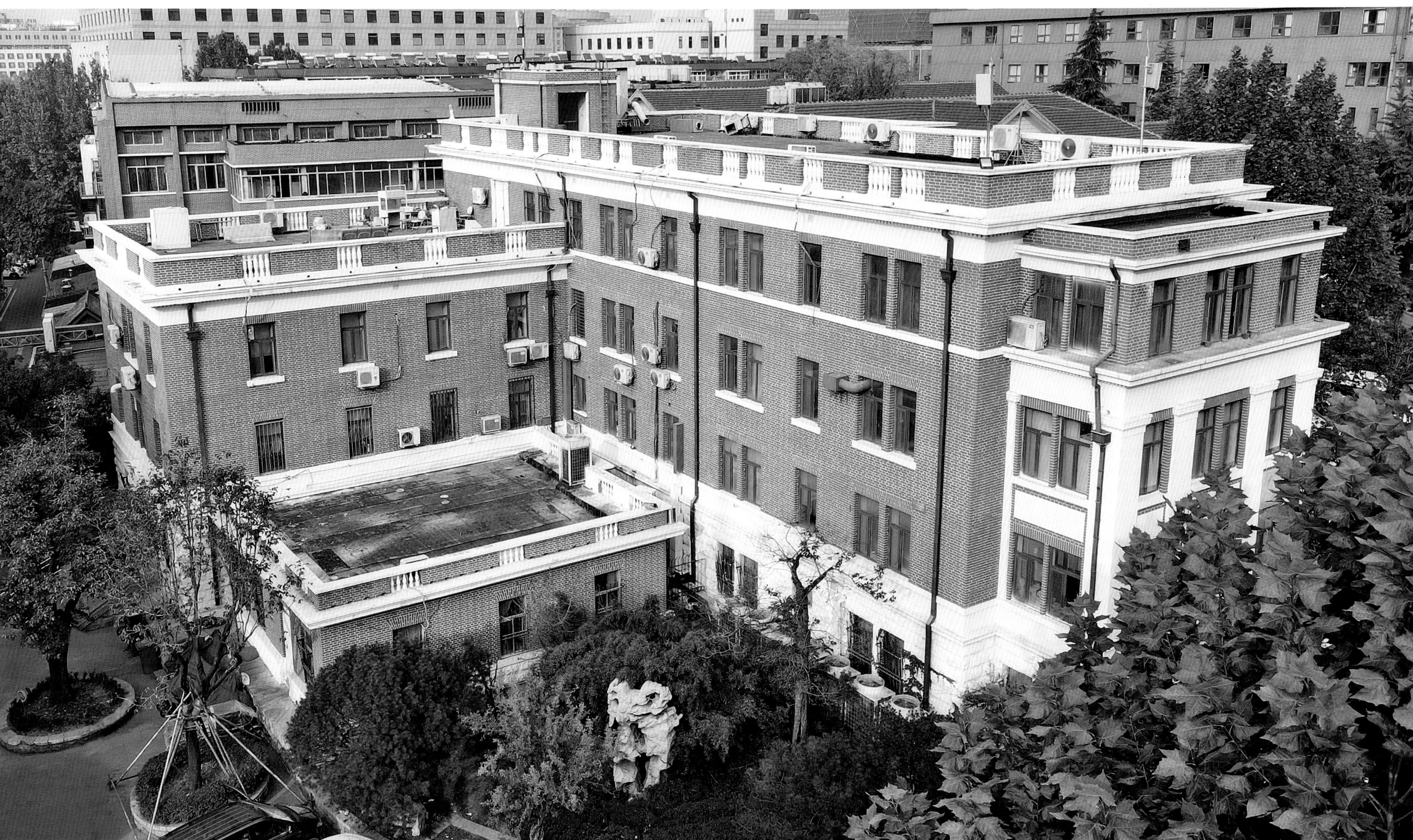

图 605 博施楼近影
Fig. 605 A recent photo of Boshi Building

57 齐鲁医院（3）

Qilu Hospital (3)

济众楼现在主要为内科病房大楼，1988 年竣工，1989 年启用，12 层，总建筑面积 20479 平方米。齐鲁医院的内科学科实力雄厚，心血管内科为国家重点学科和国家临床重点专科，血液科、消化内科、内分泌科和神经内科为国家临床重点专科。历史上涌现了高学勤、朱汉英、高德恩和张茂宏等一批名医，目前拥有中国工程院院士 1 名、教育部“长江学者”特聘教授 4 名。

高学勤 (1903 ~ 1978)，安徽蚌埠人，我国著名血液病、传染病学专家。1931 年毕业于齐鲁大学医学院，获医学博士学位，先后在南京和贵州从医。1943 年赴“陪都”重庆，任国民中央医院内科主任，兼湘雅医院教授。抗战胜利后，赴美国深造。1947 年回国，被南京大学医学院聘为教授，兼附属医院院长。1950 年应邀到齐鲁大学医学院任教授、内科教研室主任，兼山东省立第二医院内科主任。他不仅为蒋介石等达官贵人看病，也多次赴血吸虫病肆虐成灾的乡村悬壶济世，使用“老醋泡铁钉”的验方代替铁剂治疗患者，救命无数。

Being completed in 1988 and opening in 1989, the 12-storey Jizhong Building is now mainly a building of medical wards, with a total construction area of 20,479 square meters. The internal medicine of Qilu Hospital has tremendous strength. The cardiovascular medicine is the national key discipline and national clinical key specialty; hematology, gastroenterology, endocrinology and neurology are national clinical key specialties. A number of famous doctors such as Gao Xueqin, Zhu Hanying, Gao De'en and Zhang Maohong have emerged from Qilu Hospital in history. Now the hospital has one academician of Chinese Academy of Engineering and four specially appointed professors of Changjiang Scholars Program of the Ministry of Education.

Gao Xueqin (1903-1978), a native of Bengbu, Anhui Province, was a famous expert in hematology and lemology in China. In 1931, he graduated from the Medical School of Cheeloo University and got a degree of Doctor of Medicine. He successively worked as a doctor in Nanjing and Guizhou. In 1943, he went to Chongqing to serve as director of the internal medicine in the Central Hospital of the National Government of the Republic of China and held a concurrent post as professor of Xiangya Hospital. After the victory of the War of Resistance Against Japanese Aggression, he went to the United States for further education. In 1947, he returned home and was employed as a professor of the Medical School of Nanjing University and president of the affiliated hospital. In 1950, he was invited to the Medical School of Cheeloo University as a professor and director of the Teaching and Research Office of the Internal Medicine, and held a concurrent post as director of the internal medicine of Second Shandong Provincial Hospital. He not only treated Chiang Kai-shek and other dignitaries, but also went to the countryside many times where schistosomiasis was rampant to practise medicine in order to help the people. He used the proved recipe of “iron nails soaking in vinegar” to replace the chalybeate to treat patients and saved a lot of lives.

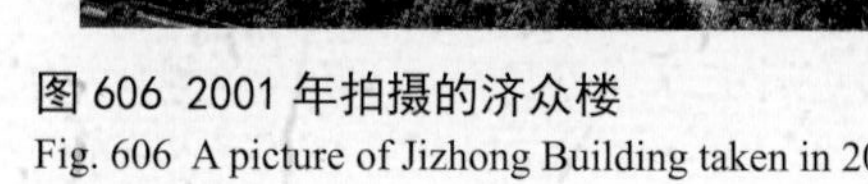

图 606 2001 年拍摄的济众楼
Fig. 606 A picture of Jizhong Building taken in 2001

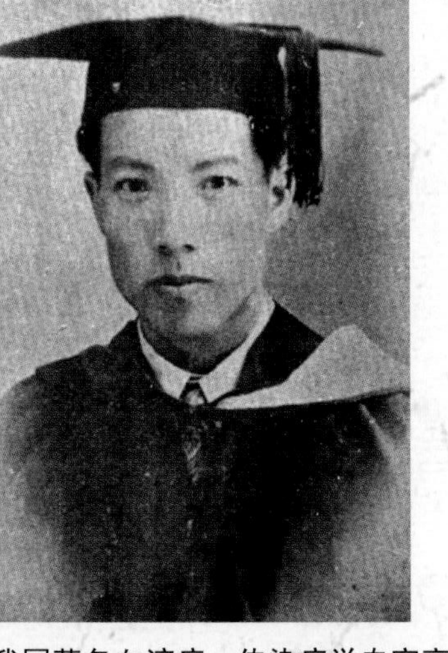

图 607 我国著名血液病、传染病学专家高学勤教授 （1903 ~ 1978）
Fig. 607 Professor Gao Xueqin (1903-1978), a famous expert in hematology and lemology in China

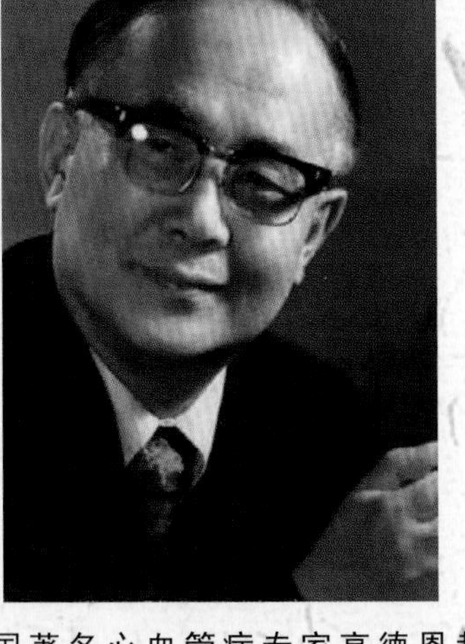

图 608 我国著名心血管病专家高德恩教授（1927 ~ 1991），张运院士的导师
Fig. 608 Professor Gao De'en (1927-1991), a famous cardiovascular expert in China and supervisor of the academician Zhang Yun

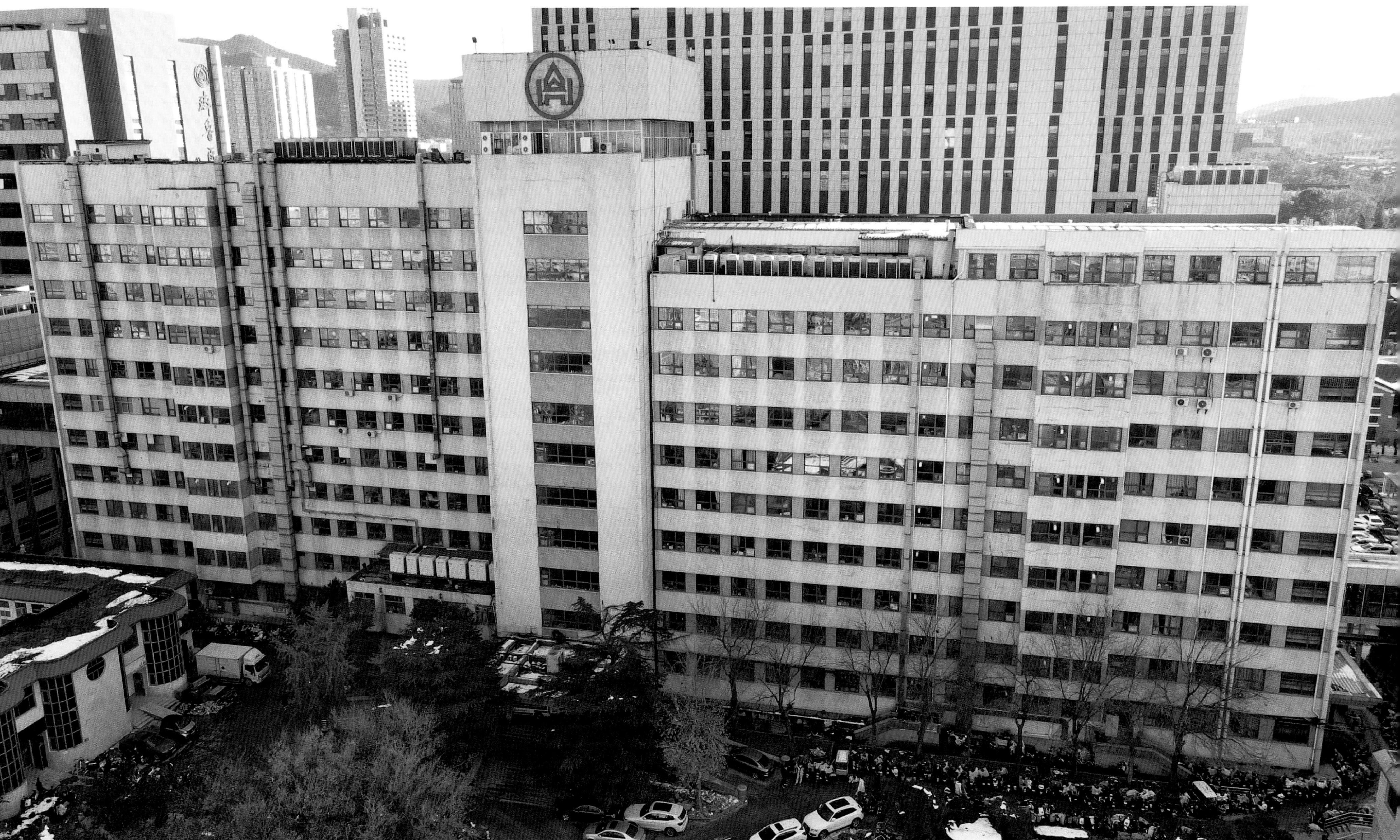

图 609 济众楼近景（北面观）
Fig. 609 A recent photo of Jizhong Building (the north view)

57 齐鲁医院（4）

Qilu Hospital (4)

心血管重构与功能研究教育部（卫健委）重点实验室由中国工程院和美国心脏病学院院士张运教授于 2002 年创建，主要研究心血管重构的调控机制、检测技术和干预策略，2009 年被评为省部共建国家重点实验室培育基地，2010 年获得国家基金委创新研究群体基金资助。实验室建筑面积近 4000 平方米，仪器设备近亿元。

张运，山东阳谷人，心血管病专家。1973 年入山东医学院医疗系学习，1981 年获山东医学院医学硕士学位并留附属医院心内科工作，1985 年获挪威奥斯陆大学博士学位。他是我国多普勒超声心动图技术的开拓者和奠基人，目前的主要研究方向是动脉粥样硬化，在国际上首次建立了动脉粥样硬化易损斑块的力学模型和多种动物模型。获国家科技进步奖二等奖 1 项、三等奖 3 项，何梁何利基金科学与技术进步奖 1 项、山东省科学技术最高奖 1 项、省部级科技进步奖一等奖 6 项。曾任山东大学副校长、医学院院长。2001 年当选中国工程院院士。

The Key Laboratory of Cardiovascular Remodeling and Function Research of Ministry of Education(National Health Commission) was founded in 2002 by Professor Zhang Yun, the academician of Chinese Academy of Engineering and the fellow of American College of Cardiology. With the emphasis on research into the regulatory mechanism, detection technology and intervention strategy of cardiovascular remodeling, it was chosen as the breeding base of the national key laboratory jointly built by the provincial and ministerial departments in 2009 and acquired the fund of Innovative Research Groups of National Natural Science Foundation in 2010. The laboratory has a construction area of nearly 4,000 square meters and the instruments and equipment are worth nearly 100 million yuan.

Zhang Yun, a native of Yanggu, Shandong Province, is an expert in cardiovascular diseases. In 1973, he joined the Medical Department of Shandong Medical College to study. In 1981, he obtained a degree of Master of Medicine from Shandong Medical College and then worked in the department of cardiology of the affiliated hospital. In 1985, he obtained a doctorate from University of Oslo in Norway. He is the pioneer and founder of Doppler echocardiography technology in China. Now his main research direction is atherosclerosis and he has established a mechanical model and a variety of animal models of atherosclerotic vulnerable plaques for the first time in the world. He has won one second prize and three third prizes of the National Science and Technology Progress Award, Ho Leung Ho Lee Foundation Prize for Science and Technology Progress, the Top Science and Technology Award of Shandong Province, and six first prizes of science and technology progress award at the provincial and ministerial levels. He once served as vice president of Shandong University and dean of the School of Medicine. He was elected academician of Chinese Academy of Engineering in 2001.

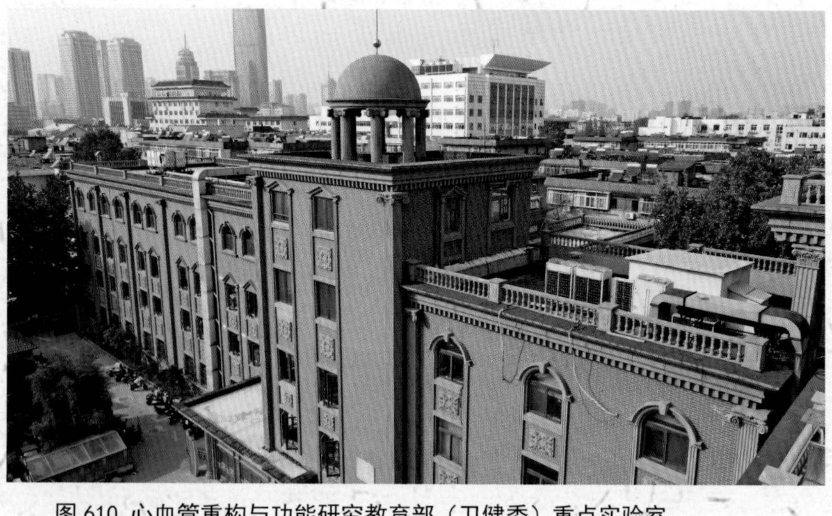

图 610 心血管重构与功能研究教育部（卫健委）重点实验室
Fig. 610 Key Laboratory of Cardiovascular Remodeling and Function Research of Ministry of Education (National Health Commission)

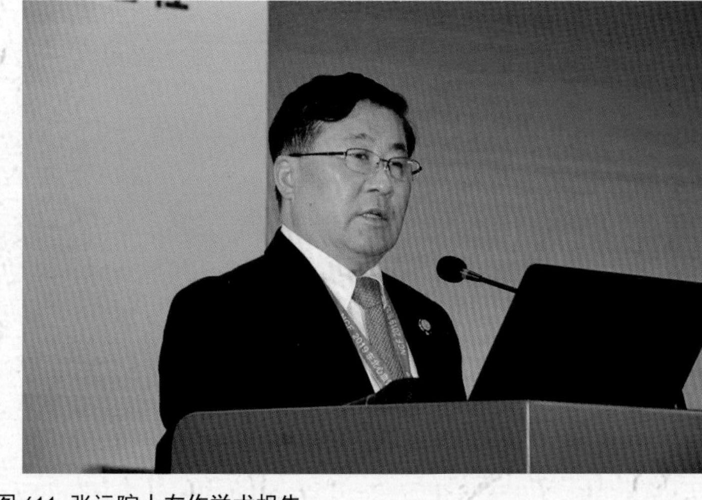

图 611 张运院士在作学术报告
Fig. 611 Academician Zhang Yun making an academic report

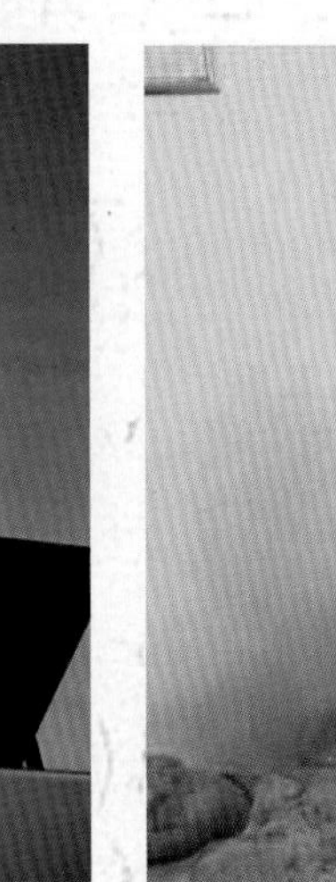

图 612 张运院士为敬老院老人看病
Fig. 612 Academician Zhang Yun treating the elderly in the nursing home

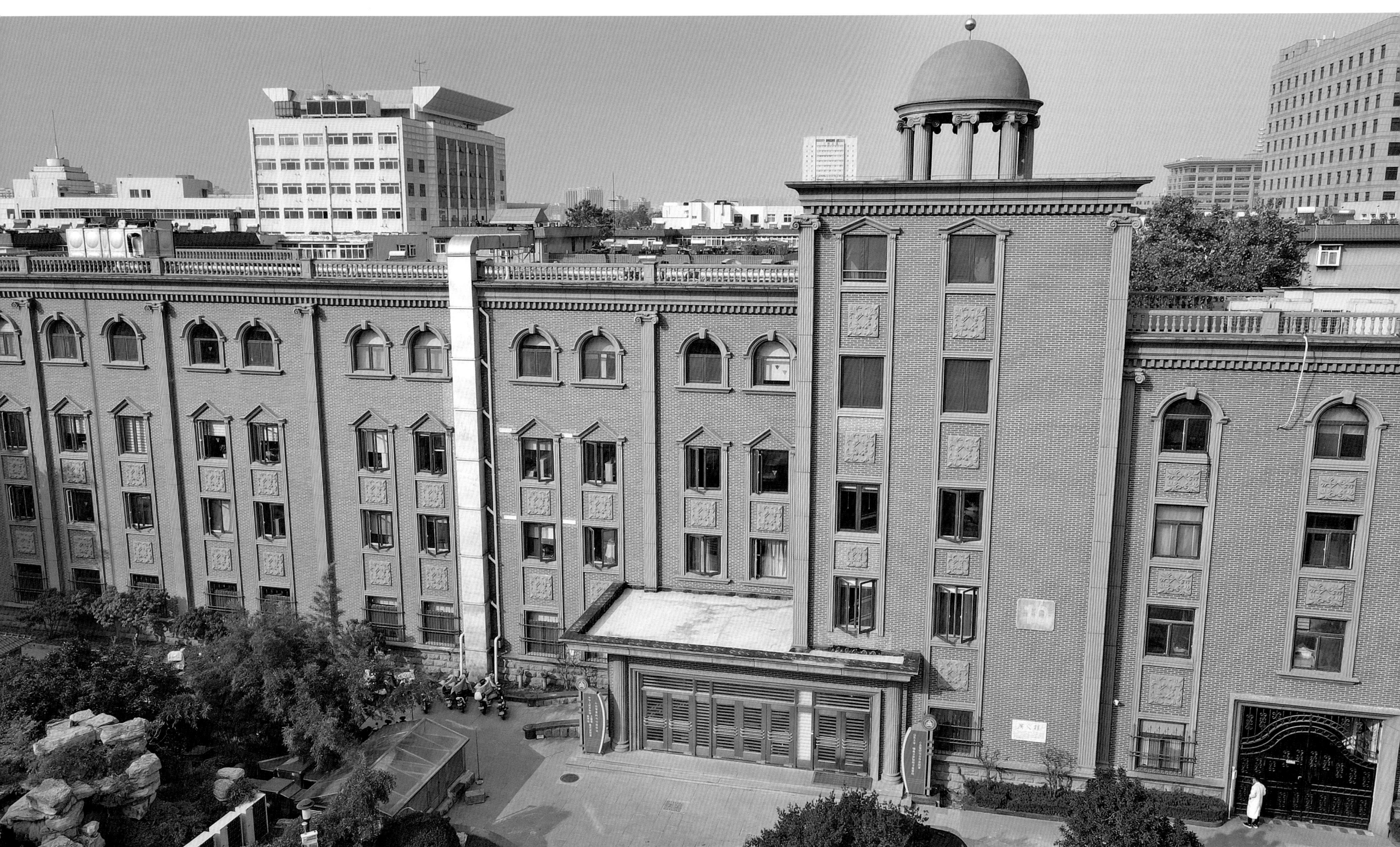

图 613 心血管重构与功能研究教育部（卫健委）重点实验室鸟瞰
Fig. 613 A bird's-eye view of the Key Laboratory of Cardiovascular Remodeling and Function Research of Ministry of Education (National Health Commission)

57 齐鲁医院（5）

Qilu Hospital (5)

华美楼于 2006 年 12 月开工，2010 年底竣工，总建筑面积为 13.6 万平方米，是目前山东省内医院中建筑面积最大的单体建筑。整栋大楼分地下两层、地上十三层和一层设备层。地下两层主要为医技检查区，一至三层为门诊，四层为 47 间层流净化手术室、CCU 监护病房，五至十三层为外科病房、保健病房等，开放床位 1700 张。齐鲁医院外科学人才济济，涌现了像赵常林、张振湘、李兆亭、寿楠海和宋惠民等名医。现已引入第 4 代达芬奇手术机器人，并自主研发智能手术器械，使外科手术实现了智能化、远程化、微创化、精准化和个性化。

赵常林（1905 ~ 1980），山东黄县人，外科学一级教授，我国骨外科学奠基人之一。1930 年毕业于齐鲁大学医学院，获医学博士学位。他对骨外科医疗技术有很深造诣，被誉为“骨科圣手”。在国家及国外刊物上发表论文 20 余篇，主编《急症外科学》等专著和教材 5 部。曾任齐鲁医院、山东医学院附属医院院长。

Being started in December 2006 and completed by the end of 2010, Huamei Building has a total construction area of 136,000 square meters, which is the largest single building among hospitals in Shandong Province. The whole building has two underground floors, thirteen floors above the ground and one floor for the equipment. The two underground floors are mainly medical examination areas, the first to third floors are sections for outpatients, the fourth floor has 47 operating rooms for laminar flow purification and CCU intensive care units, and the fifth to thirteenth floors are surgical wards and healthcare units, with 1,700 beds open. Qilu Hospital is full of talents in surgery, with famous doctors such as Zhao Changlin, Zhang Zhenxiang, Li Zhaoting, Shou Nanhai and Song Huimin. Now the hospital has introduced the fourth generation of Da Vinci Robot-assisted Surgical System and independently developed the smart surgical instruments, so that the surgical operation has become smart, remote, minimally invasive, accurate and personalized.

Zhao Changlin (1905-1980), a native of Huangxian, Shandong Province, is a first-level professor of surgery and one of the founders of bone surgery in China. In 1930, he graduated from the Medical School of Cheeloo University with a degree of Doctor of Medicine. He has deep attainments in medical skills of bone surgery and is known as the “Holy Hand of Orthopedics”. He has published more than 20 papers in national and foreign journals, and edited 5 monographs and textbooks such as *Emergency Surgery*. He once served as president of Qilu Hospital and Affiliated Hospital of Shandong Medical College.

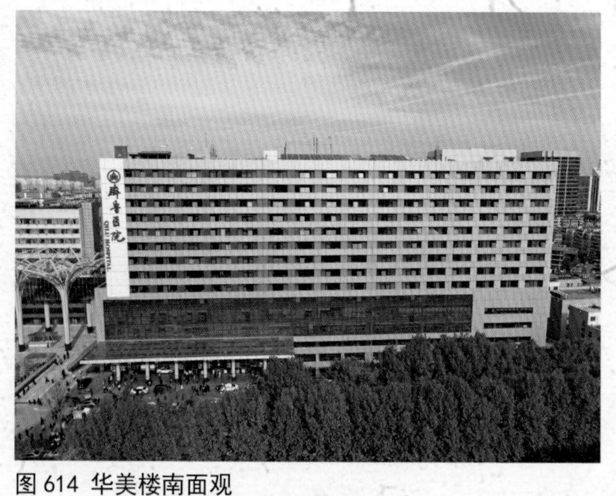

图 614 华美楼南面观

Fig. 614 The south view of Huamei Building

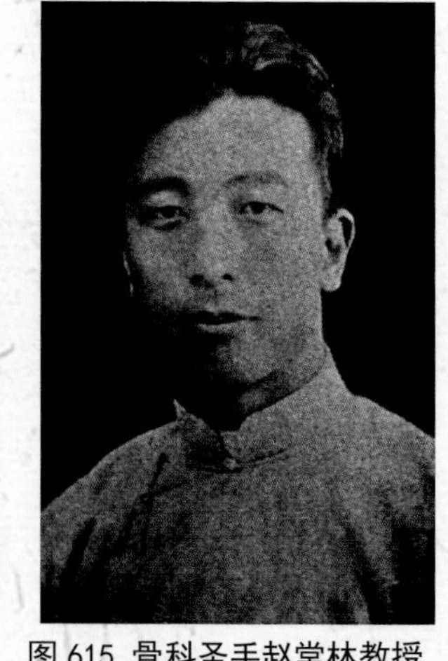

图 615 骨科圣手赵常林教授

Fig. 615 Professor Zhao Changlin, Holy Hand of Orthopedics

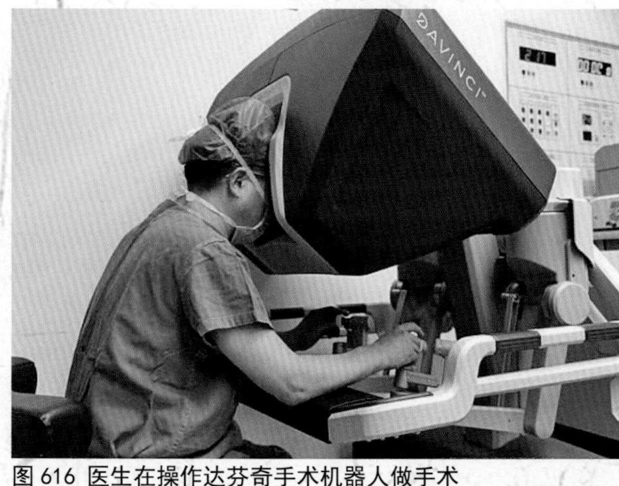

图 616 医生在操作达芬奇手术机器人做手术

Fig. 616 The doctor operating Da Vinci Robot-assisted Surgical System for surgery

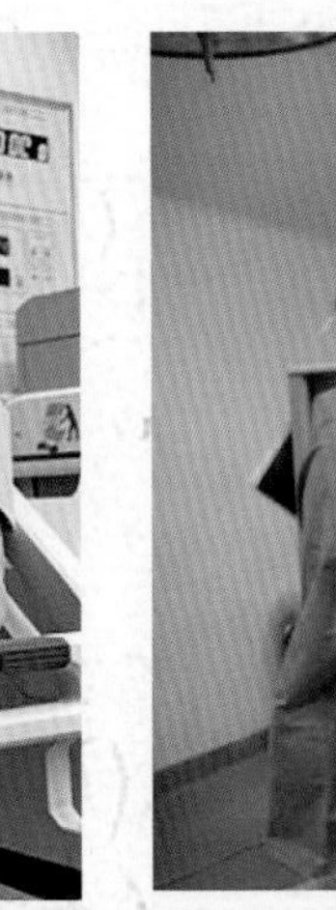

图 617 医生在用达芬奇手术机器人做手术

Fig. 617 Doctors using Da Vinci Robot-assisted Surgical System to operate

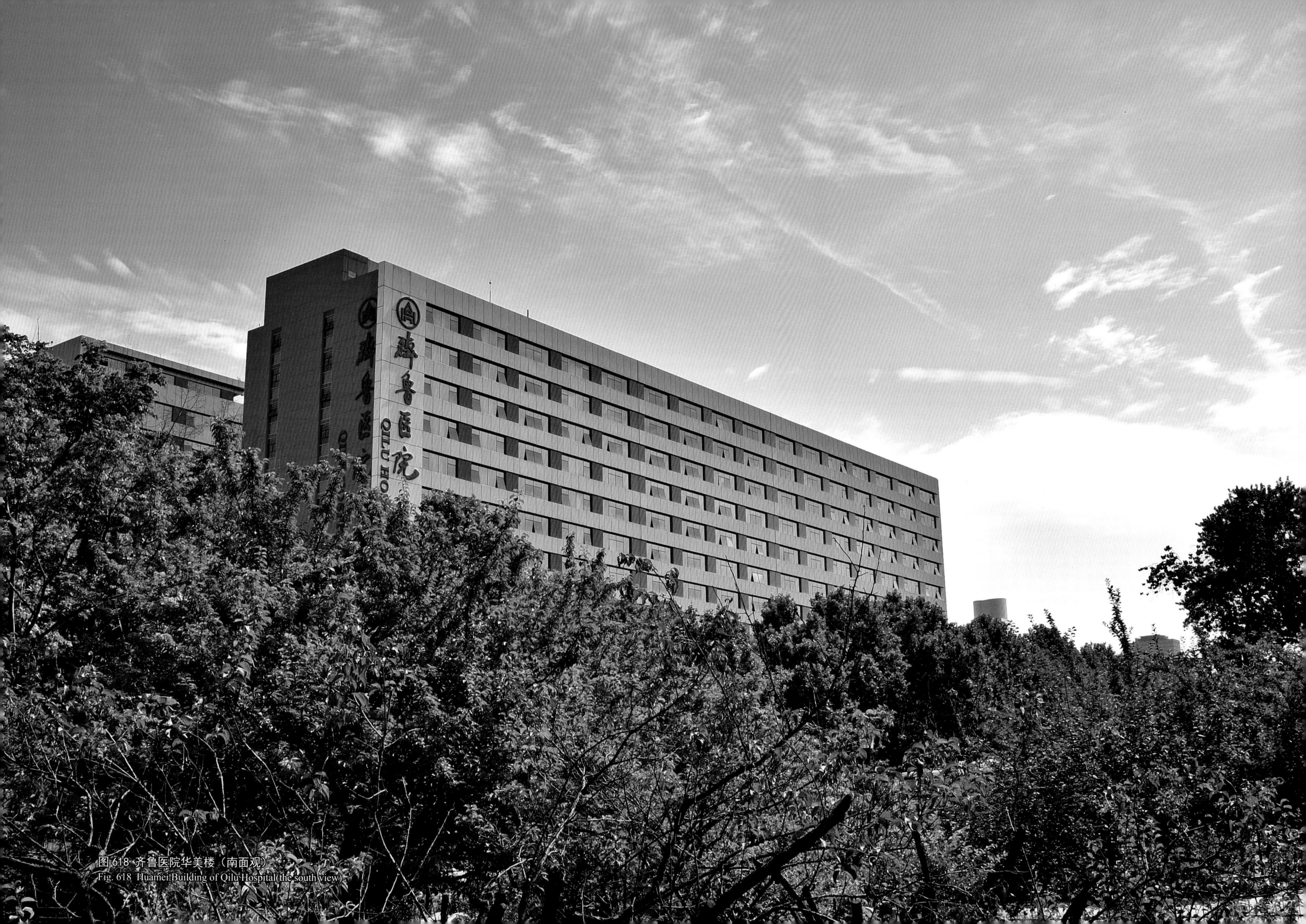

图 618 齐鲁医院华美楼（南面观）

Fig. 618 Huamei Building of Qilu Hospital(the south view)

57 齐鲁医院（6）

Qilu Hospital (6)

妇儿综合楼建成于 2020 年 7 月，总建筑面积 9.3 万平方米，设计床位 678 张，主要供妇产科和儿科使用。内部设计智能，设备先进，环境优雅，服务完善，居国内同行业前列。在江森教授领导和影响下，齐鲁医院妇产科为国家重点学科、国家临床重点专科和国家临床医学研究中心妇产科疾病领域分中心，主编普通高等教育本科国家级规划教材 2 部，主办在全国具有重要学术影响的《现代妇产科进展》杂志，妇科肿瘤研究与临床在全国享有盛誉。

江森（1921 ~ 2011），江苏南通人，著名妇产科专家、医学教育家。1948 年毕业于东南医学院（安徽医科大学前身），1949 年任职华东白求恩医学院。1952 年调往山东医学院附属医院妇产科工作，后任主任。作为主编之一的《实用妇科学》《实用产科学》为妇产科经典著作，前者获得 1978 年全国科学大会一等奖。他领导齐鲁医院妇产科长达半个多世纪，在诸多领域卓有建树，是我国妇产科学界的一面旗帜。

The Comprehensive Building for Women and Children was completed in July 2020, with a total construction area of 93,000 square meters and 678 beds mainly for the departments of gynecology and obstetrics and paediatrics. With smart design, advanced equipment, graceful environment and perfect service, this building ranks in the forefront of the same industry in China. Under the leadership and influence of Professor Jiang Sen, the Gynecology and Obstetrics of Qilu Hospital is a national key discipline and a national key clinical specialty, and the department is a sub-center in the field of Gynecology and Obstetrics of the National Clinical Medical Research Center. The department has edited two national planning textbooks for undergraduate courses of general higher education and hosts the journal *Progress in Obstetrics and Gynecology* which has important academic influence in the country. The research and clinical practice of gynecological tumors enjoy a high reputation in the country.

Jiang Sen (1921-2011), a native of Nantong, Jiangsu Province, is a famous expert in gynecology and obstetrics and medical educator. He graduated from Southeast Medical College (the predecessor of Anhui Medical University) in 1948 and worked in East China Bethune Medical College in 1949. In 1952, he was transferred to the Gynecology and Obstetrics Department of the affiliated hospital of Shandong Medical College and later served as director. He is one of the editors-in-chief of *Practical Gynecology* and *Practical Obstetrics* which are classic works of gynecology and obstetrics. Practical Gynecology won the first prize of the National Science Conference in 1978. Having led the Department of Gynecology and Obstetrics of Qilu Hospital for more than half a century and made great achievements in many fields, he is a banner of gynecology and obstetrics in China.

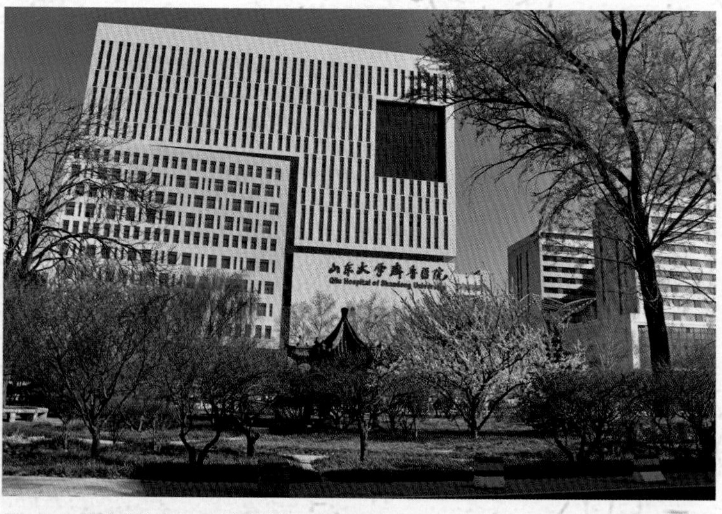

图 619 齐鲁医院妇儿综合楼（南面观）

Fig. 619 Comprehensive Building for Women and Children (the south view)

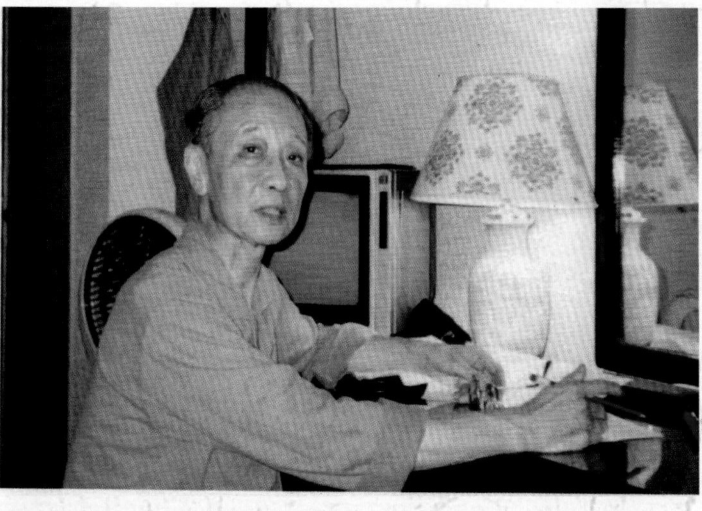

图 620 著名妇产科学家江森教授

Fig. 620 Professor Jiang Sen, an expert in gynecology and obstetrics

图 621 齐鲁医院孔北华教授担任《妇产科学》国家规划教材主编

Fig. 621 Professor Kong Beihua serving as the editor-in-chief of *Obstetrics and Gynecology*, the national planning textbook

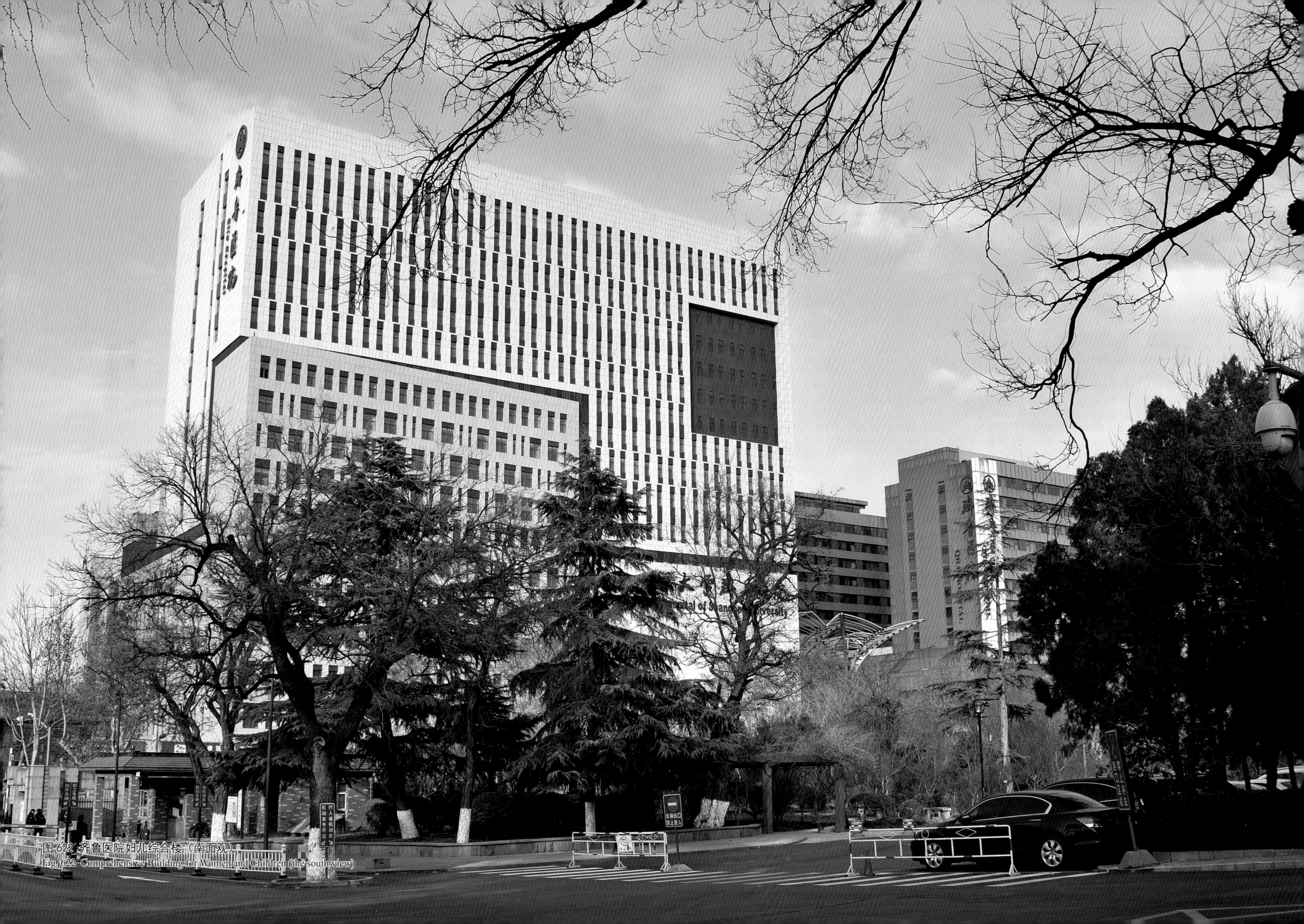

图 622 齐鲁医院妇儿综合楼（南面观）
Fig. 622 Comprehensive Building for Women and Children (the south view)

57 齐鲁医院（7）

Qilu Hospital (7)

齐鲁医院积极承担社会责任，在抗美援朝、抗震救灾和历次突发疫情应急工作中均冲锋在前，展示了国家队医院的风范。在 2020 年抗击新冠肺炎疫情中，齐鲁医院先后派出四批 150 名医疗队员驰援湖北，出色完成援鄂抗疫工作，充分彰显了“东齐鲁”的家国担当。作为援助非洲和对口帮扶的国家重要区域医疗中心，积极发挥示范、引领和带动作用，通过对口支援、管理与技术输出、远程医疗等形式，努力打造高质量医疗服务协作体系。

2021 年 8 月，医院开工建设急诊综合楼项目，预计 2023 年建成。急诊综合楼是委省共建国家区域医疗中心核心项目，位于医院东南角，总用地面积 92512 平方米，总建筑面积 18.7 万平方米。建筑主体为 5 层裙房上设置 2 栋塔楼的形式，中部裙房为配套服务用房，南侧塔楼（14 层）为急诊住院功能，北侧塔楼（13 层）为科研教学功能，地下 3 层为车库设备区。建成使用后，医院的医疗、教学、科研和服务社会工作将再上一个新台阶。

Qilu Hospital actively undertakes social responsibility and has taken the lead in the war to resist US aggression and aid Korea and in the work of earthquake relief and response to emergencies, demonstrating the style of a national hospital. In the fight against COVID-19 in 2020, Qilu Hospital successively sent four batches of 150 medical members to Hubei and successfully completed the work of assisting Hubei to fight the pandemic, fully demonstrating the strong sense of responsibility of “East Qilu”. As an important national regional medical center for aid to Africa and paired assistance, it actively plays an exemplary, leading and driving role, and strives to build a high-quality medical service cooperation system through response support, management and technology export, telemedicine and other forms.

In August 2021, the hospital started the construction of the Comprehensive Emergency Building which is expected to be completed in 2023. The Comprehensive Emergency Building is the core project of the National Regional Medical Center jointly built by National Health Commission and the province. It is located in the southeast corner of the hospital, with a total land area of 92,512 square meters and a total construction area of 187,000 square meters. The main body of the building is in the form of two towers on the 5-storey podium; the middle podium is used as supporting service rooms, the 14-storey south tower is for the emergency hospitalization, the 13-storey north tower is for scientific research and teaching, and the underground three floors are for the garage and equipment. Upon completion and putting into use, the hospital’s medical treatment, teaching, scientific research and social service work will reach a new level.

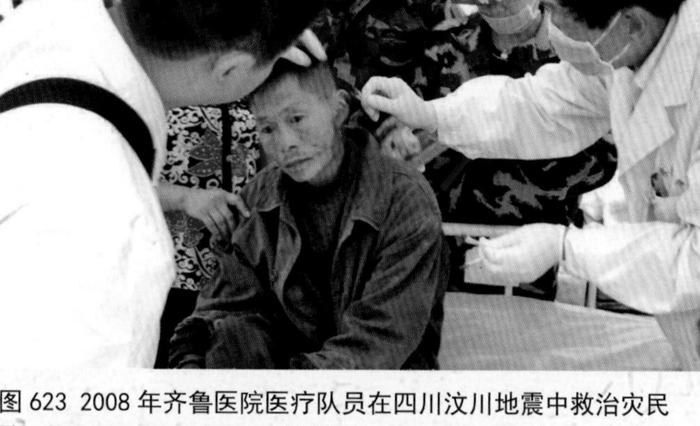

图 623 2008 年齐鲁医院医疗队员在四川汶川地震中救治灾民
Fig. 623 Members of the medical team from Qilu Hospital treating the victim in Wenchuan earthquake, Sichuan Province in 2008

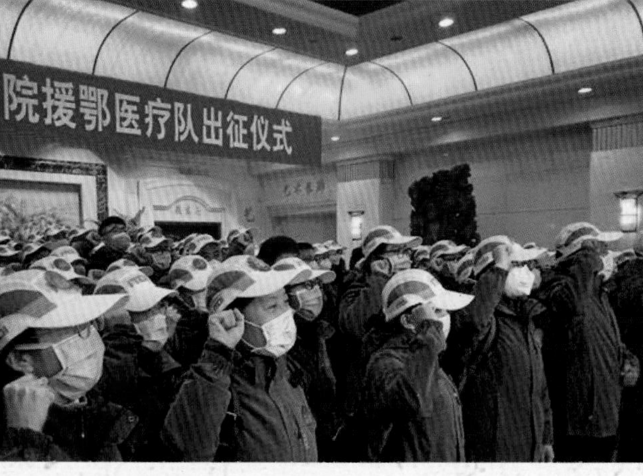

图 624 齐鲁医院援鄂抗疫国家医疗队出征仪式
Fig. 624 Departure ceremony of the national medical team from Qilu Hospital to aid Hubei Province in the fight against the epidemic

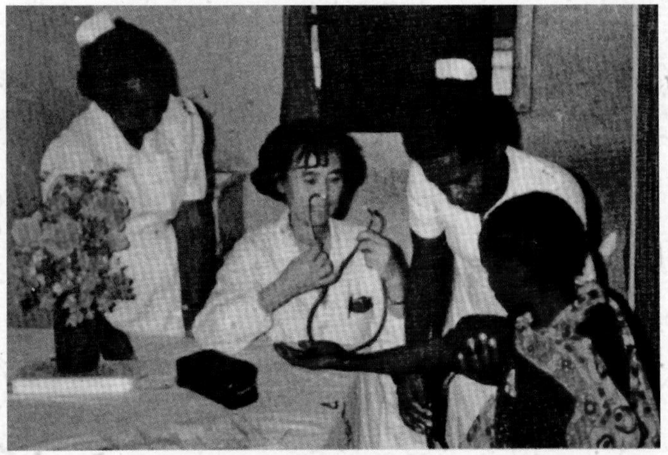

图 625 1987 年援助坦桑尼亚医疗队队员、齐鲁医院李君曼医生在门诊
Fig. 625 Li Junman, member of the medical team to aid Tanzania and doctor of Qilu Hospital, in the outpatient department in 1987

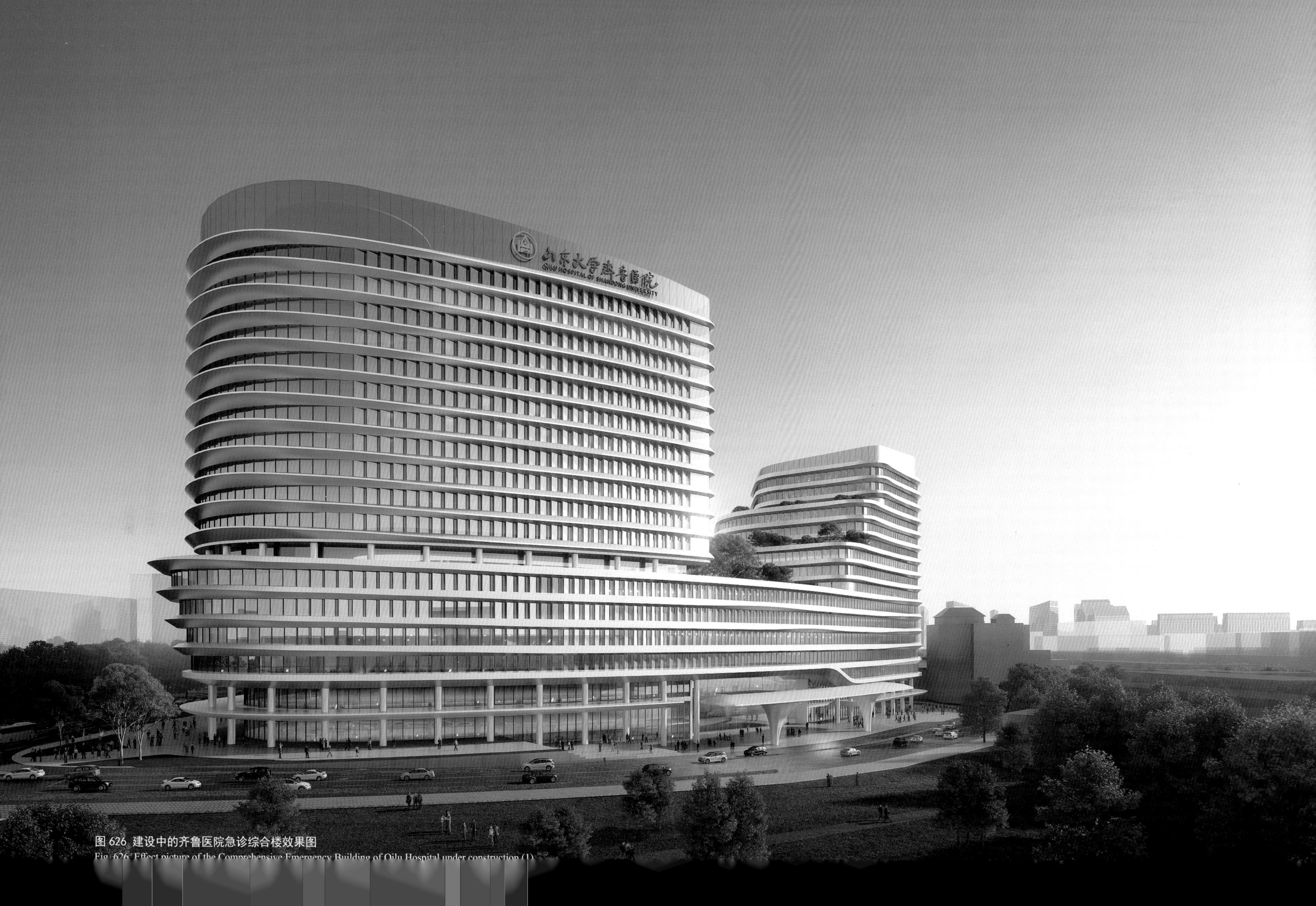

图 626 建设中的齐鲁医院急诊综合楼效果图

Fig. 626 Effect picture of the Comprehensive Emergency Building of Qilu Hospital under construction (1)

58 第二医院

The Second Hospital of Shandong University

山东大学第二医院坐落于济南北部，是国家卫生健康委委属（管）医院，2019 年入选首批委省共建国家区域医疗中心成员单位，2020 年入选山东省区域医疗中心，已形成了中心院区、南部院区、北院区“一院三区”战略发展格局。现有在院职工近 4000 人，其中院士（山东大学兼职讲席教授）、长江学者、泰山学者等高层次人才 17 人，博士生导师 49 人，硕士生导师 135 人。设立临床医技科室 69 个，其中国家临床重点专科 5 个（泌尿外科、肾脏内科、临床护理学、胸外科、乳腺外科）。建有科研机构 37 个，其中有省部级重点实验室、研究中心 10 个，科研实力日益增强。山大二院人始终奋力奔跑在国家和人民最需要的地方，先后有 8 批 162 名援鄂抗疫国家医疗队队员披甲出征，为打赢疫情防控阻击战贡献了力量。山大二院积极参加国家、地方及大学对口支援和健康扶贫项目，荣获国家卫健委“对口支援精准帮扶贡献奖”。

The Second Hospital of Shandong University is located in northern Jinan, under the administration of the National Health Commission. It was selected as member of the first batch of the national regional medical centers jointly built by the commission and the provincial governments in 2019 and regional medical center in Shandong Province in 2020. It has formed a strategic development pattern of “one hospital and three districts”, including the central district, the southern district and the northern district. The hospital has nearly 4,000 staff members, including 17 academicians (part-time chair professors of Shandong University), Changjiang Scholars, Taishan Scholars and other high-level talents, 49 doctoral supervisors and 135 master supervisors. It has 69 clinical and medical technology departments, including five national key clinical specialties (Urology, Nephrology, Clinical Nursing, Thoracic Surgery and Breast Surgery). There are 37 scientific research institutions, including 10 key laboratories and research centers at the provincial and ministerial levels, and the scientific research strength has been continuously increasing. Medical workers in the Second Hospital of Shandong University have been working hard to meet the needs of the country and the people. The hospital had sent eight batches of 162 medical workers of the national medical team to assist Hubei Province in fighting the pandemic, making its own contribution to winning the war of pandemic prevention and control. It has been actively participating in paired assistance and health and medical assistance program for poverty alleviation at the national, regional and university levels. It has received the “Accurate Paired Assistance Contribution Award” granted by the National Health Commission.

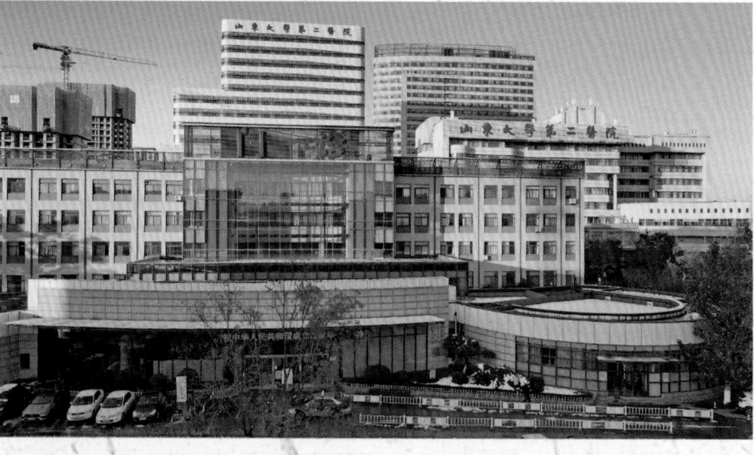

图 627 山东大学第二医院门诊大楼

Fig. 627 Outpatient Building of the Second Hospital of Shandong University

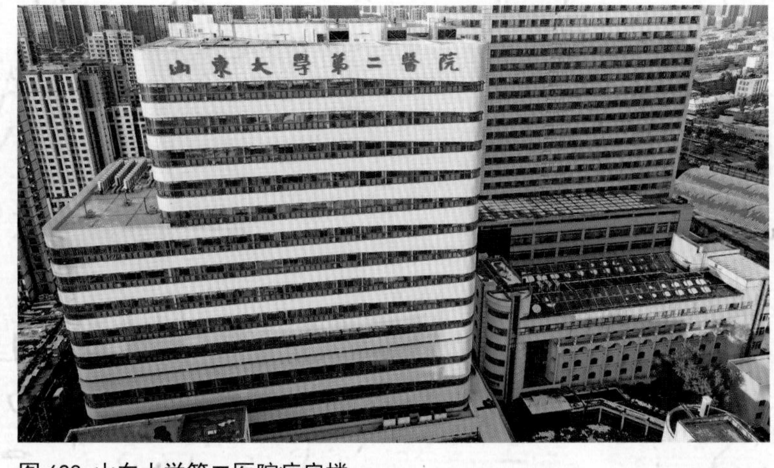

图 628 山东大学第二医院病房楼

Fig. 628 Inpatient Building of the Second Hospital of Shandong University

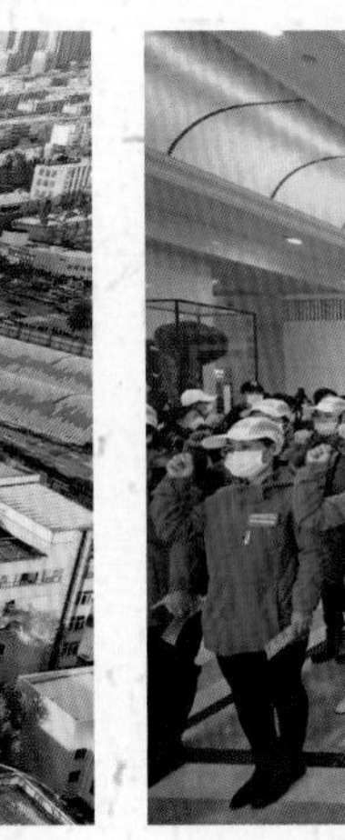

图 629 山东大学第二医院援鄂抗疫国家医疗队出征仪式

Fig. 629 Departure ceremony of the national medical team from the Second Hospital of Shandong University to aid Hubei Province in the fight against the epidemic

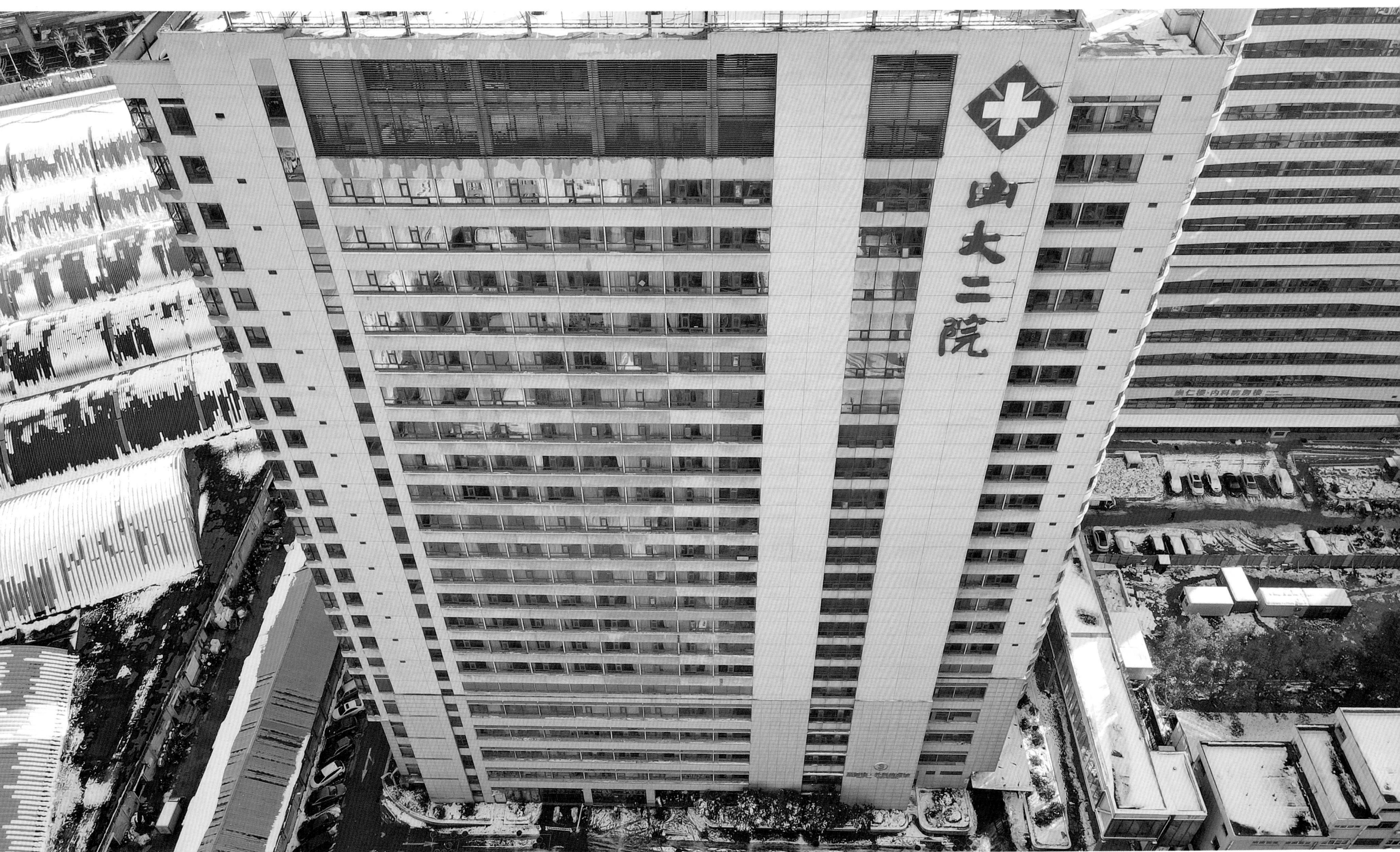

图 630 山东大学第二医院病房大楼鸟瞰（北面观）
Fig. 630 A bird's-eye view of the Inpatient Building of the Second Hospital of Shandong University (the north view)

59 口腔医院

Stomatological Hospital of Shandong University

山东大学口腔医院始建于 1992 年，首任院长为著名口腔黏膜病专家凌涤生教授。现有教职医务员工近 500 人，其中国家级人才和泰山学者 12 人、博士研究生导师 30 人、硕士研究生导师 53 人。目前，医院共有本、硕、博在校生 600 余人。医院为三级甲等口腔专科医院和山东省口腔重点专病专科医院，现有建筑面积 2 万余平方米，拥有口腔综合治疗椅 260 台，临床医技科室 21 个，其中种植科、牙周科为山东省临床精品特色专科。作为国家口腔疾病临床医学研究中心山东分中心，医院充分整合优势资源，牵头组建了中心联合体和山东省口腔医院医联体，以加大对基层口腔医疗机构的支持力度。

凌涤生，1957 年上海第二医科大学毕业后，即来山东医学院附属医院口腔科工作。一直从事口腔黏膜病研究，成果丰硕。2018 年于第十次全国口腔黏膜病学术大会上荣获口腔黏膜病学事业发展突出贡献奖。1991 年至 1995 年担任山东医科大学口腔系主任，负责筹建口腔医院并担任首任院长。

The Stomatological Hospital of Shandong University was founded in 1992. The first president was Professor Ling Disheng, a famous expert in oral mucosal diseases. At present, there are nearly 500 teaching and medical staff members, including 12 state-level talents and Taishan scholars, 30 doctoral supervisors and 53 master supervisors. Now the hospital has a total of more than 600 undergraduates, postgraduates and doctoral students. As a Class A tertiary specialized hospital of stomatology and a key stomatological hospital in Shandong Province, it covers a total construction area of more than 20,000 square meters, with 260 comprehensive oral treatment chairs and 21 clinical and medical departments. Among them, oral implantology and periodontology are excellent clinical specialties in Shandong Province. As the Shandong branch of the National Clinical Research Center for Oral Diseases, the hospital has fully integrated its advantageous resources and taken the lead in establishing the center consortium and the medical association of the Stomatological Hospital of Shandong University to increase its support to grassroots oral medical institutions.

Ling Disheng came to work in the Department of Stomatology of the Affiliated Hospital of Shandong Medical College immediately after graduating from Shanghai Second Medical University in 1957. He had been engaged in the research on oral mucosal diseases and made fruitful achievements. In 2018, he won the Outstanding Contribution Award for the research development of oral mucosal diseases at the 10th National Academic Conference on Oral Mucosal Diseases. From 1991 to 1995, he served as director of the Department of Stomatology of Shandong Medical University; he was responsible for the establishment of the Stomatological Hospital and then served as the first president.

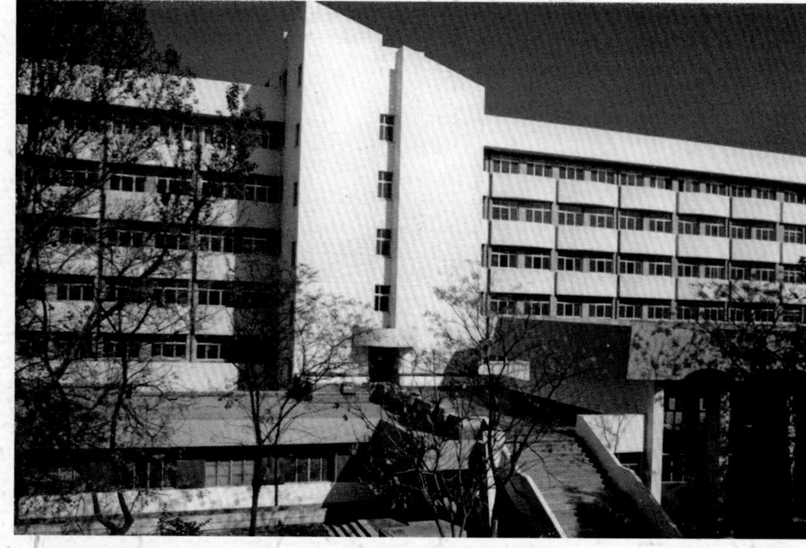

图 631 1991 年刚竣工不久的口腔医学大楼（南面观）
Fig. 631 Building of Stomatology newly completed in 1991 (the south view)

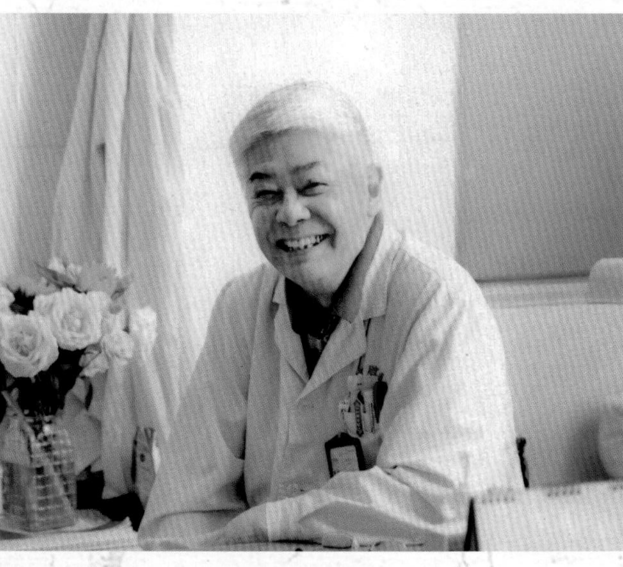

图 632 山东大学口腔医院首任院长凌涤生教授
Fig. 632 Professor Ling Disheng, the first president of Stomatological Hospital of Shandong University

图 633 新口腔大楼（南面观）
Fig. 633 New Building of Stomatology (the south view)

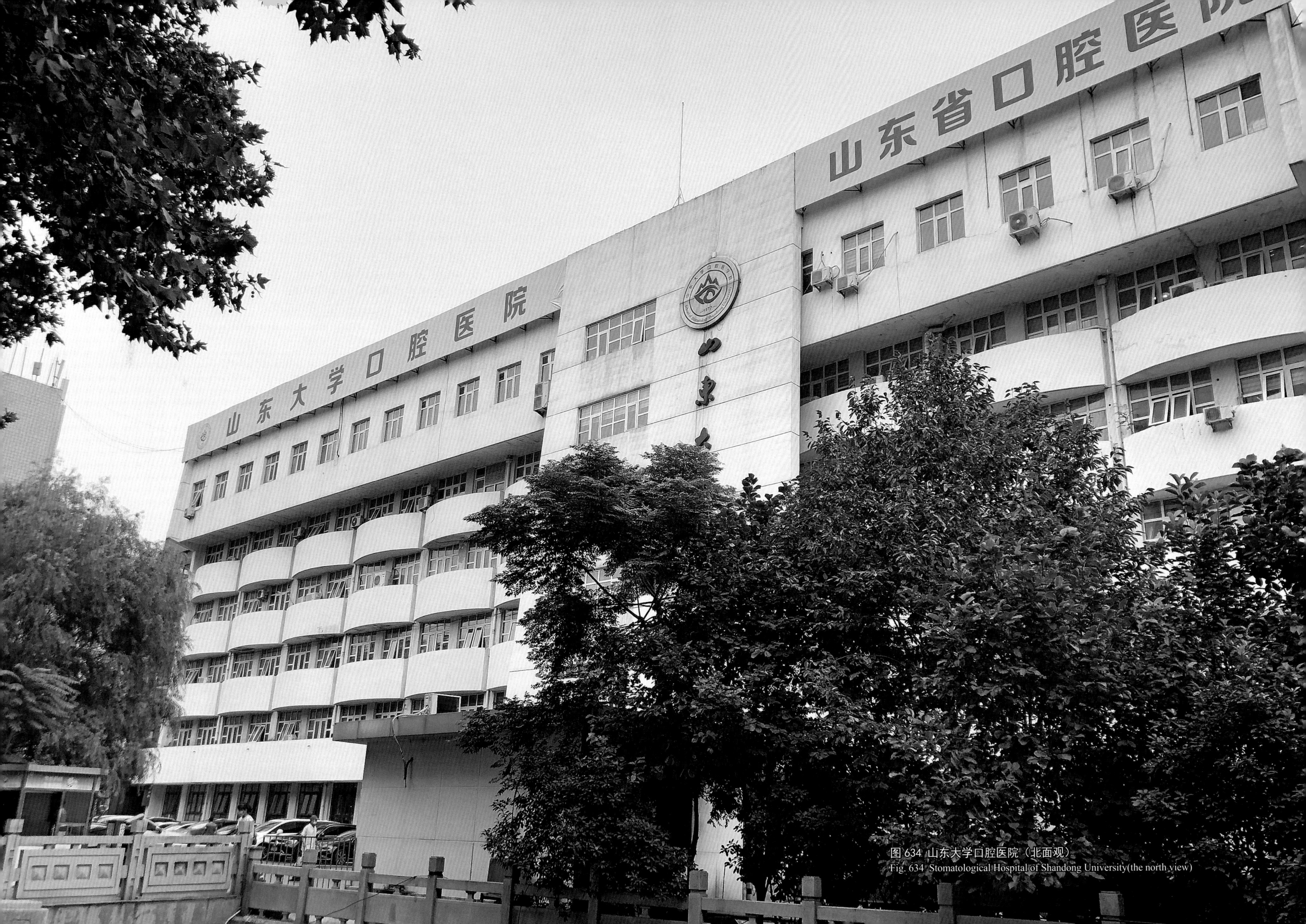

图 634 山东大学口腔医院（北面观）
Fig. 634 Stomatological Hospital of Shandong University(the north view)

60 生殖医院（1）

Hospital for Reproductive Medicine Affiliated to Shandong University (1)

山东大学附属生殖医院为国内首批通过卫生部技术准入可开展人类辅助生殖技术的十三家医疗机构之一，是全国首家三级甲等生殖健康与不孕症专科医院。目前为山东省唯一一家具有胚胎植入前遗传学诊断资质的单位，并且是人类辅助生殖技术及人类精子库培训基地。在首席科学家陈子江教授带领下，医院创立应用了一系列辅助生殖技术，其中宫腔配子移植术、PCOS 超声微创治疗术等多项技术为国际首创。每年吸引世界各地生殖障碍患者 50 余万人次，实施辅助生殖技术助孕 2 万多人次。试管婴儿技术成功率为 55% 以上，达国际先进水平。

陈子江，1959 年生于湖北武汉，1984 年山东医学院本科毕业，1989 年获得山东医科大学医学博士学位后留校任教，1993 年破格晋升教授，2001 年担任山东省立医院妇产科主任、生殖医学中心主任，2002 年担任山东省立医院副院长，曾任山东大学副校长兼齐鲁医学院院长，2019 年当选为中国科学院院士。

The Hospital for Reproductive Medicine Affiliated to Shandong University is one of the first 13 medical institutions in China that can carry out human assisted reproductive technology approved by the Ministry of Health. It is the first Class A tertiary specialized hospital of reproductive health and infertility in China. At present, it is the only unit in Shandong Province with the qualification of genetic diagnosis before embryo implantation, and it is the training base of human assisted reproductive technology and human sperm bank. Under the leadership of Professor Chen Zijiang, the Chief Scientist, the hospital has originated and applied a series of assisted reproductive technologies, among which the intrauterine gamete transplantation, the ultrasound-guided minimally invasive treatment for PCOS and other technologies are innovative in the world. More than 500,000 patients with reproductive disorders from all over the world come to the hospital for help and assisted reproductive technologies are applied to cure more than 20,000 infertile patients every year. The success rate of in vitro fertilization is more than 55%, reaching the internationally advanced level.

Chen Zijiang was born in Wuhan, Hubei Province in 1959. She graduated from Shandong Medical College with a bachelor's degree in 1984. After obtaining a doctor's degree in medicine from Shandong Medical University in 1989, she stayed to teach in the university, and she got an accelerated promotion to professor in 1993. In 2001, she served as director of the Department of Gynecology and Obstetrics and that of Reproductive Medical Center of Shandong Provincial Hospital. In 2002, she served as vice president of Shandong Provincial Hospital. She once served as vice president of Shandong University and president of Cheeloo College of Medicine. She was elected academician of Chinese Academy of Sciences in 2019.

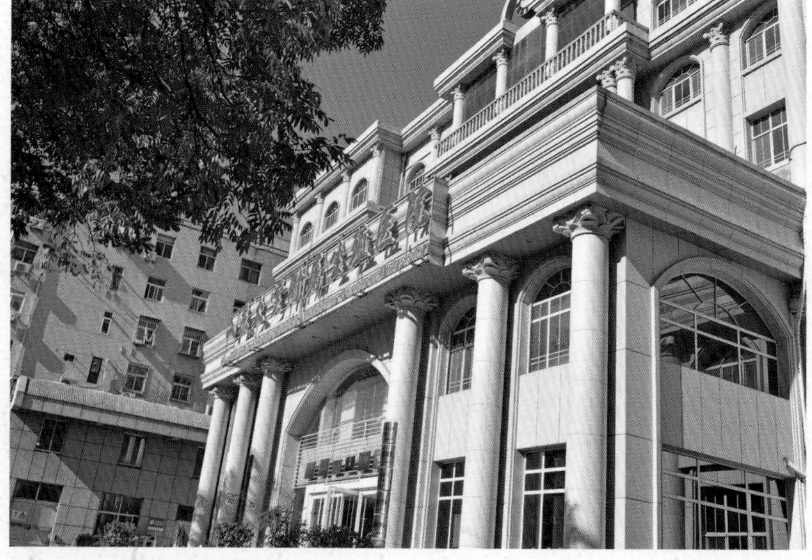

图 635 山东大学附属生殖医院大楼
Fig. 635 Building of the Hospital for Reproductive Medicine Affiliated to Shandong University

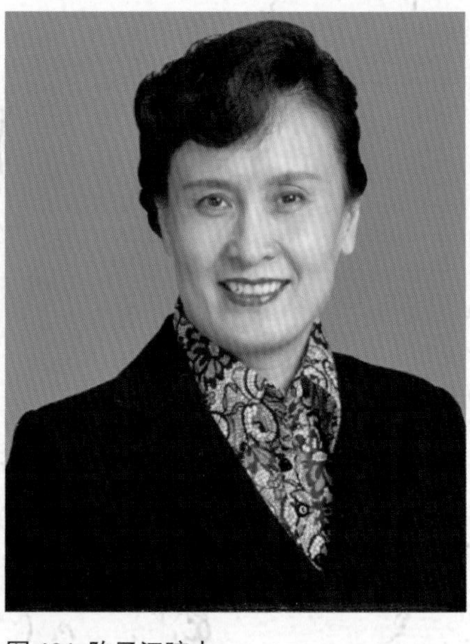

图 636 陈子江院士
Fig. 636 Academician Chen Zijiang

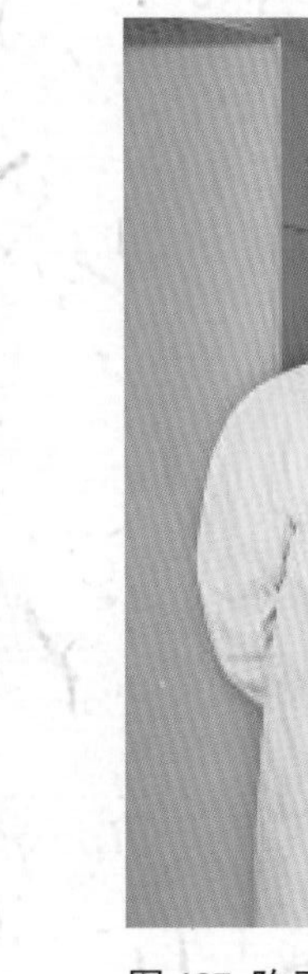

图 637 陈子江科研团队与国内首例耳聋基因 PGD 检测后健康试管婴儿合影
Fig. 637 Chen Zijiang's scientific research team taking a photo with the first healthy test-tube baby after PGD detection of deafness gene in China

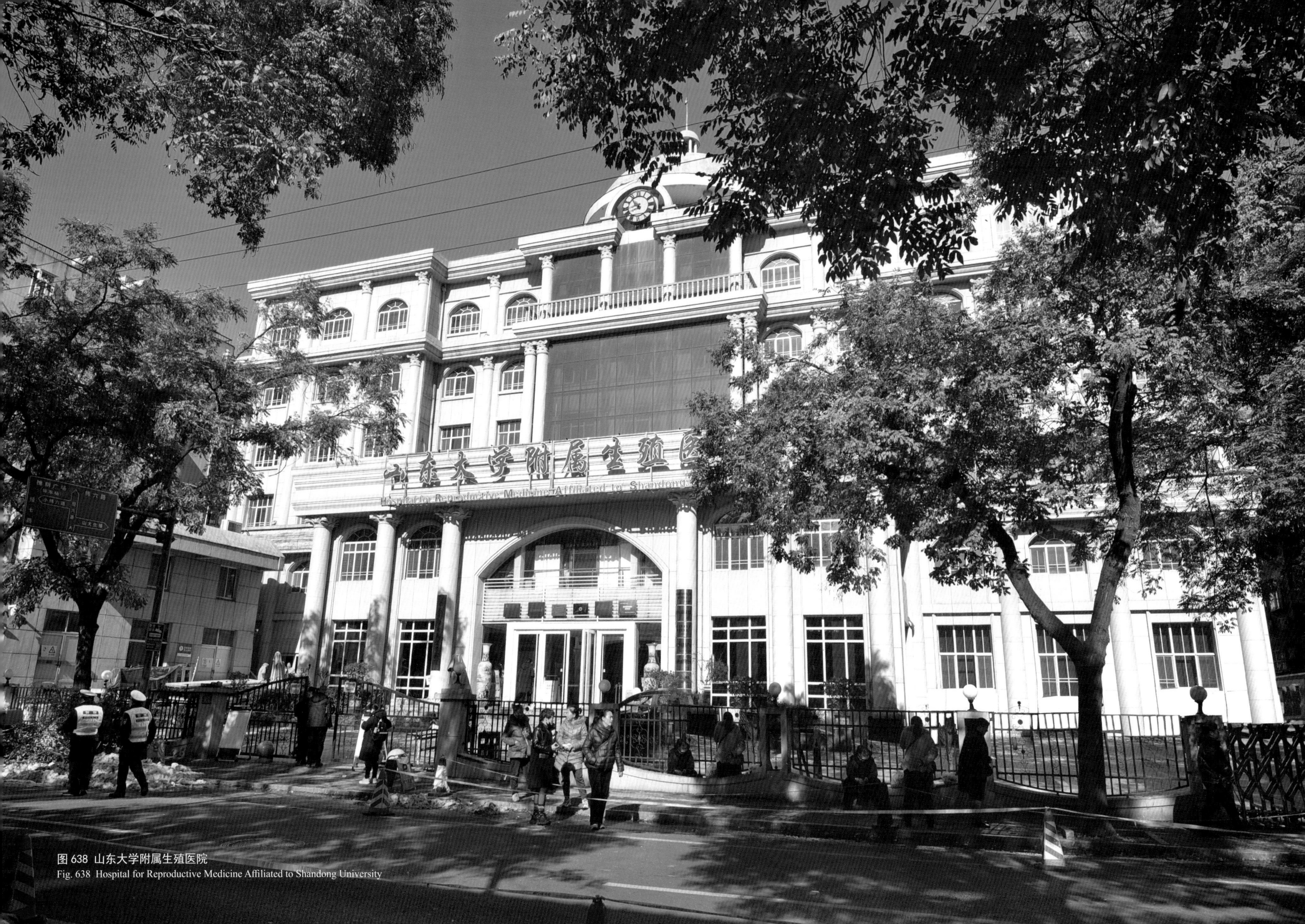

图 638 山东大学附属生殖医院
Fig. 638 Hospital for Reproductive Medicine Affiliated to Shandong University

60 生殖医院（2）

Hospital for Reproductive Medicine Affiliated to Shandong University (2)

山东大学附属生殖医院的前身为山东大学生殖医学研究中心，暨山东省立医院生殖医学中心。此中心是在我国著名妇产科专家苏应宽教授的倡导下，由其研究生陈子江教授于 1987 年创建，为全国最早开展辅助生育技术临床及科研工作的大型医疗机构之一，现在已成为山东省生殖医学重点实验室、教育部生殖内分泌重点实验室和国家辅助生殖与优生工程技术研究中心。中心牵头制定了我国生殖领域首个强制性行业标准《多囊卵巢综合征诊断》（WS 330-2011），于 2011 年 12 月 1 日正式发布实施。

苏应宽 (1918 ~ 1998)，海南人，著名妇产科专家。1943 年毕业于迁至重庆的上海医学院，1948 年来华东白求恩医学院工作。历任山东医学院副教授、教授、副院长，山东省人民医院妇产科主任、副院长。专攻宫颈癌的手术治疗和宫腔内配子移植。著有《实用妇科学》《实用产科学》等著作，前者于 1978 年获得全国科技大会一等奖。他培养的研究生陈子江，于 2019 年当选中国科学院院士。

The Hospital for Reproductive Medicine Affiliated to Shandong University was formerly the Research Center for Reproductive Medicine of Shandong University, namely the Reproductive Medical Center of Shandong Provincial Hospital. The center was established in 1987 by Professor Chen Zijiang, a postgraduate of Professor Su Yingkuan, a famous expert in gynecology and obstetrics in China and the initiator of the center. It is one of the first large-scale medical institutions in China to carry out clinical and scientific research on assisted reproductive technology. Now it has become the Key Laboratory of Reproductive Medicine in Shandong Province, the Key Laboratory of Reproductive Endocrinology of the Ministry of Education and the National Research Center for Assisted Reproductive Technology and Reproductive Genetics. The center took the lead in formulating the first mandatory industry standard in the field of reproduction in China, that is, *Diagnosis Criteria for Polycystic Ovary Syndrome*(WS 330-2011), which was officially released and implemented on 1 December 2011.

Su Yingkuan (1918-1998), a native of Hainan, is a famous expert in gynecology and obstetrics. He graduated from Shanghai Medical College in Chongqing in 1943 and came to work in East China Bethune Medical College in 1948. He successively served as associate professor, professor and vice president of Shandong Medical College, director of the Department of Gynecology and Obstetrics and vice president of Shandong Provincial People's Hospital. He specializes in the surgical treatment of cervical cancer and intrauterine gamete transplantation. The works he has edited include *Practical Gynecology* and *Practical Obstetrics*, and the former won the first prize in the National Science and Technology Conference in 1978. Chen Zijiang, his postgraduate, was elected academician of Chinese Academy of Sciences in 2019.

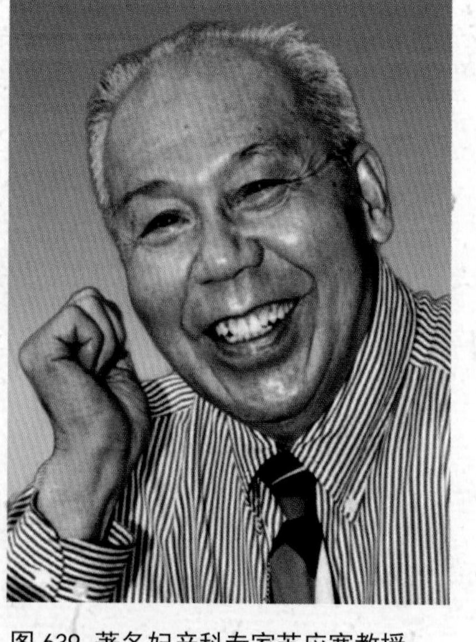

图 639 著名妇产科专家苏应宽教授
Fig. 639 Professor Su Yingkuan, a famous expert in gynecology and obstetrics

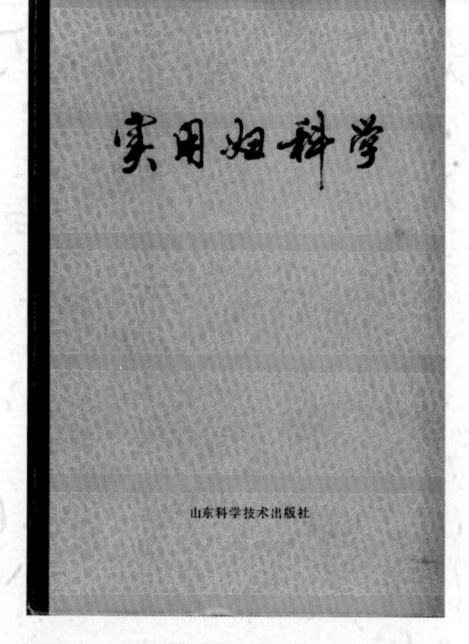

图 640 苏应宽教授等主编的《实用妇科学》
Fig. 640 *Practical Gynecology* edited by Professor Su Yingkuan and others

图 641 苏应宽教授等主编的《实用产科学》
Fig. 641 *Practical Obstetrics* edited by Professor Su Yingkuan and others

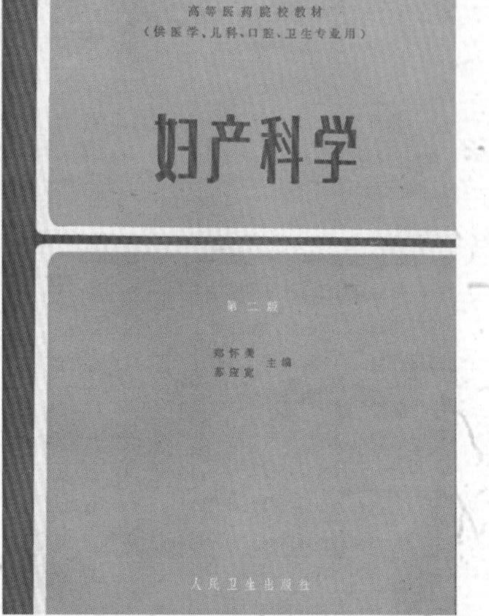

图 642 苏应宽教授参与主编的全国规划教材《妇产科学》第二版
Fig. 642 The second edition of *Gynecology and Obstetrics*, a national planning textbook with Professor Su Yingkuan as one of the chief editors

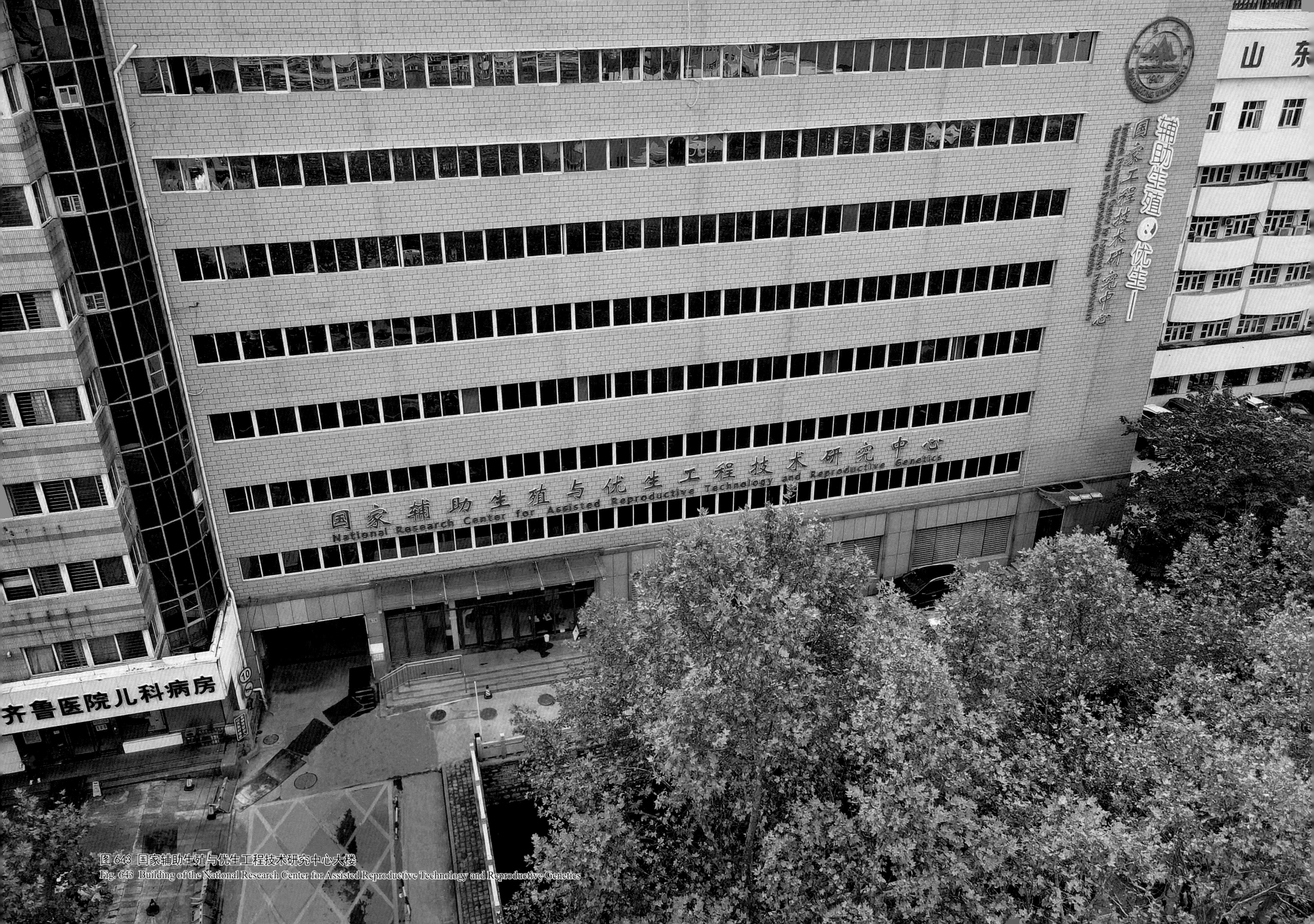

图 643 国家辅助生殖与优生工程技术研究中心大楼

Fig. 643 Building of the National Research Center for Assisted Reproductive Technology and Reproductive Genetics

参考文献

1. 陈晓阳．百年齐鲁医学史话．济南：泰山出版社，2010.
2. 岱峻．风过华西坝：战时教会五大学纪．南京：江苏文艺出版社，2013.
3. 丹尼尔·W. 费舍．狄考文传：一位在中国山东生活了四十五年的传教士．南宁：广西师范大学出版社，2009.
4. 丁宁．原齐鲁大学“考文楼”测绘与建筑风貌保护研究．美与时代（上），2012，3：20 ~ 25.
5. 董黎．中国近代教会大学建筑史研究．北京：科学出版社，2010.
6. 郭查理．齐鲁大学．珠海：珠海出版社，1999.
7. 郭大松．齐鲁大学发祥地辩证．北京教育学院学报，2018，32（1）：78 ~ 87.
8. 郭大松，陈鹏，蔡志书．文惠天下．北京：中国文史出版社，2014.
9. 郭大松，杜学霞．登州文会馆：中国第一所现代大学．济南：山东人民出版社，2012.
10. 郭大松．齐鲁大学文理医三学院渊源及英中文名称考．聊城大学学报（社会科学版），2018，5：1 ~ 14.
11. 黄培堂．纪念黄翠芬院士从事科研工作六十年暨九十华诞．北京：军事医学科学出版社，2010.
12. 李茂松．齐鲁大学前期考证：近代教育发祥青州．潍坊教育学院学报，2006，19（3）：25 ~ 29.
13. 李茂松，郝玉．青州是齐鲁大学的发祥地．春秋，2011，1：38 ~ 40.
14. 李鹏程．齐鲁大学办学模式考析．临沂师范学院学报，2002，24（4）：108 ~ 111.
15. 李耀曦．齐鲁大学校园旧影．春秋，2009，4：37 ~ 38.
16. 李耀曦．齐鲁大学麻风病疗养院旧影．春秋，2009，6：33 ~ 34.
17. 李耀曦．孔祥熙与齐鲁大学．春秋，2013，1：31 ~ 33.
18. 李耀曦，吕军．齐鲁记忆．济南：山东大学出版社，2020.
19. 刘家峰，叶大深．聂会东与齐鲁医学教育的发端（1883 ~ 1911）．山东大学学报（哲学社会科学版），2021，4：204 ~ 215.
20. 刘培平．山大第一．2 版．济南：山东大学出版社，2017.
21. 刘智鹏，刘蜀永．侯宝璋家族史．香港：和平图书有限公司，2012.
22. 鲁娜，陶飞亚．齐鲁大学的历史资料及其研究．教育评论，1994，1：54 ~ 57.

23. 吕军，曹英娟．聂会东文集．济南：山东大学出版社，2019.

24. 吕军，曹英娟．山东现代护理起源与发展．济南：山东大学出版社，2019.

25. 孟雪梅．近代中国教会大学图书馆研究．北京：国家图书馆出版社，2009.

26. 民盟山东省委员会．山东民盟贤达．北京：群言出版社，2016.

27. 宁莜．原齐鲁大学建筑遗存．济南：山东大学出版社，2021.

28. 牛胜男，宁莜．原齐鲁大学圣保罗楼雕刻装饰艺术初探．城市建筑，2019，16（321）：190 ~ 193.

29. 彭益军．近代西方基督教会与齐鲁大学．山东医科大学学报（社会科学版），1999，2：63 ~ 65.

30. 齐鲁大学校友会．齐鲁大学八十八年（1864 ~ 1952）：齐鲁大学校友回忆录．北京：现代教育出版社，2010.

31. 山东大学百年史编委会．山东大学百年史．济南：山东大学出版社，2001.

32. 山东大学药学院院志编委会．山东大学药学院院志．济南：山东大学出版社，2011.

33. 山东济南广智院．济南广智院志略．济南：齐鲁大学印刷厂，1931.

34. 山东省政协文史资料委员会．山东文史集萃·教育卷．济南：山东人民出版社，1993.

35. 山东医科大学史志编委会．山东医科大学史志．南宁：广西师范大学出版社，1991.

36. 苏慧廉．李提摩太在中国．南宁：广西师范大学出版社，2007.

37. 陶飞亚，刘家峰．哈佛燕京学社与齐鲁大学的国学研究．文史哲，1999，1：97 ~ 103.

38. 王晶．从青州博古堂到济南广智院——谈传教士怀恩光在华所创博物馆事业．艺术科技，2016，29（1）：146，241.

39. 徐保安．教会大学与民族主义：以齐鲁大学学生群体为中心（1864 ~ 1937）．南京：南京大学出版社，2015.

40. 严连生．风范（卷一、卷二）．济南：齐鲁书社，2008.

41. 于芹．二十世纪前半叶的济南广智院．春秋，2018，4：41 ~ 43.

42. 袁魁昌．齐鲁医学往事．济南：山东大学出版社，2017.

43. 张昆河，李耀曦．忆老舍在齐鲁大学．山东医科大学学报（社会科学版）1999，3：71 ~ 73.

44. 张茂宏．从医留根．济南：山东大学出版社，2017.

45. 张润武，薛立．图说济南老建筑·近代卷．济南：济南出版社，2001.

46. 赵明顺．山东大学（1901 ~ 2001）．济南：山东大学出版社，2001.

47. 赵宇．山大草木图志．济南：山东大学出版社，2021.

48. 中共平度县委党史办公室．刘谦初．北京：中共党史资料出版社，1990.

49. BALME H. A Modern School of Medicine in China. The Glasgow Medical Journal, 1921, 3: 129-137.

50. CORBETT C H. Shantung Christian University (Cheeloo). New York: United Board for Christian Colleges in China. 1955.

51. FISHER D W. Calvin Wilson Mateer: Forty-five Years a Missionary in Shantung, China. Philadelphia: The Westminster Press, 1911.

52. Tengchow College. Catalogue of Tengchow College, Tengchow, China. Shanghai: American Presbyterian Mission Press, 1891.

附录一　历史沿革图

Appendix I　Map of the Historical Evolution

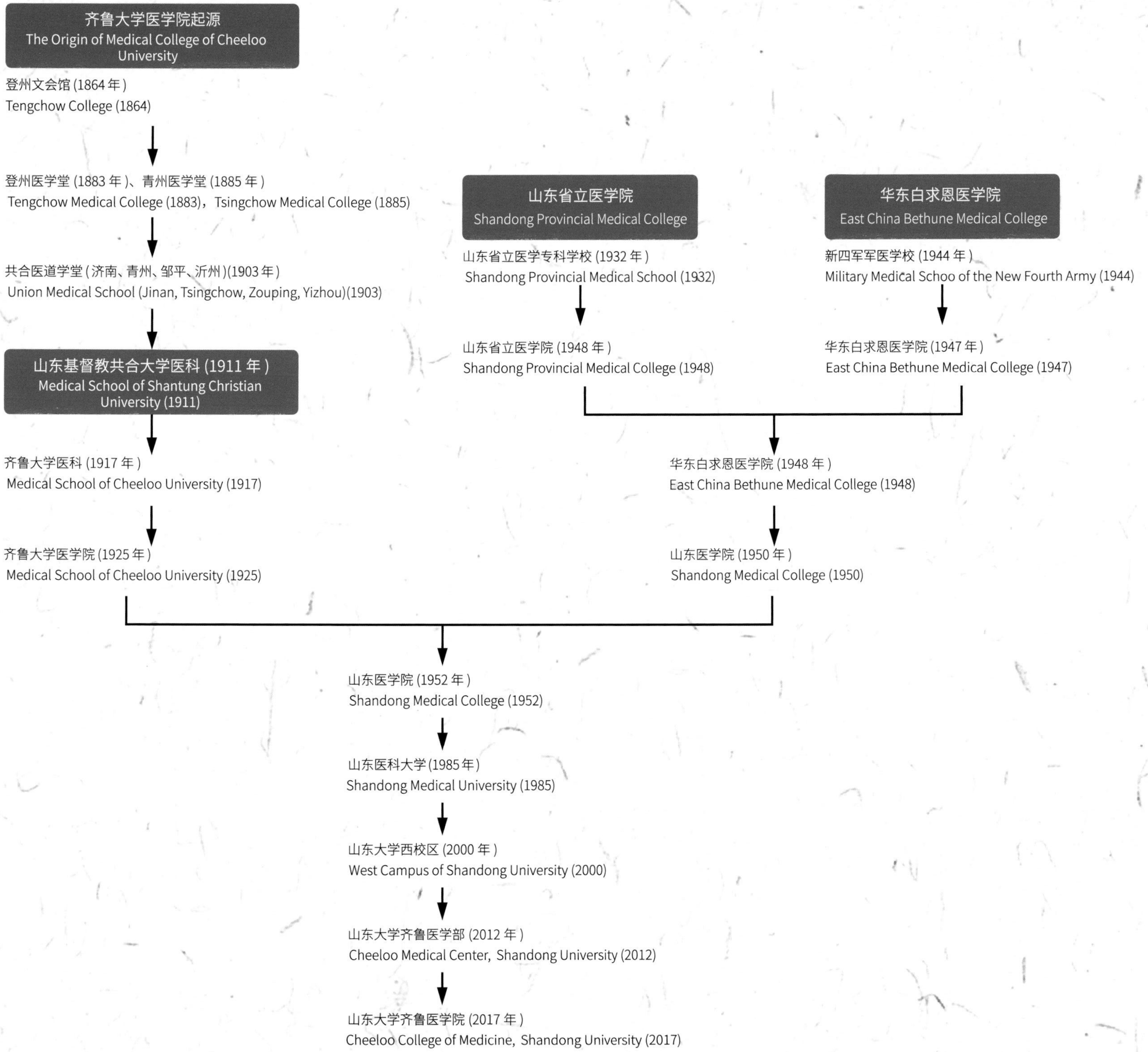

齐鲁大学医学院起源
The Origin of Medical College of Cheeloo University

登州文会馆 (1864 年)
Tengchow College (1864)

↓

登州医学堂 (1883 年)、青州医学堂 (1885 年)
Tengchow Medical College (1883)，Tsingchow Medical College (1885)

↓

共合医道学堂 (济南、青州、邹平、沂州)(1903 年)
Union Medical School (Jinan, Tsingchow, Zouping, Yizhou)(1903)

↓

山东基督教共合大学医科 (1911 年)
Medical School of Shantung Christian University (1911)

↓

齐鲁大学医科 (1917 年)
Medical School of Cheeloo University (1917)

↓

齐鲁大学医学院 (1925 年)
Medical School of Cheeloo University (1925)

山东省立医学院
Shandong Provincial Medical College

山东省立医学专科学校 (1932 年)
Shandong Provincial Medical School (1932)

↓

山东省立医学院 (1948 年)
Shandong Provincial Medical College (1948)

华东白求恩医学院
East China Bethune Medical College

新四军军医学校 (1944 年)
Military Medical Schoo of the New Fourth Army (1944)

↓

华东白求恩医学院 (1947 年)
East China Bethune Medical College (1947)

↓

华东白求恩医学院 (1948 年)
East China Bethune Medical College (1948)

↓

山东医学院 (1950 年)
Shandong Medical College (1950)

↓

山东医学院 (1952 年)
Shandong Medical College (1952)

↓

山东医科大学 (1985 年)
Shandong Medical University (1985)

↓

山东大学西校区 (2000 年)
West Campus of Shandong University (2000)

↓

山东大学齐鲁医学部 (2012 年)
Cheeloo Medical Center, Shandong University (2012)

↓

山东大学齐鲁医学院 (2017 年)
Cheeloo College of Medicine, Shandong University (2017)

附录二　山东大学齐鲁医学院要事编年

Appendix II　Chronicle of Important Events of Cheeloo College of Medicine of Shandong University

一、源头之一，齐鲁大学

I The First Source: Cheeloo University

1864 年

美北长老会传教士狄考文夫妇 1 月到达登州，9 月创建登州蒙养学堂，即登州文会馆前身。

Calvin Wilson Mateer, missionary of American Presbyterian Missions, North, arrived in Dengzhou with his wife in January, and established Tengchow Boy's Boarding School in September, the predecessor of Tengchow College.

1870 年

英国浸礼会在山东烟台开始传教活动。

The English Baptist Missionary Society began missionary activities in Yantai, Shandong Province.

1875 年

英国浸礼会将传教基地从烟台迁到青州。

The English Baptist Missionary Society moved the missionary base from Yantai to Qingzhou.

1877 年

1 月，蒙养学堂第一批 3 名学生邹立文、李秉义、李山青毕业。在毕业典礼上，狄考文取《论语》中“君子以文会友，以友辅仁”之意，将蒙养学堂正式改名为登州文会馆。此 3 人后被追认为齐鲁大学第一届毕业生。

In January, the first batch of three students, Zou Liwen, Li Bingyi and Li Shanqing graduated from Tengchow Boy's Boarding School. At the graduation ceremony, Tengchow Boy's Boarding School was renamed Tengchow College officially by Calvin Wilson Mateer, with the meaning of "The superior man on grounds of culture meets with his friends, and by friendship helps his virtue." from *The Analects of Confucius*, and the three students were later confirmed as the first graduates of Cheeloo University.

1881 年

英国浸礼会传教士仲均安和怀恩光在青州创办圣道学堂。

Alfred G. Jones and John Sutherland Whitewright, missionaries of the English Baptist Missionary Society, established the Theological Institute in Qingzhou.

1882 年

美长老会总部批准登州文会馆为登州学院，正式授权改办大学，英文名字为“Tengchow College”。

The headquarters of the American Presbyterian Missions approved Tengchow College.

1883 年

美北长老会派遣聂会东博士夫妇来山东，创办隶属于登州文会馆的医科，是为齐鲁大学医学院的发端。

The American Presbyterian Missions, North sent Dr. James Boyd Neal and his wife to Shandong to set up a medical school affiliated to Tengchow College, which was the beginning of the Medical School of Cheeloo University.

1884 年

英国浸礼会传教士库寿龄夫妇在青州以美北长老会开设的男生寄宿学校为基础创立青州中学，1986 年扩建为青州广德书院。

Samuel Couline, missionary of the English Baptist Missionary Society, founded Tsingchow Middle School with his wife in Qingzhou on the basis of the Boy's Boarding School opened by the American Presbyterian Missions, North. In 1986, it was expanded to Tsingchow Kwang Teh Shu Yun.

1885 年

4 月，英国浸礼会传教士武成献夫妇到达烟台芝罘，开始语言学习。英国浸礼会怀恩光、仲钧安和卜道成在青州府设立了神学院 (Theological Training Institute)，中文名称为培真书院。

In April, James Russell Watson, missionary of the English Baptist Missionary Society, arrived in Zhifu, Yantai with his wife to start language learning.John Sutherland Whitewright, Alfred G. Jones and Joseph Percy Bruce, missionaries of the English Baptist Missionary Society, established Theological Training Institute.

1886 年

4 月，英国浸礼会传教士武成献夫妇到达青州，开始创办广德医院和医学堂。

In April, James Russell Watson, missionary of the English Baptist Missionary Society, arrived in Qingzhou with his wife and began to set up Kwang Teh Hospital and Medical School.

1887 年

神学院增设了一所培养小学师资的师范学校 (Training School for elementary teachers)。英浸礼会怀恩光在青州培真书院前边盖展览室，称之为“博物堂”，是为广智院前身。青州广德书院增设大学班。

The Theological Training Institute established a Training School for elementary teachers. John Sutherland Whitewright of the English Baptist Missionary Society built an exhibition room in front of the institute, known as "Tsingchowfu Museum", the predecessor of Tsinanfu Institute. Tsingchow Kwang Teh Shu Yun added university classes.

1890 年

聂会东被差会调往济南，扩建文璧医院，取名华美医院，并同时筹建医校。

James Boyd Neal was sent to Jinan; he expanded McILVaine Hospital into Sino-American Hospital, and at the same time prepared for the construction of the medical school.

1893 年

青州神学院得到了一笔旨在纪念罗宾逊太太的父亲葛奇博士和罗宾逊先生的父亲伊利沙·罗宾逊的捐款，遂改名为葛奇－罗宾逊神学院 (Gotch-Robinson Theological College)，简称为葛罗神学院。

The Theological Training Institute received a donation in memory of Mrs. Robinson's father, Dr. Gotch, and Mr. Robinson's father, Elisha Robinson, and then changed its name to Gotch-Robinson Theological College.

1895 年

狄考文辞去馆主职务，赫士继任。

Calvin Wilson Mateer resigned as the president of Tengchow College and Watson Mcmillen Hayes succeeded him as president.

1900 年

义和团运动。

Yihetuan Movement

1901 年

清末新政改革。赫士应袁世凯邀创办山东大学堂，登州文会馆馆主由柏尔根接任。

New Deal Reform was carried out in the late Qing Dynasty. At the invitation of Yuan Shikai, Watson Mcmillen Hayes founded Shantung University, and Pall D. Bergen took over as the president of Tengchow College.

1902 年

6 月 13 日，北美长老会和英国浸礼会在青州开会，共同建立山东新教大学（Shantung Protestant University）。

On 13 June, the American Presbyterian Missions, North and the English Baptist Missionary Society met in Qingzhou to jointly establish Shantung Protestant University.

1903 年

济南聂会东、青州武成献和邹平巴德顺所办的医校合称为共合医道学堂（Union Medical College），武成献任校长，学制四年，四个年级的学生分别在济南、青州、邹平和沂州（今临沂）的教会医院进行教学和轮流实习。

The medical schools run by James Boyd Neal in Jinan, James Russell Watson in Qingzhou and T. C. Paterso in Zouping were jointly called Union Medical College and James Russell Watson served as the president. The college had a four-year schooling system. Students of the four grades taught and practised in turn in the church hospitals in Jinan, Qingzhou, Zouping and Yizhou (now Linyi).

1904 年

青州广德书院大学部和登州文会馆大学部的文理科合并，分别由青州和登州迁往潍县乐道院，作为山东新教大学的文理学院，取名“广文学堂”，又称“广文大学”（Wei Hsien Arts and Science College）。

The Department of Arts and Science of Tsingchow Kwang Teh Shu Yun and that of Tengchow College merged, and they moved from Qingzhou and Dengzhou to the Courtyard of the Happy Way in Weixian respectively. As the School of Arts and Science of Shantung Protestant University, it was named “Wei Hsien Arts and Science College”.

1905 年

青州的神学院“联合神道学堂”（Union Theological College）开学。

The Union Theological College opened in Qingzhou.

1906 年

校董会决定在济南建设新的医学院。

The board decided to build a new medical school in Jinan.

1908 年

齐大校董会利用阿辛顿基金（Arthington Fund) 在济南购买了医学院建院所需土地。

The Board of Cheeloo University used the Arthington Fund to buy land in Jinan for the building of the medical school

1909 年

英国圣公会加入联合，《教育工作联合准则》于 1909 年做了修订，大学英文名称由山东新教大学改为山东基督教大学（Shantung Christian University）。同年，芝加哥大学教授巴顿（Burton），作为洛克菲勒东方教育委员会主席访问中国，建议将现有的大学各学院迁到一处办学。英国浸礼会传教护士劳根来到青州广德医院工作，开创了山东的护理教育。

With the joining of the Anglican Church, the *Joint Guidelines for Education* was revised in 1909 and the English name of the university was changed from Shantung Protestant University to Shantung Christian University.In the same year, Burton, a professor at the University of Chicago, visited China as chairman of the Rockefeller Oriental Education Committee and proposed moving existing schools of the university to one place.Margaret Faiconer Logan, a missionary nurse of the English Baptist Missionary Society, came to work in Tsingchow Kwang Teh Hospital and initiated nursing education in Shandong.

1910 年

3 月 15 日，医学院在建筑尚未完全竣工时学生即已入住上课。

On 15 March, students moved into the medical school to attend classes before the building was fully completed.

1911 年

4 月 17 日，在英国利兹阿辛顿基金会的慷慨资助下，在济南修建的医学大讲堂、诊病所、宿舍等举行竣工典礼，山东巡抚孙宝琦出席并捐银千两。济南共合医道学堂正式更名为山东基督教共合大学医科，聂会东任校长，有教师 14 人。新址的竣工标志着学校开始由四地合并到济南，齐鲁大学医学院将这一天作为建院日期。

On 17 April, with the generous support of the Arthington Foundation of the United Kingdom, the dedication of the medical lecture hall, clinic and dormitory built in Jinan was held. Sun Baoqi, governor of Shandong, attended and donated 1,000 tales of silver. Jinan Union Medical College was officially renamed Medical School of Shantung Christian University, with 14 teachers and James Boyd Neal as the president. The completion of the new site marked the merger of the schools from four places to Jinan, and the Medical School of Cheeloo University set this day as the date of its establishment.

1913 年

劳根来济南工作。

Logan came to Jinan to work.

1914 年

劳根在济南创办护士养成学校，学制四年。

Logan set up a nurse training school in Jinan, with a four-year schooling.

1915 年

大学委员会决定以颇具中国传统的“齐鲁大学”作为非正式中文名字。

The University Committee decided to use the traditional “Cheeloo University” as an informal Chinese name.

1916 年

罗氏基金驻华医社（China Medical Board）带来了北京协和医院的 3 个低年级班。同年，中国博医会之医学教育委员会将金陵大学医科及汉口大同医学二校学子及诸教授一并迁到济南并入齐鲁大学医学院。

China Medical Board had brought three junior classes from Peking Union Medical College Hospital. In the same year, the Medical Education Committee of the China Medical Association moved the students and professors of the Medical School of University of Nanking and Union Medical College in Hankou to Jinan to merge into the Medical School of Cheeloo University.

1917 年

新校园建成，文理学院与神学院相继迁来济南，齐鲁大学实现了同地办学。

The new campus was completed, and the College of Arts and Science and the Theological Training Institute moved to Jinan one after another. Then Cheeloo University was run in the same place.

1919 年

五四运动爆发，齐鲁大学一些学生也走向了街头参加示威游行。

When the May 4th Movement broke out, some students from Cheeloo University also took to the streets to participate in demonstrations.

1923 年

北京协和女子医学院并入齐鲁大学医学院。9 月，齐鲁大学开始招收女生。同年，聘请李天禄任文理学院院长，自此齐鲁大学行政管理人员中终于出现了中国人的影子。

Peking Union Medical College for Women was merged into the Medical School of Cheeloo University. In September, Cheeloo University began recruiting girls. In the same year, Li Tianlu was hired as president of the College of Arts and Science, and since then the Chinese people appeared among the administrative personnel of Cheeloo University.

1924 年

7 月 19 日，加拿大授予齐鲁大学执照。齐鲁大学颁布学位授予条例，规定医学院毕业生颁发医学学士学位，同时授予美国和加拿大认可的医学博士学位。

On 19 July, the Government of Canada granted a license to Cheeloo University. Cheeloo University had issued degree-awarding regulations, which stipulated that graduates of the Medical School were award a Bachelor’s Degree of Medicine and a degree of Doctor of Medicine recognized by the United States and Canada.

1928 年

5 月，日军制造了“五三惨案”，并曾到齐鲁大学进行搜查。11 月 19 日，齐鲁大学成立了由李天禄、施尔德、程其保、罗世琦组成的立案委员会，具体负责立案事宜。

In May, the Japanese army launched Jinan Massacre and once searched Cheeloo University. On 19 November, Cheeloo University set up a Registration Committee composed of Li Tianlu, Shields, Cheng Qibao and Luo Shiqi, which was specifically responsible for registrations.

1929 年

10 月 27 日，文理学院学生开始上书、请愿、罢课、示威，在学生的冲击下，李天禄辞职，校董会中国籍董事要超过三分之二。

On 27 October, students of arts and science began to submit written statements, petition, strike and demonstrate. Under the impact of the students, Li Tianlu resigned; there should be more than two-thirds of the Chinese directors of the University Board.

1930 年

1930 年秋，在栾调甫建议下，文学院国学研究所成立。先后有老舍、顾颉刚、钱穆、严耕望、郝立权、余天庥、王敦化、范迪瑞等知名学者在所研究，齐鲁大学一时成为全国国学研究的重地。

In autumn of 1930, at the suggestion of Luan Diaofu, the Institute of National Studies of the School of Liberal Arts was established. Lao She, Gu Jiegang, Qian Mu, Yan Gengwang, Hao Liquan, Yu Tianxiu, Wang Dunhua, Fan Dirui and other well-known scholars did the research in the institute one after another, and Cheeloo University became the focus of the National Studies all over the country for a time.

1931 年

3 月，齐大请孔祥熙担任校长。秋季开学后，曾任教育部次长的朱经农来校担任校长。9 月 18 日，“九一八”事变爆发。9 月 21 日，齐大学生抗日救国团成立。12 月 17 日教育部核准齐鲁大学立案。

In March, Cheeloo University invited Kong Xiangxi to serve as president. After the university started in autumn, Zhu Jingnong, a former vice minister of the Ministry of Education, came to the university to serve as president. On 18 September, the “September 18th Incident” broke out. On 21 September, students of Cheeloo University established the group of resistance against Japanese aggression and national salvation. On 17 December, the Ministry of Education approved the registration of Cheeloo University.

1935 年

刘书铭在德位思的几番邀请下，终于来齐鲁大学就任校长之职。

Liu Shuming finally came to Cheeloo University to serve as president.

1937 年

7 月，七七事变，全面抗战爆发。10 月，大部分师生及主要教学设备迁往四川成都，与华西协和大学、金陵大学、金陵女子文理学院、燕京大学等在华西坝办学，史称“华西坝五大学”；小部分师生员工继续在原址开课。

In July, the July 7 Incident of 1937 happened and the full-scale war of resistance against aggression broke out. In October, most of the teachers and students and the main teaching equipment moved to Chengdu, Sichuan Province. The university went to run in Huaxiba with West China Union University, University of Nanking, Ginling College, Yenching University. A small number of teachers, students and employees continued to hold classes at the original site.

1939 年

9 月，顾颉刚在成都主持齐鲁大学国学研究所所务，又有钱穆、杨向奎、胡厚宣和沈镜如等加盟，使国学研究得到空前发展。

In September, Gu Jiegang presided over the work of the Institute of National Studies of Cheeloo University in Chengdu, and with the joining of Qian Mu, Yang Xiangkui, Hu Houxuan and Shen Jingru, the national studies experienced unprecedented development.

1941 年

12 月，太平洋战争爆发，济南的齐鲁大学校园被日军强占为兵站医院。外籍教师部分逃至成都、部分回国、部分被日军押送至潍县集中营，华籍人员则至济南市立医院工作。同年，在成都的齐鲁大学应国家需求，理学院增设药学系，学制四年。

In December, the Pacific War broke out, and the campus of Cheeloo University in Jinan was forcibly occupied by the Japanese army as a military station hospital. Some foreign teachers fled to Chengdu, some returned home, some were transported to the concentration camp in Weixian by the Japanese army, and Chinese personnel went to work in Jinan Hospital. In the same year, Cheeloo University in Chengdu, in response to the needs of the state, added a Department of Pharmacy to the School of Science, with a four-year schooling.

1942 年

在成都的齐鲁大学医学院与理学院合作建立寄生虫研究所，救治病人，并培养硕士研究生。

In Chengdu, the Medical School and the School of Science of Cheeloo University cooperated to set up a Parasite Research Institute to treat patients and train postgraduate students.

1943 年

10 月，因抗战需要，全国知识青年从军运动开始。华西坝上最早入伍的是医科学生，齐鲁大学学生积极应征，多人入伍。

In October, due to the War of Resistance Against Japanese Aggression, the national movement of intellectual youth joining the army began. The first to join the army in Huaxiba was medical students. Students of Cheeloo University were actively recruited and many people joined the army.

1946 年

齐鲁大学在济南复校，9 月正式开学。

Cheeloo University resumed running in Jinan and officially opened in September.

1948 年

济南解放前夕，为避战祸齐鲁大学再次迁校。文理学院迁往浙江杭州郊外的云栖寺，克服困难正常上课，实验课程借用浙江大学的仪器设备和实验室；医学院则迁往福州协和医院。

Shortly before Jinan’s liberation, Cheeloo University moved again to avoid war disasters. The Schools of Arts and Science moved to Yunqi Temple on the outskirts of Hangzhou, Zhejiang Province, and overcame difficulties to take classes normally. The experimental courses used the instruments, equipment and laboratories borrowed from Zhejiang University. The Medical School moved to Fuzhou Union Hospital.

1949 年

济南解放后，南迁的师生和仪器设备在人民政府的帮助下先后迁回济南原址。

After Jinan’s liberation, the teachers, students, instruments and equipment moved from south back to the original site in Jinan with the help of the People’s Government.

1951 年

1 月，华东军政委员会教育部接管齐鲁大学，解聘所有外籍教师的行政和董事职务，彻底收回了齐鲁大学的教育主权。

In January, the Ministry of Education of the East China Military and Political Commission took over Cheeloo University, dismissed all foreign teachers from administrative and director positions, and completely withdrew Cheeloo University’s educational sovereignty.

1952 年

9 月，全国高等院校院系调整，齐鲁大学解体。其医学院留在原址，与迁来的山东医学院合并组建新山东医学院；其它学科分别并入山东大学、山东师范学院、山东农学院、南京大学、上海财经学院、山东财经学院、华东药学院（中国药科大学）等高校和中国科学院紫金山天文台；曾经辉煌过的国学研究所被撤销。

In September, schools and departments of colleges and universities across the country were adjusted and Cheeloo University disintegrated. Its Medical School stayed in the original site and merged with the relocated Shandong Medical College to form a new Shandong Medical College. Other disciplines were merged into Shandong University, Shandong Normal University, Shandong Agricultural College, Nanjing University, Shanghai College of Finance and Economics, Shandong College of Finance and Economics, East China College of Pharmacy (China Pharmaceutical University) and Purple Mountain Observatory of Chinese Academy of Sciences. The once brilliant Institute of National Studies was abolished.

二、源头之二，山东省立医学院
II The Second Source: Shandong Provincial Medical College

1932 年
8 月，山东省立医学专科学校创建，由南京国民政府教育部和山东省教育厅领导，尹莘农任校长。校址设在济南市趵突泉前街，占地 212.84 公亩。

In August, Shandong Provincial Medical School was established, led by the Ministry of Education of Nanjing National Government and Shandong Provincial Education Department, with Yin Shennong as the president. The site is located in Baotuquanqian Street, Jinan City, covering an area of 212.84 *mu*.

1933 年
学校创办中德双语的《新医学》杂志，为季刊，1937 年停办。

The school founded the quarterly bilingual magazine *New Medicine* in Chinese and German, and closed it in 1937.

1937 年
抗日战争爆发。尹莘农校长带领学校辗转至湖北汉口、四川云阳县和万县。附属医院被国民政府改编为“军政部第十重伤医院”，后又改为“山东医院”，尹莘农兼任院长。学校的部分师生直接参加了抗日战争。

The War of Resistance Against Japanese Aggression broke out. President Yin Shennong led the school to Hankou in Hubei Province and to Yunyang County and Wanxian County in Sichuan Province. The affiliated hospital was reorganized by the National Government as “the 10th Hospital of Serious Injury of the Military and Political Department”, and later changed to “Shandong Hospital” with Yin Shennong concurrently serving as president. Some teachers and students of the school took part directly in the War of Resistance Against Japanese Aggression.

1946 年
10 月，山东省立医学专科学校从万县迁回济南，与山东省立医院合并。

In October, Shandong Provincial Medical School moved back to Jinan from Wanxian County and merged with Shandong Provincial Hospital.

1948 年
8 月 18 日，经南京国民政府教育部批准，更名为山东省立医学院，院长由山东省立医院院长王宝楹担任。9 月 24 日，济南解放，山东省立医学院被军管会接管。11 月并入华东白求恩医学院。

On 18 August, with the approval of the Ministry of Education of Nanjing National Government, it was renamed Shandong Provincial Medical College, with Wang Baoying, president of Shandong Provincial Hospital, serving as the president. On 24 September, Jinan was liberated and Shandong Provincial Medical College was taken over by the Military Control Commission. In November, it was merged into East China Bethune Medical College.

三、源头之三，华东白求恩医学院
III The Third Source: East China Bethune Medical College

1944 年
10 月 16 日，经新四军军部批准建立新四军军医学校。

On 16 October, the Medical School of the New Fourth Army was established with the approval of the headquarters of the New Fourth Army.

1945 年
3 月 18 日在淮南新浦镇招生，5 月 12 日在安徽省天长县长庄举行开学典礼。

On 18 March, the school enrolled students in Xinpu Town, Huainan, and on 12 May, it held an opening ceremony in Changzhuang, Tianchang County, Anhui Province.

1946 年
12 月新四军卫生部直属医院更名为华东国际和平医院，成为医学院的教学医院。

In December, the Hospital of the New Fourth Army directly affiliated to the Ministry of Health was renamed East China International Peace Hospital and became the teaching hospital of the Medical School.

1947 年
1 月，新四军军医学校更名为华东白求恩医学院。

In January, the Medical School of the New Fourth Army was renamed East China Bethune Medical College.

1948 年
9 月 24 日，济南解放，华东白求恩医学院从益都迁入济南，驻扎在经五路纬九路。11 月山东省立医学院并入，仍称为华东白求恩医学院。

On 24 September, Jinan was liberated. East China Bethune Medical College moved from Yidu to Jinan and was stationed on Jingwu Road and Weijiu Road. In November, Shandong Provincial Medical College was merged into it and was still known as East China Bethune Medical College.

1949 年
5 月，学院由华东野战军划归山东省人民政府领导，更名为山东省立医学院。

In May, the college was transferred by the East China Field Army to the leadership of Shandong Provincial People’s Government and renamed Shandong Provincial Medical College.

1950 年
12 月，更名为山东医学院。

In December, it was renamed Shandong Medical College.

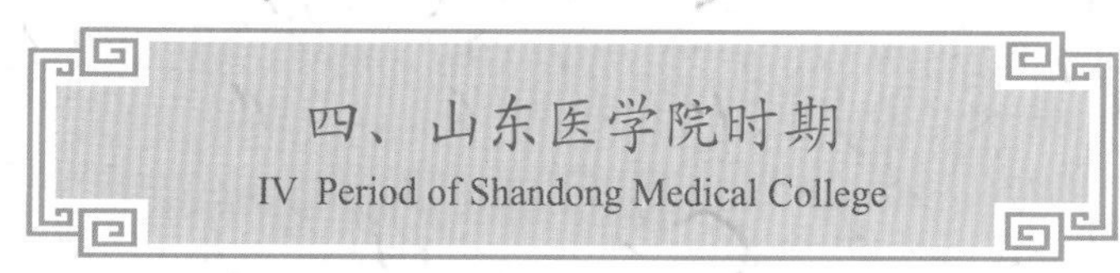

四、山东医学院时期
IV Period of Shandong Medical College

1952 年

9 月，全国高等学校院系调整。撤销齐鲁大学，其文学院、理学院等并入其它大学，医学院留在原址，与迁来的山东医学院合并组建新山东医学院。10 月 8 日，学校召开调整胜利完成大会，标志着新山东医学院正式成立。学校下设医学、药科、卫生三个专业。

In September, schools and departments of colleges and universities across the country were adjusted. Cheeloo University was abolished, and its Schools of Arts and Science were merged into other universities. The Medical School remained in its original site and merged with the relocated Shandong Medical College to form a new Shandong Medical College. On 8 October, the university held a meeting of the successful completion of the adjustment, marking the formal establishment of the new Shandong Medical College. It has three specialties, namely medicine, pharmacy and health.

1955 年

8 月，全国高等医药院校卫生专业、药学专业再次调整。山东医学院卫生系教师及 247 名学生调到了同济医学院；药学系 121 名学生及部分教师调到四川医学院。

In August, the specialties of health and pharmacy of higher medical colleges and universities across the country were adjusted again. Teachers and 247 students of the Health Department of Shandong Medical College were transferred to Tongji Medical College. 121 students and some teachers of the Department of Pharmacy were transferred to Sichuan Medical College.

1956 年

6 月，经国家批准，山东医学院成为第一批招收副博士研究生的院校之一。

In June, with the approval of the state, Shandong Medical College became one of the first colleges and universities to recruit associate doctoral students.

1959 年

1 月，学校设立基础部和临床部。

In January, the college set up a Basic Department and a Clinical Department.

1962 年

7 月，山东医学院成为第一批医疗专业五年制改六年制的 11 所院校之一。

In July, Shandong Medical College became one of the first eleven colleges and universities to change the five-year medical system to the six-year medical system.

1966 年

5 月，“文化大革命”爆发，学校受到严重冲击。

In May, the “Cultural Revolution” broke out, and the college was severely impacted.

1970 年

8 月，山东医学院与山东中医学院合并，称为山东医学院，由济南迁往泰安新泰县楼德镇办学。

In August, Shandong Medical College merged with Shandong College of Traditional Chinese Medicine to be called Shandong Medical College, which moved from Jinan to Loude Town, Xintai County, Tai’an City.

1973 年

学院主要力量撤回济南，中医系、药学系迁回济南上课。

The main strength of the college withdrew to Jinan, and the Department of Traditional Chinese Medicine and the Department of Pharmacy moved back to Jinan for classes.

1974 年

建立山东医学院楼德分院。1979 年分院迁至泰安市，更名为山东医学院泰安分院。1981 年分院独立为泰山医学院。

The Loude branch of Shandong Medical College was established. In 1979, the branch moved to Tai’an city and was renamed the Tai’an branch of Shandong Medical College. In 1981, the branch was independent as Taishan Medical College.

1977 年

山东医学院恢复和增设了卫生专业和口腔专业，共有医疗、药学、卫生、口腔 4 个专业。

Shandong Medical College has restored and added the specialties of health and stomatology, and then it has a total of four specialties, namely, medicine, pharmacy, health and stomatology.

1978 年

6 月，国务院决定对山东医学院实行卫生部和山东省双重领导、卫生部为主的领导体制。至此，山东医学院成为全国 13 所部属医学院校之一。

In June, the State Council decided to implement a dual leadership system for Shandong Medical College of the Ministry of Health and Shandong Province, with the Ministry of Health as the main body. So far, Shandong Medical College had become one of the thirteen ministerial medical colleges and universities in the country.

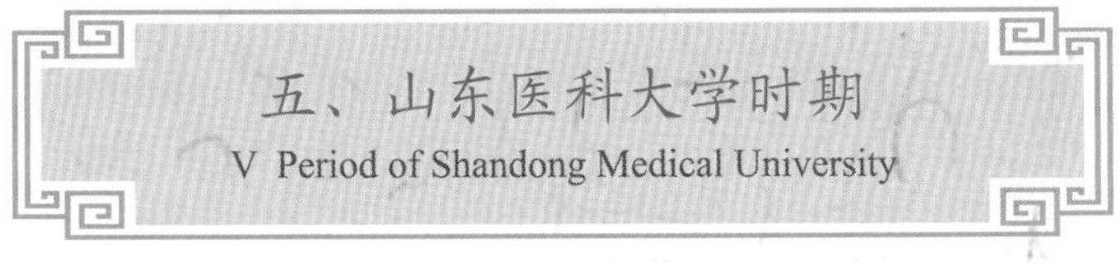

五、山东医科大学时期
V Period of Shandong Medical University

1985 年

5 月，卫生部决定山东医学院更名为山东医科大学；医学系改名为临床医学部；增设高级护理专业。

In May, the Ministry of Health decided to change the name of Shandong Medical College to Shandong Medical University. The Department of Medicine was renamed the Center for Clinical Medicine. The specialty of Advanced Nursing was added.

1987 年

卫生部批准建设第二医院。

The Ministry of Health approved the construction of the Second Hospital.

1996 年

10 月，基础医学部改组为基础医学院。

In October, the Center for Basic Medical Sciences was reorganized into the School of Basic Medical Sciences.

2000 年

合校前夕，学校下设基础医学院、临床医学部、药学院、公共卫生学院、口腔医学院、护理学院、研究生部、社会科学部、成人教育学院及附属医院、第二附属医院和口腔医院三所附属医院。

Before the integration, the university has School of Basic Medical Sciences, the Center for Clinical Medicine, School of Pharmaceutical Sciences, School of Public Health, School of stomatology, School of Nursing, Graduate Department, Department of Social Sciences, School of Adult Education, the Affiliated Hospital, the Second Affiliated Hospital and Stomatological Hospital.

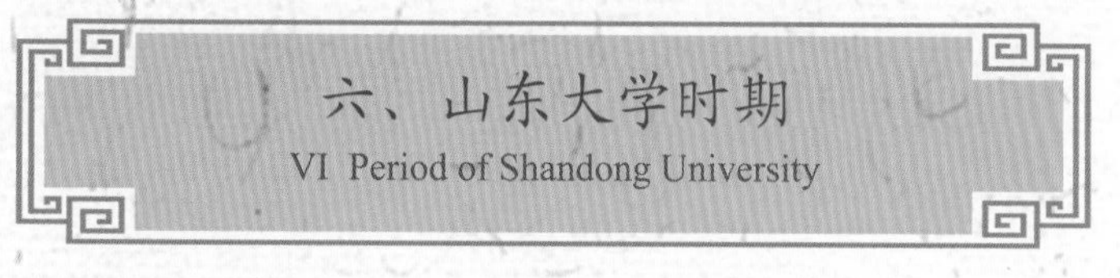

六、山东大学时期
VI Period of Shandong University

2000 年

7 月 22 日，山东大学、山东医科大学和山东工业大学合并组建新山东大学。

On 22 July, Shandong University, Shandong Medical University and Shandong University of Technology merged to form new Shandong University.

2001 年

1 月，基础医学院和临床医学部合并重组为山东大学医学院。

In January, School of Basic Medical Sciences and the Center for Clinical Medicine were merged and reorganized into the Medical School of Shandong University.

2006 年

12 月，趵突泉校区入选为第三批省级文物保护单位。

In December, Baotuquan Campus was selected as one of the third batch of Provincial Cultural Relics Protection Units.

2012 年

5 月，山东大学齐鲁医学部成立。

In May, Cheeloo Medical Center of Shandong University was established.

2013 年

5 月，趵突泉校区入选第七批全国重点文物保护单位。

In May, Baotuquan Campus was selected as one of the seventh batch of National Key Cultural Relics Protection Units.

2016 年

6 月，根据山东大学《医学教育管理体制改革实施方案》，学校决定撤销医学院建制，重新设立基础医学院和临床医学院。

In June, according to Shandong University's "Plan for the Reform of Management System of Medical Education", the university decided to abolish the organizational system of Medical School and reestablish School of Basic Medical Sciences and School of Clinical Medicine.

2017 年

9 月，齐鲁医学部更名为齐鲁医学院。至此，山东大学齐鲁医学院设有基础医学院、临床医学院、公共卫生学院、口腔医学院、护理与康复学院、药学院 6 个学院，有齐鲁医院、第二医院、口腔医院和生殖医院 4 家直属附属医院，多家非隶属附属医院，承担教学、科研及服务社会等职能。

In September, Cheeloo Medical Center was renamed Cheeloo College of Medicine. Now Cheeloo College of Medicine of Shandong Unviersity has six schools, namely School of Basic Medical Sciences, School of Clinical Medicine, School of Public Health, School of Stomatology, School of Nursing and Rehabilitation and School of Pharmaceutical Sciences; four directly affiliated hospitals, namely Qilu Hospital, the Second Hospital, the Stomatological Hospital and the Hospital for Reproductive Medicine; and many undirectly affiliated hospitals. It undertakes the functions of teaching, scientific research and serving the society.

附录三 校园导图

Appendix III Campus Map

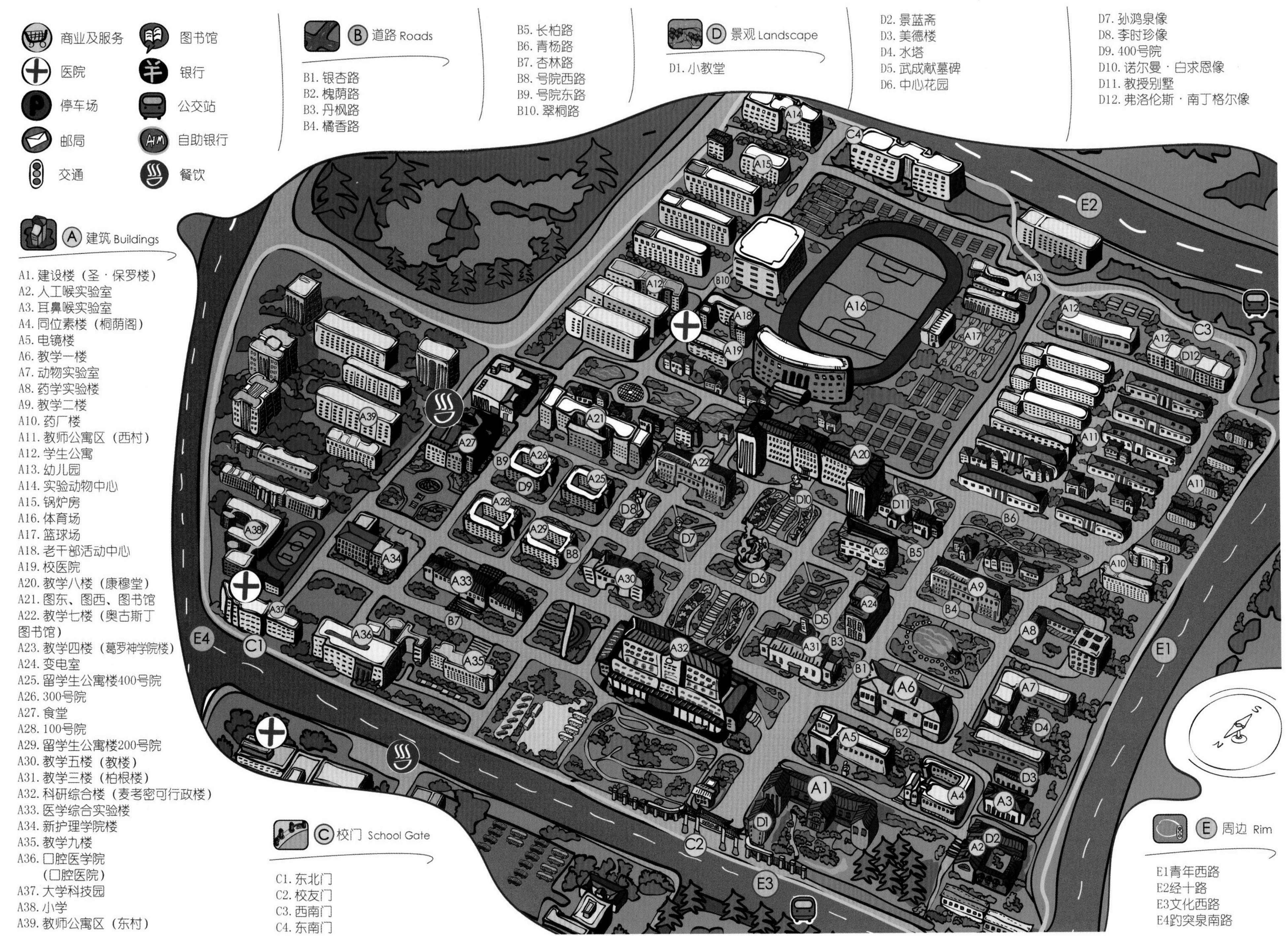

图 644 校园导图

Fig. 644 Campus Map

附录四　原齐鲁大学与山东大学齐鲁医学院培养的两院院士

Appendix IV　Academicians of the Two Academies Trained by former Cheeloo University and Cheeloo College of Medicine of Shandong University

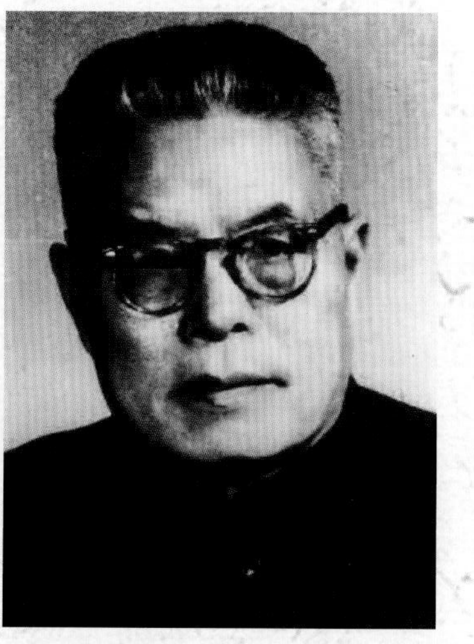

图 645 冯兰洲院士
Fig. 645 Academician Feng Lanzhou

一、冯兰洲院士

冯兰洲（(1903 ~ 1972)），山东临朐人，昆虫学家。1929 年毕业于山东济南齐鲁大学医正科，并获加拿大多伦多大学授予的医学博士学位。曾任中国医学科学院寄生虫病研究所教授、所长。1957 年选聘为中国科学院生物学部学部委员（院士）。

冯兰洲于 1929 年进入北京协和医学院工作时，就决心由媒介昆虫入手，研究解决中国的常见寄生虫病问题。当时中国在寄生虫病方面的研究极少，对医学昆虫的研究几乎是空白。北京协和医学院的寄生物学系中也没有专门研究医学昆虫的高级人员。冯兰洲凭借求学期间参加英国皇家学会工作时掌握的昆虫学知识，一面参考文献，一面在北平近郊收集按蚊成虫及幼虫，进行详细的形态观察和鉴定。他经常亲临疫区，确定了我国疟疾和丝虫病的主要蚊虫媒介，并对媒介白蛉传播黑热病的作用进行了深入研究，为防治我国主要的寄生虫病提供了科学依据和理论基础。他主编了《中国蚊虫描述汇编》和《医学昆虫学》，参与拟订了《寄生物学名词》《无脊椎动物名词》《昆虫学名词》和《蜱螨学名词》等。冯兰洲一生艰苦朴素，吃苦耐劳，热爱科研工作，努力克服困难，经常深入寄生虫病流行现场，他足迹遍及各省的代表地区，尤其是中国南方、西北和东北。他善于根据国内的实际需要选择研究课题，锲而不舍地钻研，为中国的寄生虫病防治做出了重要贡献。

Feng Lanzhou (1903-1972), a native of Linqu, Shandong Province, was an entomologist. He graduated from the Department of Medical Sciences of Cheeloo University in Jinan, Shandong Province in 1929, and received a degree of Doctor of Medicine from the University of Toronto, Canada. He once served as professor and director of the Institute of Parasitic Diseases of Chinese Academy of Medical Sciences. In 1957, he was elected member (academician) of the Department of Biology of Chinese Academy of Sciences.

When Feng Lanzhou joined Peking Union Medical College in 1929, he decided to start with vector insects to study and solve the common parasitic diseases in China. At that time, there was little research on parasitic diseases in China, and the research on medical insects was almost blank. There are also no senior staff specializing in medical insects in the Department of Parasitology at Peking Union Medical College. Feng Lanzhou, relying on his knowledge of entomology acquired from his work in the Royal Society of the United Kingdom during his study, collected Anopheles adults and larvae in the suburbs of Beijing for detailed morphological observation and identification while referring to the literature. He often visited epidemic areas, identified the main mosquito vectors of malaria and filariasis in China, and conducted in-depth research on the role of the vector sandflies in transmitting kala-azar, providing scientific basis and theoretical basis for the prevention and control of the main parasitic diseases in China. He edited *Collection of Descriptions of Chinese Mosquitoes* and *Medical Entomology*, and participated in the formulation of *Parasitology Terms*, *Invertebrate Terms*, *Entomology Terms* and *Acarina Terms*. Feng Lanzhou was plain-living and hard-working; he loved scientific research work and often went deep into the epidemic scene of parasitic diseases. He traveled all over the representative areas of various provinces, especially south China, northwest and northeast China. He selected research topics according to the actual needs of China and studied with perseverance, thus having made important contributions to the prevention and control of parasitic diseases in China.

二、周廷冲院士

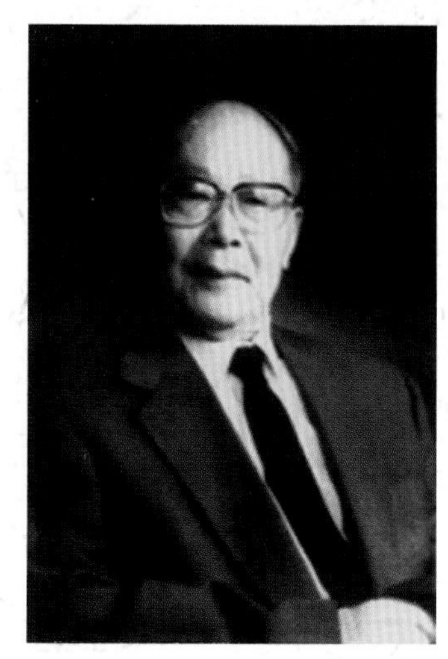

图 646 周廷冲院士
Fig. 646 Academician Zhou Tingchong

周廷冲（1917 ~ 1996），浙江富阳（新登）人，生化药理学家，1980 年当选为中国科学院学部委员（院士）。

周廷冲 1941 年从上海医学院医学系毕业后进入中央卫生实验院药理室工作，1947 年获得牛津大学药理学博士学位，1948 年赴美国康奈尔大学酶化学实验室进行博士后研究，在诺贝尔奖获得者 JB. Sumner 教授指导下进行刀豆磷酸酶的研究工作，1949 年到波士顿麻省医院生物化学实验室，在诺贝尔奖获得者 F. Lipman 教授指导下进行酶杂交完成各种乙酰化反应的研究。1950 年，他冲破各种阻挠和艰险，与夫人黄翠芬一起回国，并到华东白求恩医学院、山东医学院工作，担任药理学教研室主任、教授，创建教学及科研实验室、培养师资、技术员和进修教师，为山东医学院药理学科的发展奠定了基础。1953 年调到军事医学科学院，一直从事生物活性因子的分子生物学研究，首次阐明梭曼磷酰化乙酰胆碱酯酶的老化机制，证明梭曼磷酰化酶老化的实质是毒剂残基上特己氧基的去烷基反应，从而为毒剂防治中的药物设计指明了方向。主持完成的课题"梭曼与乙酰胆碱酯酶作用的生化"获国家自然科学奖二等奖。著有《药理学》《受体生化药理学》等 4 部专著，主编《实用药学词典》等著作。周廷冲教授信念坚定，求实创新，诲人不倦，诚挚热情，勇于献身，是一位杰出的科学家。

Zhou Tingchong (1917-1996), born in Fuyang, Zhejiang Province, was a biochemical pharmacologist. He was elected member (academician) of Chinese Academy of Sciences in 1980.

After graduating from the Medical Department of Shanghai Medical College in 1941, Zhou Tingchong entered the Pharmacy Department of the Central Hospital of Health Experiment. In 1947, he obtained his doctorate in pharmacology from Oxford University. In 1948, he went to the Laboratory of Enzyme Chemistry of Cornell University of the United States to carry out his postdoctoral research. Under the guidance of Professor J. B. Sumner, the Nobel Prize winner, he carried out the research of canavalin phosphatase. He went to the Biochemistry Laboratory of Massachusetts Hospital in Boston in 1949 and carried out the research of enzyme hybridization to complete various acetylation reactions under the guidance of Professor F. Lipman, the Nobel Prize winner. In 1950, he broke through all kinds of obstacles and dangers and returned home with his wife Huang Cuifen. Then he worked at East China Bethune Medical College and Shandong Medical College, serving as director and professor of Department of Pharmacology, established teaching and scientific research laboratories, and trained teachers, technicians and refresher teachers, laying a foundation for the development of pharmacology in Shandong Medical College. He was transferred to the Academy of Military Medical Sciences in 1953 and had been engaged in molecular biology research of bioactive factors. For the first time, he clarified the aging mechanism of Soman phosphoryl acetylcholinesterase and proved that the essence of Soman phosphoryl esterase aging was the dealkylation reaction of the special hexyloxy group on the poison residue, thus pointing out the direction for drug design in the prevention and treatment of poison. The project "Biochemistry of Soman and Acetylcholinesterase" presided over by him won the second prize of the National Natural Science Award. He had written four monographs such as *Pharmacology* and *Receptor Biochemical Pharmacology*, and edited *Practical Pharmaceutical Dictionary*. Professor Zhou Tingchong is an outstanding scientist with firm belief, realistic and innovative spirit, tireless teaching, sincere enthusiasm and courage to devote himself.

三、苗永瑞院士

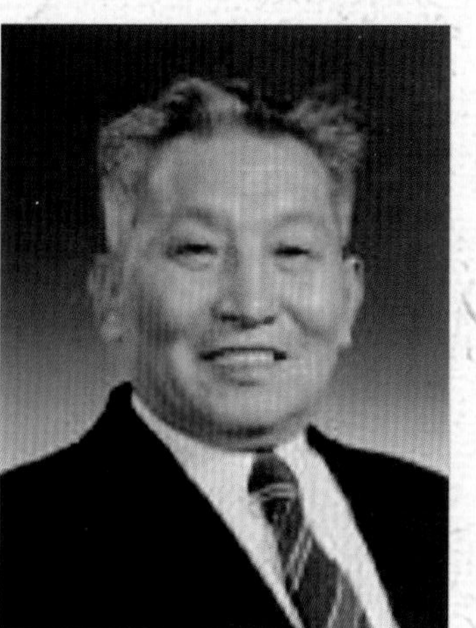

图 647 苗永瑞院士
Fig. 647 Academician Miao Yongrui

苗永瑞（1930 ~ 1999），原籍山东桓台，生于山东济南。1951 年毕业于齐鲁大学天算系，1991 年当选为中国科学院学部委员（院士）。

苗永瑞先后在紫金山天文台、上海徐家汇观象台、陕西天文台、上海天文台担任研究和技术组织等工作。1958 ~ 1961 年曾在苏联普尔科沃天文台进修。曾任上海天文台研究员，陕西天文台台长、名誉台长。在提高天文测时精度的研究方面，编制了天顶星表，测定了天顶星专门用于测时，提高了测时精度，同时改进了星位置，得到精度较高测时星表和基本星表。根据微气象理论，制定了天体测量选址方案，改进了观测室及观测位置，提高了观测精度。在提高授时技术方面，制定和研究了守时、收时、授时方法，负责建立了中国专用长、短波授时台和原子时系统，使中国授时精度进入世界先进行列。在开展日、地关系研究方面，建立了 D 电离层监测站，用 D 电离层扰动反演出太阳 X 射线爆发流量图，这是世界上第一次在地面上可以测定太阳 X 射线的方法。另外，用长波的传播特性，测定了中国大地电导率，得到了中国等效大地电导率分布图。共发表各种论文 50 余篇，培养硕士及博士生若干名。1984 年被授予国家有突出贡献专家称号。曾获得国家科技进步一等奖、中国科学院特等奖及一等奖和国家自然科学二等奖等科技奖励。

Miao Yongrui (1930-1999), a native of Huantai, Shandong Province, was born in Jinan, Shandong Province. He graduated from the Department of Astronomy and Mathematics of Cheeloo University in 1951 and was elected member (academician) of Chinese Academy of Sciences in 1991.

Miao Yongrui had successively undertaken the work of research and technical organization at Purple Mountain Observatory, Xujiahui Observatory in Shanghai, Shaanxi Observatory and Shanghai Observatory. From 1958 to 1961, he studied at the Pulkovo Observatory in the Soviet Union. He once served as a researcher of Shanghai Observatory, director and honorary director of Shaanxi Observatory. He compiled the catalogue of zenith stars, determined the zenith stars for time measurement, raised the precision of time measurement, and improved the position of stars, so that the catalogue of time measurement stars with higher precision and the basic catalogue of stars had been obtained. According to the micrometeorological theory, he formulated the scheme of the astrometry site selection, improved the observation room and position, and raised the observation precision. To improve the timing technology, he formulated and studied methods of punctuality, time receiving and timing, and was responsible for the establishment of special long and short waves stations and the atomic time system in China, which had brought China's timing precision into the advanced ranks in the world. In the study of the relationship between the sun and the earth, he established the D-ionosphere monitoring station to retrieve the flow map of the solar X-ray burst from the D-ionosphere disturbance. This is the first method in the world to measure solar X-rays on the ground. In addition, he measured the conductivity of the earth in China by using the transmission characteristics of long waves, and obtained the distribution pattern of the equivalent conductivity of the earth in China. He had published more than 50 papers and trained many masters and doctoral students. In 1984, he was awarded the title of "National Expert with Outstanding Contributions". He once won the first prize of the National Science and Technology Progress Award, the special prize and the first prize of Chinese Academy of Sciences, and the second prize of the National Natural Science Award and other scientific and technological awards.

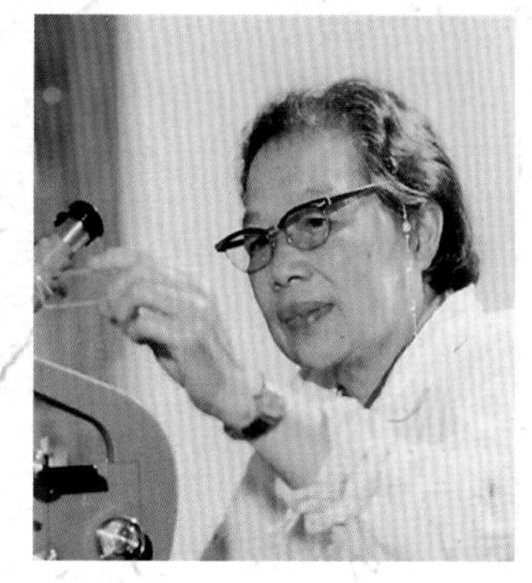

图 648 黄翠芬院士
Fig. 648 Academician Huang Cuifen

四、黄翠芬院士

黄翠芬（1921～2011），广东台山人，微生物、免疫及遗传工程专家，我国基因工程创始人之一，1996年当选为中国工程院院士。

黄翠芬1944年毕业于广州私立岭南大学化学系，毕业后来到重庆，在前中央卫生实验院流行病研究所细菌研究室工作。1948年1月，黄翠芬赴美国康奈尔大学农学院细菌系攻读硕士学位。1949年获得美国康奈尔大学理学硕士学位后，与丈夫周廷冲一起冲破重重障碍回到祖国。1950年，两人一起来到华东白求恩医学院、山东医学院。黄翠芬在微生物教研室，从事医学微生物方面的教材编写和教学工作。1954年被调到军事医学科学院。20世纪50～60年代，研制成功四联创伤类毒素、高效甲、乙型肉毒类毒素和“354装置”，为我国的国防建设做出了突出贡献。70年代，在国内率先采用分子生物学技术开展细菌毒素的结构与功能研究及基因工程疫苗研究，研制出高保护率的幼畜大肠菌腹泻预防基因工程疫苗及人用腹泻预防基因工程疫苗。80年代后，开展了基因工程多肽药物研究，首先在国内获得尿激酶原（Pro-UK）基因克隆及表达，并对人组织型纤溶酶原激活剂结构改造，提高其性能，是当前溶血栓特效的多肽药物。2000年后开展分子肿瘤研究。黄翠芬院士的伟大之处在于她总能站在医学科学的最前沿，洞察医学科学发展趋势，准确把握科研的大方向。

Huang Cuifen (1921-2011), a native of Taishan, Guangdong Province, is an expert in microbiology, immunology and genetic engineering. She is one of the founders of genetic engineering in China and was elected academician of Chinese Academy of Engineering in 1996.

Huang Cuifen graduated from the Department of Chemistry of Lingnan University in Guangzhou in 1944. After graduation, she came to Chongqing to work in the Bacterial laboratory of the Institute of Epidemiology of the former Central Hospital of Health Experiment. In January 1948, Huang Cuifen went to the United States to study for a master's degree in the Department of Bacteria, School of Agriculture, Cornell University. In 1949, after obtaining a degree of Master of Science from Cornell University, Huang Cuifen and her husband Zhou Tingchong broke through many obstacles and returned to the motherland. In 1950, they came to work in East China Bethune Medical College and Shandong Medical College. Huang Cuifen worked in the Department of Microbiology and was engaged in the compilation of textbook and teaching work of Medical Microbiology. In 1954, she was transferred to the Academy of Military Medical Sciences. From the 1950s to the 1960s, she successfully developed quadruple trauma toxoid, high-efficiency botulinum toxins A and B and "354 device", which made outstanding contributions to the national defense construction in China. In the 1970s, she took the lead in carrying out the research on the structure and function of bacterial toxins and the research on genetic engineering vaccines by using molecular biology technology in China, and developed the genetic engineering vaccines for preventing diarrhea of young livestock and human with high protection. After 1980s, she carried out the research on genetic engineering polypeptide drugs. First, she obtained the gene cloning and expression of pro-UK in China, and modified the structure of human tissue plasminogen activator to improve its performance. They are currently polypeptide drugs with specific thrombolytic effect. After 2000, she carried out the research on molecular tumor. The greatness lies in her ability to always stand at the frontier of the medical science, fully perceive its development trend, and accurately grasp the general direction of the scientific research.

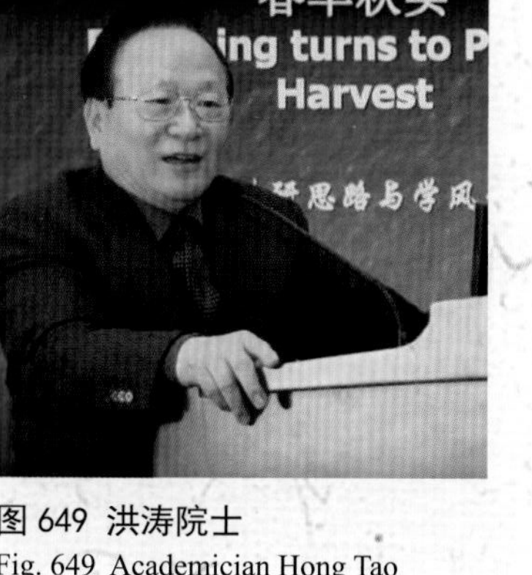

图 649 洪涛院士
Fig. 649 Academician Hong Tao

五、洪涛院士

洪涛（1931 ～ ），山东荣成人，医学超微结构及病毒学专家，1996 年当选为中国工程院院士；2001 年当选为第三世界科学院院士。

洪涛于 1947 年至 1949 年间担任华东白求恩医学院生理解剖实验室技术员，1955 年山东医学院医疗系毕业，1955 年至 1960 年间在罗马尼亚科学院病毒学研究所病毒学专业学习，获得副博士学位。现任中国疾病预防控制中心首席专家，病毒病预防控制所研究员，院士实验室主任，曾兼任《中华实验和临床病毒学杂志》主编，太平洋科协公共卫生和医学委员会主席。洪涛院士是我国医学电镜技术领域的主要开创者之一和病毒形态学主要奠基人，中华医学会病毒学会会刊《中华实验和临床病毒学杂志》主要创建人和总编辑。首次发现了人类 B 组轮状病毒，查明了水源爆发流规律，提出有效控制措施，集中研究该病毒的分子生物学，建立了全基因文库。首次发现了肾病综合征出血热病毒的形态，认定该病原为新的布尼亚病毒，获得了世界学术界的验证和公认，其研究成果被世界卫生组织作为鉴定汉坦病毒形态的标准。获 WHO 奖、国家自然科学奖、国家科学技术进步奖等 18 项。洪涛院士在疾控领域探索耕耘，成果卓著，耄耋之年仍孜孜不倦，作为一位浸润了母校精神并坚守终身的标志性校友，他行进在“上医”之途不知疲倦的身影，已成为这所百年学府经典的文化符号。

Hong Tao (1931-), a native of Rongcheng, Shandong Province, is an expert in medical ultrastructure and virology. He was elected academician of Chinese Academy of Engineering in 1996 and academician of the World Academy of Sciences in 2001.

From 1947 to 1949, Hong Tao served as a technician in the laboratory of physiology and anatomy of East China Bethune Medical College. He graduated from the Medical Department of Shandong Medical College in 1955. From 1955 to 1960, he studied virology in the Institute of Virology of Romanian Academy of Sciences and obtained an associate doctor's degree. He is currently the chief expert of Chinese Center for Disease Control and Prevention, researcher of the National Institute for Viral Disease Control and Prevention, and director of the Academician Laboratory. He once served as editor-in-chief of the *Chinese Journal of Experimental and Clinical Virology*, and chairman of the Committee of Public Health and Medicine of the Pacific Association for Science and Technology. Academician Hong Tao is one of the main founders in the field of medical electron microscope and the main founder of viral morphology in China. He is also the main founder and editor-in-chief of the *Chinese Journal of Experimental and Clinical Virology*, a journal of the Virology Society of the Chinese Medical Association. He discovered the human rotavirus Group B for the first time, ascertained the rule of water burst flow, and put forward the effective control measures. He studied the molecular biology of the virus intensively, and established the whole gene library. He discovered the morphology of the hemorrhagic fever virus of nephrotic syndrome for the first time, and identified the pathogen as a new Bunya virus which had been verified and recognized by the academic circles in the world, and his research results have been taken as the standard for identifying the morphology of Hantaan virus by the World Health Organization. He has won 18 awards, including that granted by WHO, the National Natural Science Award and the National Science and Technology Progress Award. Academician Hong Tao has made outstanding achievements in the field of disease control and prevention and he still works diligently in his 80s. As an outstanding alumnus who has followed the spirit of his alma mater and adhered to it in his life, he has been tireless on the road to medicine, which has already become a classic cultural symbol of this century-old university.

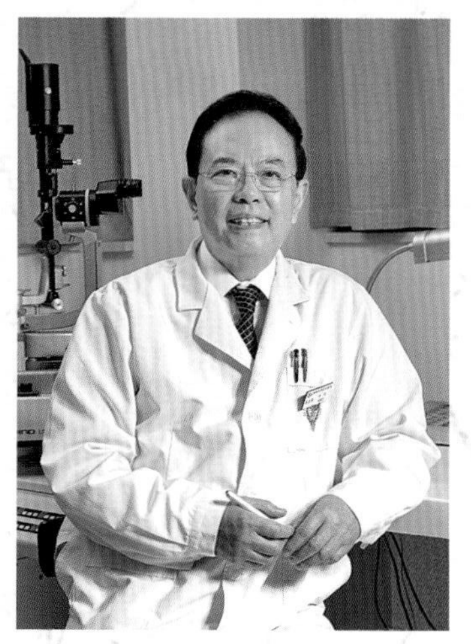

图 650 谢立信院士
Fig. 650 Academician Xie Lixin

六、谢立信院士

谢立信(1942～)，山东莱州人，眼科学专家。1965 年毕业于山东医学院医疗系。现任山东省眼科研究所名誉所长、青岛眼科医院院长、亚太角膜病学会名誉主席、中华医学会眼科学分会荣誉主任委员。第八、九届全国人大代表，中共十六大代表，全国劳动模范。2001 年当选为中国工程院院士。

谢立信于 1965 年毕业后到潍坊医学院眼科任教，1987-1988 年赴美国路易斯安那州立大学眼科中心从事角膜病博士后研究。回国后于 1991 年在青岛创建山东省眼科研究所，现已拥有青岛眼科医院、山东省眼科医院(济南)两个三级甲等专科医院，是教育部眼科学国家重点学科、卫计委国家临床重点专科建设单位，目前已成为集科研、医疗、教学为一体的我国主要眼科中心之一。谢立信教授是我国角膜病专业的领军者和白内障超声乳化手术的开拓者，现每年仍主刀完成约 1000 例复明手术。获国家科技进步奖二等奖 3 项、山东省科技进步奖一等奖 4 项和山东省科学技术最高奖。出版专著和主编、主译书籍 30 部。发表学术论文 500 余篇。先后获得中美眼科学会“金钥匙奖”、中华眼科杰出成就奖、美国眼科学会成就奖、亚太地区眼科学会“Arthur Lim 奖”、何梁何利基金科学与技术进步奖。在 2015 年中华医学会眼科学分会发布的“我国眼科科研人员近 15 年国内学术影响力”排名榜中居榜首。

Xie Lixin (1942-), a native of Laizhou, Shandong Province, is an expert in ophthalmology. He graduated from the Medical Department of Shandong Medical College in 1965. He is currently honorary director of Shandong Eye Institute, president of Qingdao Eye Hospital, honorary chairman of Asia-Pacific Keratopathy Society, and honorary chairman of Ophthalmology Branch of Chinese Medical Association. He is the deputy to the Eighth and Ninth National People's Congresses, deputy to the 16th National Congress of the Communist Party of China, and national model worker. He was elected academician of Chinese Academy of Engineering in 2001.

After graduating in 1965, Xie Lixin came to Weifang Medical College to teach in the Department of Ophthalmology. From 1987 to 1988, he carried out his postdoctoral research on keratopathy in the Ophthalmology Center of Louisiana State University in the United States. After returning to China, he established Shandong Eye Institute in Qingdao in 1991, and now has Qingdao Eye Hospital and Shandong Eye Hospital (Jinan), two Class A tertiary specialized hospitals. The institute is the construction unit for the National Key Discipline of Ophthalmology of the Ministry of Education and the National Key Clinical Specialty of the National Health Commission, and it has become one of the main ophthalmology centers integrating scientific research, medical treatment and teaching in China. Professor Xie Lixin is a leader in keratopathy and a pioneer in phacoemulsification in China, and he still performs about 1,000 cases of vision recovery operations every year. He has won three second prizes of National Science and Technology Progress Award, four first prizes of Shandong Provincial Science and Technology Progress Award and the top prize of Shandong Provincial Science and Technology Award. He has published 30 monographs, edited and translated books and more than 500 academic papers. He has successively won the "Golden Key Award" of Chinese-American Ophthalmological Society, the Outstanding Achievement Award of Chinese Ophthalmological Society, the Achievement Award of the American Academy of Ophthalmology, Arthur Lim Award of Asia-Pacific Academy of Ophthalmology, and Ho Leung Ho Lee Foundation Prize for Science and Technology Progress. He ranked first in the ranking list of academic impacts of Chinese ophthalmologists in the past 15 years as announced by Chinese Ophthalmological Society in 2015.

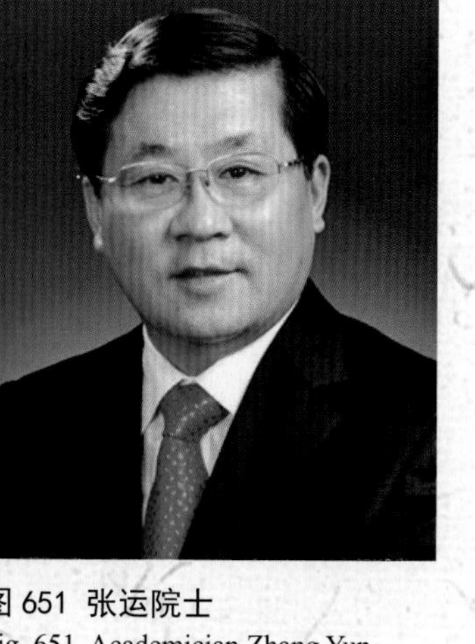

图 651 张运院士
Fig. 651 Academician Zhang Yun

七、张运院士

张运(1952 ~),山东阳谷人,心血管疾病专家。1973 年入山东医学院医疗系学习，1981 年获山东医学院医学硕士学位，1985 年获挪威奥斯陆大学博士学位，曾任山东大学副校长兼医学院院长，2001 年当选为中国工程院院士。

张运一直在山东大学齐鲁医院心内科工作，现任心血管重构与功能研究教育部（卫健委）重点实验室主任、山东省心血管病临床医学中心主任。他是我国多普勒超声心动图技术的开拓者和奠基人，他在国际上首先建立了多普勒超声定量诊断瓣膜性和先天性心脏病的系列新方法，使这些患者避免了创伤性的心导管检查；他与国际同步开展了多平面经食管超声心动图诊断技术，自行研制了我国第一台三维超声心动图软件系统，建立了三维超声诊断心血管病的系列新技术；他在国际上首次建立了动脉粥样硬化易损斑块的力学模型和多种动物模型，阐明了斑块易损的炎症机制，建立了以斑块体积应变和冠脉循环炎症和凝血因子浓度梯度预测易损斑块的新方法，筛选出可预防斑块破裂的多个新的基因和药物疗法；发现促血管生长因子和促动脉生成因子可协同诱导生成有功能的血管网络，改善心肌局部血流量和收缩功能，为缺血心肌的促血管生成治疗提供了新方法。获国家科技进步奖二等奖 1 项、三等奖 3 项，何梁何利基金科学与技术进步奖 1 项。

Zhang Yun (1952-), a native of Yanggu, Shandong Province, is an expert in cardiovascular diseases. In 1973, he joined the Medical Department of Shandong Medical College to study. In 1981, he obtained a degree of Master of Medicine from Shandong Medical College. In 1985, he obtained a doctorate from University of Oslo in Norway. He once served as vice president of Shandong University and dean of the School of Medicine. He was elected academician of Chinese Academy of Engineering in 2001.

Zhang Yun has been working in the Department of Cardiology of Qilu Hospital of Shandong University. He is now the director of the Key Laboratory of Cardiovascular Remodeling and Function Research of Ministry of Education(National Health Commission), and the director of Shandong Clinical Medical Center for Cardiovascular Diseases. He is the pioneer and founder of Doppler echocardiography technology in China. He was the first to establish a series of new methods for quantitative diagnosis of valvular and congenital heart diseases by Doppler ultrasound in the world, which enables these patients to avoid traumatic cardiac catheterization. He carried out the multi-plane transesophageal echocardiography diagnosis technology in the world, developed the first three-dimensional echocardiography software system in China, and established a series of new technologies for three-dimensional ultrasound diagnosis of cardiovascular diseases. He established a mechanical model and a variety of animal models of atherosclerotic vulnerable plaques for the first time in the world, clarified the inflammatory mechanism of vulnerable plaques, developed a new method for predicting vulnerable plaques by plaque volume, coronary circulation inflammation and the concentration and gradient of coagulation factors, and found out a number of new genes and drug therapies that can prevent plaque rupture. He found factors that trigger angiogenesis and arteriogenesis can synergistically induce the formation of functional vascular networks and improve the blood flow and systolic function of local myocardium, which provides a new method for the angiogenic therapy of ischemic myocardium. He has won one second prize and three third prizes of the National Science and Technology Progress Award, and Ho Leung Ho Lee Foundation Prize for Science and Technology Progress.

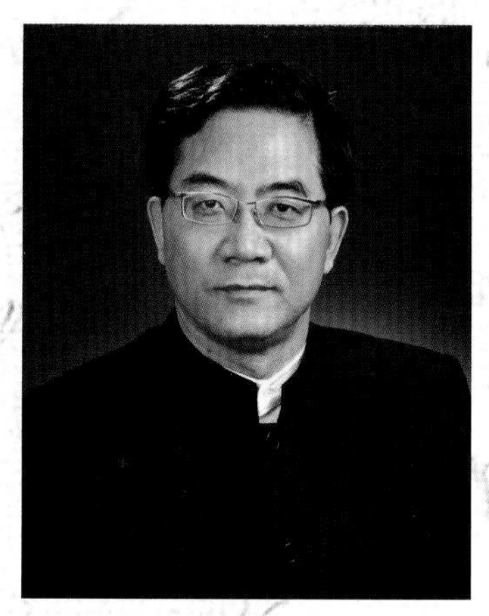

图 652 葛均波院士
Fig. 652 Academician Ge Junbo

八、葛均波院士

葛均波（1962～），山东五莲人，心血管病学家。1984 年毕业于青岛医学院医疗系，1987 年获山东医科大学医学硕士学位，1990 年毕业于上海医科大学并获医学博士学位，1993 年获德国美因茨大学医学博士学位。2011 年当选为中国科学院院士。

葛均波主要从事介入性心脏病学及血管内超声研究，现为复旦大学附属中山医院教授、上海市心血管病研究所所长、亚太介入心脏病学会主席和美国心脏病学会国际顾问。他在国际上首次发现心肌桥特异性超声影像学诊断指标“半月现象”和“指尖现象”；主持研制了我国首例可降解涂层新型冠脉支架；作为首位国内学者在美国 TCT 会议上首创“逆行钢丝对吻技术”；成功实施国内首例经皮主动脉瓣置入术、经皮二尖瓣修复术及经皮肺动脉成形术。他先后发表 SCI 收录的通讯、第一作者论文 150 余篇，以第一完成人获国家科技进步奖、国家技术发明奖等省部级以上科技奖励 10 余项；主编卫生部《内科学》全国统编教材、*Intravascular Ultrasound* 等中英文学术著作 6 部。葛均波长期致力于推动中国心血管疾病临床技术革新和科研成果转化，创造了多个心脏病诊治上的“全国首例”和“上海第一”；他在血管内超声研究、新型冠脉支架研发、支架内再狭窄防治等领域取得一系列突破性成果，为提升中国心血管病学领域的国际学术地位做出了突出贡献。

Ge Junbo (1962-), a native of Wulian, Shandong Province, is an expert in cardiovascular diseases. He graduated from the Medical Department of Qingdao Medical College in 1984, and obtained a master's degree in medicine from Shandong Medical University in 1987. He graduated from Shanghai Medical University in 1990 and obtained a doctorate in medicine. He obtained a doctorate in medicine from Johannes Gutenberg University of Mainz in Germany in 1993. In 2011, he was elected academician of Chinese Academy of Sciences.

Ge Junbo is mainly engaged in interventional cardiology and intravascular ultrasound research. He is currently a professor at Zhongshan Hospital affiliated to Fudan University, the director of Shanghai Institute of Cardiovascular Diseases, president of Asia-Pacific Society of Interventional Cardiology and international consultant of American College of Cardiology. For the first time in the world, he discovered the "half-moon phenomenon" and "fingertip phenomenon", diagnostic indicators of myocardial bridge ultrasound imaging. He presided over the development of the first new coronary stent with degradable coating in China. As the first Chinese scholar, he first created "Retrograde Kissing Wire Technique" in TCT Conference in the United States. He successfully performed the first case of percutaneous aortic valve implantation, percutaneous mitral valvuloplasty and percutaneous pulmonary angioplasty in China. He has successively published more than 150 papers included in SCI as the corresponding author and the first author, and won more than ten scientific and technological awards at or above the provincial and ministerial levels such as the National Science and Technology Progress Award and the National Technological Invention Award as the first person in charge. He edited six Chinese and English academic works such as *Internal Medicine*, the state-compiled textbook of the National Health Commission, and *Intravascular Ultrasound*. Ge Junbo has been committed to promoting the innovation of clinical technology and the transformation of scientific research achievements in cardiovascular diseases, creating "the first case in China" and "the first in Shanghai" in the diagnosis and treatment of heart diseases many times. He has made a series of breakthrough achievements in intravascular ultrasound research, research and development of new coronary stents, and prevention and treatment of in-stent restenosis, thus having made outstanding contributions to enhancing the international academic status of China's cardiovascular disease research.

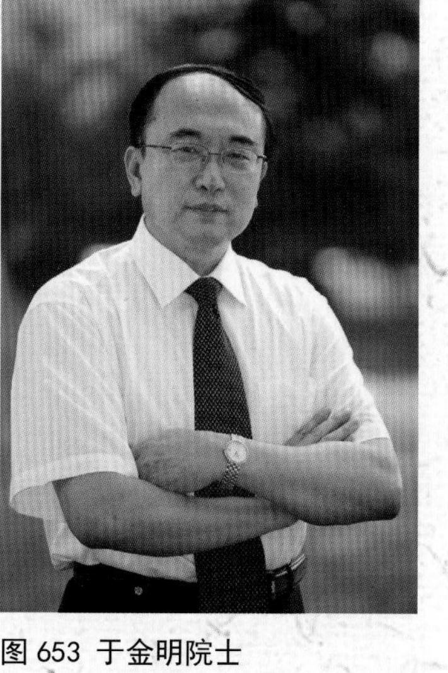
图 653 于金明院士
Fig. 653 Academician Yu Jinming

九、于金明院士

于金明（1958 ~ ），山东潍坊人，放射肿瘤学家。1983 年毕业于潍坊医学院医疗系，1988 年至 1993 年在美国弗吉尼亚大学和哈佛大学从事肿瘤放射治疗研究，2003 年毕业于山东大学医学院影像医学与核医学专业并获医学博士学位。2011 年当选为中国工程院院士。

于金明本科毕业后被分配到山东省肿瘤医院从事肿瘤放射治疗工作，现任山东省医学科学院名誉院长、山东省肿瘤医院院长，中国抗癌协会副理事长、中华医学会放射肿瘤治疗学分会名誉主任委员、山东省高层次人才发展促进会会长。他是我国精确放射治疗技术的主要开拓者之一，在突破制约放疗疗效的两大瓶颈——靶区精确勾画和射线精确施照方面做出了突出贡献，研究成果修改了美国、欧洲、加拿大和中国等多个国家肿瘤治疗指南，造福于广大恶性肿瘤患者。近年来在 SCI 杂志发表论文 200 余篇，被引用 500 余次，出版专著 20 余部。2006 年和 2009 年分别为首获国家科技进步奖二等奖 2 项、2017 年为主获国家科技进步奖二等奖 1 项、2003 年和 2004 年分别为首获山东省科技进步一等奖 3 项，2010 年荣获山东省科学技术最高奖，2015 年获得何梁何利科学与技术进步奖。当选首批山东省“泰山学者”特聘专家，入选第一批“泰山学者攀登计划”。其率领的团队被山东省委、省政府评为“山东省十大优秀创新团队”，并授予集体一等功。

Yu Jinming (1958-), a native of Weifang, Shandong Province, is a radiation oncologist. He graduated from the Medical Department of Weifang Medical College in 1983. From 1988 to 1993, he engaged in the research on tumor radiotherapy at the University of Virginia and Harvard University in the United States. In 2003, he graduated from the School of Medicine of Shandong University with a doctorate in imaging medicine and nuclear medicine. In 2011, he was elected academician of Chinese Academy of Engineering.

After graduating from his undergraduate course, Yu Jinming was assigned to Shandong Cancer Hospital to engage in tumor radiotherapy. He is currently honorary president of Shandong Academy of Medical Sciences, president of Shandong Cancer Hospital, vice chairman of China Anti-cancer Association, honorary chairman of Radiation Oncology Branch of Chinese Medical Association, and president of Shandong Promotion Association of High-level Talents Development. He is one of the main pioneers of precision radiotherapy technology in China. he has made outstanding contributions to breaking through the two bottlenecks that restrict the curative effect of radiotherapy, namely, accurate delineation of target volume and accurate irradiation of radiography. His research results made the cancer treatment guidelines of many countries such as the United States, those in Europe, Canada and China revised, benefiting the vast number of patients with malignant tumors. In recent years, he has published more than 200 papers in journals included in SCI which have been cited more than 500 times, and published more than 20 monographs. He has won two second prizes of the National Science and Technology Progress Award in 2006 and 2009 respectively as the first person in charge, one second prize of the National Science and Technology Progress Award in 2017 as the chief person in charge, three first prizes of Shandong Provincial Science and Technology Progress Award in 2003 and 2004 respectively as the first person in charge, the top prize of Shandong Provincial Science and Technology Award in 2010, and Ho Leung Ho Lee Foundation Prize for Science and Technology Progress in 2015. He was elected as one of the first batch of special experts of “Taishan Scholars” in Shandong Province and the first batch of “Taishan Scholars Scaling Plan”. The team led by him was rated as “top ten excellent innovation teams in Shandong Province” by the Shandong Provincial Party Committee and Shandong Provincial Government, and was awarded first-class collective merit.

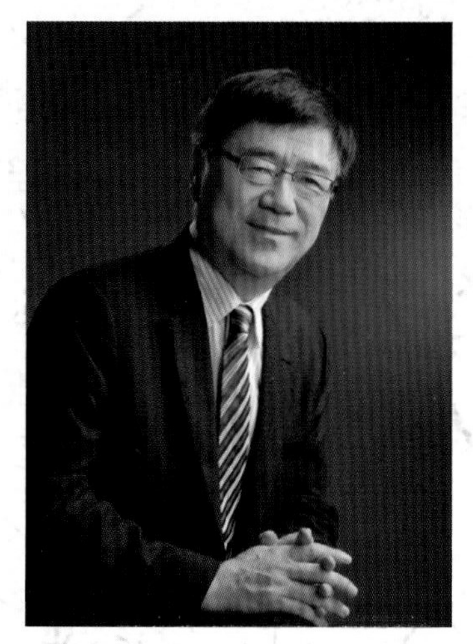

图 654 宁光院士
Fig. 654 Academician Ning Guang

十、宁光院士

宁光（1963～），山东滨州人，内分泌代谢病学专家。1987 年毕业于山东医科大学医学系，1994 年毕业于上海第二医科大学并获临床医学博士学位。获国家自然科学基金委国家杰出青年科学基金资助，并被聘为教育部“长江学者奖励计划”特聘教授。2015 年当选为中国工程院院士。

宁光本科毕业后进入山东滨州市人民医院内科工作两年，1989 年 9 月赴上海第二医科大学攻读博士学位，毕业后留校工作。1997 年 10 月至 1999 年 11 月，在美国贝勒医学院从事博士后研究。现任上海交通大学医学院附属瑞金医院院长，上海市内分泌研究所所长、山东第一医科大学校长。他长期致力于内分泌代谢病临床与科研工作，在内分泌肿瘤及糖尿病的诊治与研究领域取得创新性成果。发现多发性内分泌腺瘤病Ⅰ型、胰岛细胞瘤与肾上腺库欣综合征发病机制及致病基因，规范并优化诊疗方案，显著提升内分泌肿瘤基础研究与临床诊治整体水平；致力于通过大型队列创建生物样本库的研究模式，全面阐述中国代谢性疾病严峻形势，深入探索危险因素及防治新方案。先后主持国家科技支撑计划、国家自然科学基金委创新研究群体、国家重点基础研究发展计划（973 计划）等课题 20 余项，近年在 *Science*、*JAMA* 等 *SCI* 收录杂志发表论文 300 余篇，三次获国家科技进步二等奖（2 项排名第一，1 项排名第二）。

Ning Guang (1963-), a native of Binzhou, Shandong Province, is an expert in endocrinology and metabolism. He graduated from the Medical Department of Shandong Medical University in 1987, and graduated from Shanghai Second Medical University in 1994 with a doctorate in clinical medicine. He was awarded the National Science Fund for Distinguished Young Scholars of the National Natural Science Foundation of China, and was elected the special professor of the “Chang Jiang Scholars Program” of the Ministry of Education. In 2015, he was elected academician of Chinese Academy of Engineering.

Ning Guang had worked in the Department of Internal Medicine of Binzhou People’s Hospital in Shandong Province for two years after graduation. In September 1989, he went to Shanghai Second Medical University to study for a doctor’s degree and he stayed to work in the university after graduation. From October 1997 to November 1999, he was engaged in postdoctoral research at Baylor College of Medicine in the United States. He is currently president of Ruijin Hospital affiliated to the School of Medicine of Shanghai Jiao Tong University, director of Shanghai Institute of Endocrinology and President of Shandong First Medical University. He has been committed to the clinical and scientific research of endocrine and metabolic diseases, and has made innovative achievements in the diagnosis, treatment and research fields of endocrine tumors and diabetes. He has discovered the pathogenesis and pathogenic genes of multiple endocrine neoplasia type I, islet cell adenoma and adrenal Cushing syndrome, and standardized and optimized the diagnosis and treatment plan, which has significantly improved the overall level of the basic research and clinical diagnosis and treatment of endocrine tumors. He has been committed to the research mode of establishing a biological sample bank through a large cohort, comprehensively described the severe situation of metabolic diseases in China, and deeply explored risk factors and new prevention and treatment schemes. He has successively presided over more than 20 projects such as the National Science and Technology Support Program, the program of the Innovative Research Group of the National Natural Science Foundation, and the National Key Basic Research Program (973 Program). In recent years, he has published more than 300 papers in journals included in SCI such as *Science* and *JAMA*. He has won the second prize of National Science and Technology Progress Award three times (2 ranked first and 1 ranked second).

十一、陈子江院士

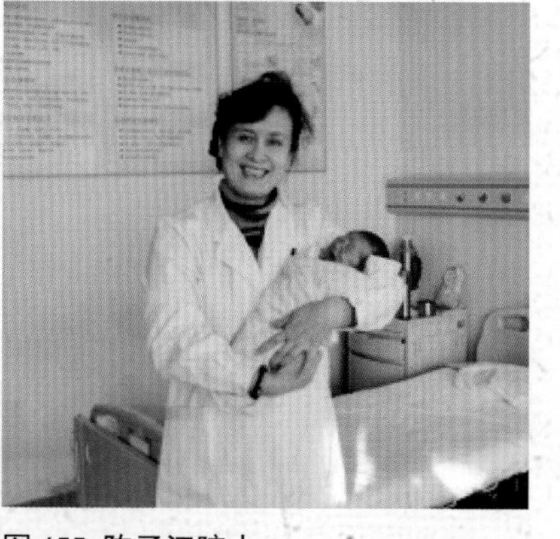

图 655 陈子江院士
Fig. 655 Academician Chen Zijiang

陈子江（1959 ~ ），祖籍湖南浏阳，出生于湖北武汉，妇产科学与生殖医学家。1984 年毕业于山东医学院医疗系，1989 年毕业于山东医科大学妇产科专业并获医学博士学位。曾任山东大学副校长兼齐鲁医学院院长，2019 年当选为中国科学院院士，2021 年当选为发展中国家科学院院士。

陈子江为山东大学附属生殖医院首席专家、国家辅助生殖与优生工程技术研究中心主任和生殖内分泌教育部重点实验室主任。她带领团队，主要围绕不孕症等生殖障碍疾病及出生缺陷重大科学问题，在生殖医学理论创新、疾病机制解析和辅助生殖临床研究等方面取得了系列创新性成果；发现生殖障碍疾病的多个致病基因，系统阐释了其发病机制和早期胚胎发育染色质开放的时空调控规律。完成系列多中心、前瞻性、随机对照临床试验（RCTs）研究，牵头制定了《不孕症诊断指南》和《多囊卵巢综合征中国诊疗指南》等 10 项诊疗规范，推动了我国生殖疾病临床诊疗的规范化发展。她还研发了多项基于辅助生殖的优生技术，建立了安全有效的优生技术体系并应用于临床，辅助诞生了我国首例阻断重度遗传性耳聋的 PGD 健康婴儿等，为降低我国出生缺陷提供了技术保障。她以通讯作者在《新英格兰医学杂志》《柳叶刀》《自然》和《细胞》等著名期刊发表论文 200 多篇。她注重人才培养，多人已成长为国家"四青"人才。

Chen Zijiang (1959-), a native of Liuyang, Hunan Province, was born in Wuhan, Hubei Province. She is an expert in gynecology and obstetrics and reproductive medicine. She graduated from the Medical Department of Shandong Medical College in 1984, and graduated from Shandong Medical University with a doctorate in gynecology and obstetrics in 1989. She once served as vice president of Shandong University and head of Cheeloo College of Medicine. She was elected academician of Chinese Academy of Sciences in 2019 and academician of the World Academy of Sciences in 2021.

Chen Zijiang is the chief expert of Hospital for Reproductive Medicine Affiliated to Shandong University, director of the National Research Center for Assisted Reproductive Technology and Reproductive Genetics and director of the Key Laboratory of Reproductive Endocrinology of the Ministry of Education. With her leading in major scientific issues such as infertility and reproductive disorders and birth defects, her team has made a series of innovative achievements in theoretical innovation of reproductive medicine, analysis of disease mechanisms and clinical research on assisted reproduction. She discovered a number of pathogenic genes of reproductive disorders and systematically explained the pathogenesis and the space-time regulation of chromatin opening in early embryonic development. She completed a series of multicenter, prospective and randomized controlled trials (RCTs) , and took the lead in formulating ten diagnosis and treatment standards such as *Guidelines for Infertility Diagnosis* and *Chinese Guidelines for the Diagnosis and Treatment of Polycystic Ovary Syndrome*, which promoted the standardized development of clinical diagnosis and treatment of reproductive diseases in China. She has also developed a number of eugenic technologies based on assisted reproduction, established a safe and effective system of the eugenic technology and applied it to clinical practice, which helps the birth of the first healthy baby to block severe hereditary deafness after PGD detection in China, providing technical guarantee for reducing birth defects in China. She has published more than 200 papers as a correspondent in *The New England Journal of Medicine*, *The Lancet*, *Nature* and *Cell*. She attaches importance to talent training; under her training, many people have grown into the country's outstanding talents.